CURRENT THERAPY IN PEDIATRIC INFECTIOUS DISEASE-2

Current Therapy Series

Bayless:
    Current Therapy in Gastroenterology and Liver Disease
Bayless, Brain, Cherniack:
    Current Therapy in Internal Medicine
Brain, Carbone:
    Current Therapy in Hematology–Oncology - 3
Callaham:
    Current Therapy in Emergency Medicine
Cameron:
    Current Surgical Therapy
Charles, Hurry:
    Current Therapy in Obstetrics
Cherniack:
    Current Therapy of Respiratory Disease
Dubovsky, Shore:
    Current Therapy in Psychiatry
Ernst, Stanley:
    Current Therapy in Vascular Surgery
Fazio:
    Current Therapy in Colon and Rectal Surgery
Eichenwald, Stroder:
    Current Therapy in Pediatrics
Foley, Payne:
    Current Therapy of Pain
Fortuin:
    Current Therapy in Cardiovascular Disease
Garcia, Mastroianni, Amelar, Dubin:
    Current Therapy of Infertility
Garcia, Mikuta, Rosenblum:
    Current Therapy in Surgical Gynecology
Gates:
    Current Therapy in Otolaryngology—Head and Neck Surgery
Glassock:
    Current Therapy in Nephrology and Hypertension
Grillo, Austen, Wilkins, Mathisen, Vlahakes:
    Current Therapy in Cardiothoracic Surgery
Jeejeebhoy:
    Current Therapy in Nutrition
Johnson:
    Current Therapy in Neurologic Disease
Kass, Platt:
    Current Therapy in Infectious Disease
Krieger, Bardin:
    Current Therapy in Endocrinology and Metabolism
Lichtenstein, Fauci:
    Current Therapy in Allergy, Immunology and Rheumatology
Long:
    Current Therapy in Neurological Surgery
Marsh:
    Current Therapy in Plastic and Reconstructive Surgery
McGinty, Jackson:
    Current Therapy in Orthopaedic Surgery
Nelson:
    Current Therapy in Neonatal–Perinatal Medicine
Nelson:
    Current Therapy in Pediatric Infectious Disease
Parrillo:
    Current Therapy in Critical Care Medicine
Provost, Farmer:
    Current Therapy in Dermatology
Resnick, Kursh:
    Current Therapy in Genitourinary Surgery
Rogers:
    Current Practice in Anesthesiology
Spaeth, Katz:
    Current Therapy in Surgical Ophthalmology
Trunkey, Lewis:
    Current Therapy of Trauma
Welsh, Torg, Shephard:
    Current Therapy in Sports Medicine

CURRENT THERAPY IN PEDIATRIC INFECTIOUS DISEASE-2

JOHN D. NELSON, M.D.

Department of Pediatrics
The University of Texas
Southwestern Medical Center at Dallas

1988

B.C. Decker Inc • Toronto • Philadelphia

Publisher

B.C. Decker Inc
3228 South Service Road
Burlington, Ontario   L7N 3H8

B.C. Decker Inc
320 Walnut Street
Suite 400
Philadelphia, Pennsylvania   19106

Sales and Distribution

United States
and Possessions

The C.V. Mosby Company
11830 Westline Industrial Drive
Saint Louis, Missouri   63146

Canada

The C.V. Mosby Company, Ltd.
5240 Finch Avenue East, Unit No. 1
Scarborough, Ontario   M1S 4P2

United Kingdom, Europe
and the Middle East

Blackwell Scientific Publications, Ltd.
Osney Mead, Oxford OX2 OEL, England

Australia

Harcourt Brace Jovanovich
30–52 Smidmore Street
Marrickville, N.S.W. 2204
Australia

Japan

Igaku-Shoin Ltd.
Tokyo International P.O. Box 5063
1–28–36 Hongo, Bunkyo-ku, Tokyo 113, Japan

Asia

Info-Med Ltd.
802–3 Ruttonjee House
11 Duddell Street
Central Hong Kong

South Africa

Libriger Book Distributors
Warehouse Number 8
''Die Ou Looiery''
Tannery Road
Hamilton, Bloemfontein 9300

South America
(non-stock list
representative only)

Inter-Book Marketing Services
Rua das Palmeriras, 32
Apto. 701
222–70 Rio de Janeiro
RJ, Brazil

Printed and bound in Canada

Current Therapy in Pediatric Infectious Disease–2

ISBN 1–55664–038–2

10 9 8 7 6 5 4 3 2 1

DONALD C. ANDERSON, M.D.

Professor of Pediatrics, Microbiology and Immunology, and Cell Biology, Baylor College of Medicine, Houston, Texas
Leptospirosis

ELIA M. AYOUB, M.D.

Professor of Pediatrics, University of Florida College of Medicine, Gainesville, Florida
Rheumatic Fever

NANCY A. AYRES, M.D.

Assistant Professor of Pediatrics, The University of Texas Southwestern Medical Center, Dallas, Texas
Myocarditis

ROBERT S. BALTIMORE, M.D.

Associate Professor of Pediatrics and Epidemiology, Yale University School of Medicine; Attending Physician in Pediatrics, Yale-New Haven Hospital, New Haven, Connecticut
Catheter-Associated Infections

JAMES W. BASS, M.D., M.P.H.

Professor of Pediatrics, Uniformed Services University of the Health Sciences, Bethesda, Maryland; Clinical Professor of Pediatrics, University of Hawaii John A. Burns School of Medicine and Chairman, Department of Pediatrics, Tripler Army Medical Center, Honolulu, Hawaii
Tonsillopharyngitis and Scarlet Fever
Gas Gangrene

THOMAS A. BELL, M.D., M.P.H.

Assistant Professor of Pediatrics and Epidemiology, University of Washington School of Medicine, School of Public Health and Community Medicine, Seattle, Washington
Infection of the Female Genital Tract
Chancroid

FRANK E. BERKOWITZ, M.B., B.Ch., F.C.P.(Paed)(SA)

Senior Pediatrician, Department of Pediatrics, University of the Witwatersrand and Baragwanath Hospital, Johannesburg, Republic of South Africa
Typhoid Fever

JOHN G. BIRCH, M.D., F.R.C.S.(C)

Assistant Professor of Orthopaedic Surgery, The University of Texas Southwestern Medical Center; Staff Orthopaedist, Texas Scottish Rite Hospital for Crippled Children, Dallas, Texas
Decubitus Ulcer

WILLIAM BORKOWSKY, M.D.

Associate Professor of Pediatrics and Director of Pediatric Infectious Diseases and Immunology, New York University Medical Center, New York, New York
Viral Hepatitis

KENNETH M. BOYER, M.D.

Associate Professor of Pediatrics and Immunology/Microbiology, Rush Medical College; Director, Section of Infectious Diseases, Department of Pediatrics, Rush-Presbyterian-St.Luke's Medical Center, Chicago, Illinois
Neonatal Sepsis

ARTHUR E. BROWN, M.D., F.A.C.P.

Associate Professor of Clinical Medicine and Pediatrics, Cornell University Medical College; Assistant Attending Physician, Memorial Hospital for Cancer and Allied Diseases and Associate Attending Pediatrician, The New York Hospital, New York, New York
Fever and Infection in the Child with Cancer

ORVAL E. BROWN, M.D., F.A.C.S., F.A.A.P.

Assistant Professor of Otorhinolaryngology, Department of Otorhinolaryngology, The University of Texas Southwestern Medical Center; Attending Staff, Children's Medical Center, Dallas, Texas
External Otitis
Mastoiditis

JACK H. T. CHANG, M.D.

Attending Surgeon, The Children's Hospital, Denver, Colorado
Surgical Infections

THOMAS G. CLEARY, M.D.

Associate Professor of Pediatrics, Program in Infectious Diseases and Clinical Microbiology, University of Texas Medical School, Houston, Texas
Antibiotic-Associated Diarrheal Syndromes

DALE COLN, M.D.

Associate Professor of Surgery, The University of Texas Southwestern Medical Center; Chief of Pediatric Surgery, Baylor University Medical Center and Director, Pediatric Trauma Unit, Parkland Memorial Hospital, Dallas, Texas

Necrotizing Fasciitis
Thrombophlebitis

J. CARL CRAFT, M.D.

Associate Director, Clinical Research, Pharmaceutical Products Division, Abbott Laboratories, Abbott Park, Illinois

Protozoan Infections

JAMES C. CUNNINGHAM, M.D.

Clinical Instructor of Pediatrics, Pediatric Pulmonology Section, University of Arizona College of Medicine, Arizona Health Sciences Center, Tucson, Arizona

Acute Pulmonary Exacerbations in Cystic Fibrosis

ALICE H. CUSHING, M.D.

Professor, Department of Pediatrics, University of New Mexico School of Medicine, Albuquerque, New Mexico

Plague

ADNAN S. DAJANI, M.D.

Professor of Pediatrics, Wayne State University School of Medicine; Director, Division of Infectious Diseases and Attending Staff, Children's Hospital of Michigan, Detroit, Michigan

Cervical Adenitis

GAIL J. DEMMLER, M.D.

Assistant Professor, Departments of Pediatrics and Microbiology and Immunology, Baylor College of Medicine, Houston, Texas

Cytomegalovirus Infections

HUGH C. DILLON Jr., M.D.

Professor of Microbiology and Professor and Chairman, Department of Pediatrics, University of Alabama School of Medicine, Birmingham, Alabama

Impetigo and Pyoderma

DUANE L. DOWELL, M.D.

Associate Professor of Pediatrics, The University of Texas Southwestern Medical Center at Dallas; Attending Physician, Children's Medical Center and Parkland Memorial Hospital, Dallas, Texas

Tetanus
Ectoparasitic Infections

MORVEN S. EDWARDS, M.D.

Associate Professor of Pediatrics, Baylor College of Medicine; Attending Physician, Texas Children's Hospital, Ben Taub General Hospital, and Jefferson Davis Hospital, Houston, Texas

Necrotizing Enterocolitis
Infection Following a Bite

HANS E. EINSTEIN, M.D., F.A.C.P.

Professor of Clinical Medicine, University of Southern California School of Medicine; Medical Director, Barlow Hospital, Los Angeles, California

Coccidioidomycosis

KEITHA FARMER, M.B., Ch.B., F.R.C.P.(U.K.), F.R.A.C.P., Ph.D.

Clinical Teacher, Auckland Medical School; Pediatrician, Neonatology, National Women's Hospital and Infectious Disease Section, Princess Mary Hospital, Auckland, New Zealand

Funisitis and Omphalitis
Neonatal Breast Abscess
Listeriosis

RALPH D. FEIGIN, M.D.

J. S. Abercrombie Professor and Chairman, Department of Pediatrics, Baylor College of Medicine; Physician-in-Chief, Texas Children's Hospital and Harris County Hospital District and Chief, Pediatric Service, The Methodist Hospital, Houston, Texas

Brain Abscess

WILLIAM E. FELDMAN, M.D., M.S.

Associate Professor of Family Medicine, Eastern Virginia Medical School, Norfolk, Virginia

Acute Pericarditis

GREGORY A. FILICE, M.D.

Assistant Professor of Medicine, University of Minnesota Medical School; Staff Physician, Infectious Disease Section, Veterans Administration Medical Center, Minneapolis, Minnesota

Actinomycosis

JOSEPH F. FITZGERALD, M.D.

Professor of Pediatrics, Indiana University School of Medicine; Gastroenterologist, James Whitcomb Riley Hospital for Children, Indianapolis, Indiana

Acute Diarrheal Disease of Unknown Etiology

WILLIAM S. FOSHEE, M.D.

Associate Professor of Pediatrics, Medical College of Georgia School of Medicine; Education Coordinator, Pediatrics, University Hospital, Augusta, Georgia

Sporotrichosis

BISHARA J. FREIJ, M.D.

Clinical Assistant Professor of Pediatrics, Georgetown University School of Medicine, Washington, D.C.; Visiting Fellow, Infectious Diseases Branch, National Institute of Neurological and Communicative Disorders and Stroke, National Institutes of Health, Bethesda, Maryland
Acute Epiglottitis and Uvulitis
Pneumonia of Known Etiology

ANNE A. GERSHON, M.D.

Professor of Pediatrics, Columbia University College of Physicians and Surgeons; Attending Physician, Babies Hospital, New York, New York
Varicella-Zoster Virus Infection

CHARLES M. GINSBURG, M.D.

Robert L. Moore Professor of Pediatrics, The University of Texas Southwestern Medical Center, Dallas, Texas
Purulent Rhinitis
Molluscum Contagiosum

LAURENCE B. GIVNER, M.D.

Assistant Professor of Pediatrics, Bowman Gray School of Medicine of Wake Forest University; Attending Physician, North Carolina Baptist Hospitals, Winston-Salem, North Carolina
Anthrax

W. PAUL GLEZEN, M.D.

Professor of Microbiology and Pediatrics, Influenza Research Center, Baylor College of Medicine, Houston, Texas
Bronchiolitis and Bronchitis
Influenza

JOHN R. GRAYBILL, M.D.

Department of Internal Medicine, University of Texas Health Science Center, San Antonio, Texas
Cryptococcosis
Zygomycosis and Phaeohyphomycosis

MOSES GROSSMAN, M.D.

Professor and Vice Chairman, Department of Pediatrics, University of California School of Medicine; Chief of Pediatric Services, San Francisco General Hospital, San Francisco, California
Pertussis

STANLEY HELLERSTEIN, M.D.

Professor of Pediatrics, University of Missouri School of Medicine; Chief, Section of Pediatric Nephrology, Children's Mercy Hospital, Kansas City, Missouri
Cystitis and Pyelonephritis

WALTER T. HUGHES, M.D.

Professor of Pediatrics, University of Tennessee Center for the Health Sciences; Chairman, Department of Infectious Diseases, Saint Jude Children's Research Hospital, Memphis, Tennessee
Aspergillosis

GEORGE E. HURT Jr., M.D.

Associate Professor of Urology, The University of Texas Southwestern Medical Center; Private Practice, Dallas, Texas
Epididymitis and Orchitis

JOHN L. HUNT, M.D.

Professor of Surgery, The University of Texas Southwestern Medical Center, Dallas, Texas
Infections in Burn Patients

MARY ANNE JACKSON, M.D.

Assistant Professor of Pediatrics, University of Missouri School of Medicine; Pediatrician in Infectious Diseases, Children's Mercy Hospital, Kansas City, Missouri
Cerebrospinal Fluid Shunt Infection

RICHARD F. JACOBS, M.D., F.A.A.P.

Associate Professor of Pediatrics, Division of Infectious Diseases, University of Arkansas for Medical Sciences and Arkansas Children's Hospital, Little Rock, Arkansas
Tuberculosis

DOUGLAS H. JONES, M.D.

Instructor, Department of Pediatrics and Research Fellow, Leukocyte Biology Section, Department of Pediatrics, Baylor College of Medicine, Houston, Texas
Leptospirosis

DAVID B. JOSEPH, M.D.

Assistant Professor of Surgery, Divison of Urology, The University of Alabama School of Medicine; Chief of Pediatric Urology, The Children's Hospital of Alabama, Birmingham, Alabama
Urethritis, Meatitis, and Balanitis
Renal and Perirenal Abscess
Prostatitis

SHELDON L. KAPLAN, M.D.

Associate Professor, Department of Pediatrics, Baylor College of Medicine; Chief, Infectious Disease Service, Texas Children's Hospital and Attending Pediatrician, Ben Taub General Hospital, Houston, Texas
Liver Abscess
Suppurative Arthritis and Osteomyelitis

JAY S. KEYSTONE, M.D., M.Sc.(CTM), F.R.C.P.(C)

Associate Professor, Department of Medicine, Medical Microbiology and Pharmacology, University of Toronto Faculty of Medicine; Director, Tropical Disease Unit, Toronto General Hospital, Toronto, Ontario, Canada
Larval Tapeworm Infections

BRUCE S. KLEIN, M.D.

Clinical Instructor, Infectious Disease Section,
Departments of Pediatrics and Internal Medicine,
University of Wisconsin Medical School,
Madison, Wisconsin
Blastomycosis

JEROME O. KLEIN, M.D.

Professor of Pediatrics, Boston University School of
Medicine; Director, Division of Pediatric Infectious
Diseases, Boston City Hospital, Boston, Massachusetts
Antibiotic Prophylaxis

STEVE KOHL, M.D.

Professor of Pediatrics, Department of Pediatrics and
Program of Infectious Diseases and Clinical
Microbiology, University of Texas Medical School;
Attending in Pediatrics, University Children's Center and
Hermann Hospital and Consultant, Pediatric Infectious
Diseases, M.D. Anderson Hospital and Tumor Institute,
Houston, Texas
Herpes Simplex Virus Infection

KEITH KRASINSKI, M.D.

Assistant Professor of Pediatrics, New York University
Medical Center; Assistant Epidemiologist, Bellevue
Hospital Center, New York, New York
Nontuberculous (Atypical) Mycobacterial Disease

THOMAS L. KUHLS, M.D.

Assistant Professor of Pediatrics, Division of Infectious
Diseases, University of Oklahoma College of Medicine;
Attending Physician, Oklahoma Children's Memorial
Hospital, Oklahoma City, Oklahoma
Cholangitis and Bacterial Hepatitis

PHILIP S. LaRUSSA, M.D.

Assistant Professor of Pediatrics, Columbia University
College of Physicians and Surgeons; Attending Physician,
Babies Hospital, Columbia-Presbyterian Medical Center,
New York, New York
Infections Associated with International Travel

EDGAR O. LEDBETTER, M.D.

Professor of Pediatrics, Texas Tech University Health
Sciences Center School of Medicine, Lubbock, Texas
Nocardiosis

MYRON J. LEVIN, M.D.

Professor of Pediatrics and Medicine and Chief of
Pediatric Infectious Diseases, University of Colorado
Health Sciences Center School of Medicine,
Denver, Colorado
Viral Meningitis and Encephalitis

JACOB A. LOHR, M.D.

McLemore Birdsong Professor, Department of Pediatrics,
University of Virgina School of Medicine; Director,
Children's Medical Center Clinics and Chief, Division of
General Pediatrics, Children's Medical Center,
Charlottesville, Virginia
Rickettsial Diseases

SARAH S. LONG, M.D.

Professor of Pediatrics, Temple University School of
Medicine; Chief, Section of Infectious Diseases,
St. Christopher's Hospital for Children,
Philadelphia, Pennsylvania
Botulism

SCOTT C. MANNING, M.D.

Assistant Professor, Department of Otolaryngology, The
University of Texas Southwestern Medical Center,
Dallas, Texas
Retropharyngeal and Lateral Pharyngeal Space Infections

COLIN D. MARCHANT, M.D.

Associate Pediatrician, Division of Infectious Diseases,
Floating Hospital for Infants and Children, Tufts-New
England Medical Center and Biologic Laboratories of the
Center for Disease Control of the Massachusetts
Department of Public Health, Boston, Massachusetts
Immunizations

S. MICHAEL MARCY, M.D.

Clinical Professor of Pediatrics, University of Southern
California School of Medicine, Los Angeles; Staff
Pediatrician, Kaiser Foundation Hospital,
Panorama City, California
Infection of the Salivary Glands (Sialadenitis)

ANDREW M. MARGILETH, M.D.

Professor and Vice Chairman of Pediatrics, F. Edward
Hébert School of Medicine, Uniformed Services
University of the Health Sciences; Senior Consultant,
Bethesda Naval Hospital, Walter Reed Army Medical
Center, Bethesda, Maryland
Cat Scratch Disease

EDWARD K. MARKELL, M.D., Ph.D.

Clinical Professor of Family, Community, and Preventive
Medicine, Emeritus, Stanford University School of
Medicine, Stanford and Clinical Professor of Medicine
and Tropical Medicine, University of California School of
Medicine, San Francisco; Attending Physician (retired),
Kaiser-Permanente Medical Center, Oakland, California
Trematode Infections

LAURENE MASCOLA, M.D., M.P.H.

Staff Physician, Children's Hospital and Medical
Epidemiologist, Los Angeles County Department of
Health Services, Los Angeles, California
Syphilis

WILBERT H. MASON, M.D.

Associate Professor of Clinical Pediatrics, University of Southern California School of Medicine; Associate Attending in Pediatrics, Childrens Hospital of Los Angeles, Los Angeles, California
Kawasaki Syndrome

ALICE MATOBA, M.D.

Assistant Professor of Ophthalmology, Yale University School of Medicine, New Haven, Connecticut and Baylor College of Medicine, Houston; Chief, Ophthalmology Service, Veterans Administration Medical Center, Houston, Texas
Conjunctivitis and Keratitis
Endophthalmitis

GEORGE H. McCRACKEN Jr., M.D.

Professor of Pediatrics, The University of Texas Southwestern Medical Center; Attending Physician, Children's Medical Center and Parkland Memorial Hospital, Dallas, Texas
Aspiration Pneumonia and Lung Abscess
Bacterial Meningitis

ANTHONY B. MINNEFOR, M.D.

Clinical Associate Professor, Preventive Medicine and Community Health, University of Medicine and Dentistry, New Jersey Medical School, Newark; Chief, Division of Infectious Disease, Saint Joseph's Hospital and Medical Center, Paterson, New Jersey
Acquired Immunodeficiency Syndrome

F. KEVIN MURPHY, M.D., F.A.C.P.

Clinical Associate Professor of Internal Medicine, The University of Texas Southwestern Medical Center, Dallas, Texas
Leprosy

TRUDY V. MURPHY, M.D.

Assistant Professor, Department of Pediatrics, The University of Texas Southwestern Medical Center, Dallas, Texas
Leprosy

PISESPONG PATAMASUCON, B.Sc.(Med), M.D.

Assistant Professor, Department of Pediatrics, Prince of Songkla University, Haadyai, Songkla, Thailand and Adjunct Assistant Professor, Department of Pediatrics, Georgetown University School of Medicine, Washington, D.C.
Diphtheria
Pyomyositis

ZBIGNIEW S. PAWLOWSKI, M.D., D.T.M.&H.

Professor of Medical Parasitology and Tropical Diseases, Academy of Medicine, Poznan, Poland
Roundworm Infections (Nematodiases)

RONALD M. PERKIN, M.D.

Director, Pediatric Critical Care, Children's Hospital, Orange, California
Toxic Shock Syndrome
Septic Shock

LARRY K. PICKERING, M.D.

Professor of Pediatrics, Program in Infectious Diseases and Clinical Microbiology; Director, Pediatric Infectious Diseases, The University of Texas Medical School, Houston, Texas
Specific Diarrheal Diseases

PHILIP A. PIZZO, M.D.

Professor of Pediatrics, Uniformed Services University of the Health Sciences; Chief of Pediatrics and Head, Infectious Disease Section, National Cancer Institute, National Institutes of Health, Bethesda, Maryland
Candidiasis

CHARLES G. PROBER, M.D.

Associate Professor of Pediatrics, Stanford University School of Medicine; Co-Director, Division of Pediatric Infectious Diseases, Stanford University Medical Center, Stanford, California
Cellulitis

GARY F. PURDUE, M.D.

Assistant Professor, Department of Surgery, The University of Texas Southwestern Medical Center, Dallas, Texas
Infections in Burn Patients

ANTHONY J. REID, M.D., C.C.F.P.

Assistant Professor of Family Practice and Community Medicine, University of Toronto Faculty of Medicine; Staff Physician, Family Practice Unit and Tropical Disease Unit, Toronto General Hospital, Toronto, Ontario, Canada
Adult Tapeworm Infections

PHILIP J. RETTIG, M.D.

Associate Professor of Pediatrics and Director, Division of Pediatric Infectious Diseases, University of Oklahoma Health Sciences Center; Attending Physician, Oklahoma Children's Memorial Hospital, Oklahoma City, Oklahoma
Gonorrhea
Lymphogranuloma Venereum

LYNNE J. ROBERTS, M.D.

Assistant Professor of Dermatology and Pediatrics, The University of Texas Southwestern Medical Center; Co-Director of Dermatology, Children's Medical Center, Dallas, Texas
Acne

WILLIAM J. RODRIGUEZ, M.D., Ph.D.

Professor of Child Health and Development, George Washington University School of Medicine and Associate Professor of Microbiology, Georgetown University School of Medicine; Chairman, Department of Infectious Diseases and Chief, Microbiology Research, Children's Hospital National Medical Center, Washington, D.C.
Otitis Media with Effusion
Travelers' Diarrhea

HARLEY A. ROTBART, M.D.

Assistant Professor of Pediatrics, Infectious Diseases Section, University of Colorado School of Medicine, Denver, Colorado
Viral Meningitis and Encephalitis

RAUL C. RUDOY, M.D., M.P.H.

Professor of Pediatrics and Chief, Pediatric Infectious Disease, University of Hawaii John A. Burns School of Medicine, Honolulu, Hawaii
Sinusitis

ANDREA J. RUFF, M.D.

Associate, Department of International Health, The Johns Hopkins School of Hygiene and Public Health, Baltimore, Maryland
Protozoan Infections

PABLO J. SÁNCHEZ, M.D.

Research Fellow, Pediatric Infectious Disease, The University of Texas Southwestern Medical Center, Dallas, Texas
Nosocomial Infections in the Nursery

JAY P. SANFORD, M.D.

Professor of Internal Medicine and Dean, F. Edward Hébert School of Medicine and President, Uniformed Services University of the Health Sciences; Attending Physician, Walter Reed Army Medical Center and Naval Hospital, Bethesda, Maryland
Brucellosis
Clostridial Sepsis
Melioidosis

URS B. SCHAAD, M.D.

Associate Professor of Pediatrics, Division of Pediatric Infectious Diseases, Department of Pediatrics, University of Berne, Berne, Switzerland
Periorbital and Orbital Cellulitis

PENELOPE G. SHACKELFORD, M.D.

Associate Professor of Pediatrics and Microbiology and Immunology, Washington University School of Medicine, Saint Louis, Missouri
Rat-Bite Fever
Relapsing Fever

KEVIN M. SHANNON, M.D.

Instructor in Pediatrics, University of California School of Medicine, San Francisco, California
Suppurative Bursitis

EUGENE D. SHAPIRO, M.D.

Assistant Professor of Pediatrics and Epidemiology, Yale University School of Medicine; Director of the Pediatric Emergency Room, Yale-New Haven Hospital, New Haven, Connecticut
Fever Without Focal Infection in Infants and Toddlers

KATHLEEN A. SHEERIN, M.D.

Fellow, Pediatric Allergy Immunology, Duke University School of Medicine, Durham, North Carolina
Brain Abscess

ZIAD M. SHEHAB, M.D.

Assistant Professor, Department of Pediatrics, University of Arizona College of Medicine; Assistant Professor, University Medical Center, Tucson, Arizona
Herpangina

STANFORD T. SHULMAN, M.D.

Professor of Pediatrics, Northwestern University Medical School; Chief, Infectious Diseases, Children's Memorial Hospital, Chicago, Illinois
Infective Endocarditis

JANE D. SIEGEL, M.D.

Associate Professor of Pediatrics, The University of Texas Southwestern Medical Center; Attending Physician, Children's Medical Center and Parkland Memorial Hospital, Dallas, Texas
Intra-Abdominal Sepsis

BARBARA W. STECHENBERG, M.D.

Assistant Professor of Pediatrics, University of Massachusetts Medical School, Worcester; Director, Pediatric Infectious Disease, Baystate Medical Center, Springfield, Massachusetts
Bartonellosis
Lyme Disease

RUSSELL W. STEELE, M.D.

Professor of Pediatrics, University of Arkansas College of Medicine; Division Head, Infectious Diseases, Immunology, and Allergy, Arkansas Children's Hospital, Little Rock, Arkansas
Tularemia

MAXWELL STILLERMAN, M.D.

Professor of Clinical Pediatrics and Medicine, Division of Infectious Diseases, State University of New York Health Science Center, Stony Brook, New York
Childhood Exanthems

CIRO V. SUMAYA, M.D., M.P.H.T.M.

Professor of Pediatrics and Pathology, The University of Texas Health Science Center; Consultant, Diagnostic Virology Laboratory, Medical Center Hospital, San Antonio, Texas
Epstein-Barr Virus Infection (Infectious Mononucleosis)

MASATO TAKAHASHI, M.D.

Attending Staff, Children's Hospital of Los Angeles,
Los Angeles, California
Kawasaki Syndrome

LYNN M. TAUSSIG, M.D.

Professor and Head, Department of Pediatrics, University
of Arizona Health Sciences Center, Tucson, Arizona
Acute Pulmonary Exacerbations in Cystic Fibrosis

PAUL P. TAYLOR, D.D.S., M.S.

Professor Emeritus, Department of Pediatric Dentistry,
Baylor College of Dentistry, Dallas, Texas
Infections of the Oral Cavity

MUTHAYIPALAYAM C. THIRUMOORTHI, M.B.,
B.S.

Associate Professor of Pediatrics, Wayne State University
School of Medicine; Attending Physician, Division of
Infectious Diseases, Children's Hospital of Michigan,
Detroit, Michigan
Subdural, Epidural, and Subgaleal Infections

JAMES K. TODD, M.D.

Professor of Pediatrics and Microbiology/Immunology,
University of Colorado Health Sciences Center School of
Medicine; Director of Infectious Disease, Children's
Hospital, Denver, Colorado
Staphylococcal Scalded Skin Syndrome

THEODORE P. VOTTELER, M.D.

Clinical Professor of Surgery and Pediatrics, The
University of Texas Southwestern Medical Center;
Director of Surgical Services, Children's Medical Center,
Dallas, Texas
Mediastinitis

ELLEN R. WALD, M.D.

Associate Professor of Pediatrics, University of Pittsburgh
School of Medicine; Associate Medical Director of
Ambulatory Care and Member, Division of Infectious
Disease, Children's Hospital of Pittsburgh,
Pittsburgh, Pennsylvania
Acute Pneumonia of Unknown Etiology

RICHARD L. WASSERMAN, M.D., Ph.D.

Assistant Professor of Pediatrics and Microbiology, The
University of Texas Southwestern Medical Center;
Director, Division of Pediatric Allergy and
Immunology, Children's Medical Center and Attending
Physician, Parkland Memorial Hospital, Dallas, Texas
Antibody Deficiency States
Chronic Granulomatous Disease

DAVID A. WHITING, M.D., M.Med.(Derm),
F.A.C.P., F.R.C.P.

Clinical Associate Professor, Departments of Dermatology
and Pediatrics, The University of Texas Southwestern
Medical Center, Dallas, Texas
Warts
Erythrasma
Dermatophytosis

RAOUL L. WIENTZEN Jr., M.D.

Associate Professor of Pediatrics, Georgetown University
School of Medicine; Chief, Division of Pediatric
Infectious Diseases, Georgetown University Hospital,
Washington, D.C.
Infections of the Larynx and Trachea

H. DAVID WILSON, M.D., F.A.A.P.

Professor of Pediatrics and Director, Pediatric Infectious
Diseases, Albert B. Chandler Medical Center, University
of Kentucky College of Medicine, Lexington, Kentucky
Ludwig's Angina
Histoplasmosis

JOHN M. WRIGHT, D.D.S., M.S.

Professor, Department of Pathology, Baylor College of
Dentistry, Dallas, Texas
Infections of the Oral Cavity

TERRY YAMAUCHI, M.D.

Professor and Vice Chairman, Department of Pediatrics;
Chief of Infectious Diseases, University of Arkansas for
Medical Sciences and Arkansas Children's Hospital,
Little Rock, Arkansas
Nosocomial Pneumonia

PREFACE

The aims and format of this book are explained in the Preface to the first edition. The second edition is extensively revised and considerably expanded. Of the 116 topics carried over from the first edition only the five chapters on parasitic diseases and ten other chapters retain the same authors. The new authors of the remaining 101 chapters bring different perspectives and, in situations in which there have been advances in knowledge during the past 2 years, new information about treatment. If you own a copy of the first edition, do not discard it. Keep it by the side of the new edition and consult both of them. Getting a second opinion is a good clinical precept to follow.

Eighteen new chapters have been added to the book. Four rare conditions (uvulitis, suppurative bursitis, phaeohyphomycosis, and epidural and subgaleal infections) were not included in the first edition, and that oversight has been corrected. Recommendations about cytomegalovirus and Epstein-Barr virus infections and acquired immunodeficiency syndrome were scattered about in appropriate chapters, but each of the three is now covered comprehensively in separate chapters.

The first edition of this book focused on specific diseases and syndromes. In an attempt to increase the utility of the book, I have expanded to broader areas by adding 11 chapters: *Fever Without Focal Infection in Infants and Toddlers; Antibiotic Prophylaxis; Immunization; Infections Associated with International Travel; Antibody Deficiency States; Chronic Granulomatous Disease; Surgical Infections; Catheter-Associated Infections; Infections in Burn Patients; Nosocomial Pneumonia;* and *Nosocomial Infections in the Nursery*.

Another change in this book is the addition of a Suggested Reading list at the end of each chapter. The authors were told to present their approaches to specific and supportive management without the need to document every statement with a citation to the medical literature. However, many readers have said that they would like to have guides to further reading. The authors have selected a handful of references which they consider to be the best expositions of their subjects.

In editing this book, I kept two things paramount in my mind to distinguish it from other pediatric textbooks: scope and currency. Every infectious condition that you are likely—or even unlikely—to encounter should be covered in sufficient detail for you to feel comfortable in managing it (or to know when to refer the patient to an expert!). The currency depends on two factors: the cooperation of the authors and the efficiency and technologic expertise of the publisher's staff. The authors were marvelously cooperative in meeting the deadlines for their manuscripts, and the copy editor and production staff of B.C. Decker worked diligently and rapidly. If the printers do their job well, and I am sure they will, this book should be available to you within five months of the time that I am writing these words. That is truly remarkable for a multiauthored medical book. The greatest credit goes to the authors, whom I salute. Without their cooperation we could not achieve the goal of currency of the material.

John D. Nelson, M.D.

PREFACE TO THE FIRST EDITION

Infections are such a pervasive part of childhood that illness seems at times to be the norm. This is particularly true during the early years when the world of the infant or toddler expands to large numbers of his peers in day care or preschool settings and there is the inevitable exchange of microbes that is part of those new experiences.

The physician who treats children spends more time managing infections than all other types of diseases combined. It seemed strange, therefore, that there was no textbook devoted exclusively to therapy of infections in children. This vacuum was perceived by the publisher, Brian C. Decker, who invited me to serve as editor of *Current Therapy of Pediatric Infectious Diseases*.

The premise of this book is simple and the format is straightforward. Each author was told to make the assumption that the doctor has already made the diagnosis before reaching for this book. Therefore, detailed discussions of signs, symptoms, and differential diagnosis are not presented. This is not a textbook of infectious diseases, and so discussions of pathophysiology, epidemiology, and pathology are left to those texts where they rightfully belong.

The authors were asked to present their personal approach to management without having to document every opinion or choice with literature citations. In fact, there are no references cited in this book. Why? Because I realize that most thinking physicians choose a course of action for treating a specific disease that is based on their past instruction, their critical evaluation of the medical literature, and their experiences. This is the magical part of medicine called art. Controlled clinical trials give us statistically evaluable information, but many common problems are not easily evaluable by the hallowed randomized, prospective, double-blind approach to therapy because the denominator would have to be vast. Most investigators—or their research grants—do not last long enough to accumulate those numbers. It is comparatively easy to show whether or not a new therapeutic intervention is effective in a disease such as typhoid fever or meningitis. But in common illnesses such as streptococcal pharyngitis, urinary tract infection, or otitis media, many drugs work, and in order to show significant differences, the "n" has to be immense.

In this book the authors tell you their preferred management in detail rather than present a group of options. Thus, it is a highly personal approach. We recognize that alternative approaches could be equally effective. In future biennial revisions of this book, new authors will be chosen for each subject in order to bring you new perspectives.

John D. Nelson, M.D.

CONTENTS

DISEASES OF THE HEART AND BLOOD VESSELS

DISEASES OF THE CENTRAL NERVOUS SYSTEM

DISEASES OF THE GENITOURINARY TRACT

DISEASES CAUSED BY FUNGI

DISEASES OF THE EARS AND PARANASAL SINUSES

EXTERNAL OTITIS

ORVAL E. BROWN, M.D., F.A.C.S., F.A.A.P.

External otitis is inflammation of the skin of the external auditory canal. This inflammation can be divided into six classifications: acute, fungal, acute circumscribed, eczematous, chronic, and progressive necrotizing or "malignant" external otitis. The usual cause of external otitis is water in the ear canal, which causes loss of the ceruminous protective skin surface barrier. This changes the normally slightly acid pH of the ear canal to an alkaline pH, and predisposes to infection. As surface barriers are removed, organisms are able to colonize the skin and produce an inflammatory reaction. The most common clinical signs of acute external otitis are ear canal edema, erythema, and pain. *Pseudomonas aeruginosa* is the most common infecting organism, followed by *Staphylococcus aureus* and gram-negative enterics such as *Escherichia coli, Proteus* species, and others.

ACUTE OTITIS EXTERNA

Early acute otitis externa is characterized by mild edema and erythema of the ear canal without significant swelling or purulent debris. This can be treated with Otic Domeboro solution (2 percent acetic acid in a modified Burow's solution), VoSol solution (2 percent acetic acid in a 3 percent propylene glycol vehicle), or acid–alcohol solution (half white vinegar and half 70 percent isopropyl alcohol) 3 to 5 drops in the ear canal three times a day. This is followed by drying of the ear canal with a hair dryer. In moderate disease with a greater degree of edema of the ear canal, VoSol HC (which contains hydrocortisone) can be used to reduce the edema more rapidly. Severe acute otitis externa is characterized by marked edema of the ear canal with copious purulent secretions. The ear canal may be swollen shut. The ear is examined and cleaned under microscopic control with Frazier tip suctions. Patients who are unable to cooperate are carefully restrained. I usually use Cortisporin otic suspension (which contains polymixin, neomycin, and hydrocortisone) 3 drops three times daily for 5 to 7 days, until the patient is markedly improved. Ophthalmic Cortisporin, gentamicin, or tobramycin drops may be used as an alternative for patients who develop severe pain from Cortisporin otic suspension. After the patient is markedly improved, either Otic Domeboro or VoSol solution is administered for a 10- to 14-day total course. If the ear canal is swollen closed, the ear canal is carefully suctioned to clear secretions before placement of an ear wick. Iodoform gauze or a Pope Otowick is used. Cortisporin otic suspension drops are applied to the wick three times a day. These patients are seen daily, or every 2 days, for aural hygiene and replacement of the wick until the ear canal is patent for administration of drops.

Occasionally cellulitis of the periauricular area may complicate acute otitis externa. Cellulitis is usually caused by gram-positive cocci, not the gram-negative enteric bacilli that usually infect the ear canal skin. In these cases, a specimen for culture is taken from the ear canal. Although an aspiration for culture from the leading edge of the cellulitis can be attempted, this procedure has not been very productive in my hands. If the cellulitis is minimal and the patient is reliable, therapy is begun with oral Augmentin (amoxicillin and clavulanic acid), 40 mg per kilogram of body weight per day in three divided doses, or cefaclor, 40 mg per kilogram per day in three divided doses. The ear canal is treated as described previously. The patients are seen daily in follow-up. Patients with severe cellulitis, those with failure to improve on therapy, and those with complicating medical problems are hospitalized for intravenous antibiotic therapy. The initial drugs of choice pending culture results are cefuroxime, 75 to 120 mg per kilogram per day in three divided doses, and either gentamicin, 6 mg per kilogram per day in three divided doses, or tobramycin, 5 mg per kilogram per day in three divided doses. Nafcillin, 150 mg per kilogram per day in four divided doses, may be used as an alternative to cefuroxime. The patients are followed in the hospital with daily or twice-daily cleaning of the ear canal under microscopic control. Antibiotic therapy is adjusted based on the culture results.

Other supportive measures are used to control symptoms related to the ear canal infection. Pain is treated with acetaminophen or aspirin. If the pain is severe, acetaminophen with codeine elixir is administered. Severe, persistent pain raises the suspicion of a complication, such as progressive necrotizing otitis externa. I do not generally use otic drops with topical lidocaine or benzocaine, because these have not been effective in my hands. Itching is usually relieved with topical therapy. If severe itching persists, hydroxyzine, 1 to 2 mg per kilogram per day in four divided doses, or cyproheptadine, 0.25 mg per kilogram per day in three divided doses, is administered.

"SWIMMER'S EAR"

Certain simple preventive measures may be recommended for children with recurrent otitis externa related to swimming. The ear conchae are painted with petrolatum, custom ear plugs are fitted, and then the ears are covered with a bathing cap. I recommend that these children avoid getting their heads under water. The effectiveness of this therapy varies with the cooperativeness of the child in keeping water out of the ear canals. After swimming, the ear canals should be rinsed with acid–alcohol solution or Otic Domeboro drops.

FUNGAL OTITIS EXTERNA

The most common cause of fungal otitis externa is *Aspergillus* sp. This usually presents as a dark velvety lining of the external auditory canal. The diagnosis is made by physical examination. This can be confirmed with a potassium hydroxide (KOH) prep or a fungal culture, but these are rarely needed. Initial treatment consists of cleaning the external auditory canal, using the microscope. After all fungal elements are removed, the ear canal is treated with acid–alcohol or Otic Domeboro solution three times a day, as described earlier. This is continued for 7 to 14 days, three times a day, depending on the patient's response. If the response is poor, the ear canal is painted daily or every other day with 2 percent gentian violet or 25 percent *m*-cresyl-acetate (Cresylate) until the patient improves. Gentian violet stains clothes. Patients who do not respond to this treatment are seen daily for ear cleaning and administration of "gold dust" powder. This consists of equal portions of amphotericin B, sulfanilamide, and chloramphenicol powder. This is also used occasionally for patients with refractory bacterial external otitis.

Systemic antifungals such as amphotericin B are reserved for patients with invasive fungal disease. These are usually immunosuppressed patients. A culture and susceptibility tests are required, and therapy is individualized (see chapter on *Aspergillosis*). These patients require daily ear canal hygiene, and may require surgical debridement of necrotic tissue.

ACUTE CIRCUMSCRIBED OTITIS EXTERNA

Acute circumscribed otitis externa results from an infected hair follicle in the outer external auditory canal. A pustule results, which is usually caused by *Staphylococcus aureus*. An antistaphylococcal antibiotic such as cloxacillin, 50 mg per kilogram per day in four divided doses, or cephalexin, 50 mg per kilogram per day in four divided doses, is administered. Incision and drainage are often required; use of the operating microscope makes this procedure less painful. Acetaminophen with codeine elixir usually suffices for pain. Severe pain raises the suspicion of abscess formation. If periauricular cellulitis is present, it is treated as described previously.

ECZEMATOUS OTITIS EXTERNA

Eczematous otitis externa occurs in association with eczema, seborrhea, psoriasis, and other skin diseases. It often extends to the pinna with scaling, weeping fissures, vesicles, and inflammation. Secondary infection is a common complication. Itching can be severe, and the lesions are worsened by children's tendency to scratch and pick at them. Initial therapy is the application of topical solutions such as Otic Domeboro on a wet to dry dressing, two to four times per day. If the acid pH is not tolerated, Burow's solution (2 Domeboro tablets in 16 oz of warm water) is used as an alternative. Wet to dry dressings are continued until the inflammation subsides. Then topical creams or ointments, usually with a steroid such as 1% hydrocortisone cream, or 0.1% topical betamethasone cream or lotion, are applied twice daily until healing is complete. Boric acid and lanolin ointment are helpful in cases in which steroids are not used. The patient must be prevented from scratching the pruritic areas. Antipruritics may be used as outlined earlier. Some children require mittening of the hands or elbow restraints with "no-nos" to prevent picking at the lesions.

CHRONIC OTITIS EXTERNA

Chronic otitis externa is a result of long-term inflammation of the ear canal. It is often secondary to chronic otitis media or cholesteatoma with purulent discharge into the ear canal (see the chapter on *Mastoiditis*). The ear canal lumen is narrow because of thickening and cicatricial scarring of the canal skin. The predisposing condition must be remedied before the chronic ear canal inflammation can be managed. Once this is done, the ear canal must be cleaned frequently using the operating microscope. Otic drops such as VoSol HC are administered three times daily. If there is no response after long-term aural hygiene measures, surgical therapy is considered. A rare patient may require excision of the ear canal skin, enlargement of the bony canal, and application of a split thickness skin graft. This removes the cerumen glands of the ear canal, and the result can be unsatisfactory because of continued infection of the grafted canal skin. These patients require continual preventive measures, as described earlier.

PROGRESSIVE NECROTIZING OR "MALIGNANT" OTITIS EXTERNA

Progressive necrotizing otitis externa was previously labeled malignant otitis externa. This terminology should be abandoned, as this is not a malignant disease. The condition is uncommon in children. It is usually reported in diabetic or immunosuppressed adults. Progressive necrotizing otitis externa is usually caused by *Pseudomonas aeruginosa*. Infection spreads from the external auditory canal skin to the cartilaginous and bony ear canal. If not controlled, infection then spreads to the adjacent soft tissues, parotid, and temporal bone. Osteomyelitis of the base of the skull can ensue, with multiple cranial nerve palsies and intracranial complications. Severe, constant pain is an early symptom. Granulation tissue in the external auditory canal floor is a diagnostic sign.

Treatment is primarily nonsurgical. Patients are hospitalized for a 6-week course of ticarcillin, 200 to 300 mg per kilogram per day in four divided doses, and tobramycin, 5 mg per kilogram per day in three divided doses. A specimen for culture is taken from the ear canal to assess antibiotic efficacy. Ceftazidime, 100 to 150 mg per kilogram per day in three divided doses, can be used as an alternative, but single-drug therapy is not usually recommended. Antibiotic therapy is continued for a 6-week course, but may be longer if pain persits. Persistent pain indicates ongoing uncontrolled infection. Aural hygiene with ear canal debridement is performed daily while the patient is hospitalized. Mastoidectomy and exenterative procedures are rarely required. Antibiotic concentrations in serum are monitored, and audiometric tests are administered periodically and after therapy.

The technetium 99m disodium methylene diphosphonate (Tc-99mMDP) scan is useful in determining the presence of skull base osteomyelitis in early cases. A negative Tc-99 scan indicates infection limited to the ear canal, and a briefer course of therapy can be used. A gallium-67 citrate scan detects inflammation by uptake in granulocytes. This scan returns to normal when inflammation ceases, and it is used to detect osteomyelitis after a course of treatment. A positive scan indicates the necessity for further treatment. In patients who can be monitored closely, home administration of intravenous antibiotics by a professional home care team is considered.

SUGGESTED READING

Bergstrom L. Diseases of the external ear. In: Bluestone CD, Stool SE, eds. Pediatric otolaryngology. Philadelphia: WB Saunders, 1983; 347.

Casissi N, Davidson T, Cohn A, Witten BR. Diffuse otitis externa: clinical and microbiologic findings in the course of a multicenter study on a new otic solution. Ann Otol Rhinol Laryngol 1977; 86(Suppl 39):1–16.

Chandler JR. Malignant external otitis. Laryngoscope 1968; 78:1257–1294.

Parisier SC, Lucente FE, Hirschman SZ, et al. Nuclear scanning in necrotizing progressive "malignant" external otitis. Laryngoscope 1982; 92:1016–1019.

Senturia, BH. Diseases of the external ear. Springfield, IL: Charles C Thomas, 1957.

OTITIS MEDIA WITH EFFUSION

WILLIAM J. RODRIGUEZ, M.D., Ph.D.

Acute otitis media is one of the most common infectious diseases of childhood. It has been defined as an inflammation of the mucoperiosteal lining of the middle ear cleft that includes the eustachian tube, tympanic cavity, mastoid antrum, and mastoid air cells. Generally, otitis media represents a continuum of pathologic conditions, and defining them individually may be helpful to the clinician's therapeutic approach. A diagnosis of acute otitis media is logically followed by the prescription of antimicrobial therapy in the hope of speeding the resolution of acute symptoms and preventing sequellae. A reliable diagnosis of acute otitis media is critical, and for this, the physician needs a dependable source of brilliant light in the otoscope, such as the new halogen bulb. All debris must be removed from the external ear canal to ensure an unimpeded view of the tympanic membrane.

DEFINITIONS*

Acute Otitis Media with Effusion (AOME)

Acute otitis media with effusion encompasses acute inflammation of the middle ear with suppuration, loss of ossicular landmarks, a tympanic membrane that is yellow or gray, bulging or segmented, and with poor mobility of the eardrum on pneumatic otoscopy; fever and malaise may also be present.

Persistent Otitis Media with Effusion (POME)

Persistent otitis media with effusion is seen in 50 to 70 percent of patients following antimicrobial

---

* Some categories are arbitrary and may reflect my bias.

treatment for AOME. The tympanic landmarks are diminished, the tympanic membrane is opaque, there is poor or no mobility of the tympanic membrane to pneumomassage, and the patient is asymptomatic except for hearing impairment.

Acute Otitis Media with Effusion, Persistent (AOMEP)

AOMEP is a condition seen in approximately 10 percent of patients who have been treated for acute otitis media with effusion. Symptoms of AOMEP are usually noted within 7 days of completion of therapy. This diagnosis does not apply to the patient with OME.

Acute Otitis Media with Effusion, Recurrent (AOMER)

AOMER is a recrudescence, or reappearance, of symptoms of acute otitis media detected more than 1 week after therapy is completed.

Otitis-Prone (OP)

The otitis-prone patient is one who has experienced three or more episodes of AOME in the preceding 6- to 12-month period. Diagnostic criteria include a medical history and physical findings in the middle ear similar to those noted in AOME.

Chronic Otitis Media with Effusion (COME)

Chronic otitis media with effusion is persistent effusion in the middle ear cleft behind an intact eardrum and lasting for 3 months or more. The physical findings may be similar to those described for POME.

Chronic Suppurative Otitis Media (CSOM)

CSOM is chronic inflammation of the middle ear and the mastoid. The tympanic membrane is not intact, either because it has perforated or because tympanostomy tubes have been implanted; otorrhea, or discharge, is also present.

MICROBIOLOGY

For appropriate treatment, the epidemiology and the microbiology of the causative agents in each of the preceding conditions must be considered. *Streptococcus pneumoniae* is recovered in approximately 30 percent of AOME, and *Haemophilus influenzae* in 20 to 30 percent (20 percent of these organisms are ampicillin-resistant in our locale); and Group A streptococci constitute 5 percent or fewer. A most important agent of the 1980s is *Branhamella catarrhalis,* a microbe that can be recovered in 7 to 27 percent of cases of AOME (depending on locale),

with a reported incidence of beta-lactamase production ranging from 0 to 70 percent. Currently, the overall incidence of ampicillin resistance in middle ear pathogens ranges from 18 to 27 percent. In many locales, resistance in this range affects the status of amoxicillin as the first line of defense for acute otitis media. In about 30 percent of cases, no pathogens are recovered from the middle ear, occasionally mixed flora of traditional middle ear pathogens are found, and rarely gram-negative enteric bacteria are seen. Viruses have also been detected in middle ear fluid (see following).

THERAPEUTICS

Antibiotics are prescribed with the expectation of symptomatic relief. Information from the preantibiotic era suggests that many patients with acute otitis media heal without them. In spite of antibiotics, some patients may still require myringotomy, and others perforate spontaneously. With the use of antibiotics, however, the incidence of intracranial complications has apparently dropped from the approximately 3 percent reported in the preantibiotic era to less than 1 percent.

Antimicrobial Treatment

Inappropriate, or Usually Inappropriate, Therapy

Tetracyclines are not indicated in the treatment of acute otitis media because their use yields middle ear antibiotic concentrations insufficient to inhibit the growth of *H. influenzae.* Penicillin G and penicillin V may give adequate concentrations for *S. pneumoniae,* and *Streptococcus pyogenes,* but are effective against only 50 percent of *H. influenzae,* primarily those that produce no beta-lactamase. Ampicillin, in a dosage of 50 to 75 mg per kilogram daily, gives antimicrobial concentrations in the middle ear ranging between 1.6 and 12 μg per milliliter, which should be sufficient to inhibit non-beta-lactamase producing *H. influenzae* and other susceptible pathogens. The incidence of diarrhea, however, makes it second best to its congener, amoxicillin (see following section). Erythromycin by itself has excellent activity against *S. pneumoniae* and *S. pyogenes,* but does not reliably cover all *H. influenzae* strains. Even the estolate form, whose superior kinetics result in higher concentrations in the middle ear, fails to cover all strains of *H. influenzae.* Lincomycin and clindamycin have no role in the treatment of acute otitis media because their activity against *H. influenzae* is poor. Cephalexin does not perform well against *H. influenzae;* in addition, it is affected by dietary factors such as milk ingestion. The same can be said of cefradine.

Logical Therapy

Penicillin derivatives (with and without 6-beta-lactamase inhibitors) are appropriate for treatment.

Amoxicillin, in a dosage of 30 to 40 mg per kilogram per day in three divided doses administered for a 10-day period, still constitutes an excellent first choice for patients with AOME in geographic areas where beta-lactamase–producing organisms are in the minority. Its era may quickly be coming to an end, however. The advantages of amoxicillin include a convenient dosage schedule and less diarrhea with its use than with ampicillin. Amoxicillin is effective against *S. pneumoniae* and *H. influenzae,* and even against an occasional strain of beta-lactamase–producing *B. catarrhalis.* Problems with this antimicrobial agent include rashes and unreliable activity against beta-lactamase–producing organisms.

Other beta-lactam antimicrobials that are available include cyclacillin and bacampicillin. These ampicillinlike compounds are known to give good blood concentrations; however, they cost more than amoxicillin, and there is no evidence they are clinically superior to amoxicillin for treatment of acute otitis media. In addition, they are susceptible to beta-lactamase.

Augmentin is an antimicrobial formulation that contains amoxicillin and potassium clavulanate in a ratio of 4 to 1. It is administered in a dosage of 40 mg per kilogram per day and is effective against *S. pneumoniae, H. influenzae, B. catarrhalis,* and *S. pyogenes.* The clavulanate component inhibits beta-lactamase activity. Hypersensitivity and side effects are similar to those of amoxicillin; however, a high incidence of diarrhea (10 to 20 percent) is associated with the use of this preparation.

Of the cephalosporin preparations, the most widely used is cefaclor. In a dosage of 40 mg per kilogram per day in three divided doses, it has proved to be effective in most cases of AOME. Cefaclor has improved activity in vitro against *H. influenzae* and appears not to be inactivated by its penicillinase; however, it is susceptible to the phenomenon of the inoculum effect. Because of the number of failures noted with *H. influenzae* and *S. pneumoniae,* recommendations regarding the use of cefaclor in dosages as large as 60 mg per kilogram per day, or at least a minimum of 15 mg per kilogram per dose, have appeared in the literature. A recent publication by Marchant and colleagues raises even more doubts about the effectiveness of cefaclor in sterilizing the middle ear fluid. Therapy with cefaclor has been associated not only with diarrhea but with erythema multiforme, serum-sickness–like reaction, and various other rashes as well.

Cefuroxime axetil, the oral formulation of cefuroxime, has been evaluated by several investigators and it appears promising; however, its final usefulness in pediatric acute otitis media remains to be elucidated.

Sulfa Combinations

Trimethoprim–sulfamethoxazole constitutes a rather effective treatment for acute otitis media caused by most agents, with the exception of Group A beta-hemolytic streptococci. The dosage recommended is 40 mg per kilogram per day, based on the sulfamethoxazole component. Side effects include the potential for Stevens–Johnson syndrome with sulfamethoxazole (however, this seldom occurs in practice) and the possibility of hemolytic crisis in patients severely deficient in glucose-6-phosphate dehydrogenase (G6PD).

The other sulfa combination is erythromycin and sulfisoxazole, or Pediazole. This combination has synergistic activity in vitro against *H. influenzae* strains, including those that produce beta-lactamase. The recommended dosage, based on the erythromycin component, is 40 mg per kilogram per day in four divided doses. Problems with this combination include the potential for gastrointestinal irritation attributed to erythromycin and the possibility for Stevens–Johnson syndrome associated with the use of sulfonamides.

AOMEP

At the end of therapy, AOME symptoms persist in approximately 10 percent of patients. In our experience, 70 percent of the middle ear fluid of these patients yields microorganisms. Of patients with middle ear pathogens, one-third are ampicillin-resistant and the other two-thirds are ampicillin-susceptible strains, such as *S. pneumoniae* or *H. influenzae.* Thus, in approximately 50 percent of cases of AOMEP, ampicillin-susceptible strains can be recovered. In at least 30 percent of cases of AOMEP, no pathogen is recoverable from the middle ear exudate. With AOMEP, one can either prescribe the original course of therapy (and risk missing a number of ampicillin-resistant strains), or use an alternative antimicrobial agent effective against beta-lactamase–producing strains. Regardless of the antimicrobial agent used, however, in 50 percent of cases of AOMEP, otitis media with effusion persists at the end of therapy.

Other reasons for failure, after presumptively effective antimicrobial therapy, are bacteria still susceptible to ampicillin, and also, as was recently shown by various investigators, either pure or synergistic infections with viruses such as influenzae A, respiratory syncytial virus, parainfluenza, and adenoviruses. These viral agents have been detected both singly and in combination with bacteria. The presence of viral agents should be suspected, particularly at that time of the year when these viruses are prevalent in the community. Hence, the practitioner must examine the possibility of viral prevalence when deciding on subsequent treatment in antimicrobial failure, and use this information when counseling parents.

AOME in Patients Older than 5 Years of Age

It is important to remember that the prevalence of *H. influenzae* does not cease after children reach 5 or even 8 years of age. Several investigators, including myself, have actually treated teenagers with *H. influenzae*. In fact, in a study my colleagues and I performed, *H. influenzae* was recovered from the middle ear of one-third of these older pediatric patients. Hence, antimicrobial therapy of the older child and adolescent should take into consideration *H. influenzae* and other potentially beta-lactamase–producing agents such as *Branhamella*.

For practical purposes, if one uses amoxicillin as a first-line drug and the patient responds poorly, one may presume that this particular episode of acute otitis media is caused by agents not susceptible to amoxicillin. I recommend considering trimethoprim-sulfa, erythromycin-sulfisoxazole, Augmentin, or cefaclor as alternatives.

AOME in the First Weeks of Life

Several conditions make it likely that a neonate will develop acute otitis media with effusion: cleft palate, hypotonia, mental retardation (such as Down syndrome), prematurity, and a family history of otitis media. Babies up to 3 months of age with acute otitis media were traditionally considered at high risk for middle ear infection caused by enteric agents, and therefore needed to be treated with ampicillin and an aminoglycoside. This recommendation unquestionably applies to patients whose stay in a neonatal nursery has been prolonged or who have recently been discharged after a prolonged stay. For all practical purposes, however, patients who are discharged within the first 3 days of life are less likely to have enteric pathogens in the middle ear, and, in fact, tend to have a pattern of pathogens similar to that of older infants.

Neonates with *nosocomial* acute otitis media should have a tympanocentesis to diagnose and/or exclude gram-negative enteric pathogens or Group B streptococci. Babies in the first 4 to 8 weeks of life who were discharged from the nursery after 3 days without complications and who are afebrile, stable, and relatively asymptomatic (except for fussiness) can be treated with oral therapy and followed closely for the first 24 to 48 hours. If they fail to improve and/or become febrile, these babies should be considered candidates for tympanocentesis and hospitalization for parenteral therapy. If febrile initially, the child should be considered for in-house treatment, as would a neonate with presumed sepsis. In such cases, lumbar puncture and antimicrobial therapy with ampicillin/gentamicin are appropriate management.

Follow-up Visits after AOME

The traditional follow-up scheme in treating a patient with acute otitis media includes a recheck, by telephone, at 36 to 48 hours after therapy is started. If the patient's symptoms are worse, a reevaluation for meningitis, mastoiditis, sinusitis, or bacteremia is in order. Patients whose condition is improved should be seen at 10 to 14 days after therapy is begun. If purulent otitis media is persistent after 10 to 14 days, an alternative antimicrobial therapy is started and myringotomy is considered. A reevaluation is done again in about 10 days.

Although follow-up visits are traditionally scheduled at 10 to 14 days after the beginning of therapy, reevaluation visits could be scheduled 4 to 6 weeks after diagnosis and treatment for AOME. However, this scheme may apply only to patients with reliable parents, who can be counseled to return promptly if symptoms (earache, fussiness, or fever) persist or recur after therapy is ended. We expect most symptomatic recurrences to occur within a week after antibiotic therapy has been discontinued. With this scheme, AOME is found in a small number of patients who are reevaluated 4 to 6 weeks after the initial episode of AOME. We have noted no deleterious effects using this scheme; because it was developed in a middle-class practice setting, however, it may be applicable only to this group. We do not recommend it for patients who are otitis-prone. This scheme ignores the issue of POME for approximately 4 weeks awaiting spontaneous resolution of a significant number of cases.

Persistent Otitis Media with Effusion (POME)

At the conclusion of appropriately treated acute otitis media with effusion, approximately 60 percent of patients have middle ear effusions (POME). The natural history is for resolution to occur gradually; by 3 months, effusion persists in 10 percent or fewer of cases. POME occurs regardless of initial antimicrobial therapy, and we have observed it after administration of amoxicillin, ampicillin, erythromycin-sulfa, trimethoprim–sulfamethoxazole, and cefaclor. The incidence of middle ear effusion seems not to be affected by the causative agent.

Several therapeutic options are available. One option is to prescribe an antihistamine or decongestant for a 2- to 4-week period, although the evidence for effectiveness is anecdotal. Another option is to allow spontaneous resolution without any further therapy. A third option is to give a course of prophylaxis with an antibacterial agent, administered preferably at bedtime, and reevaluate the patient at 2 to 4 weeks. The fourth alternative is to retreat the patient with another full course of antimicrobial agent and reevaluate after 10 to 14 days. This last approach has been justified by investigators who state that in some patients with effusion bacterial agents have been recovered from middle ear fluid. Although we have not previously noted improvement in the speed of resolution of POME using antimicrobials, primarily sulfas (sulfamethoxazole, TMP/SMZ), other investigators have noted a modest increase in resolution of POME with a course of amoxicillin and decongestants. Patients so treated were primarily those with a history of previous middle ear disease, and some had had effusion for 1 month or longer. (See section on chronic otitis media with effusion.) In patients who are otitis-prone, we have seen a reduction in the incidence of recurrent acute otitis media with effusion in those who received either TMP/SMZ, or sulfamethoxazole alone, compared with that of untreated controls.

Acute Otitis Media with Effusion, Recurrent (AOMER)

Some patients develop recurrence of AOME symptoms after a satisfactory response to antimicrobial therapy. These symptoms are indistinguishable from those that originally brought them to the physician. Recurrence can be caused by either a new pathogen or persistence of the initial pathogen. The practitioner must consider either repeating the course with the previous antibiotic or using another first-line antimicrobial agent.

Other Supportive Treatment for Acute Otitis Media

Patients with intractable or more persistent pain may be candidates for myringotomy, as are those who have failed on antibiotic therapy or who have persistent conductive hearing loss. Myringotomy could also be recommended for patients who have failed to improve, or who have not defervesced after 48 hours of antimicrobial therapy. Phenylephrine hydrochloride at 1.4 percent may be used, or oral decongestants such as pseudoephedrine or antihistamines, although the published support for their efficacy in AOM is virtually nonexistent. They may be used for 3 to 5 days and only in children who are older than 4 months of age. Oral decongestants for symptomatic relief may have a potential role for patients with severe rhinorrhea. It is important to remember that studies with oral decongestants have failed to show significant improvement of POME in treated patients versus controls when patients are followed *beyond* the acute 2-week phase (i.e., at the 4- to 6-week follow-up).

Whenever AOME is treated in children who have gastrointestinal manifestations such as vomiting, the first antibiotic dose may be given intramuscularly if the physician is ensured that the patient does not have central nervous system (CNS) complications.

OTITIS-PRONENESS (OP)

Twenty-six percent of children have had six or more episodes of AOME by the time they are 6 years of age; they have these factors in common: (1) they started having acute otitis media when they were younger than 1 year of age and (2) whenever tym-

panocentesis was done, pneumococci were more commonly recovered. In approximately 20 percent of patients, there was a family history of AOME. This seems to be a more common problem among Eskimos, in whom a high risk for hearing loss has been reported.

Children who have suffered three or more episodes of AOM in the previous 12 months should be called otitis-prone. These patients are candidates for therapeutic intervention and may benefit from prophylactic antibiotic therapy. Prophylactic therapy could consist of administration of either sulfa agent, such as a bedtime dose of sulfamethoxazole (20 mg per kilogram), or sulfisoxazole (30 mg per kilogram). We have used both of these preparations as well as TMP/SMZ, calculated at 20 to 40 mg per kilogram of the sulfa component at bedtime. (This use of TMP/SMZ is not approved by the FDA.) In this type of therapy, we have noted a decrease in the incidence of AOME in patients followed prospectively over a 3-month period. Other prophylactic options include administration of either a penicillin or amoxicillin (10 mg per kilogram) preferably at bedtime or at most twice a day.

In general, the principle to be observed in calculating antimicrobial prophylaxis for otitis media is to use one-half the therapeutic dose once or twice a day, and preferably in the evening. Regardless of the approach, prophylactic use comes with a challenge. This type of therapy, although it appears effective in reducing the episodes of AOME, does not seem to affect persistence of fluid, and therefore the auditory morbidity may still be there. Prophylactic therapy may be more effective during the "otitis media season," i.e., during the cooler months of December through April. For children with a history of POME, tympanograms should be considered. None of the sulfa preparations is indicated for children younger than 2 months of age. An audiogram should be done in children old enough to cooperate during the procedure.

CHRONIC OTITIS MEDIA WITH EFFUSION (COME)

Despite various maneuvers, approximately 10 percent of patients have persistence of otitis media with effusion for 3 months. This diagnosis is made by noting an opaque tympanic membrane, which appears neutral and retracted in position with poor or no mobility and decreased landmarks, in a patient who is generally asymptomatic except for hearing impairment. In some groups, chronic middle ear effusion has been blamed for conductive hearing loss secondary to decreased auditory perception, delayed development and impaired speech and language, with lower scores on tests of cognitive ability, and poor performance in school. When the effusion has persisted for 3 months or more, it is important to enlist the help of an otorhinolaryngologist; patients who have a history of recurrent otitis media with effusion may actually be referred to this specialist earlier. It is our practice to offer at least one additional course of full antimicrobial therapy before any surgical procedure is performed; this is done more with hope than conviction. Additionally, it is known that when middle ear effusions from patients with chronic persistent otitis media with effusion are cultured, approximately one-third contain bacterial pathogens, primarily *H. influenzae.*

As one considers the most cogent etiologies for POME or COME, eustachian tube dysfunction with or without allergy, the possibility of using intranasal topical steroids becomes more appealing. No solid guidelines are available in this regard. The use of systemic steroids such as prednisone in short courses has been advocated by some to promote drainage of mucoid fluid, either with or without an antimicrobial agent such as sulfa. I do not recommend the use of these steroidal preparations.

Ventilation tubes offer probably the last resort for the patient with COME. The few patients under consideration should be selected carefully. Usually, the medical prophylactic approach takes care of most cases. The role of ventilatory tubes is limited to patients who have failed medical management, who have recurrent acute otitis media or persistent atelectasis, or who are otitis-prone. These tubes are by no means a panacea and in themselves are associated with complications such as otorrhea, obstruction of the tube lumen, premature extrusion (normally, they would extrude between 6 and 9 months after insertion), problem with retention of tube, myringosclerosis, atrophic scar, retraction pockets, persistent perforation of tympanic membrane, cholesteatoma, bleeding, and displacement of tube into the middle ear cavity.

CHRONIC SUPPURATIVE OTITIS MEDIA (CSOM)

Occasionally, chronic otitis media is associated with chronic otorrhea and evidence of suppurative reaction. The microbiology of the fluid recovered includes *Pseudomonas aeruginosa,* and beta-lactamase–producing *S. aureus,* but primarily gram-negative enteric microbes. The ear canal and tympanic membrane should be examined otomicroscopically and the middle ear fluid cultured directly through the perforation or ventilating tubes. Audiograms, tympanograms, mastoid radiographs, and appropriate susceptibility testing of the microbe should be done.

Because the causative agents in CSOM differ widely and radically from those traditionally associated with acute otitis media, the therapy is predicated on the susceptibility pattern of the microbe. In patients with no gross abnormalities (e.g., cholesteatoma), the therapy should be given parenterally at least until the patient's ear has been dry by otomicroscopic examination on three consecutive days. Therapy could be completed on an outpatient basis, and individualized prophylactic therapy continued thereafter to prevent recurrence. Hence, barring the presence of cholesteatoma or other structural abnormality, medical management may be sufficient to effect a cure. Because *P. aeruginosa* and *S. aureus* are the most common agents recovered, initial antibiotic therapy should be directed to cover at least these two agents until identification is made. Surgical management is dictated by the presence of such conditions as cholesteatoma.

SUGGESTED READING

Barriga F, Schwartz R, Hayden GF. Adequate illumination for otoscopy. Am J Dis Child 1986; 140:1237–1240.

Mandel E, Rochette HE, Bluestone CD, et al. Efficacy of amoxicillin with and without decongestant antihistamine for otitis media with effusion in children. N Engl J Med 1987; 316:432–437.

Marchant CD, Shurin P, Johnson C. A randomized controlled trial of amoxicillin plus clavulanate compared with cefaclor for treatment of acute otitis media. J Pediatr 1986; 109:891–896.

Marchant CD, Shurin PA, Turcyzk VA, et al. A randomized controlled trial of Ceclor® compared with trimethoprim-sulfamethoxazole for treatment of acute otitis media. J Pediatr 1984; 105:633–637.

Schwartz RH, Rodriguez WJ, McAveney W, et al. Cerumen removal: how necessary is it to diagnose acute otitis media? Am J Dis Child 1983; 137:1064–1065.

Schwartz R, Rodriguez W, Grundfast K. Duration of middle ear effusion after acute otitis media. Pediatr Infect Dis 1983; 3:204–207.

MASTOIDITIS

ORVAL E. BROWN, M.D., F.A.C.S., F.A.A.P.

ACUTE MASTOIDITIS

Acute mastoiditis is an infection of the air cell complex of the temporal bone. This air cell complex connects with the middle ear space through the aditus ad antrum, creating one continuum of mucosa-lined air spaces. Effusion in the middle ear space is therefore almost invariably accompanied by effusion in the mastoid air cells. Mastoiditis is a general term encompassing a spectrum of diseases, including acute mastoiditis, which includes the stages of mastoiditis with periostitis and coalescent mastoid abscess, and chronic mastoiditis. The stage of mastoiditis with periostitis is characterized by infection of the mastoid periosteum, and the stage of coalescent mastoid abscess is characterized by destruction and lysis of the bony septa of the mastoid air cells. The bacteriology is similar to that of acute otitis media, with *Streptococcus pneumoniae, Haemophilus influenzae,* and *Streptococcus pyogenes* being the most frequently isolated microorganisms. Immunosuppressed patients and infants have a higher incidence of gram-negative organisms such as *Klebsiella pneumoniae, Pseudomonas aeruginosa,* and *Staphylococcus aureus.*

Clinical Evaluation

An infant with mastoiditis is usually ill with low-grade fever. It is unusual to see sepsis in the absence of central nervous system complications or other underlying problems. The pinna is classically displaced anteriorly and inferiorly. The retroauricular area is inflamed and may be fluctuant in the presence of a subperiosteal abscess. Otoscopic examination may reveal sagging of the posterior superior aspect of the external auditory canal, which obscures examination of the tympanic membrane. The tympanic membrane is thickened and inflamed, and a small perforation may be present. This is identified by a small nipple of granulation tissue at the site of the perforation and purulent otorrhea exuding from the middle ear space. Almost invariably a purulent middle ear effusion exists, except in cases in which the mastoid air cell complex is blocked at the aditus ad antrum and the middle ear space is cleared through the eustachian tube. Radiographs in acute mastoiditis with periostitis reveal clouding of the mastoid air cell system as a result of effusion and mucosal edema of the air cells. Coalescent mastoid abscess is indicated by loss of the delicate bony septa of the mastoid air cells and demineralization or loss of mastoid cortex. These radiographic findings are essential to the diagnosis of coalescent mastoid abscess.

Medical Therapy

Patients with mastoiditis are hospitalized and volume deficits are repleted by intravenous fluids. Material for Gram stain, culture, and antibiotic susceptibility tests is obtained by means of a tympanocentesis or myringotomy before antibiotic therapy is instituted. If the postauricular area is fluctuant, fluid for culture is obtained by needle aspiration. My initial antibiotic of choice is cefuroxime, 75 to 100 mg IV per kilogram of body weight per day, in three divided doses. Alternatively, nafcillin, 100 to 200 mg IV per kilogram per day in four divided doses, may be administered. Initial antimicrobial therapy is continued until culture and susceptibility results are available, and is modified based on these results. When the patient has been afebrile for 48 hours, and pain, retroauricular swelling, and constitutional symptoms are resolving, oral antimicrobial therapy is started. Usually amoxicillin/potassium clavulanate (Aug-

mentin), 40 mg per kilogram per day in three divided doses, or cefaclor, 40 mg per kilogram per day in three divided doses, is administered, depending on the culture and susceptibility results. Oral therapy is continued for a total course of 10 to 14 days or longer, depending on the patient's response. If unusual organisms are suspected, broader antibiotic coverage can be obtained with combinations such as nafcillin, (150 mg per kilogram per day in four divided doses) and ceftazidime (100 to 150 mg per kilogram per day in three divided doses) or with ampicillin (100 to 200 mg per kilogram per day in four divided doses) and an aminoglycoside such as amikacin (15 to 20 mg per kilogram per day in three divided doses).

Surgical Therapy

Surgical therapy is not undertaken until the patient is stable, volume deficits are replaced, and antibiotic therapy has been initiated. In patients with acute mastoiditis with periostitis, a wide myringotomy for drainage is performed. A tympanostomy tube is placed, but not in the wide myringotomy incision, because early extrusion of the tube may result. Patients with coalescent mastoid abscess undergo drainage through a retroauricular incision, and a complete mastoidectomy is performed to remove the mastoid empyema.

The temporal bone of the infant lacks a mastoid process; this begins to develop during the second year of life and nears completion by age 6 years. The facial nerve is in a lateral and unprotected position until this development is completed. Accordingly, the postauricular incision is made 1 cm behind the postauricular crease to protect the facial nerve. The cortex of the mastoid is removed, and the mastoid air cells are exenterated until the aditus ad antrum is opened widely and irrigation fluid flows freely into the middle ear from the mastoid cavity. The posterior bony canal wall is not removed; "radical" exenterative surgical procedures are almost never indicated. The wound is closed, and drains are left in the mastoid cavity. Postoperative mastoid dressings are changed daily, and the drain is removed when the disease is controlled.

Complications

Intratemporal complications of mastoiditis include petrositis, labyrinthitis, facial paralysis, and Bezold's abscess. Bezold's abscess is an extension of infection through the mastoid tip into the superior sternocleidomastoid muscle and neck. Cervical drainage is required in addition to otologic management. Petrositis and labyrinthitis require appropriate surgical drainage. Facial paralysis caused by acute otitis media and mastoiditis is treated with wide myringotomy, removal of the purulent effusion from the middle ear space, and complete mastoidectomy. Facial nerve decompression is not acutely indicated. Intracranial complications include epidural and subdural abscess, meningitis, and brain abscess. Neurologic evaluation arouses suspicion of these entities, and computed tomography provides radiographic diagnosis. Appropriate neurosurgical consultation and management are mandatory.

CHRONIC MASTOIDITIS

Chronic mastoiditis is invariably associated with chronic suppurative otitis media, defined as chronic inflammation of the middle ear and mastoid with tympanic membrane perforation. Physical examination reveals purulent otorrhea draining from the tympanic membrane perforation. The eardrum remnant and middle ear space are inflamed. The middle ear mucosa may be polypoid and extrude through the eardrum perforation into the ear canal. Occasionally cholesteatoma is associated with chronic otitis media. The retroauricular area is almost always normal. Mastoid radiographs reveal a small, poorly pneumatized, or sclerotic mastoid. The microbiology of the otorrhea is usually *Pseudomonas aeruginosa*, *Proteus* species, *Staphylococcus aureus,* or anaerobes.

Medical Therapy

Initial medical management is directed at drying the ear with topical preparations. After careful cleaning of the ear, using the microscope and suction, a short course of otic drops such as Cortisporin Otic Suspension, which contains neomycin, polymyxin B, and hydrocortisone, is administered three times a day for no more than 5 to 7 days. Although aminoglycosides administered in the middle ear space have the potential to cause ototoxicity and sensorineural hearing loss, I have never seen a case caused by short-term administration of these agents. At 1 week, if the patient has not responded, a culture and antibiotic susceptibility test is performed.

Often a resistant *Pseudomonas* is the responsible pathogen. This may respond to gentamicin ophthalmic drops, given into the external ear canal three times a day, or to a regimen of ear canal irrigation using Otic Domeboro solution three times a day. This solution is administered using a Monoject curved-tip syringe for gently flushing the ear canal and middle ear. The commercially available Otic Domeboro solution may be used, or a solution can be made using 1 cup of water, 1 cup of white vinegar, and 2 Domeboro tablets.

For patients who do not respond to a course of gentamicin drops or Otic Domeboro irrigations, intensive outpatient therapy is tried. Patients are seen at least daily, preferably twice a day, for aural suctioning to remove all purulent debris. The ear is powdered with "gold dust" powder, which consists of chloramphenicol, amphotericin B, and sulfadiazine powder mixed in equal proportions. For patients who do not

respond, I consider hospitalization for 10 to 14 days with administration of intravenous antibiotics based on the culture and susceptibility results. This usually consists of ticarcillin (200 to 300 mg per kilogram per day in four divided doses) and tobramycin (3 to 5 mg per kilogram per day in three divided doses), with twice-a-day aural hygiene. Most patients respond to this regimen.

Surgical Therapy

When otorrhea is controlled by medical therapy, surgical therapy is not urgent. In older children, a tympanoplasty for repair of the tympanic membrane perforation is not recommended until after an observation period of a minimum of 6 to 12 months, to ensure that the ear remains dry. A mastoidectomy is usually unnecessary if the ear is dry with healthy middle ear mucosa. Very young children are usually not candidates for early surgical repair, because eustachian tube dysfunction and resultant otitis media with effusion can complicate repair of the perforation. These patients are followed until at least age 5 or 6 years, and the status of the opposite ear is a good indicator of improved eustachian tube function. When the opposite ear has been clear for 1 year, surgical repair is confidently recommended.

Patients who respond poorly to medical therapy and have continued otorrhea undergo complete mastoidectomy with tympanoplasty to repair the tympanic membrane perforation. The mastoid air cells are completely exenterated. They are often filled with granulation tissue with softening of the air cell septae from osteitis. The posterior external ear canal wall is preserved in most cases; rarely is this removed to convert the mastoidectomy to an open cavity procedure. Radical mastoidectomy, with removal of the tympanic membrane and ossicular chain, is not indicated.

Occasionally acquired cholesteatoma accompanies chronic mastoiditis. Mastoidectomy with tympanoplasty is indicated to remove the cholesteatoma from the mastoid and middle ear and to repair the tympanic membrane defect. The choice of procedure, whether intact posterior external ear canal wall or open cavity, is controversial. The decision is individualized and based on the extent and location of the cholesteatoma, among other factors.

SUGGESTED READING

Bluestone CD, Klein JO. Intratemporal complications and sequelae to otitis media. In: Bluestone CD, Stool SE, eds. Pediatric otolaryngology. Philadelphia: WB Saunders, 1983; 513.

Ginsburg CM, Rudoy R, Nelson JD. Acute mastoiditis in infants and children. Clin Pediatr 1980; 19(8):549–553.

Kenna M, Bluestone CD, Reilly JS, Lusk RP. Medical management of chronic suppurative otitis media without cholesteatoma in children. Laryngoscope 1986; 96 (2):146–151.

SINUSITIS

RAUL C. RUDOY, M.D., M.P.H.

ACUTE SINUSITIS

Acute sinusitis is an infection of the paranasal sinuses, which is usually preceded by an acute viral respiratory infection. Malfunction of the sinus ciliary apparatus and obstruction of the sinus ostia result in retention of sinus secretions and subsequent infection. The microbiology of sinus infections in pediatric patients has been recently delineated. *Streptococcus pneumoniae,* nontypable *Haemophilus influenzae,* and *Branhamella catarrhalis* are the organisms responsible for more than 70 percent of the cases of acute maxillary sinusitis. Occasionally Group A streptococcus and peptostreptococcus have been isolated from infected maxillary sinuses. *Staphylococcus aureus* is not a common pathogen of acute sinusitis except for cases of ethmoiditis, in which it is the second most commonly isolated organism, after *H. influenzae.*

For acute uncomplicated sinusitis I usually begin treatment with amoxicillin (40 mg per kilogram per day in three divided doses for 10 days). Most patients respond rapidly to this treatment with improvement of symptoms within 48 to 72 hours. No response by that time indicates poor compliance in taking the medication, lack of effective sinus drainage, or infection with bacteria resistant to amoxicillin such as a beta-lactamase–producing *H. influenzae* or *B. catarrhalis.* I usually assume the latter and change therapy to an antibiotic resistant to beta-lactamases. Suitable choices include Augmentin (amoxicillin and potassium clavulanate, 40 mg per kilogram per day in three divided doses) and the erythromycin–sulfisoxazole combination (40/120 mg per kilogram per day in four divided doses) for 10 days. Trimethoprim–sulfamethoxazole is also effective against beta-lactamase–producing bacteria, but it is ineffective against group A streptococci.

Patients with worsening clinical conditions or those with presenting symptoms that include periorbital swelling, generalized toxicity, or evidence of intraorbital or intracranial dissemination of the infection should be hospitalized and treated with parenterally administered antibiotics. A combination of methicillin or nafcillin (150 to 200 mg per kilogram per day in four divided doses) and chloramphenicol (50 to 75 mg per kilogram per day in four divided doses) provides adequate antimicrobial coverage until blood, sinus, and (if indicated) cerebrospinal fluid (CSF) culture results are available. Duration of treatment depends on the severity of the disease, but in most cases it is 10 to 14 days. If intracranial complications have been ruled out and improvement is rapid after parenteral antibiotics are given, the rest of the treatment course can be completed with one of the oral antibiotics effective against beta-lactamase–producing bacteria.

Aspiration of the infected sinus is indicated when culture material is needed to guide the choice of antimicrobials used and when clinical failure is a result of deficient sinus drainage. Removal of infected material results in better ventilation and oxygenation of the sinus, provides material for culture and promotes effective drainage. Aspiration is recommended for severely ill children, those with suppurative complications, those who fail to respond to antimicrobial treatment, and selected immunocompromised patients.

The role of antihistamines and decongestants (oral or topical) has not been studied critically, but from the limited available studies they do not seem to be beneficial and are perhaps even detrimental by producing inspissated secretions (antihistamines) or by decreasing ciliary function and blood flow to the sinus mucosa (decongestants).

CHRONIC SINUSITIS

Sinusitis lasting longer than 3 months is considered to be chronic. The etiologic agents of chronic sinusitis include a large number of anaerobic bacteria, staphylococci, streptococci, and other bacterial species capable of producing acute sinusitis. Medical treatment consists of using antibiotics effective against beta-lactamase–producing bacteria for prolonged periods of time (3 to 6 weeks).

Possible contributing factors such as polyps, cysts, and nasal septum deviation should be evaluated by careful examination and by obtaining sinus radiographs. The chances that medical treatment will be successful are reduced if the anatomic abnormalities are not corrected. Sinus aspiration with or without sinus lavage or antrostomy should be considered for patients who fail to respond to antimicrobial treatment.

COMPLICATIONS

The proximity of the sinuses to intracranial and intraorbital structures occasionally results in orbital or periorbital cellulitis and rarely in intracranial infections such as cavernous sinus thrombosis, meningitis, or brain abscess. Parenteral antimicrobial therapy is indicated, and it should be tailored to the bacteria isolated from cultures. Intraorbital suppuration is usually the result of an infection with *Staphylococcus aureus, H. influenzae,* or *Streptococcus pneumoniae.* Sinus aspiration and lavage are recommended, particularly for cases with intracranial complications. Initial antibiotic treatment for cases with intracranial suppuration should include coverage against staphylococci, *H. influenzae,* group A streptococcus, and anaerobic bacteria. A combination of an antistaphylococcal penicillin (methicillin or nafcillin 150 to 200 mg per kilogram per day in four divided doses) and chloramphenicol (75 to 100 mg per kilogram per day in four divided doses) provides adequate initial coverage. Cefotaxime (200 mg per kilogram per day in four divided doses) or cefuroxime (240 mg per kilogram per day in four divided doses) can be used for patients with less severe complications, such as periorbital cellulitis.

SUGGESTED READING

Bluestone CH. The diagnosis and management of sinusitis in children: proceedings of a closed conference. Pediatr Infect Dis 1985; 4:549–581.

Brook I. Bacteriological features of chronic sinusitis in children. JAMA 1981; 246:947–969.

Hawkins DB, Clark RW. Orbital involvement in acute sinusitis: lessons from 24 childhood patients. Clin Pediatr 1977; 16:464–471.

Ward ER, Reilly JS, Casselbrant M, et al. Treatment of acute maxillary sinusitis in childhood: a comparative study of amoxicillin and cefaclor. J. Pediatr 1984; 104:297–302.

DISEASES OF THE EYE

CONJUNCTIVITIS AND KERATITIS

ALICE MATOBA, M.D.

CONJUNCTIVITIS

The most frequently identified etiologic agent in infectious neonatal conjunctivitis is *Chlamydia trachomatis.* Bacterial agents that are commonly isolated include *Streptococcus* sp., *Staphylococcus aureus,* and *Haemophilus influenzae.* Gonococcal ophthalmia neonatorum is now rare, but its association with systemic infection and its potential for serious ocular complications, including corneal ulceration, make this a significant entity. Viral conjunctivitis is rare and usually is associated with systemic infection.

In older infants and children, bacterial and viral agents are the predominant etiologic agents of conjunctivitis. *H. influenzae* and *S. pneumoniae* are the most commonly diagnosed bacteria. Viral conjunctivitis may occur as an ocular manifestation of systemic disease (secondary to varicella, rubella, measles, or Epstein-Barr virus) or as relatively localized infection (resulting from adenovirus, herpes simplex virus, or enterovirus 70). Chlamydial conjunctivitis is rare in older infants and children; consideration of workup for other sexually transmitted infections and for evidence of sexual abuse is appropriate in children with chlamydial or gonococcal conjunctivitis.

Infectious conjunctivitis is characterized by diffuse conjunctival injection, variable degrees of chemosis and lid edema, and ocular discharge. In older infants and children, evaluation of presence or absence of conjunctival follicles (lymphoid hyperplasia), quality of the discharge, and preauricular lymphadenopathy help to distinguish the major groups of etiologic agents (Table 1). These clinical features are not helpful in neonates. Both chlamydia and bacteria give rise to purulent-appearing discharge in the newborn. Follicular hypertrophy and preauricular lymphadenopathy are usually absent. The time of onset is variable.

Patients with suspected infectious conjunctivitis should undergo microbiologic investigation. Collection of a specimen by scraping with a platinum spatula is slightly more productive than swabbing with an applicator stick.

Treatment

I treat neonatal chlamydial conjunctivitis with oral erythromycin suspension, either erythromycin estolate or the ethylsuccinate ester, 40 mg per kilogram per day given in four divided doses for 14 days (Table 2). Therapy is aimed at eradication of systemic infection and nasopharyngeal colonization, which is associated with significant risk of development of pulmonary infection. Topical therapy is not necessary. After therapy is completed, nasopharyngeal swabs are evaluated by culture or fluorescein-conjugated monoclonal antibody staining. If persistent infection is noted, a second course of treatment is initiated. The mother and her sex partner(s) are treated with erythromycin base, 500 mg given orally four times daily for 7 days. Chlamydial conjunctivitis in children is treated with erythromycin, 40 mg per kilogram per day in four divided doses up to 2 per day.

Gonococcal conjunctivitis is treated with intravenous penicillin G, 100,000 U per kilogram per day in four divided doses for 7 days. Frequent ocular irrigation with saline and topical penicillin treatment are used as adjunctive measures (see Table 2). Treatment for other bacterial infections is determined by the Gram stain of the smear and the severity of infection (see Table 2).

Prevention of neonatal conjunctivitis is not achieved completely by any of the measures currently employed. Silver nitrate solution is not effective in prophylaxis of chlamydial conjunctivitis. Erythromycin is effective in preventing gonococcal conjunctivitis and possibly chlamydial conjunctivitis (there are conflicting reports). However, none of the topically applied agents affect nasopharyngeal chlamydial colonization.

Viral conjunctivitis associated with systemic disease caused by varicella, varicella-zoster, rubella, measles, or Epstein-Barr virus is usually self-limited and requires no specific treatment. If pain or photophobia is marked, however, the patient should be evaluated by an ophthalmologist, because keratitis or iritis rarely coexists with conjunctivitis. For adenoviral infection, no specific therapy is available. Patients should be treated conservatively with suppor-

TABLE 1 Signs of Conjunctivitis[a]

Stage of Disease	Infant and Child			Neonate		
	Viral	Chlamydial	Bacterial	Viral	Chlamydial	Bacterial
Discharge	Serous	Mucoid or mucopurulent	Purulent	Serous	Purulent	Purulent
Conjunctival follicles	+	+	−	−	−	−
Preauricular lymphadenopathy	+	+	−[b]	−	−	−

[a] + = present; − = absent.
[b] Exceptions: Severe conjunctivitis, classically gonococcal.

tive measures such as cold compresses. If inflammation is marked or subepithelial corneal infiltrates causing blurring of vision develop, the patient should be referred to an ophthalmologist for evaluation and consideration of topical corticosteroid therapy. I treat patients with herpes simplex conjunctivitis with topical vidarabine, 3 percent ointment used five times a day, or trifluridine, 1 percent solution used five to eight times a day for 4 to 5 days, to minimize the risk of development of herpetic keratitis. Ocular infection with enterovirus 70 or Coxsackie virus type A24 (acute hemorrhagic conjuncti-

TABLE 2 Treatment of Conjunctivitis

Infection	Drug	Systemic Therapy	Topical Therapy	Adjunctive Therapy
Gonococcal Neonate	Penicillin G	100,000 U/kg/day IV in 4 doses for 5–7 days. If penicillin-resistant, IV cefotaxime 100 mg/kg/day in 4 doses or IV ceftriaxone, 50 mg/kg/day once daily	100,000 U/ml solution[a] One drop every hour	Saline irrigation every 1–2 hours Treat parents
Infant and child	Penicillin G	Same. Give adult dose if child weighs 100 lb or more. If penicillin-resistant, IV cefotaxime 150 mg/kg/day in 2–3 divided doses or Ceftriaxone 50 mg/kg/day once daily up to 1 g/day	Same as above	Consider possibility of sexual abuse
Bacterial[b] Gram positive cocci	Erythromycin[c]		Ointment, every 2 hours	
	Cefuroxime[d]	Treatment tailored to extraocular disease (orbital or preseptal cellulitis, etc)	50 mg/ml solution[a] one drop every hour	
Gram negative rods	Gentamicin	None if disease localized to the eye. If evidence of extraocular involvement, tailor regimen to nature of disease	0.3 mg/ml solution, one drop every 1–2 hours	
	Cefuroxime[e]			
Chlamydia trachomatis Neonate	Erythromycin	Suspension, 40 mg/kg/day in 4 doses for 14 days	Ointment, every 2 hours. Optional	Saline irrigation every 2 hours; treat parents
Infant and child	Erythromycin	40 mg/kg/day up to 2 g/day in 4 doses for 14 days	Same as above	Consider possibility of sexual abuse

[a] Mix in artificial tears. Refrigerate or keep on ice at bedside.
[b] In older children mild bacterial conjunctivitis can be treated with erythromycin or bacitracin/polymyxin ointment without Gram stain evaluation.
[c] Mild disease.
[d] Severe disease or extraocular involvement.
[e] Add if suspected *H. influenzae* infection.

vitis) is generally self-limited, and only supportive treatment is necessary.

KERATITIS

Keratitis is characterized by variable degrees of pain, blurring of vision, and photophobia. The quality of the pain can range from foreign-body sensation (suggestive of epithelial disease) to aching or throbbing (suggestive of ciliary body irritation associated with stromal or epithelial keratitis or secondary iritis).

Most cases of keratitis associated with infection are secondary to active microbial replication or are immunologically mediated. Entities classified as immunologically mediated are so designated based on lack of response to antimicrobial therapy and favorable response to steroid therapy. However, in most cases the exact pathogenesis has not been defined and the antigen and antibodies or effector cells not identified.

Immunologically mediated, infection-associated keratitis is generally nonulcerative and may be classified by the pattern of corneal involvement. Subepithelial or anterior stromal infiltrates are classically seen sequential to adenoviral conjunctivitis. But similar infiltrates may be seen following chlamydial, Epstein-Barr viral, or herpes simplex viral (HSV) infection. Disciform keratitis, characterized by full-thickness stromal edema and iritis is seen in association with recurrent herpes simplex infection. Less commonly, it may be noted in association with varicella-zoster virus (VZV), adenovirus, and mumps virus infection. Interstitial keratitis (IK) is classically seen in patients with congenital syphilis and in a small percentage of patients with acquired syphilis. Although spirochetes have been identified in the corneas of a few neonates with syphilitic IK, interstitial keratitis is considered to be primarily immunologic. Stromal infiltration associated with deep vascularization is also seen in patients with herpes simplex virus and Epstein-Barr virus infection.

Keratitis associated with active replication of organisms may involve the epithelium or stroma. Infectious epithelial keratitis is secondary to viral infection and is manifested in a dendritic pattern with varying degrees of underlying stromal infiltration. Herpes simplex virus is the primary etiologic agent. Very rarely varicella-zoster virus may cause dendritic keratitis while Epstein-Barr virus has been linked to

TABLE 3   Treatment of Infection-Associated Immunologically Mediated Keratitis

Stage of Disease	Type of Disease	Corticosteroid Therapy	Antimicrobial Therapy
Inflammation mild and no involvement of visual axis	Subepithelial infiltrates (SEI)	None	If ADV, EBV—none. If associated with active chlamydial infection, treat as for chlamydial conjunctivitis. If active HSV ocular infection (conjunctivitis, blepharitis, dendritic keratitis) treat with vidarabine 3% ointment 5 times per day or trifluridine 1% 1 drop 8 times per day.[a]
	Disciform keratitis	None	If VZV, ADV, EBV, mumps—none. If HSV, consider vidarabine ointment 5 times a day or trifluridine solution one drop 5–8 times per day if associated conjunctivitis is marked.[a]
	Interstitial keratitis (IK)	Prednisolone acetate 1%, one drop every 2 hours while awake.[a] Consider observation prior to initiation of therapy	If syphilis: treat with appropriate systemic regimen for syphilis. See chapter on *Syphilis*. No topical antimicrobial therapy necessary. If VZV—none except as necessary for extraocular site or dissemination. If HSV treat with vidarabine or trifluridine at doses recommended above I-SEI.[a] If EBV—none.
Inflammation moderate to severe or visual axis involvement	Subepithelial infiltrates	Prednisolone acetate one drop 4–6 times per day. Taper to minimal amount needed to maintain response within 2–4 weeks[a]	If ADV, EBV—none. If chlamydial—see I-SEI. If HSV—vidarabine or trifluridine in doses recommended above I-SEI. Taper along with corticosteroid.[a]
	Disciform keratitis	See II-SEI	If ADV, VZV, mumps—none. If HSV—see II-SEI
	Interstitial keratitis	Prednisolone acetate 1% one drop every 1–2 hours while awake[a]	See I-IK

[a] Should be carried out under guidance of an ophthalmologist.

one documented case of dendritic keratitis. Stromal keratitis associated with microbial replication is caused by a variety of organisms. Bacterial keratitis is associated with ulceration and suppuration, which can rapidly lead to corneal perforation if not treated. *Pseudomonas aeruginosa, S. pneumoniae,* and *S. aureus* are the most commonly identified etiologic agents. Fungal keratitis is most often caused by *Candida, Aspergillus,* or *Fusarium* species. HSV and VZV are probably capable of replication in stromal keratocytes and are believed to produce necrotizing keratitis through that mechanism. The pathogenesis of diffusely scattered punctate epithelial keratitis, which is seen transiently in patients with adenoviral, herpes simplex, molluscum, chlamydial, varicella-zoster, and measles conjunctivitis is not well-defined. This pattern may be a result of a combination of mechanisms, including epithelial infection.

Factors that predispose to development of infectious keratitis include dry eyes, exposure, generalized immunosuppression, corneal denervation, injury, and contact lens wear. *P. aeruginosa* is the bacterial agent most commonly implicated in contact lens-associated corneal ulceration. In recent years, *Acanthamoeba* has also been identified with increasing frequency as a pathogenic organism in contact lens wearers.

Cultures should be taken from patients with suspected keratitis by scraping with a platinum spatula and direct inoculation of culture media. This procedure is most effectively performed by slit lamp examination and should be performed by an ophthalmologist. In patients with deep stromal infection or suspected *Acanthamoeba* keratitis, corneal biopsy may be necessary to identify the infecting organism.

Treatment

Patients with immunologically mediated keratitis should be evaluated by an ophthalmologist to determine the severity of the inflammation and the degree of visual impairment and to exclude concomitant active infection. Patients with mild inflammation with little or no visual impairment can be treated conservatively, with observation. Patients with more marked disease should be treated with topical corticosteroids under the supervision of an ophthalmologist (Table 3). Frequent slit-lamp biomicroscopic evaluations are crucial to gauge response to therapy and

TABLE 4   Initial Medical Therapy of Infectious Keratitis

Etiology	Topical Therapy	Subconjunctival Therapy[a]	Systemic Therapy[b]
Bacterial			
Gram-positive cocci	Cefazolin or cefuroxime 50 mg/ml 1 drop every hour[c,d]	Cefazolin or cefuroxime 100 mg in ½ cc	Cefazolin IV 50–100 mg/kg/day divided every 6 or 8 hours or Cefuroxime IV 75–100 mg/kg/day divided every 6–8 hours
Gram-negative rods	Tobramycin 13.6 mg/ml one drop every 15–30 min around the clock[c,e,f]	Tobramycin 20 mg in ½ cc[f]	Tobramycin IV 3.0–7.5 mg/kg/day divided every 8 hours[b]
No organisms seen or multiple organisms	Cefuroxime plus tobramycin[c]	Cefuroxime plus tobramycin	Cefuroxime plus tobramycin
Acid-fast bacilli	Amikacin 10–20 mg/ml one drop every 30 min while awake	Amikacin 20 mg in ½ cc	
Fungal	Natamycin 1% one drop every hour around the clock[c] or Amphotericin B 0.25% one drop every hour	Miconazole 10 mg (polyenes too toxic to inject sunconjunctivally)	Consider ketoconazole, miconazole, amphotericin
Viral			
HSV—necrotizing stromal keratitis	Prednisolone acetate 1% one drop every 1–2 hours while awake. Consider addition of trifluridine 1% one drop 8 times per day	None	Inadequate data available to justify systemic corticosteroid or antiviral therapy in ocular infection

[a] Reserve for severe keratitis.
[b] If cornea perforated or scleral extension.
[c] May be treated while awake rather than around the clock if infection is mild.
[d] Mix in artificial tears. Refrigerate or keep on ice at bedside.
[e] One vial intravenous formulation 80 mg per 2 cc + 1 bottle ophthalmic formulation 15 mg in 5 ml.
[f] If *H. influenzae* suspected add cefuroxime.

assess development of side effects of topical corticosteroid therapy such as glaucoma (reversible) and cataract (nonreversible). Patients with interstitial keratitis should be evaluated for lues and treated with appropriate doses of systemic penicillin and topical corticosteroid.

Patients with infectious keratitis are treated with topical antimicrobial agents (Table 4). Subconjunctival antimicrobial therapy is reserved for severe infection and systemic therapy is reserved for patients with perforation or imminent perforation. In patients with bacterial corneal ulcers, I add topical corticosteroid therapy 24 to 48 hours following response to antibiotic therapy. Corticosteroid therapy is withheld in the setting of fungal keratitis and its role is controversial for active stromal keratitis caused by *Acanthamoeba*. HSV necrotizing stromal keratitis is treated primarily with topical corticosteroids, although the condition is believed to be associated with viral replication within the cornea. Topical antiviral agents and moderate amounts of systemic antiviral therapy have not proven to be of benefit. If corneal perforation occurs during the course of therapy, penetrating keratoplasty is performed to restore the integrity of the eye.

Evaluation of Response to Therapy

If clinical response is not seen within 24 to 48 hours, modification of therapy should be considered. Choice of antibiotic should be based on culture results and susceptibility testing. If identification of an organism is not available, rescraping or corneal biopsy should be considered. Signs of favorable response to therapy include reepithelialization of the ulcer or breakup of dendrite, decrease in suppuration, and change in the morphology of the edge of the stromal infiltrate to a more discrete or granular appearance. These signs should be evaluated by an ophthalmologist and modification of therapy carried out with his consultation.

SUGGESTED READING

Matoba A. Ocular viral infections. Pediatr Infect Dis 1984; 3:358–368.

Morbidity and Mortality Weekly Report (suppl) 1985; 34:75S–108S.

Omerod LD, Murphree AL, Gomes DS, et al. Microbial keratitis in children. Ophthalmology 1986; 93:449–455.

PERIORBITAL AND ORBITAL CELLULITIS

URS B. SCHAAD, M.D.

Acute erythematous swelling of the periorbital area requires immediate and aggressive diagnostic workup and management. Trivial causes such as trauma, insect bite, allergic reaction, or localized pyogenic infection (hordeolum, dacrocystitis, conjunctivitis) are usually readily diagnosed by a careful history and clinical examination. The remaining majority of cases of red and swollen eyes represent a spectrum of serious, potentially invasive infections with important differences in pathogenesis, bacterial etiology, clinical presentation, and consequently appropriate therapy. The identified route of infection especially has essential implications for the need for diagnostic procedures and type of antibacterial therapy.

Bacteriologic diagnosis always includes cultures of blood and conjunctiva and if applicable, of needle aspirate from the infected area or of pus from the primary local infection. Bacterial antigen testing in the urine increases the rate of bacteriologic diagnosis.

The potential and often asymptomatic association with bacterial meningitis implies that lumbar puncture should be performed not only when objective signs of meningeal irritation occur, but also in each patient younger than 2 years of age with suspected acute bacteremic facial cellulitis, based on typical clinical presentation or positive urinary antigen test. Once a relevant specific etiologic diagnosis has been established, antimicrobial therapy is adapted according to the bacterial isolate and in vitro susceptibility tests.

Whenever there is any question of orbital (postseptal) involvement because of the presence of proptosis, ophthalmoplegia, or decreased visual acuity, computerized tomography is indicated to demonstrate subperiosteal or intraorbital abscess formation. The diagnostic value of sinus radiographs is limited, especially in infants, who often have radiographically opaque sinuses with simple upper respiratory tract infections.

PRIMARY SKIN INFECTION

Periorbital (preseptal) cellulitis that has clearly spread from an infected wound or injury is usually caused by either *Staphylococcus aureus* or *Streptococcus pyogenes*. My first choice in these cases is clindamycin, 30 to 40 mg per kilogram per day in four divided intravenous doses, for 8 to 10 days; oral administration of the drug is feasible after definite clinical response, usually after 4 to 5 days of parenteral therapy. Clindamycin-associated pseudomembranous enterocolitis is extremely rare in children.

Alternative regimens are a penicillinase-resistant penicillin such as flucloxacillin (not available in the United States) or nafcillin (not available in Europe), 150 to 200 mg per kilogram per day divided into four intravenous doses, or vancomycin, 40 mg per kilogram per day divided into four intravenous doses, administered as 60-minute infusions.

For patients in whom there is any uncertainty whether or not the pathogenesis of infection is based on bacteremic spread, especially in those younger than 2 years of age, the antimicrobial therapy must include not only the gram-positive skin organisms mentioned earlier, but also *Haemophilus influenzae* type b and *Streptococcus pneumoniae*. In these cases my recommended initial therapy consists of administration of cefuroxime, 240 mg IV per kilogram per day in four divided doses. When meningitic involvement has been excluded by negative cerebrospinal fluid (CSF) culture, the dosage of cefuroxime can be reduced to 120 mg per kilogram per day divided into four doses, administered intravenously every 6 hours.

In older children, if the periorbital cellulitis spreading from an infected wound or injury near the eye is mild, outpatient management is possible. Close follow-up is essential and any progression requires immediate hospitalization. My choice for these cases is clindamycin, 30 to 40 mg per kilogram per day in four divided oral doses.

BACTEREMIC FACIAL CELLULITIS

Patients with acute bacteremic (idiopathic) periorbital (preseptal) cellulitis are typically between 6 and 24 months of age, and their disease is characterized by an abrupt onset of fever, toxicity, and swelling and discoloration of the area around the eye, often with symptoms of an upper respiratory tract infection. The principal etiologic agents are *H. influenzae* type b and *S. pneumoniae*. My first choice in these cases is ceftriaxone, 100 mg per kilogram per day, administered in a single intravenous dose. An alternative regimen is cefuroxime, 240 mg per kilogram per day in four divided intravenous doses. As stated before, after meningitis is excluded by a negative CSF culture result, these dosages can be reduced by half. Parenteral therapy is given for a minimum of 4 to 5 days. If outpatient management is acceptable after prompt clinical response to intravenous treatment, either our patients are continued on ceftriaxone therapy, once daily intravenously or intramuscularly, or therapy is switched to cefaclor, 50 to 60 mg per kilogram per day, divided into three doses administered orally every 8 hours. The total duration of antimicrobial therapy should be 8 to 10 days.

PERIORBITAL CELLULITIS SECONDARY TO SINUSITIS

The majority of these cases are actually inflammatory edema in the periorbital (preseptal) area secondary to ethmoid or maxillary sinusitis. Affected children may be of any age, but only rarely are they infants. The disease is characterized by subacute onset and low-grade fever. Treatment is directed against the bacteria that commonly cause acute sinusitis in children: *Streptococcus pneumoniae, Branhamella catarrhalis,* nontypable *H. influenzae,* and various streptococci. A significant number of *B. catarrhalis* and *H. influenzae* strains are beta-lactamase positive, and hence ampicillin and amoxicillin resistant. Staphylococci and respiratory anaerobes are rarely isolated from the sinuses of children with acute infection. My first choice in these cases is cefuroxime, 120 mg per kilogram per day in four divided intravenous doses. An alternative regimen is parenteral amoxicillin-potassium clavulanate (Augmentin), 200 mg per kilogram per day of the amoxicillin part divided into four doses administered intravenously every 6 hours (not available in the United States). Oral therapy is possible after definite clinical response to the intravenous treatment administered over a minimum of 4 to 5 days.

Immune deficiency and progression of acute sinusitis despite seemingly appropriate antibiotic therapy are indications for diagnostic and therapeutic sinus aspiration (percutaneous or transantral). (For detailed information about treatment of sinusitis, see the chapter on *Sinusitis.*)

ORBITAL CELLULITIS

Infection of the deep structures of the orbit (postseptal) is the rarest but most serious of the periocular infections. This is because the orbital contents are extremely close to the cavernous sinus and the optic nerve. This entity is usually seen in school-age children and teenagers, and is virtually always secondary to advanced purulent frontal or maxillary sinusitis, penetrating ocular injury, or foreign body. The organisms most frequently involved are penicillinase-producing *Staphylococcus aureus,* streptococci and anaerobes, less frequently gram-negative bacteria, and even fungi. My recommended initial therapy consists of flucloxacillin (nafcillin in the United States) (200 mg per kilogram per day intravenously in four divided doses) or vancomycin (40 mg per kilogram per day intravenously in four divided doses) plus a third-generation cephalosporin compound (ceftazidime, cefotaxime, or moxalactam, 150 mg per kilogram per day intravenously in three or four divided doses, or ceftriaxone, 50 mg per kilogram per day intravenously in a single dose). An alternative to flucloxacillin or nafcillin when anaerobic infection is suspected is clindamycin (30 to 40 mg per kilogram per day in four divided doses). These patients are usually treated for 2 to 3 weeks. Change to oral therapy is not recommended.

In addition to antimicrobial therapy, most cases require surgical intervention to decompress the orbit and prevent damage to the optic nerve and intracranial spread. In these cases, Gram stain of surgically obtained material (especially drainage fluid) is never reliable to narrow the antimicrobial regimen, and also the culture results of such material must be carefully interpreted before single-drug therapy is continued against a specific organism. In my experience, contamination of such specimens by skin and/or respiratory tract bacteria is quite common. Unequivocal culture results from initial blood or aspirate specimens are, of course, reliable, but available only in fewer than 50 percent of cases of orbital cellulitis.

SUGGESTED READING

Baker RC, Bausher JC. Meningitis complicating acute bacteremic facial cellulitis. Pediatr Infect Dis 1986; 5:421–423.
Goldberg F, Berne AS, Oski FA. Differentiation of orbital cellulitis from preseptal cellulitis by computed tomography. Pediatrics 1978; 62:1000–1005.
Shapiro ED, Wald ER, Brozanski BA. Periorbital cellulitis and paranasal sinusitis: a reappraisal. Pediatr Infect Dis 1982; 1:91–94.
Teele DW. Management of the child with a red and swollen eye. Pediatr Infect Dis 1983; 2:258–262.

ENDOPHTHALMITIS

ALICE MATOBA, M.D.

The etiologic agent in exogenous endophthalmitis, whether traumatic or postoperative, is most commonly a gram-positive organism. *Staphylococcus epidermidis* is the most frequently cultured agent, accounting for 18 to 50 percent of the culture-proven cases of endophthalmitis for series combining adult and pediatric patients. *S. aureus* is the second most frequently identified agent, accounting for approximately 15 percent of cases. Streptococcal species account for 13 to 27 percent, and other gram-positive organisms account for another 10 percent. Gram-negative bacteria are cultured in 7 to 23 percent of the cases, with no single predominant agent. Fungal agents account for 3 to 11 percent of the pathogens.

Endogenous endophthalmitis is seen primarily in immune-compromised hosts. Fungal agents account for a much higher percentage of the total number of cases than in exogenous endophthalmitis. *Candida albicans* is the most common yeast and *Aspergillus* the most common filamentous organism identified in endogenous fungal endophthalmitis.

The major complaints of patients with endophthalmitis are acute loss of vision and pain in the eye. The signs of microbial endophthalmitis (injection, chemosis of the conjunctiva, and intraocular inflammation with loss of or change in the funduscopic red reflex) should be evaluated by an ophthalmologist as soon as the diagnosis is suspected. Upon confirmation of the clinical diagnosis, laboratory diagnosis should be sought by obtaining samples of aqueous and vitreous. The anterior chamber aspiration and vitreous aspiration or vitrectomy should be performed by an ophthalmologist in an operating room as soon as possible after the diagnosis is suspected. Even if no organisms are seen on Gram-stained slides, antimicrobial therapy should be initiated immediately, as delay in therapy of even a few hours can lead to irreversible damage to the retina with loss of vision.

TREATMENT

My preferred initial therapy for suspected bacterial endophthalmitis consists of cefazolin or cefuroxime and gentamicin or tobramycin given by the intravenous, subconjunctival, topical, and intravitreal routes (Table 1). Although clinical experience with cefuroxime in the treatment of ocular infection is limited, cefuroxime is recommended as an alternative to cefazolin because it has significant activity against *Haemophilus influenzae* while retaining activity against group B streptococcus, *Staphylococcus,* and most anaerobic organisms excluding *Bacteroides fragilis.* Tobramycin is suggested as an alternative to gentamicin because it may be slightly less toxic to the retina than gentamicin and because its minimum inhibitory concentration for *Pseudomonas aeruginosa* is lower.

Intravenous administration of gentamicin and cefazolin leads to aqueous and vitreous drug concentrations that compare favorably with other antibiotics in their classes. Subconjunctival injection of either drug leads to a marked gradient within the eye with high antibiotic concentrations in the aqueous and those in the vitreous that are significantly lower but nevertheless may inhibit most susceptible pathogens. The subconjunctival dosage of gentamicin should be adjusted for children weighing less than 40 kg to be no more than half of a single dose given by the intravenous route. Subconjunctival injection may be repeated at 12- or 24-hour intervals, but if there is clinical response to therapy, I discontinue subconjunctival injections in children within 24 hours because the injections are quite painful. Intravenous

TABLE 1 Initial Therapy of Infectious Endophthalmitis

Suspected Organism	Drug	Intravenous	Subconjunctival	Topical	Intravitreal
		Dosages of Drugs			
Bacteria	Gentamicin or Tobramycin	3.0–7.5 mg/kg/24 hr divided every 8 hrs	20 mg in 0.5 cc[a]	13.6 mg/ml 1 drop q½h–q1h[b]	100 μg in 0.1 ml[c]
Bacteria	Cefazolin	50–100 mg/kg/day divided every 6 or 8 hours	100 mg in 0.5 cc	50 mg/ml 1 drop q½h–q1h[d]	2.25 mg in 0.1 ml[c]
Bacteria	Cefuroxime	75–100 mg/kg/day divided every 6 or 8 hours	100 mg in 0.5 cc	50 mg/ml 1 drop q½h–q1h[d]	250 μg in 0.1 ml[c]
Fungus	Miconazole	20–40 mg/kg/day in children	5 mg in 0.5 cc	10 mg/ml 1 drop q1h	20 μg in 0.1 ml[c]
Fungus	Amphotericin B	Follow guidelines	[e]	1.5 mg/ml 1 drop q1h	5 μg in 0.1 ml[c]

[a] In children weighing less than 40 kg, give no more than ½ of a single intravenous dose.
[b] One vial intravenous formulation 80 mg per 2 cc + 1 bottle ophthalmic formulation 15 mg in 5 ml.
[c] Children aged 3 or older. No established guidelines for neonates and infants.
[d] Refrigerate. Change bottle every 3 days.
[e] Reported to cause conjunctival sclerosis.

therapy is continued for approximately 7 to 10 days until approximately 5 to 7 days of progressive improvement is seen.

Topical drug administration, though inadequate as the sole route for the treatment of deep ocular infection, can add significantly to the aqueous drug concentrations. It is important to remember that the average eye drop size (50 μl) far exceeds the capacity of the inferior cul de sac of the eye, so that the drop is rapidly lost from the preocular tear film either by spillage or drainage through the lacrimal sac. Drug absorption through mucous membrane is extremely efficient, and most of the drug draining through the lacrimal system can be considered to be absorbed systemically. In neonates or patients in renal failure, the potential for systemic toxicity because of medication absorbed by this route is not insignificant (Table 2). Drainage through the lacrimal system can be minimized by placing a finger against the medial canthal area to occlude the puncta for several seconds following administration of an eye drop. Topical therapy is tapered as the infection resolves. Intravitreal injection of antibiotic can be carried out at the time of the vitreous aspiration or vitrectomy. Intravitreal administration of drug leads to a high concentration of the drug within the eye with little potential for systemic toxicity. However, improper injection technique could lead to local toxicity with retinal necrosis or to mechanically induced problems such as intraocular hemorrhage, cataract formation, or retinal detachment. All intravitreal injections should be performed by an ophthalmologist.

The recommended dosage of gentamicin for intravitreal injection in adults is 100 to 200 μg in 0.1 ml. I prefer to use 100 μg for adults and children 3 years of age or older. In infants and neonates, guidelines for intravitreal antibiotic use are not well established. The dosage can be decreased to 25 to 50 μg based on estimates of the size of the eye and the vitreous volume, but I prefer to avoid intravitreal injec-

tions in neonates and infants. Animal studies in rabbits and primates indicate that the half-life of gentamicin in the noninflamed eye is approximately 25 to 33 hours. In rabbit eyes, inflammation resulting from intraocular injection of *S. aureus* led to a decrease in the half-life to 10 hours. However, because antibiotic is delivered to the eye by several other routes, a second injection is often not necessary and is not considered before 48 hours. I recommend a dose of 2.25 mg in 0.1 ml for intravitreal injection of cefazolin in children 3 years of age or older. The dosage is adjusted for infant eyes. The half-life of intravitreal cefazolin in noninflamed eyes is reported to be approximately 7 hours. Use of systemic probenecid to prolong the half-life of cefazolin is recommended by some authors, but the results of animal studies have not been consistent, and I do not routinely administer probenecid with cefazolin. No studies are available to indicate a nontoxic dose of cefuroxime for intravitreal use. Cephaloridine, another cephalosporin that has been well studied, has been reported to induce retinal toxicity at dosages of 500 μg or greater. The recommended intravitreal dosage of cephaloridine is 250 μg, and cefuroxime, if given intravitreally, should be given at dosages not exceeding 250 μg in 0.1 ml. The potential toxicity of intravitreal drug injection must be weighed against the risk of retinal

TABLE 2 Potential Cumulative Dose of Drug After 24 Hours of Topical Delivery

Drug	Concentration (mg/ml)	Total drug (mg) given one drop q½h	Total drug (mg) given one drop qh
Gentamicin	13.6	32.6	16.3
Cefazolin	50	120	60
Cefuroxime	50	120	60

necrosis, which occurs with uncontrolled intraocular infection.

Fungal Endophthalmitis

For suspected fungal endophthalmitis, the two major treatment options are amphotericin B and miconazole (see Table 1). The advantages of miconazole are the relatively low toxicity both systemically and locally, the greater penetration of the intraocular compartments by all routes, and the fact that larger dosages can be safely administered by all routes. The advantage of amphotericin B is its superior spectrum of activity against fungal agents. For the therapy of fungal endophthalmitis, I prefer to begin treatment with miconazole and to convert at a later time to amphotericin B if necessary.

Vitrectomy

The role of vitrectomy in the treatment of endophthalmitis is not clearly defined. The concept that vitrectomy accomplishes surgical drainage of an intraocular abscess is an attractive one. However, vitrectomy can be complicated by retinal hole formation and retinal detachment. Furthermore, it has been shown that patients who are infected with indolent organisms such as *S. epidermidis* have the most favorable visual outcome when treated medically without invasive intraocular procedures. Nevertheless, toxins produced by virulent bacteria are clearly toxic to the retina, and inflammation can destroy neurosensory cells even if the infection is controlled. I favor early vitrectomy in patients who appear to be infected by a virulent organism, based on the rapidity of onset of signs and symptoms and the clinical appearance of the eye. In patients who have had a relatively slow evolution of signs (3 to 4 days or longer, without loss of the red reflex). I prefer to initiate medical therapy and to observe for 24 to 36 hours.

For suspected fungal endophthalmitis, I prefer early vitrectomy for exogenous endophthalmitis with suspected intraocular foreign body and for eyes with extensive intravitreal inflammation. If the endophthalmitis is endogenous in origin with minimal-to-moderate vitreous reaction overlying areas of chorioretinitis, I prefer to initiate medical therapy and close observation.

Corticosteroids

The need for the addition of steroid therapy to antimicrobial therapy in the treatment of endophthalmitis is widely accepted, but the time of initiation of steroid therapy is somewhat controversial. When dealing with indolent organisms, the initiation of steroid therapy may be delayed without adversely affecting final visual outcome. However, virulent organisms such as *Bacillus cereus, Pseudomonas aeruginosa,* or beta-hemolytic streptococci can cause

TABLE 3 Corticosteroid Therapy in Endophthalmitis

Systemic	Subconjunctival	Topical	Intravitreal
Prednisone 30–60 mg/day	Dexamethasone 2 mg in ½ cc	Prednisolone acetate 1% 1 drop q1h	[a]

[a] Although dexamethasone 360 μg in 0.1 ml is advocated by some authors, I do not routinely administer intravitreal corticosteroid.

extensive retinal damage within 24 hours of onset of signs.

For suspected exogenous bacterial endophthalmitis, I generally initiate early treatment with topical, subconjunctival, and systemic corticosteroids (Table 3). Subconjunctival injection can be given at the time of aqueous and vitreous sampling. Thereafter, steroids can be given through topical and systemic routes. Once the infection is controlled, systemic and topical therapy is tapered over 1 to 2 weeks. If the infection has extended to the sclera, however, subconjunctival steroid injection should be avoided because of the danger of perforation. If the endophthalmitis is believed to be endogenous in origin, systemic steroid therapy should be withheld until the original focus of infection has been identified and a fungal etiology ruled out.

In suspected fungal endophthalmitis, I withhold corticosteroid therapy. Fungal endophthalmitis is usually a relatively indolent process with less acute inflammation than bacterial endophthalmitis. Fungal endophthalmitis may be more difficult to control than bacterial infection, and the risk of adverse effect on outcome by the premature addition of steroid therapy is relatively high.

MONITORING RESPONSE TO THERAPY AND MODIFICATION OF THERAPY

If clinical response is not seen within 24 to 36 hours, modification of therapy should be considered. Choice of antibiotic should be based on culture results and susceptibility testing. If identification of an organism is not available, a diagnostic and therapeutic vitrectomy should be considered.

Signs of favorable response to therapy include retraction and breakup of intraocular fibrin clots, improvement in the quality of the red reflex, and decrease in the number of inflammatory cells in the anterior chamber and vitreous. These signs should be evaluated by an ophthalmologist.

SUGGESTED READING

Barza M, Kane A, Baum J. Pharmacokinetics of intravitreal carbenicillin, cefazolin and gentamicin in Rhesus monkeys. Invest Ophthalmol Vis Sci 1983; 24:1602–1606.

Forster RK, Abbott RL, Gelender H. Management of infectious endophthalmitis. Ophthalmology 1980; 87:313–319.

O'Day D, Jones DB, Patrinely J, Elliot JH. *Staphylococcus epidermidis* endophthalmitis. Ophthalmology 1982; 89:354–360.

DISEASES RELATED TO THE MOUTH AND NASOPHARYNX

CERVICAL ADENITIS

ADNAN S. DAJANI, M.D.

Enlargement of cervical lymph nodes is a very common finding in children. Frequently, these enlarged lymph nodes represent physiologic, age-related changes or are a response to local or systemic infections originating in the upper respiratory tract or skin. Occasionally cervical lymphadenopathy heralds serious reticuloendothelial system diseases such as a malignancy, histiocytic infiltration, or an altered immune reaction.

Localized, tender cervical lymph node enlargement (adenitis) usually affects the tonsillar or submandibular nodes. Acute-onset cervical adenitis is most often caused by *Staphylococcus aureus* or, less commonly, by group A beta-hemolytic streptococci. These organisms account for at least 75 percent of all cases. Occasionally, anaerobic bacteria, either alone or mixed with aerobic bacteria, are responsible. In neonates, group B streptococci are sometimes encountered.

Less acute or chronic adenitis is most often caused by atypical mycobacteria (*Mycobacterium avium-intracellularis-scrofulaceum*), cat-scratch disease, or toxoplasmosis.

Other bacteria, fungi, and *Toxoplasma gondii* can cause cervical adenitis, particularly in immunocompromised children.

To establish the etiology of cervical adenitis, needle aspiration is a simple, definitive method that can be accomplished easily in an office or clinic setting. I prefer a 20-gauge needle attached to a 10- or 20-ml syringe and do not recommend the injection of saline or distilled water. Aspiration of a few drops of tissue fluid, or pus if present, frequently yields a pathogen in stained specimens and culture. Skin testing with purified protein derivative (PPD) is often helpful in the diagnosis of mycobacterial adenitis. In some instances (in the presence of group A streptococci, toxoplasmosis, certain fungal infections) serologic tests are helpful for the retrospective diagnosis of cervical adenitis.

Initial therapy for cervical adenitis should be directed against *S. aureus* and group A streptococci. Systemic antibiotics, usually by the oral route, should be given for 10 to 14 days. Among the oral agents, I prefer dicloxacillin (50 mg per kilogram per day in 3 to 4 divided doses). Dicloxacillin suspension is unpalatable, and in young children cloxacillin (50 to 100 mg per kilogram per day in three to four divided doses) is more readily accepted. Oral cephalosporins are more palatable but also more expensive. Cephalexin, cephradine (50 mg per kilogram per day divided every 6 hours), and cefadroxil (30 mg per kilogram per day divided every 12 hours) are adequate agents. I do not recommend cefaclor because of its relatively high minimal inhibitory concentration for most staphylococci and because of possible side effects. In penicillin-allergic patients, clindamycin (30 mg per kilogram per day in four equal doses) is my choice. Clindamycin offers the additional advantage of activity against most anaerobic bacteria.

Intravenous antibiotics are usually not necessary except in toxic patients or ones with severe infection. I prefer cefazolin (100 mg per kilogram per day in three equal doses) until oral therapy can be started, usually in about 3 days. Methicillin (200 mg per kilogram per day given every 6 hours) or nafcillin (150 mg per kilogram per day given every 6 hours) is also acceptable, but nafcillin more often causes phlebitis.

With any therapeutic modality, the response of cervical adenitis is often not dramatic. Lymph nodes may remain tender for a few days, and enlargement may persist for many days. This should not lead to a change in therapeutic approach. I usually instruct parents not to get alarmed and impress on them the slow resolution of this infection.

It is not unusual for cervical adenitis caused by *S. aureus* to suppurate. In this situation surgical drainage is recommended. I usually wait until the node is fluctuant before asking for surgical intervention. Such a surgical procedure is accomplished easily on an outpatient or same-day surgery basis.

For treatment of adenitis caused by atypical mycobacteria, cat-scratch disease, toxoplasmosis and other conditions, see the relevant chapters.

SUGGESTED READING

Barton LL, Feigin RD. Childhood cervical lymphadenitis: a reappraisal. J Pediatr 1974; 84:846–852.

Dajani AS, Garcia RE, Wolinsky E. Etiology of cervical lymphadenitis in children. N Engl J Med 1963; 268:1329–1333.

Yamauchi T, Ferrieri P, Anthony BF. The aetiology of acute cervical adenitis in children: serological and bacteriological studies. J Med Microbiol 1980; 13:37–43.

INFECTIONS OF THE ORAL CAVITY

JOHN M. WRIGHT, D.D.S., M.S.
PAUL P. TAYLOR, D.D.S., M.S.

A variety of infections affect the teeth, bone, and soft tissues of the oral cavity. The most common oral infections in pediatric patients are tooth decay (dental caries) and periodontal disease. Despite the fact that these are primarily "dental problems," they are infectious diseases that influence the overall health of the patient. Less commonly, specific bacterial, viral, and fungal infections also occur. We describe only those infections we encounter frequently and the therapeutic measures that we use to treat them.

DENTAL CARIES

Dental caries is a nonspecific infection caused by bacteria that colonize the surfaces of the teeth. These acidogenic bacteria produce acids as metabolic products of carbohydrate metabolism. Over time, these acids slowly demineralize the enamel and dentin of the teeth. Early dental caries cannot be detected visually, but can be discovered by the use of radiographs and a well-developed tactile sense, using a dental probe.

The normal oral flora contains several bacteria that are capable of colonizing the surfaces of the teeth; among the most common is *Streptococcus mutans.* These bacteria establish their colonies by excreting a sticky substance called dextran, which is manufactured from carbohydrates in the child's diet. These polysaccharides allow the bacteria to adhere to the tooth surface and to each other. These bacterial colonies are known as plaque and, if not disrupted, continue to build up until they are visible clinically. Plaque serves as a storage area where bacteria proliferate while their metabolic by-products destroy the teeth.

As an infection, dental caries is preventable. Preventive therapy is directed toward physical disruption of plaque and diet modification. Both require patient education and compliance. Daily oral hygiene—flossing and brushing—can significantly reduce the incidence of decay by physically removing dental plaque. In addition, dental caries is fueled by bacterial acid production from dietary carbohydrate metabolism. Restricting the quantity and frequency of carbohydrate intake is also important in controlling acid production.

Early dental caries is treated by removing the decayed area of the tooth and restoring the resultant defect with a dental material. If untreated, dental caries progresses and eventually leads to bacterial invasion of the dental pulp. The resultant pulpitis is irreversible and then must be treated by either tooth extraction or removal of the inflamed pulp by endodontic procedures.

Untreated dental caries will eventually spread beyond the confines of the involved tooth. Once the soft tissues of the dental pulp are reached, the infection spreads into the bone around the tooth root(s). The intrabony infection can remain localized or spread into the adjacent soft tissues as a sinus tract or cellulitis. At this point, a broad-spectrum antibiotic is often required; penicillin is the drug of choice for most odontogenic infections. Erythromycin is a good alternative. Although antibiotics can produce dramatic resolution of the soft tissue infection, they alone are not curative because the infection invariably returns when antibiotic therapy ceases. The condition can be resolved satisfactorily only by treating the source of the infection, the offending tooth, with extraction or root canal therapy.

Occasionally, odontogenic infections are life-threatening. This is especially true when the cellulitis involves the floor of the mouth, producing Ludwig's angina (see the chapter on *Ludwig's Angina*).

PERIODONTAL DISEASE

The most common periodontal diseases affecting children and adolescents are gingivitis and periodontitis. Both are nonspecific bacterial infections and represent tissue reactions to bacterial plaque that accumulates around the necks or cervical areas of the teeth. Initially, the plaque induces a marginal gingivitis, but if untreated, the infection is progressive, resulting in resorption of the underlying bone (periodontitis) and eventually tooth loss.

Even though periodontal disease causes the greatest loss of teeth after the age of 30, the process starts in childhood. Treatment of the early stages of periodontal disease in children includes meticulous oral hygiene, professional cleaning of the tissues and teeth, and patient education by providing the child and parent with good instruction for home care. As an infection, periodontal disease is preventable.

Although periodontal disease is essentially a tissue reaction to local irritants, it is important to remember that the reaction is influenced by a wide variety of systemic factors such as inadequate nutrition and hormonal imbalance. Periodontal disease also progresses very slowly because of normal host defenses and the low virulence of the infecting microorganisms. What is normally a painless, indolent infection can become rapidly progressive in a patient with congenital or acquired immunodeficiency. We have seen many cases of atypical gingivitis or advanced periodontitis in young male homosexuals who have been infected with acquired immunodeficiency syndrome (AIDS) virus. A child or young adult with rapidly advancing periodontal disease should alert the clinician to the possibility of an underlying systemic disorder, such as diabetes mellitus or immunodeficiency.

A specific type of acute gingivitis deserves special mention because of its occurrence in adolescents and young adults. Acute necrotizing ulcerative gingivitis (ANUG, or trench mouth) is a fusospirochetal infection characterized by pain and necrosis of the interdental papillae. The necrotic areas can be covered by a pseudomembrane. The tongue may be coated, a fetid odor is present, and the patient sometimes has a low-grade fever. The infection is commonly seen in patients whose resistance is lowered. Most cases can be managed with local debridement and hourly rinses with warm water, whereas more severe cases may require systemic antibiotic therapy with penicillin V, 250 mg, four times a day for a week. We do not recommend oxygenating mouth rinses (hydrogen peroxide) because hydrogen peroxide has been shown to retard wound healing.

BACTERIAL INFECTIONS

Syphilis

Acquired primary intraoral syphilis results from direct orogenital contact. The chancre presents as an indurated, raised ulcer, often accompanied by regional lymphadenitis. Chancres are found most often on the lips or tongue. Secondary syphilis often follows, commencing as a skin and mucosal rash. Intraorally, a whitish coating may overlie shallow ulcers. Split papules may be found at the corners of the mouth. Tertiary syphilis produces areas of gummatous necrosis intraorally but is rarely seen today. Early syphilis responds well to benzathine penicillin G, 2.4 million units intramuscularly. For penicillin-allergic patients, tetracycline, 500 mg four times daily for 15 days, is an alternative. After starting therapy, some patients experience a self-limiting Herxheimer's reaction.

Gonorrhea

Oral manifestations of gonorrhea are rare. The anterior mouth is relatively resistant, and when infection occurs, the oropharynx is usually involved. The oropharynx is infected by direct contact, usually deep fellatio. Most oral infections are asymptomatic and are characterized by erythema. Vesicles, ulcers, and pseudomembranes have also been described. Diagnosis is established by throat culture.

Penicillin is the drug of choice. Although some claim that pharyngeal infections are more difficult to control than genital infections, the drug regimen is the same. Ideally, 4.8 million units of aqueous procaine penicillin G are injected intramuscularly at one visit in at least two doses at different sites with 1.0 g of probenecid, given orally, just before the injections. Beta-lactamase–producing strains can be treated with spectinomycin, 2.0 g IM, or a cephalosporin (cefoxi-tin, 2.0 g IM with 1.0 g probenecid orally or cefotaxime, 1.0 g IM). Because many pharyngeal infections are asymptomatic, we recommend posttreatment cultures.

Aphthous Ulcers (Canker Sores)

Recurrent aphthous ulcerations are included for completeness, because they are perhaps the most common oral condition misdiagnosed as an infectious lesion and are often thought to be herpetic ulcers. Aphthae are currently thought to have an autoimmune pathogenesis. The ulcers can be single or multiple and occur only on mucosa that does not overlie bone—that is, cheek, tongue, lips, and soft palate. The ulcer is painful and covered by a fibrinous exudate and surrounded by an erythematous border.

Aphthous ulcers are self-limiting and heal within a week to 10 days without scarring. For most patients, the disease is, at worst, a nuisance we do not treat. The patient can be reassured about the local nature of the condition and informed that the number of outbreaks tends to decrease slowly with time, although this normally takes years.

The number of remedies for aphthae that have been reported over the years is limitless. This is understandable considering the fact that the condition is common and most patients want treatment. Claims for success must be kept in perspective by remembering that healing can be achieved by placing almost anything on a self-limiting condition.

We have had limited success with topical application of corticosteroids on the area, covered with a vehicle that will not dissolve in saliva (Orabase), four to five times daily. This decreases pain and hastens healing. Topical steroids are effective only when applied during the prodromal symptoms of the condition, in the preulcerative stage. Once ulceration occurs, the damage is done and treatment affords little relief. The condition can be managed successfully with systemic corticosteroids. Although the dosage varies according to the severity of the condition, we generally start with 40 mg of prednisone and taper the dosage over about 5 days. Tapering Dosepaks are convenient. We must stress that the severity and frequency of outbreaks of aphthae are extremely variable. We consider systemic steroids aggressive therapy, and reserve its use for only the most severe and debilitating cases. The usual contraindications for steroid therapy must be considered. The normal side effects of steroid therapy are minimal when treating for this period of time. Patients with aphthae are not curable. Although some relief can be attained with corticosteroids, treatment does not affect the incidence of future outbreaks.

The success reported by some for tetracycline mouth rinses is probably a result of the control of secondary bacterial infection after ulceration has occurred. Tetracycline seems to work best with the herpetiform type of aphthae. Although chemical cauterization of the ulcer reduces pain, we are cautious to recommend its use, because we have seen severe tissue destruction from the injudicious use of compounds such as silver nitrate. Hydrogen peroxide is contraindicated.

VIRAL INFECTIONS

Herpes Simplex

The most common intraoral viral infections are caused by the herpes simplex virus (HSV). Most intraoral infections are caused by HSV-1. The initial exposure to the virus in most patients results in subclinical infection. Some patients develop primary herpetic gingivostomatitis; this is usually seen in children or young adults.

Primary herpetic gingivostomatitis is a symmetrical, vesicular eruption of the mouth, lips, and perioral skin. The vesicles quickly break, leaving painful ulcers and erosions. The gingivae are often red and swollen, and most patients have a low-grade fever. Lymphadenitis is common.

Treatment for the primary infection remains supportive. An antipyretic and analgesic are prescribed for fever and pain. The mouth is sufficiently painful for some patients that dehydration can be a serious complication. Maintaining adequate fluid intake is important, and we often recommend popsicles for young children. The frozen ice is soothing and provides fluids and some nutrition. Topical anesthetics can relieve pain. Dyclonine hydrochloride, 0.5 percent, or Benadryl elixir, 12.5 mg per 5 ml, mixed with equal parts of Kaopectate, works well to relieve pain and make eating more comfortable. This solution should be used as a mouth rinse and is intended for topical effect. It should be held in the mouth for about 2 minutes and spit out.

After initial exposure to the virus, the HSV is not destroyed, but remains dormant in sensory ganglia where it can be reactivated in some patients to produce recurrent or secondary infections. The most common recurrent infection is herpes labialis (cold sores, fever blisters). Rarely, recurrent infections occur intraorally where they present as multiple, small ulcers that characteristically affect the attached gingiva or hard palate (anatomic sites that are rarely affected by aphthae).

Because recurrent oral herpetic infections are self-limited, no treatment is needed for most patients. As for aphthae, the remedies proposed are endless. In selected patients, we have found topically applied antiviral drugs such as acyclovir or idoxuridine to be beneficial. These drugs are effective only when applied during the prodromal, prevesicular stages. When using these drugs, the patient must not apply the medication with an uncovered finger because of the possibility of autoinnoculating the finger, with the subsequent development of herpetic whitlow. We must emphasize that we do not routinely prescribe antiviral medications for most patients because of the danger of developing drug-resistant strains of the virus. It is also known that a course of systemic acyclovir does not destroy latent virus in the trigeminal ganglion.

Patient education is an important aspect in the management of patients with herpetic infections. Patients should understand that their lesions are caused by a virus that is infectious. Other family members can be infected by direct contact. Instruct patients to refrain from touching their own lesions, to prevent innoculating other sites such as the eye.

Other Herpes Viruses

The varicella-zoster virus produces chicken pox in children. Oral lesions are common, but there is no specific treatment. Analgesics or topical anesthetics relieve pain.

In some patients, exposure to the Epstein–Barr virus produces infectious mononucleosis. The most common intraoral manifestations are palatal petechiae and exudative tonsillitis. There is no specific treatment.

Coxsackievirus

The most common intraoral coxsackieviral infection is herpangina, which often occurs as summertime epidemics in children. The onset is acute, and patients develop fever, malaise, anorexia, and a sore throat. The lesions start as vesicles that are usually bilaterally symmetrical and affect the posterior mouth: palate, tonsils, and oropharynx. The vesicles break, leaving shallow erosions and ulcers. The disease is usually mild and self-limited. There is no specific therapy but analgesics are sometimes helpful (see the chapter on *Herpangina*).

Human Papilloma Virus (HPV)

There are more than 40 types of HPV that produce clinically distinctive wartlike growths of the skin and mucous membranes. The common wart, or verruca vulgaris, is a papillary skin tumor affecting children and young adults. Lesions of the fingers can innoculate mucous membranes and cause warty growths. These are particularly common on the lips but are also well documented intraorally. It is now known that many of the other intraoral papillary epithelial tumors are caused by different HPV types.

Warty tumors of the anogenital region are known as condyloma acuminatum (HPV 6). These can occur on the lips, tongue, and buccal mucosa. Any young patient with multiple wartlike intraoral growths and no hand lesions should be examined for genital condylomata and questioned about sexual abuse.

Although some of the lesions induced by HPV are self-limited, there is presently no way to predict which lesions will progress and which might regress. Therefore, papillary growths in the mouth should be removed. This has usually been accomplished by surgical excision, but electro-, cryo-, and laser surgery are equally effective. Chemical destruction of the lesion has been much more difficult for intraoral tumors. Removal ensures the virus will not spread to other mucosal surfaces. Once removed, the lesion should be submitted for microscopic examination and pathologic confirmation of the diagnosis.

FUNGAL INFECTIONS

The only intraoral fungal infection seen in pediatric patients with any frequency is that caused by *Candida* species. Although oral involvement by other fungi has been documented, their rarity in young individuals precludes their inclusion. (See the related chapters on systemic fungal infections.)

Candidosis (candidiasis) is one of the most prevalent fungal diseases. The candidal species live as commensals in the mouths of many normal, healthy individuals. They usually produce clinical disease as an opportunistic infection in debilitated or otherwise predisposed individuals.

Although there are several pathogenic species of *Candida* for man, *Candida albicans* is by far the most prevalent. The fungus is biphasic; it was once thought that the yeast phase was relatively noninfectious while the hyphal phase was responsible for invasiveness and disease. Oral smears from more than 2,000 newborns showed *Candida* yeasts in 3.8 percent. Several days later, when clinical thrush was evident, the smears showed both yeasts and hyphae. Although the yeast form is now speculated to be involved in the pathogenesis of candidosis, the presence of hyphae is still an indication of active growth and probably enhanced virulence.

C. albicans has been isolated from the oral cavities of up to 50 percent of healthy individuals. Isolation rates from hospitalized patients are usually greater. The quantities and types of yeasts vary from day to day and from hour to hour in some individuals.

Factors predisposing to candidosis include antibiotic or steroid therapy and endocrine disorders such as diabetes mellitus, hypoparathyroidism, and Addison's disease. Nutritional deficiencies, particularly iron, are also seen in some patients with infections. One of the most common opportunistic infections in cancer patients is candidosis.

Oral manifestations of candidosis are varied. The following classification provides a workable and clinically applicable approach: acute pseudomembranous candidosis (thrush), acute atrophic candidosis (antibiotic sore mouth), chronic hyperplastic candidosis, and chronic atrophic candidosis (denture sore mouth). It should be pointed out that numerous inflammatory conditions of the oral mucosa are not infectious in nature. We see numerous patients in consultation for noninfectious types of stomatitis, who are referred only when the condition does not respond to antifungal medication.

Acute Pseudomembranous Candidosis (Thrush)

Thrush is the most common type of candidosis seen in children and young adults. Most cases of neonatal disease are exogenous infections contracted from vaginal yeasts during birth, but the clinical features often are not manifest until after the first week. Thrush is more common in bottle-fed than in breast-fed babies.

The lesions are white, curdlike plaques that can occur on all mucosal surfaces. The plaques consist mostly of desquamated surface epithelial cells, matted together by the pseudohyphae of *C. albicans*. The plaques can be scraped off with some difficulty, leaving an erythematous or bleeding base and, if untreated, the infection rarely extends into the pharynx, esophagus, and bronchi. The clinical features are usually distinctive, but the diagnosis is confirmed by cytologic smear of a plaque and demonstration of the organism by potassium hydroxide wet mount or Gram stain.

In children and young adults, acute pseudomembranous candidosis usually occurs as an opportunistic infection. The most common predisposing factor in this age group is use of broad-spectrum antibiotics. Oral candidosis is also a common manifestation of patients infected with the human immunodeficiency virus. Management of patients with oral candidosis involves identifying and correcting any predisposing factors and specific antifungal medication.

Acute pseudomembranous candidosis can generally be controlled with topically applied antifungal medications. Infections in infants can usually be controlled with nystatin oral suspension (100,000 units per milliliter). Sixty-milliliter bottles are available with a calibrated dropper, and 1 ml can be placed in each corner of the mouth four times daily. For children and young adults, the usual dosage is about 500,000 units (1 tsp) held in the mouth for 3 to 4 minutes four times daily. Nystatin oral tablets (500,000 units) can also be allowed to dissolve slowly in the mouth four times daily. Although patients occasionally complain of the taste of nystatin, it has the advantage of being relatively inexpensive as a generic drug and is relatively nontoxic, with few side effects. The severity of infection influences the length of treatment, however, we treat patients for an average of 10 to 14 days.

Other antifungal medications have been equally effective. Clotrimazole is available in a 10-mg troche (Mycelex). One troche should be allowed to dissolve slowly in the mouth five times daily for 2 weeks.

Although abnormal liver function tests have been reported (usually increased serum aspartate aminotransferase, most oral infections can be controlled within 2 weeks. The safety and effectiveness of clotrimazole in children younger than 3 years has not been determined. Success has also been reported using amphotericin B and miconazole. We do not recommend gentian violet because it is messy, stains tissue and clothing, and can irritate tissue.

For most patients with candidosis, we recommend topical treatment. However, in selected cases, we have had success with ketoconazole. For adults, a single 200-mg tablet is taken once a day with a meal for 2 weeks. Children between 20 and 40 kg are given ½ tablet (100 mg) once daily, and children under 20 kg are given ¼ tablet (50 mg) once daily. Hepatotoxicity has been associated with ketoconazole use, and liver function should be monitored. Anaphylaxis has also been reported following the initial dose.

Some patients experience recurrence of their candidosis following treatment. This often results from the patient completing the course of medication before the fungus is totally eradicated. We treat patients for a minimum of 2 to 3 days after symptoms have abated and the mucosa appears healthy. We have had some success managing recalcitrant cases by treating until posttreatment cultures are negative.

Acute Atrophic Candidosis

The infection can evolve from the desquamation of the plaques in thrush or it can occur de novo. As a de novo infection, it usually follows antibiotic therapy and has been referred to as antibiotic sore mouth, particularly affecting the tongue. The mucosa appears thin, atrophic, and somewhat erythematous. It responds well to topical antifungal agents.

Chronic Hyperplastic Candidosis

This is generally a condition of adulthood, but cases have been described in the second decade of life. The lesion is either a solitary white plaque or speckled red and white lesion that occurs most commonly in the cheek, especially at the corner of the mouth. Unlike the pseudomembranous type, the lesion does not rub off. Because of this fact, it has also been called candidal leukoplakia. There is nothing clinically distinctive about this white plaque, and the diagnosis can be established only by biopsy. Ultrastructural studies have shown that the hyphae invade the deeper layers of epithelium, which probably accounts for the concomitant epithelial hyperplasia. There have been documented cases of chronic hyperplastic candidosis eventuating in carcinoma, but the frequency of this evolution is unknown. The treatment is surgical excision, but lesions can recur; recurrence is higher in smokers who continue to smoke. Antifungal medications can produce some clinical improvement, particularly in the speckled lesions, but lesions rarely disappear completely.

Chronic Atrophic Candidosis

Chronic atrophic candidosis is rarely seen in pediatric patients. It occurs under dentures and is characterized by an erythematous mucosa confined to areas in contact with the denture. The condition may or may not be painful. When seen in pediatric patients, this form of candidosis usually occurs under an orthodontic retainer. Although the mucosal infection responds well to topical antifungal medications, the fungus is also found within the porosity of the plastic prosthesis, which must also be disinfected. The prosthesis can be soaked in nystatin oral suspension and the intraoral infection treated. We have also had some success with coating the fitting surface of the prosthesis with an antifungal ointment or powder and inserting it into the mouth.

Other forms of candidal infection that do not fall readily into the foregoing classification should be mentioned. Angular cheilitis (angular cheilosis, perleche) is a term used to describe an inflammatory condition at the corners of the mouth, characterized by erythema, erosions, fissures, and often crusting. The condition can be seen accompanying any of the other types of candidal lesions or as the only manifestation of oral disease. *Candida* can usually be isolated from the lesions, but its exact etiologic significance is debatable because pathogenic bacteria can also be isolated in some cases. When angular cheilitis occurs with an intraoral candidal infection, controlling the intraoral infection usually results in resolution of the angular cheilitis. If the patient complains only of angular cheilitis, an antifungal ointment rubbed into the corners of the mouth usually suffices. Recalcitrant cases can be managed by changing antifungal medication or by using an antibacterial ointment.

SUGGESTED READING

Budnik SD. Handbook of Pediatric Oral Pathology. Chicago: Year Book Medical Publishers, 1981.

Lynch MA, Brightman VJ, Greenberg MS. Burket's Oral Medicine: Diagnosis and Treatment. Philadelphia: JB Lippincott, 1984.

McDonald RE, Hurt WC, Gilmore HW, et al. Current Therapy in Dentistry, Vol. 7. St. Louis: CV Mosby, 1980.

Megran DW, Scheifele DW, Chow AW. Odontogenic infections. Pediatr Infect Dis 1984; 3:257–265.

Wright JM, Taylor PP, Allen EP, et al. A review of the oral manifestations of infections in pediatric patients. Pediatr Infect Dis 1984; 3:80–88.

LUDWIG'S ANGINA

H. DAVID WILSON, M.D., F.A.A.P.

Ludwig's angina, first described in 1836 by von Ludwig, is a rapidly spreading cellulitis involving the sublingual and submandibular spaces. It is usually a complication of an abscess involving the second and third molar teeth with extension of the infection through thin alveolar bone into the submandibular and sublingual spaces. It also occurs following lacerations of the floor of the mouth or compound fractures of the mandible. Children with immunodeficiencies or malignancies (especially when associated with marked neutropenia) and patients undergoing bone marrow or other organ transplantation are at special risk. Although the condition is rare in childhood, it is recognized by the tender swelling of the floor of the mouth with marked upward displacement of the swollen and hard tongue and the "bull-neck" swelling under the mandible extending to the level of the hyoid bone. These children present with fever, malaise, extreme toxicity, and often symptoms of dysphagia, drooling, and difficulty in speaking. The greatest risk is complete airway obstruction.

This infection is caused by organisms found in the mouth and is frequently a mixed infection with both aerobes and anaerobes such as peptococci, peptostreptococci, *Bacteroides melaninogenicus, Fusobacterium* species, and spirochetes. Gram-negative enteric organisms, *Pseudomonas aeruginosa, Staphylococcus aureus, Candida albicans,* and a host of other organisms may be the causative agent(s), especially in debilitated patients and those who have been receiving antibiotic therapy for other conditions.

Successful treatment includes maintaining the child's airway, establishing the microbial etiology, delivering an effective antibiotic, draining any accumulated pus, and providing supportive treatment until recovery.

If any significant impairment of the airway is caused by the swollen and displaced tongue, an orotracheal tube, or preferably a nasotracheal tube, should be inserted immediately. This is best done under general anesthesia. A tracheostomy should be done only when intubation is impossible. This step is essential in the severely ill patient because, when death occurs, it is usually a result of airway obstruction. Other rare complications are usually the result of extension of the infection into the mediastinum or involvement of the major neck vessels with hemorrhage or thrombosis.

Identification of the pathogen(s) is usually accomplished by extraoral aspiration of the submental region using a syringe and large-bore needle. Blood cultures should also be done. If panorex radiographs of the mandible disclose diseased teeth as the cause, the teeth should be removed and the tooth sockets cultured. The use of computed tomography (CT) and ultrasound techniques may aid in locating deep abscesses or extension beyond the submandibular and sublingual spaces. When infected material is aspirated by syringe and needle, Gram stain and other stains may disclose the characteristic morphology of some anaerobic organisms or other rare causes such as fungi. All specimens should be cultured under both aerobic and anaerobic conditions.

Unless I have reason to suspect unusual organisms, I begin treatment with penicillin G, 250,000 U per kilogram per day divided into six equal doses, given every 4 hours and infused over a period of 10 to 20 minutes. If the patient is allergic to penicillin, I begin treatment with clindamycin, 40 mg per kilogram per day divided into four equal doses, given every 6 hours, and infused over a 20-minute period. One should be aware of the uncommon complication of pseudomembranous enterocolitis associated with clindamycin treatment. If I am dealing with a debilitated or immunologically compromised patient, I give clindamycin as just described, and ceftazidime, 150 mg per kilogram per day divided into three equal doses, given every 8 hours and infused over 20 minutes. Antibiotic choice may be altered according to the results of cultures and susceptibility tests.

If loculated abscesses are identified, the surgeon should place bilateral penrose drains into the various compartments to allow for any drainage. Supportive care would include the usual intravenous fluids, blood, nutritional support, and liberal use of narcotic or other strong pain medications.

The majority of these patients should show clinical improvement within 24 to 48 hours. If they fail to improve, complete reassessment should follow, with CT scan of the neck to evaluate for extension to other areas of the deep neck and for undrained abscesses or foci of infection by resistant organisms. The length of therapy varies, but most patients require at least 1 to 2 weeks of parenteral therapy, sometimes followed by oral treatment with penicillin V, clindamycin, or other appropriate antibiotics selected on the basis of culture and susceptibility testing.

SUGGESTED READING

Barkin RM, Bonis SL, Elghammer RM, Todd JK. Ludwig angina in children. J Pediatr 1975; 87:563–565.

Goldberg MH, Topazian RG. Odontogenic infections and deep fascial space infections of dental origin. In: Topazian RG, Goldberg MH, eds. Management of infections of the oral and maxillofacial regions. Philadelphia: WB Saunders, 1981; 173–231.

Gross SJ, Nieburg PI. Ludwig angina in childhood. Am J Dis Child 1977; 131:291–292.

HERPANGINA

ZIAD M. SHEHAB, M.D.

Herpangina is a clinical entity manifested by fever (usually 102 to 104°F), anorexia, sore throat, and an enanthem, which consists of up to 20 vesicles or ulcers distributed over the soft palate, uvula, or anterior tonsillar pillars. The illness is self-limited, usually lasting 3 to 6 days. It tends to occur in the summer and fall and results from infection with Coxsackie A virus. Coxsackie B and echoviruses have also been implicated. Herpangina affects children between the ages of 1 and 10 years, but it has been reported only rarely in neonates. Herpangina is readily diagnosed clinically, and diagnostic confirmation by viral culture is usually not required except for epidemiologic considerations. The main differential diagnosis is that of herpetic gingivostomatitis, which also involves the gums, tongue, and buccal mucosa.

THERAPY

There is no specific therapy for herpangina. Treatment is supportive, with attention to maintenance of good hydration. The prognosis is excellent except in the rare cases in which other organ systems are involved (e.g., encephalitis, myocarditis).

SUGGESTED READING

Cherry JD, John LL. Herpangina: the etiological spectrum. Pediatrics 1965; 36:632–634.
Parrott RH, Ross S, Burke FG, et al. Herpangina: clinical studies of a specific infectious disease. N Engl J Med 1951; 245:275–280.

INFECTION OF THE SALIVARY GLANDS (SIALADENITIS)

S. MICHAEL MARCY, M.D.

ACUTE VIRAL SIALADENITIS

Acute viral infection of the salivary glands usually affects the parotids; involvement of the submandibular and sublingual gland(s) is less common. Despite the dramatic success of vaccination programs over the past 20 years, mumps virus is probably still the preeminent cause of this condition. Other viral agents causing acute parotitis include parainfluenza types 1 and 3, influenza A, coxsackie A, echovirus, lymphocytic choriomeningitis virus, and human immunodeficiency virus (HIV).

The propensity of the mumps virus to invade virtually any tissue can result in widespread involvement of organs such as the meninges, brain, testicles, epididymis, ovaries, and pancreas. Such infections should be regarded as manifestations of a systemic disease rather than "complications." They may occur before, during, after, or without salivary gland involvement.

Therapy

There is no specific therapy for sialadenitis caused by mumps or other viral agents. Treatment is symptomatic.

The association of parotitis with influenza A infection suggests that acetaminophen rather than aspirin, which may predispose to Reye syndrome, should be used for relief of fever and pain. Hot or cool compresses also provide comfort. Opium alkaloids, which may cause spasm of the sphincter of Odi, should not be used when pancreatitis is suspected.

Providing a liquid or soft diet minimizes discomfort caused by chewing. Sour foods such as citrus fruits, highly seasoned foods, or other mucous membrane irritants such as peppermint aggravate pain by inducing rapid salivary flow, and these should be avoided.

The treatment of infection of organs other than the salivary glands can be found elsewhere in this book (see chapters on *Viral Meningitis and Encephalitis,* and on *Epididymitis and Orchitis*) and in other general references.

Failure to Respond to Therapy

Mumps sialadenitis generally worsens for 1 to 3 days, persists for an equal length of time, and then subsides over the next week. Children with prolonged swelling and tenderness should be evaluated for other causes of salivary gland enlargement, including tumors or cysts, obstruction of the salivary duct(s), drugs, and metabolic and immunologic disorders (see Marcy and Kibrick for detailed information). Rarely, suppurative parotitis (see following) occurs as a complication of viral salivary gland infection.

Prevention

Live attenuated mumps virus vaccine, usually given in combination with measles and rubella vaccine (MMR) at 15 months of age, provides effective and durable immunity. Children who fail to receive vaccine at the recommended age can be immunized at any time unless vaccination is contraindicated.

Children with viral sialadenitis should be isolated until swelling and pain have subsided. Virus has been recovered from the saliva of patients with mumps from 7 days before to 9 days after the onset of illness. The period of communicability is, however, probably somewhat shorter.

There is no reliably effective means of protecting exposed, susceptible persons. I give live mumps vaccine to such patients up to 72 hours after exposure. Because adverse reactions are uncommon, this poses little risk and may be of value in preventing or attenuating the disease—if not immediately, at least at a time of subsequent exposure. The incubation period of mumps is about 14 to 25 days.

ACUTE SUPPURATIVE SIALADENITIS

Suppurative sialadenitis occurs in neonates, particularly premature infants, as well as in older children with salivary gland obstruction, dehydration, or immunosuppression. The parotid gland is involved in most cases. *Staphylococcus aureus* is by far the predominant cause. Streptococci (*viridans streptococci, S. pyogenes, S. pneumoniae*), gram-negative organisms (*Escherichia coli* and other coliforms, *Pseudomonas*), and anaerobic bacteria have also been associated with this condition. Rare causes include *Haemophilus influenzae, Actinomyces* species, the agent of cat-scratch disease, typical and atypical *Mycobacteria,* and histoplasmosis.

Antimicrobial therapy should be guided by Gram stain and culture of pus expressed from the salivary ducts by massage of the affected gland(s). Because the common etiologic agents are part of the normal mouth flora, Gram stain is important in determining the predominant organism(s) and the significance of duct secretion cultures. Blood cultures should be obtained from all patients and a complete septic workup performed on neonates with suppurative sialadenitis.

Hospitalization for parenteral antibiotic therapy, vigorous hydration, and active salivary gland massage are indicated during the first days of treatment. If staphylococci predominate in secretions expressed from the gland, therapy should be initiated with oxacillin (150 to 200 mg per kilogram per day, up to 12 g, in four divided intravenous doses for older children; 25 mg per kilogram every 12 to 6 hours, depending on birthweight and age, for neonates). Anaerobic bacteria, as well as staphylococci and streptococci, are usually susceptible to clindamycin (25 to 40 mg per kilogram per day, up to 2.7 g, in three or four divided intravenous doses). Gram-negative bacilli can be treated with either ceftazidime (125 to 150 mg per kilogram per day, up to 6 g, in three divided intravenous doses for older children; 50 mg per kilogram

every 12 to 8 hours, depending on birthweight and age, for neonates) or gentamicin (6 to 7.5 mg per kilogram per day in three divided intravenous doses in older children, using serum levels to determine dosage after 24 hours; 2.5 mg per kilogram every 12 to 8 hours, depending on birthweight, age, and serum levels in neonates). A combination of clindamycin and gentamicin is appropriate initial therapy when no organisms can be identified on Gram stain.

Children allergic to penicillin can be treated with either cefazolin (100 to 150 mg per kilogram per day, up to 6 g, in three divided doses) or clindamycin in place of oxacillin.

Salivary gland massage is an important part of therapy. The parotid gland is best emptied using the flat of the hand to apply a wavelike compressive motion from the mastoid process to the nasolabial fold. The submandibular gland is emptied using two or three fingers, starting at the angle of the mandible and sliding forward to the chin.

After discharge from hospital, oral therapy with cloxacillin, cephalexin, or cephradine (all 50 mg per kilogram per day, up to 4 g, in four divided doses) is adequate for staphylococcal infection. Clindamycin (15 to 20 mg per kilogram per day, up to 1.8 g, in four divided doses) can be used if anaerobes were isolated. Appropriate oral therapy for gram-negative bacillary infection must be guided by the results of culture and susceptibility studies.

Failure to Respond to Therapy

Persistent fever, inflammation, or toxicity despite seemingly appropriate medical treatment may indicate the need for surgical drainage. Evaluation by ultrasonography or computed tomography can be helpful in determining the presence of abscesses; sialography with retrograde injection of contrast material should be avoided.

The dense fascia and septation of the parotid cause multiple small loculations of pus and prevent fluctuance in all but the most advanced stages of suppuration. Thus, incision and drainage with complete surgical exposure of the gland is generally recommended, particularly if extension of infection into the parotid space is suspected. Percutaneous needle aspiration guided by ultrasonography can be used when only a few abscesses are present.

RECURRENT ACUTE SIALADENITIS

Recurrent sialadenitis, almost always affecting the parotid gland, may occur from once every few years to several times a year. The condition usually resolves during adolescence. Alpha-hemolytic streptococci are sometimes cultured from expressed purulent saliva. No other organism has been consistently associated with this condition.

Therapy

Evaluation with Gram stain and culture should be performed as for suppurative sialadenitis. Oral penicillin V (50 mg per kilogram per day, up to 4 g, in four divided doses) or erythromycin ethylsuccinate (40 mg per kilogram per day in four divided doses with food, up to 1.6 g), good hydration, parotid massage, and use of sialagogues such as chewing gum are usually adequate to bring about a prompt remission.

Failure to Respond to Therapy

Infection caused by an organism unresponsive to penicillin V or erythromycin can be ascertained through the results of pretreatment cultures. A search for causes of obstruction such as a stricture or stone should be pursued through ultrasonography, plain radiography, computerized tomogrpahy, or sialography.

Frequent incapacitating episodes of swelling should be referred to an otolaryngologist for evaluation; however, because resolution at puberty is common, conservative management is indicated in almost all cases.

SUGGESTED READING

David RB, O'Connell EJ. Suppurative parotitis in childhood. Am J Dis Child 1970; 119:332–335.

Kaban LB, Mulliken JB, Murray JE. Sialadenitis in childhood. Am J Surg 1978; 135:570–576.

Leake D, Leake R. Neonatal suppurative parotitis. Pediatrics 1970; 46:203–207.

Marcy SM, Kibrick S. Mumps. In: Hoeprich PD, ed. Infectious diseases, 3rd ed. Philadelphia: Harper & Row, 1983; 733–744.

Rice DH. Advances in diagnosis and management of salivary gland diseases. West J Med 1984; 140:238–249.

Work WP, Johns ME, eds. Symposium on salivary gland diseases. Otolaryngol Clin North Am 1977; 10:259–465.

ACUTE TONSILLOPHARYNGITIS AND SCARLET FEVER

JAMES W. BASS, M.D., M.P.H.

The primary care clinician's major concern in the management of patients with acute tonsillopharyngitis is to determine whether the infection is bacterial or nonbacterial in etiology and therefore amenable or nonamenable to antimicrobial therapy. Treatment of nonbacterial tonsillopharyngitis is symptomatic. Treatment of specific bacterial infections of the tonsillopharyngeal area including diphtheria, epiglottitis, and retropharyngeal and lateral pharyngeal space infections are detailed in other chapters. This discussion is limited to the treatment of streptococcal tonsillopharyngitis and scarlet fever. Treatment of these infections involves the use of specific antimicrobial drugs.

BACKGROUND AND CURRENT CONSIDERATIONS

Since the classic studies of Denny et al and Wannamaker et al in the early 1950s when it was shown that early antimicrobial treatment of patients with streptococcal pharyngitis resulted in prevention of rheumatic fever, this principle has remained foremost in treating physicians' concerns. Although these and other studies conducted since have clearly shown that other clinical benefits from early treatment can be achieved, the importance of the prevention of rheumatic fever initially so overshadowed these benefits that they became regarded as inconsequential. Subsequently, many authorities have come to teach that the prevention of rheumatic fever is the only clinical benefit from early treatment.

Several recently reported studies clearly refute this. Although prevention of rheumatic fever remains important, these studies have shown other significant clinical benefits from early treatment of children with streptococcal pharyngitis. In one of these studies children treated early were afebrile within 24 hours, had significant improvement in their symptoms, and their throat cultures became negative, so that they were presumably noncontagious and could return to school. In contrast, children who received a placebo for 72 hours had persistence of fever and other symptoms for 48 hours; because their throat cultures remained positive, they were presumably contagious for the 72-hour period of observation, and obviously should not return to school during this period. Early treatment should decrease the incidence of suppurative complications, limit the spread of the disease in the family and community, and permit an earlier return of the child to school. With both parents in many households in the United States currently working outside the home, early treatment of children with streptococcal pharyngitis clearly offers significant clinical, public health, social, educational, and economic benefits.

During the past four decades throat culture has been the standard test to confirm the diagnosis of streptococcal pharyngitis. Because a delay in treatment of up to several days does not incur the risk of rheumatic fever, and many authorities taught that early treatment does not significantly alter the acute clinical course of the disease, this delay has been considered acceptable. Recently, commercially available tests that permit rapid diagnosis of streptococcal pharyngitis by detecting group A carbohydrate-specific antigen directly in the throat swab have become available. These tests require only minutes to perform, and in most studies results correlate well with the throat culture, or as well as a second throat culture correlates with the reference first throat culture taken at the same time. If these tests can be perfected and remain cost-effective, they may soon replace the throat culture for laboratory-confirmed diagnosis of streptococcal pharyngitis. Until this is achieved these tests should be used selectively to establish presumptive diagnosis at the initial clinic visit and permit early antimicrobial treatment with the inherent benefits that have been outlined. A throat culture taken at the same time provides information to guide subsequent management of the patient.

ANTIMICROBIAL TREATMENT

Since penicillin first became available for general use in the late 1940s, it has been the drug of choice for treatment of streptococcal infections. All strains of group A beta-hemolytic streptococci (GABHS) remain exquisitely susceptible to penicillin, and there has been no indication of emerging resistance to this drug. The optimal preparation and route of administration varies with the clinical circumstances.

Oral Penicillin

In private practice settings, good compliance with oral treatment and results equal to those with intramuscular administration of benzathine penicillin G can be achieved with parental counseling that emphasizes the need for the medication to be given for a full 10 days to eliminate the infecting organisms and prevent rheumatic fever. The small risk of rheumatic fever in private practice settings, the desire to avoid giving a painful injection, the inherent greater risk of penicillin allergy and other untoward reactions, plus a relatively lower cost compared with that of parenteral treatment have led primary care physicians in the United States to prefer oral therapy.

Oral penicillin G and penicillin V are equally effective, but the latter is preferred because it is acid stable, is better absorbed, and produces predictably higher blood concentrations of penicillin. For children younger than 12 years of age optimal oral penicillin treatment of streptococcal pharyngitis is achieved with doses of 250 mg given twice daily for 10 days. For children older than 12 years of age, adolescents, and adults, doses of 500 mg twice daily for 10 days (a treatment regimen approved by the Food and Drug Administration [FDA]) are recommended. Because compliance in taking oral medications decreases with the frequency of dosing and duration of treatment, dose intervals of more than twice daily and treatment periods for longer than 10 days should probably not be prescribed. In addition, twice-daily treatment are more realistically achieved in school children with working parents. A rational exception might be in the first 24 to 48 hours of treatment, when doses may be given every 6 to 8 hours while the child remains sick and at home, in an effort to ensure an early bacteriologic cure and render the child noncontagious as soon as possible.

Intramuscular Penicillin Preparations

Intramuscular benzathine G should be given to patients with streptococcal pharyngitis in areas where rheumatic fever is prevalent, particularly in poor and crowded inner-city populations, where medical care is episodic and compliance in taking oral penicillin cannot be relied on. These conditions apply in many pediatric populations in the United States and for most children in developing countries. In such circumstances intramuscular penicillin G benzathine in a dosage of 600,000 U for children weighing less than 27 kg (60 lb) and 900,000 to 1,200,000 U for those weighing more than 27 kg is recommended.

A significantly less painful and better accepted intramuscular preparation that contains 900,000 U of penicillin G benzathine and 300,000 U of procaine penicillin G within 2-ml volume has been shown to be effective. In addition to reducing pain at the injection site, the procaine component results in larger penicillin blood concentrations, although this does not effect a more rapid clinical response than benzathine penicillin G. It produces an earlier bacteriologic cure rate, approaching 100% after 24 hours, presumably rendering the patient noncontagious and able to return to school.

Extended-spectrum oral penicillins, including ampicillin and ampicillinlike penicillins (amoxicillin, cyclacillin, and bacampicillin) as well as oral penicillinase-resistant penicillins (cloxacillin, dicloxacillin, oxacillin, and nafcillin), are all effective for treatment of streptococcal pharyngitis. Their use should be reserved for situations in which they afford added benefit. Ampicillin or ampicillinlike penicillins may be preferred for treatment of individuals who have concomitant acute otitis media because these drugs provide additional coverage for *Haemophilus influenzae*. Penicillinase-resistant penicillins may be preferred for treating patients with concomitant suppurative cervical lymphadenitis to provide additional coverage for penicillinase-resistant *Staphylococcus aureus*. In these and similar circumstances these drugs appear to be as effective as penicillin V for treating streptococcal pharyngitis, but they offer no other advantages. They are generally more expensive and are associated with more untoward reactions, including skin rashes, gastrointestinal disturbances, and emergence of antimicrobial-resistant organisms.

Alternatives to Penicillin

For individuals who cannot take penicillin, erythromycin is the first alternative for oral treatment of streptococcal pharyngitis. The recommended dosage for erythromycin estolate is 20 to 40 mg per kilogram per day in two to four divided doses, and for erythromycin ethylsuccinate it is 40 mg per kilogram per day in two to four doses, both given for 10 days. Erythromycin estolate in a dosage of 20 mg per kilogram per day in two divided doses has been shown to be well tolerated and equally effective as 250 mg of penicillin V given three or four times daily. To be equally effective, erythromycin ethylsuccinate must be given in a dosage of 40 to 50 mg per kilogram per day, and at this dosage it is better tolerated when given in four divided doses daily. Both of these oral erythromycin preparations are better absorbed and better tolerated when given with food rather than during fasting. Although the incidence of resistance of GABHS to erythromycin has been reported to be as high as 60 percent in Japan, fewer than 5 percent of isolates from several areas across the United States are resistant to erythromycin.

Oral first-generation cephalosporins have been shown to be equally effective alternatives for individuals who cannot take penicillin or erythromycin. Cephalexin or cephradine (25 to 50 mg per kilogram per day in two divided doses for children and 500 mg twice daily for adolescents and adults) or cefadroxil (30 mg per kilogram per day in two divided doses) is as effective as penicillin V for treatment of streptococcal pharyngitis. Some studies have even shown that these drugs produce greater cure rates than penicillin, allegedly because of their resistance to penicillinase-producing anaerobes and staphylococci in the tonsillopharyngeal flora, which may inactivate penicillin. Cefaclor, an oral second-generation cephalothin given in a dosage of 40 mg per kilogram per day in three divided doses, may be used to treat individuals with streptococcal pharyngitis who also have otitis media because of its additional activity against *H. influenzae.* Erythromycin–sulfisoxazole, 40 mg per kilogram per day of the erythromycin component, in four divided doses, is an alternative under these circumstances, but trimethoprim–sulfamethoxazole is inadequate for treatment of GABHS infections. Although oral cephalosporins are generally more expensive than oral penicillins, cephalosporin suspensions taste better and they are significantly better accepted. Clindamycin, 25 to 40 mg per kilogram per day in three to four divided doses, is an acceptable alternative for individuals who cannot take penicillins, cephalosporins, or erythromycin.

As in the case of penicillin V treatment regimens, using twice-daily dosage schedules, alternative antimicrobial treatment regimens listed here, with twice-daily dosage schedules appear to be optimal because they employ the lowest drug dosage in the fewest number of doses over the shortest duration of time that achieves the best results. These regimens also reduce cost and untoward reactions to a minimum and enhance compliance to a maximum.

RESPONSE TO TREATMENT

Clinical response of children with streptococcal pharyngitis to appropriate antimicrobial treatment is nearly always evident within 24 hours. Most children are fully recovered and have become culture negative within 1 to 2 days after initiation of treatment and can return to school. Persistence of high fever and severe symptoms beyond this period suggests the development of a suppurative complication or some other underlying disease.

FOLLOW-UP

Posttreatment Follow-Up Throat Cultures

Routine posttreatment follow-up throat cultures are not recommended for individuals who remain asymptomatic. Exception to this policy should be made for patients who have had rheumatic fever or when other family members in the household have had rheumatic fever. Every attempt should be made to eradicate GABHS from these patients and other household members in an effort to prevent further episodes of rheumatic fever.

Chronic Carriers

Nearly all treated individuals are culture-negative during the 10 days of treatment. However, if follow-up cultures are done during the 6-week period after treatment is completed, about 10 to 15 percent of patients are seen to develop positive cultures for GABHS, regardless of the type of treatment given. Most of these isolates are the same serotype as the initial isolate made before treatment was given, and they represent the "asymptomatic chronic convalescent carrier state." This chronic carrier state usually persists for several months regardless of whether the patient is treated again or not. In contrast to children who have classic streptococcal pharyngitis, whose throat cultures grow a heavy or almost pure culture of GABHS, who are highly contagious and are at significant risk of developing rheumatic fever if left untreated, chronic carriers usually have throat cultures that yield only a scant growth or a few colonies of GABHS, and it is generally agreed that these children are not a significant source of infection or at risk of developing rheumatic fever. There is therefore no need to detect individuals who manifest only the asymptomatic chronic convalescent carrier state of GABHS.

Relapses and Reinfections

Patients who develop symptomatic illnesses suggestive of streptococcal pharyngitis during the first 2 to 3 months posttreatment and again have throat cultures positive for GABHS should be considered to have relapses or reinfections. Those with GABHS of the same serotype as the initial isolate before treatment should be considered to have relapses and should be retreated. Those with a serotype different from the initial isolate should be considered to have reinfections; these children should also be retreated. Serotype information on GABHS isolates is difficult to obtain, and not practical as a help in deciding on management of these patients. It is not possible to differentiate by clinical evaluation posttreatment symptomatic patients who are treatment failures or reinfections from those who are chronic convalescent carriers of GABHS who might be symptomatic because of a coincidental nonstreptococcal pharyngitis. One study of patients whose throat cultures grew only a few colonies of GABHS (fewer than 10 colonies) showed that one-third of them had a significant rise in GABHS antistreptococcal antibodies in their serum, indicating serologic evidence of infection. Accordingly, all individuals who have symptomatic illnesses suggestive of streptococcal pharyngitis whose throat culture yields any GABHS growth should probably be treated.

CONTACTS

Household members of index cases have a substantial incidence of secondary infection. From 30 to 50 percent of siblings and 10 to 20 percent of parents or adult household contacts are culture positive for GABHS, and as many as one-half of the siblings develop symptoms of streptococcal pharyngitis within several weeks. These observations have led some physicians in the past to get throat cultures from all household members at the outset and treat those who are culture positive to prevent "ping-pong" infection and reinfection in the household during and after treatment of the index case. Most primary care physicians today, however, prefer to obtain throat cultures only from symptomatic household contacts and to treat only those whose cultures are positive.

RECURRENT STREPTOCOCCAL PHARYNGITIS

Children who have frequent and recurrent bouts of culture-proved streptococcal pharyngitis are special management problems. If oral antibiotics were prescribed, compliance should be questioned, and the use of intramuscular benzathine penicillin G should be considered. If other family members (usually siblings) are involved, intrafamiliar spread of infection in a ping-pong fashion might be suspected; in this case obtaining throat cultures from all household members and treating those with positive cultures for GABHS simultaneously in an effort to eradicate the organism from the household should be considered.

Recent studies present convincing evidence that beta-lactamase–producing organisms in tonsillar tissue inactivate penicillin drugs and promote survival and persistence of GABHS in these tissues, which leads to recurrent infection. If this situation is suspected, a trial of treatment with antimicrobials that are not inactivated by beta-lactamases, such as erythromycin, a cephalosporin, or clindamycin, should be considered.

NON-GROUP A STREPTOCOCCAL PHARYNGITIS

Persons with symptoms of streptococcal pharyngitis whose throat cultures yield a significant growth of non-group A streptococci (usually group C and G) pose a problem to the treating physician. Although it is agreed that these patients are not at risk of developing rheumatic fever if they do not receive antimicrobial treatment, there is controversy as to whether these organisms actually cause symptomatic streptococcal pharyngitis. There is also controversy over whether the clinical illnesses in these patients are responsive to antimicrobial therapy. More than 80 percent of responding physicians in a recent survey of pediatricians, internists, and family practitioners indicated that they considered non-group A streptococci a significant cause of streptococcal-like pharyngitis and believed the clinical illness in these individuals was responsive to penicillin treatment. Although clinical data specifically substantiating these claims are lacking, antimicrobial treatment is recommended for individuals with symptoms of streptococcal pharyngitis whose throat culture yields a significant growth of non-group A streptococci. Because these organisms are usually susceptible to antimicrobial drugs that are effective against group A streptococci, the same treatment regimens recommended for streptococcal pharyngitis caused by group A organisms are recommended.

SUGGESTED READING

Arthur JD, Bass JW, York WB. How is suspected streptococcal pharyngitis managed? A study of what physicians actually think and do. Postgrad Med 1984; 75:241–248.

Bass JW. Treatment of streptococcal pharyngitis revisited. JAMA 1986; 256:740–743.

Bass JW, Crast FW, Knowels CR, et al. Streptococcal pharyngitis in children: a comparison of four treatment schedules with intramuscular penicillin G benzathine. JAMA 1976;235:1112–1116.

Breese BB, Disney FA. Factors influencing the spread of beta hemolytic streptococcal infections within the family group. Pediatrics 1956; 17:834–841.

Brook I. Role of beta-lactamase-producing bacteria in the failure of penicillin to eradicate group A streptococci. Pediatr Infect Dis 1985; 5:491–495.

Colcher IS, Bass JW. Penicillin treatment of streptococcal pharyngitis: a comparison of schedules and the role of specific counseling. JAMA 1972; 222:657–659.

Denny FW, Wannamaker LW, Brink WR, et al. Prevention of rheumatic fever: treatment of the preceding streptococcic infection. JAMA 1950; 143:151–153.

Gerber MA, Spadaccini LJ, Wright LL, et al. Twice daily penicillin in the treatment of streptococcal pharyngitis. Am J Dis Child 1985; 139:1145–1148.

Kaplan ED. The group A streptococcal upper respiratory tract carrier state: an enigma. J Pediatr 1980; 97:337–345.

Kaplan EL, Top FH Jr, Dudding BA, et al. Diagnosis of streptococcal pharyngitis: differentiation of active infection from the carrier state in symptomatic children. J Infect Dis 1971; 123:490–501.

Krober MS, Bass JW, Michells GN. Streptococcal pharyngitis: placebo controlled double-blind evaluation of clinical response to treatment. JAMA 1985; 253:1271–1274.

Stillerman M. Comparison of oral cephalosporins with penicillin therapy for group A streptococcal pharyngitis. Pediatr Infect Dis 1985; 5:649–654.

RETROPHARYNGEAL AND LATERAL PHARYNGEAL SPACE INFECTIONS

SCOTT C. MANNING, M.D.

RETROPHARYNGEAL SPACE INFECTIONS

Retropharyngeal space infections usually present in children under the age of 6 years as sequelae of upper respiratory infections or local trauma. The retropharyngeal space lies deep to the pharyngeal constrictor muscles and extends from the base of the skull to the superior mediastinum. The space contains lymphatic chains of two to four nodes on either side of the midline, which drain the pharynx, nose, nasopharynx, paranasal sinuses, and ears. Upper respiratory infections can therefore lead to retropharyngeal adenitis, with the potential for cellulitis or abscess formation. Classically, children present with fever, cervical adenopathy, neck rigidity, difficulty swallowing, noisy breathing, muffled voice, and at times progressive airway obstruction. Initial presentation may be subtle, especially if oral antibiotics were previously administered.

The presence of pronounced swelling of the posterior pharyngeal wall is strong evidence for retropharyngeal inflammation; however, oral examination can be difficult in small children. Palpation of a fluctuant mass just lateral to the midline of the posterior pharynx is diagnostic of abscess, but the clinician must be cautious and avoid any manipulation that could further compromise a borderline airway. The diagnosis of retropharyngeal inflammation is confirmed when a lateral neck radiograph, taken in inspiration with the neck extended, demonstrates widening of the retropharyngeal space. Abscess formation is strongly suggested by demonstration of gas or by discrete dramatic bulging of the retropharyngeal soft tissue. Most often, however, plain radiographs do not distinguish abscess from cellulitis. Computed tomography or ultrasonography can be helpful in delineating abscess from cellulitis in questionable cases.

When the diagnosis of retropharyngeal space infection is considered, the initial concern should be for the airway. Most patients have minimal airway compromise and are treated with careful observation, intravenous fluid rehydration, antibiotics, and possibly cool oxygen mist. Carbon dioxide monitoring and oximetry can be considered when significant stridor is present. The rare child with severe upper airway obstruction manifested by increasing inspiratory stridor, exhaustion, and carbon dioxide retention should be taken to the operating room as soon as possible for control of the airway by means of intubation or, rarely, tracheotomy prior to abscess drainage.

Although older reports in the literature emphasized *Streptococcus pyogenes* and *Staphylococcus aureus,* modern culture techniques have demonstrated the polymicrobial nature of most of these infections. Mouth anaerobes such as *Fusobacterium nucleatum, Bacteriodes melaninogenicus,* and anaerobic streptococci predominate. Initial antibiotic therapy should therefore be targeted at both aerobic and anaerobic oral flora. Classically, penicillin has been the initial drug of choice; however, concern is growing over increasing reports of penicillin-resistant *Bacteroides* and *Clostridium* species. Clindamycin, 25 to 40 mg per kilogram per day in divided doses, is a good first choice in that it is effective against the usual anaerobes and gram-positive aerobic organisms.

In cases of penicillin or clindamycin sensitivity, a broad-spectrum cephalosporin such as cefuroxime (75 to 150 mg per kilogram per day intravenously in divided doses every 8 hours) can be considered. Some authors have recommended additional coverage against gram-negative enteric bacilli; however, these organisms are rarely encountered in neck infections. Antibiotics are generally continued for 10 to 14 days, depending on the response to therapy. Patients can be switched to oral antibiotics such as clindamycin, 20 mg per kilogram per day in divided doses every 6 hours, when they are afebrile and tolerate fluids by mouth.

Most patients with retropharyngeal inflammation present during the initial stages of cellulitis-adenitis, and they respond adequately to appropriate antibiotics. If abscess is strongly suspected on the basis of initial workup, or by the patient's failure to improve with antibiotics over a 24- to 48-hour period, surgical drainage is indicated. After oxygenation and anesthetic induction, the patient is carefully intubated in the Trendelenburg head-down position to prevent aspiration, should insertion of the endotracheal tube cause rupture of the abscess. Prior to incision and drainage, pus is aspirated through a syringe for Gram stain and cultures. Small abscesses can be drained transorally by incising vertically just lateral to the midline over the area of greatest fluctuance. The patient is maintained in the Trendelenburg position to prevent aspiration. The abscess cavity is opened widely with blunt dissection and then emptied with suction and irrigation.

For larger abscesses extending low in the hypopharynx or laterally into the lateral pharyngeal space, an external approach is used to obtain adequate drainage. A horizontal incision is made at the level of the hyoid bone so as to expose the anterior border of the sternocleidomastoid muscle. The muscle is retracted laterally, and the carotid artery and jugular vein are located. These are then retracted laterally, and the lateral pharyngeal space is entered with blunt dissection between the carotid sheath and inferior constrictor muscles. It is sometimes necessary to ligate and divide the middle thyroid vein for adequate exposure. Finger dissection is used to open the lateral pharyngeal and retropharyngeal spaces to drain the abscess. The wound is closed loosely, and a large penrose drain is left in place. The abscess cavity is irrigated daily through the drain tract, and the drain is gradually advanced as the wound discharge diminishes.

LATERAL PHARYNGEAL SPACE INFECTIONS

The lateral or parapharyngeal space is shaped like an inverted cone with its apex at the hyoid and its base at the skull. The space is bounded medially by the superior constrictor muscle and laterally by the pterygoid muscles and mandible. It communicates posteriorly with the retropharyngeal space and it can therefore become involved with infections originating in that area. In addition, dental and tonsillar infections can spread directly to the lateral pharyngeal space. Trismus, medial bulging of the tonsillar area, and swelling at the angle of the mandible are diagnostic clues. Bacteriology and antibiotic therapy are similar to those of retropharyngeal space infections in that oral flora is the primary concern. Drainage of the space is identical to that described in the external neck approach to the retropharyngeal space. Transoral drainage should never be attempted because of the danger of injury to the great vessels.

COMPLICATIONS

Patients are left intubated and observed in the intensive care unit (ICU) for at least 24 hours after drainage of all but the smallest abscesses, to allow for resolution of edema and to avoid upper airway obstruction. The clinician must keep in mind that, in addition to loss of airway, deep neck abscess is rarely complicated by mediastinitis, jugular vein thrombosis, sepsis, and major vessel hemorrhage. A high index of suspicion and prompt aggressive treatment are therefore necessary in managing these potentially lethal infections.

SUGGESTED READING

Baratt GE, Koopman CF, Coulthard SW. Retropharyngeal abscess —a ten-year experience. Laryngoscope 1984; 94:455–463.
Bartlett JG, Gorbach SL. Anaerobic infections of the head and neck. Otolaryngol Clin North Am 1976; 9:655–675.
Edson RS, Rosenblatt JE, Lee DT, McVey EA. Recent experience with antimicrobial susceptibility of anaerobic bacteria—increasing resistance to penicillin. Mayo Clin Proc 1982; 57:737–741.
Levitt GW. Cervical fascia and deep neck infections. Otolaryngol Clin North Am 1976; 9:703–716.
Seid AB, Cotton RT. Retropharyngeal abscess in children revisited. Laryngoscope 1979; 89:1717–1724.

PURULENT RHINITIS

CHARLES M. GINSBURG, M.D.

Purulent rhinitis, a syndrome that occurs in otherwise healthy appearing children, is characterized by opaque, usually yellowish green, bilateral nasal discharge. Although there are no age-specific epidemiologic data on the precise incidence of this condition, purulent rhinitis appears to be most common in preschool and early school-aged children. Anecdotally, day care workers report a large incidence of this condition in toddlers during the winter and spring.

Information available on the microbiology of purulent rhinitis is limited. Todd and coworkers studied 107 children with purulent rhinitis and correlated the results of aerobic cultures with those of Gram-stained smears of the purulent secretions. (Neither viral nor anaerobic cultures were obtained from these patients.) Strains of *Streptococcus pneumoniae, Branhamella catarrhalis,* and *Haemophilus influenzae* were the predominant organisms recovered. They were present in 46 percent, 41 percent, and 38 percent of patients, respectively. Although the percentage of *H. influenzae* type b isolates (as opposed to nontypable *Haemophilus*) in children with purulent rhinitis was larger (20 percent) than would be expected from normal children of the same age, it is not possible to determine whether these or any of the other organisms isolated from a permissive culture site are pathogens or are merely normal nasopharyngeal flora. Species of streptococcus were isolated from 25 percent of patients; however, strains of *S. pyogenes* accounted for only 8 percent of all isolates. Many other aerobic organisms, including strains of *Staphylococcus aureus* (8 percent) and *Corynebacterium* species (20 percent), were also isolated from these patients, but these were considered to be normal flora of the upper respiratory tract.

Despite the perceptions of many experienced clinicians that antimicrobials are effective for therapy of purulent rhinitis, there are no data from controlled studies to confirm or refute this. In the only controlled study that compared an antimicrobial agent, cephalexin, to placebo, Todd concluded that there were no differences between the two groups of study patients in the clinical outcome (Todd et al, 1984). Unfortunately, the antibiotic, cephalexin, that was used in this study has limited activity against strains of *H. influenzae*. Since these strains are present in approximately one-fourth of patients with purulent rhinitis, it is possible that an antimicrobial agent active against this organism would be effective for treatment. Furthermore, purulent rhinitis may be a manifestation of subacute maxillary or ethmoid sinusitis, conditions for which antimicrobials are justified and have proved efficacy. Antimicrobials such as amoxicillin, cefaclor, erythromycin–sulfisoxazole or amoxicillin–potassium clavulanate should be effective for treatment.

Two other conditions, intranasal foreign body and group A streptococcal nasopharyngitis, are occasionally confused with purulent rhinitis. Children with intranasal foreign bodies generally have chronic unilateral nasal discharge with a marked fetid odor. Careful examination of the involved nasal passage with a nasal speculum or a large-diameter otic speculum will generally reveal the foreign material; in most instances the object can be extricated with alligator-type forceps. In contrast to intranasal foreign bodies, the nasal discharge associated with group A streptococcal infection is generally bilateral and, unlike purulent rhinitis, is serous to serosanguineous. There is often erythema, tenderness, and edema of the skin of the nasolabial fold and prolabium. Therapy of this condition consists of warm compresses and either penicillin V or erythromycin estolate.

SUGGESTED READING

Todd JK, Todd N, Damato J, Todd W. Bacteriology and treatment of purulent nasopharyngitis: a double-blind, placebo controlled evaluation. Pediatr Infect Dis 1984; 3:226–232.

DISEASES OF THE MID AND LOWER RESPIRATORY TRACT

INFECTIONS OF THE LARYNX AND TRACHEA

RAOUL L. WIENTZEN Jr., M.D.

Laryngitis and laryngotracheitis (infectious croup) are common pediatric illnesses. Although most episodes are mild and self-limited viral processes, a significant percentage progress to life-threatening airway obstruction, because of the anatomy of the subglottic area in infants. In addition, epiglottitis and bacterial tracheitis, two rapidly progressive disorders with a high likelihood of airway obstruction, may be confused early in their courses with the more benign viral processes mentioned here.

LARYNGITIS

Laryngitis is seen in older children and adolescents as a complication of viral upper respiratory infection. Occasionally *Streptococcus pyogenes* infection can be associated with laryngitis. Consequently, I obtain a throat culture in older children with laryngitis to rule out this possibility. If the throat culture is positive, I treat with antibiotics as for any pharyngitis caused by group A streptococcus. In the majority of instances the culture is negative and therapy for this benign and self-limited illness is exclusively symptomatic. I recommend a period of several days of voice rest and the breathing of humidified air, preferably provided by a cool mist vaporizer. Mild analgesics and antipyretics such as acetaminophen should be used to alleviate discomfort and fever. Gargling with a saline solution at times offers some additional symptomatic relief. I see no role for the use of corticosteroids in the therapy of this usually trivial illness, and there are few data to support any such approach. In patients whose laryngeal symptoms do not resolve within a period of 2 weeks, laryngoscopic examination is indicated to exclude the presence of a foreign body, tumor, polyps, and the like.

LARYNGOTRACHEITIS

Table 1 lists the treatment modalities available for laryngotracheitis. Many of these modalities are conventional therapies untested by controlled clinical trials. They seem to work, nonetheless, and are to be recommended.

The first consideration in my therapy of a child with laryngotracheitis is to determine whether or not hospitalization is indicated. Children who have persistent significant inspiratory stridor or tachypnea at rest are candidates for hospital admission and more intensive therapy. Children who do not have significant stridor or tachypnea may bc managed as outpatients. For these mildly ill patients the only modalities of therapy that need be used are reassurance for the parents that this is a benign and self-limited condition, and mist therapy for the child in an effort to liquify his tracheobronchial secretions to avoid their inspissation. I do not use sedation with chloral hydrate or other pharmacologic agents in outpatients. One of the most important components to this outpatient management is instructing the parents to observe the child for the onset of progressive respiratory difficulty, especially an increased respiratory rate and more labored inspirations. I notify parents that such changes in the child's condition should prompt a call to their primary caretaker. Last, I believe there is no place for the use of racemic epinephrine nebulization in the treatment of children with croup who are to be managed as outpatients.

Children who are ill enough to require hospitalization for croup require more intensive therapy. Still, the mainstay of therapy is humidification, which reduces the viscosity of their tracheobronchial exudate, but also stimulates nasal and laryngeal receptors, thereby slowing the respiratory rate. Mist in conjunction with a reassuring parent and occasionally the use of chloral hydrate for sedation benefits the child by diminishing the force of inspiration and thereby diminishing the collapse of the extrathoracic airway and the ensuing obstruction. In addition to mist, oxygen therapy is almost always used. Recent studies show that a significant number of hospitalized children with this disease have mild hypoxia, which may not be clinically appreciated. Consequently, oxygen in a concentration of 25 to 30 percent is added to the mist tent.

In children who have persistent, significant, inspiratory stridor after mist, antianxiety medicines, and oxygen are applied, I begin racemic epinephrine nebulization treatment.

Table 2 gives the recommended dosage of racemic epinephrine per treatment. A marked reduction in acute upper airway obstruction is seen in most

TABLE 1 Therapies for Laryngotracheitis

Outpatient	Inpatient
Reassurance	Reassurance/sedation
Mist	
Parental education	Mist tent
	25–30% oxygen
	Racemic epinephrine nebulization
	Steroids
	Mechanical airway
	Antibiotics

patients following a treatment. This effect, however, is frequently short-lived and symptoms return within a few hours. (It is because of this that racemic epinephrine should not be used in the outpatient setting.) In hospitalized patients the use of racemic epinephrine may be needed as frequently as every hour to relieve obstruction. I monitor the patient's heart rate and continue to give treatments as needed until the pulse exceeds 200 per minute or an arrythmia occurs.

It has been shown that this modality of treatment, although temporarily effective in the acute situation, does not change the course of the illness. However, the need for the insertion of an artificial airway has been substantially reduced since the era of racemic epinephrine treatments.

In patients who progress with illness even in the face of oxygen, mist, reassurance, sedation, and racemic epinephrine therapy, it is important to reassess the diagnosis, and to consider whether the patient may in fact have progressive viral laryngotracheitis heading toward airway obstruction, or epiglottitis, bacterial tracheitis, or foreign body aspiration. Lateral radiographic views of the soft tissue of the neck, a chest radiogram and an otolaryngology consultation may then be indicated.

In my approach to the patient with laryngotracheitis, the final step in treatment is the decision to insert a mechanical airway. This is seldom necessary, but it is far better to have planned for this contingency in advance than to execute such a step at the last moment under emergency conditions. The preferred method of establishing a mechanical airway is by nasotracheal intubation. Once inserted, the airway need be maintained for 3 to 5 days, during which time oxygen and mist therapy is continued with aggressive suctioning of secretions. Usually by 5 days the patient can be successfully extubated.

The most controversial aspect of the management of infectious croup is the use of steroids. Several studies have advocated, and many have denied, the effectiveness of steroids in patients with laryngotracheitis. It is my practice not to use steroids on a routine bases. Rather, I use steroids (dexamethasone, 0.3 mg per kilogram every 12 hours for 2 to 3 days) in those patients who appear to be progressing to more severe forms of upper airway obstruction, which might eventuate in the need for an artificial airway. It

is important to be very certain that one is not dealing with bacterial tracheitis or epiglottitis when the decision is made to use corticosteroids.

Two antiviral antibiotics have activity against the agents causing laryngotracheitis. Amantadine has been approved for use in treating infection caused by influenza A virus, and ribavirin is active against respiratory syncytial virus as well as parainfluenza virus and influenza A and B viruses. Although there are few trials of amantadine in pediatric populations, I would use this drug in the dosage of 5 to 8 mg per kilogram per day in two divided doses in patients with severe tracheobronchitis during an epidemic of influenza A infection, especially if the patients are known to be at high risk for influenza infection (such as those with underlying bronchopulmonary dysplasia or cardiac disease). I would use ribavirin aerosol for 12 to 18 hours per 24 hours in patients who have proven respiratory syncytial virus laryngotracheitis and who are sick enough to be hospitalized. Again, high-risk groups (babies with bronchial pulmonary dysplasia and children with underlying cardiac disease) are optimal candidates for treatment.

It cannot be stated too forcefully that the management of a child with severe laryngotracheitis must always be concerned with the possibility of a missed diagnosis of epiglottitis or bacterial tracheitis. If patients continue to progress to more serious forms of respiratory failure during the course of treatment for infectious croup, evaluation for these other two entities must be carried out.

BACTERIAL TRACHEITIS

Though not a new disease, bacterial tracheitis has been rediscovered in the last decade, during which several reports of this entity have been published. It is probably a bacterial superinfection of viral tracheitis, and the infecting organisms are usually *Staphylococcus aureus, Streptococcus pneumoniae,* and *Haemophilus influenzae.*

When patients have progressive laryngotracheitis that is unresponsive to the modalities of treatment outlined earlier, I consider the diagnosis of bacterial tracheitis. I obtain an anterior-posterior neck roentgenogram and a routine chest radiograph to evaluate for a shaggy, irregular border of the tracheal

TABLE 2 Racemic Epinephrine Treatment

Weight of Patient (kg)	Amount of Drug (2.25% Solution) (ml)	Amount of Saline (ml)	Total Volume (ml)
<10	0.50	2.50	3.0
10–15	0.75	2.25	3.0
15–20	1.00	2.00	3.0
20–25	1.25	1.75	3.0
>25	1.50	1.50	3.0

**TABLE 3 Alternative Antibiotic Therapies
for Bacterial Tracheitis**

Drugs	Dose (mg/kg/day)	Interval
Cefuroxime	100–150	q8h
Cefotaxime	100–150	q6h
Nafcillin and	150	q6h
chloramphenicol*†	75	q6h

* Discontinue if cultures exclude *Haemophilus influenzae.*
† Follow peak and trough serum concentrations.

wall. At the same time I obtain tracheal secretions for Gram stain and culture and a blood culture, and then I institute antimicrobial therapy with cefuroxime (150 mg per kilogram per day in three divided doses) or an alternative regimen (Table 3).

An important part of the treatment program for bacterial tracheitis is the maintenance of an adequate airway. The majority of patients with this entity require intubation. After this has been accomplished, tracheal suctioning to remove the copious thick purulent secretions is important to preserve the patency of the artificial airway. Mist treatment and supplemental oxygen are essential in the first several days of therapy, but racemic epinephrine and steroids usually play no part in my approach. Usually 3 to 5 days after the institution of an artificial airway and appropriate antibiotic therapy, the patient can be safely extubated.

SUGGESTED READING

Cherry JD. Croup (laryngitis, laryngotracheitis, spasmodic croup and laryngotracheobronchitis). In: Feigin RD, Cherry JD, eds. Textbook of pediatric infectious diseases. Philadelphia: WB Saunders, 1987; 237–250.

Jones R, Santos JI, Overall JC Jr. Bacterial tracheitis. JAMA 1979; 242:721–726.

Koren G, Frand M, Barzilay Z, et al. Corticosteriod treatment of laryngotracheitis *vs.* spasmodic croup in children. Am J Dis Child 1983; 137:941–944.

Liston SL, Gehrz RC, Siegel LG, et al. Bacterial tracheitis. Am J Dis Child 1983; 137:764–767.

ACUTE EPIGLOTTITIS AND UVULITIS

BISHARA J. FREIJ, M.D.

Infection of the epiglottis and its contiguous soft tissues, collectively referred to as supraglottitis, is responsible for about 5 percent of pediatric hospital admissions for upper airway obstruction. This condition is typically abrupt in onset, worsens rapidly over a few hours, and may even be fatal if inappropriately managed. Its early differentiation from the more common viral laryngotracheobronchitis (see chapter on *Infections of the Larynx and Trachea*) is therefore critical. Whenever possible, these patients should be managed by a multidisciplinary team consisting of a pediatrician, anesthesiologist, otolaryngologist, radiologist, and intensivist. The availability of a carefully prepared written protocol as a guide to management allows these patients to be approached in a controlled, time-efficient manner that maximizes their chances for a good outcome.

EPIGLOTTITIS

Overview

The inflammatory process in this condition usually involves, in addition to the epiglottis, the arytenoids, aryepiglottic folds, ventricular bands, and, rarely, the uvula or subglottic area. The extent to which any of these structures is affected varies from sparing of the epiglottis per se to the formation of an epiglottic abscess. Epiglottitis has been described in individuals of all ages, including newborns and the elderly, but about 75 percent of patients are between 1 to 5 years of age. *Haemophilus influenzae* type b is by far the most common etiologic agent and can be isolated from the blood of about 75 percent of patients. A variety of other bacteria have been sporadically implicated, including, *Streptococcus pneumoniae,* groups A, B, and C beta-hemolytic streptococci, *Staphylococcus aureus,* and *H. parainfluenzae.* An etiologic role for influenza and parainfluenza viruses has recently been suggested but not conclusively demonstrated.

Certain features of the history and the child's physical appearance should alert the physician to the possibility of acute epiglottitis. Patients classically present with an illness of short duration characterized by sudden onset of fever and sore throat, followed by dysphagia and excessive drooling; onset of stridor and other signs of respiratory distress occurs shortly thereafter. The children are typically ill-appearing, irritable, anxious, and have a muffled voice. Patients usually refuse to lie down, preferring to sit upright in a parent's lap with their neck extended and mouth open, a position favoring maximum airway patency. It should be emphasized, however, that many patients present with an atypical history or milder symptomatology, thereby necessitating a high index of suspicion. Missing the diagnosis can be disastrous, because rapid progression of the disease to complete upper airway obstruction is likely, resulting in death or hypoxic brain damage.

Initial Management

When the first contact with a child suspected of having epiglottitis occurs in an office setting, the physician should refrain from any attempts to establish the diagnosis by direct visualization of the epiglottis because this may precipitate a respiratory arrest. Instead, every effort should be made not to disturb the child while arrangements are being made for transport to a nearby hospital. Oxygen should be administered by face mask or an oxygen-delivery tube; this may reduce their restlessness and anxiety by partially correcting hypoxemia. Some children, however, resist placement of the face mask. In such instances I prefer to discontinue its use rather than risk aggravating their condition. An individual skilled in resuscitation should remain with the patient at all times, including during the ambulance ride to the hospital. The emergency department should be alerted that a patient with possible epiglottitis is being transported so that all necessary personnel can be mobilized.

Should the patient precipitously worsen before arrival at a hospital, positive-pressure ventilation using bag and mask is effective in reversing this deterioration. This procedure can be repeated as often as necessary until an artificial airway can be inserted. Intubating these patients can be difficult even for skilled personnel and should not be attempted outside the hospital setting. The glottic opening may be obscured by inflammation and its position only inferred by noting the appearance of small air bubbles.

In the event that the initial contact with the patient is made over the telephone and the diagnosis of epiglottitis is suspected, the child should be immediately transported to the hospital by ambulance. Paramedics should be forewarned not to force the patient to lie flat on a stretcher and to follow the same guidelines outlined previously.

When the patient arrives at the emergency department, a rapid assessment of the severity of upper airway obstruction is made. If this represents the first evaluation by a physician, emergency department personnel should proceed in the same cautious manner described earlier. Disturbances to the child should be kept to a minimum and supplemental oxygen provided until the patient can be taken to the operating room. Blood should not be drawn or intravenous catheters inserted at this time to avoid distressing the child further.

Diagnosis

A definitive diagnosis of epiglottitis is made only by direct inspection of the epiglottis and the surrounding soft tissues. This is usually done just before an artificial airway is placed. Certain patients may be cooperative, however, and agree to open their mouths if asked to do so by the examiner. It is sometimes possible to see the red, swollen epiglottis under such circumstances.

Children in whom the diagnosis of epiglottitis is in question can be approached in one of two ways. The first is careful direct laryngoscopic examination in the emergency department as long as the child is comfortable in the supine position and willing to cooperate. The examiner should avoid touching the epiglottis and be prepared to intervene in the unlikely event that complete airway obstruction and cardiac arrest occurs. If a physician skilled at performing flexible fiberoptic laryngoscopy is available, this procedure might be better tolerated by the child because it is done transnasally after application of a topical anesthetic and can be performed with the patient in any position.

The second, and safer, approach is to obtain portable lateral neck roentgenograms with the patient sitting and the attending physician present. In spite of numerous potential pitfalls in their interpretation, roentgenographic studies are helpful in confirming or excluding the diagnosis of epiglottitis. The epiglottis is typically enlarged in this infection, approximating the size and shape of the child's thumb, and there is associated thickening of the aryepiglottic folds. However, epiglottic enlargement is a nonspecific roentgenographic finding that can be seen in association with other conditions including Stevens–Johnson syndrome, angioneurotic edema, caustic ingestion, hemophilia, and supraglottic tumors; it may also represent a normal variant (omega epiglottis). Furthermore, overinterpretation (false-positive) of roentgenographic findings is common. To complicate matters further, some cases of supraglottitis (as in group A streptococcal disease) may not involve the epiglottis itself and the only finding may be thickening of the aryepiglottic folds. If an anteroposterior projection is also obtained, some patients may be found to have localized subglottic edema similar to what is found in croup. With these caveats, correlation of the clinical and roentgenographic findings still provides an accurate diagnosis in most instances. It should be emphasized that roentgenography should be done only when the diagnosis is in doubt. In more certain cases, these studies are unnecessary and only contribute to delays in the initiation of appropriate therapy.

Anesthesia

Parents should be allowed to remain with their child until all preparations for anesthesia, nasotracheal intubation, and possible tracheostomy have been completed in the operating room. Induction of anesthesia is usually started with the child in the sitting position and is accomplished by inhalation of halothane and 100 percent oxygen. An intravenous catheter should be inserted during induction. Intravenous atropine (0.01 mg per kilogram) can be given to decrease oral secretions and reduce the risk of bradycardia or even cardiac arrest from vagal stimulation during instrumentation of the airway. Once a sufficiently deep level of anesthesia is achieved, direct laryngoscopy can be performed to establish the diagnosis of epiglottitis and to insert an endotracheal tube.

Intubation

An artificial airway should be secured as soon as the diagnosis of epiglottitis is confirmed. Although some children with this disease are managed successfully with antibiotics and careful monitoring in an intensive care unit, this practice is potentially dangerous. As many as half of all patients with epiglottitis develop complete upper airway obstruction requiring an artificial airway, and this can occur suddenly. It is also not possible to predict accurately who will develop life-threatening obstruction. Furthermore, emergency intubation of the obstructed airway is more difficult than that performed electively under controlled conditions.

The preferred method for maintaining an airway in epiglottitis is nasotracheal intubation. The internal diameter of the endotracheal tube should be 0.5 to 1 mm smaller than what would normally be used for a child of that age. Orotracheal intubation is comparable to the nasotracheal approach except that the tube's proper position is more difficult to maintain and accidental extubation is more likely. Tracheostomy should be reserved for the occasional child for whom attempts at endotracheal intubation are unsuccessful. Children with endotracheal tubes are at a lower risk for complications and have a shorter duration of hospitalization than those managed with tracheostomies, but nursing care of the latter is easier.

Postintubation Management

Once an artificial airway is securely in place, cultures of the blood and epiglottis can be obtained. Following this, antibiotics can be given (see section on Antibiotic Therapy). A chest roentgenogram should be obtained to ensure proper placement of the endotracheal tube and to detect pulmonary infiltrates or pulmonary edema. Patients should be closely monitored in an intensive care unit. Respiratory care consists of providing (1) humidified gas to avoid airway blockage by inspissated secretions, (2) at least 4 cm of water of continuous positive airway pressure (CPAP) to the airway, and (3) chest physiotherapy and endotracheal suctioning. Arterial pH and blood gas tensions should be measured at least once after intubation and then again as warranted by the patient's condition. Supplemental humidified oxygen may be needed for correction of hypoxemia. Antipyretics and intravenous fluids at daily maintenance levels are also needed. Steroids and racemic epinephrine are not beneficial and should not be used.

To minimize the risk of accidental extubation, I prefer to keep these patients sedated at all times in addition to using extremity restraints. Sedation also helps reduce the anxiety generated by the disease and its therapy. Morphine sulfate (0.1 to 0.2 mg per kilogram), administered intravenously or intramuscularly every 4 hours, is effective and does not depress respiration. If necessary, this can be combined with hydroxyzine (1 mg per kilogram), administered intramuscularly every 4 to 6 hours, diazepam (0.1 to 0.2 mg per kilogram), intravenously every 4 hours, or chloral hydrate (25 mg per kilogram), rectally every 8 hours. If need for sedation increases, then it is necessary to determine whether this is due to hypoxemia, in which case administration of oxygen rather than sedatives is the proper therapy.

Antibiotic Therapy

Several antimicrobial agents have been successfully used in the treatment of epiglottitis. The traditional ampicillin and chloramphenicol combination, still the initial therapy of choice for many physicians, has some limitations that should be recognized. About 25 percent of *H. influenzae* type b strains in the United States produce beta-lactamase and are resistant to ampicillin. This is as high as 50 percent in certain locales. Some strains are beta-lactamase negative but still resistant to ampicillin. One must therefore await the results of in vitro susceptibility tests before altering therapy. Other *H. influenzae* type b strains are resistant to both ampicillin and chloramphenicol. These strains are uncommon at the present time but are being increasingly recognized in other countries such as Spain. My personal preference is to initiate therapy with one of the newer cephalosporins such as cefuroxime, cefotaxime, or ceftriaxone because the aforementioned strains are susceptible to these agents. In addition, the dosing interval for these antibiotics is longer, thereby reducing the nursing load.

The dosage schedule for the various intravenous antibiotics is as follows: ampicillin 25 to 50 mg per kilogram every 6 hours, chloramphenicol 20 to 25 mg per kilogram every 6 hours, cefuroxime 50 to 80 mg per kilogram every 8 hours, cefotaxime 50 mg per kilogram every 6 to 8 hours, and ceftriaxone 25 to 50 mg per kilogram every 12 hours. For each of these antibiotics, the larger dosage should be used if a concomitant meningitis is present. If there is no central nervous system involvement, the smaller dosage provides adequate therapy. Patients should be treated for 5 to 7 days. Longer treatment may be needed if there is an associated infection at another site.

Antibiotic therapy does not need to be given parenterally for the duration of the illness. Once the bacteremia has cleared and the child is extubated and tolerating oral intake, a suitable oral antibiotic can be used for the remainder of the treatment course. Patients with beta-lactamase–negative *H. influenzae* strains can be treated with amoxicillin (15 mg per kilogram every 8 hours), whereas those whose infection was caused by beta-lactamase–positive strains can be treated with cefaclor (15 to 20 mg per kilogram every 8 hours) or the combination of amoxicillin and potassium clavulanate (Augmentin) in a dosage of 15 mg per kilogram of the amoxicillin component every 8 hours. Penicillin V at 25 mg per kilogram every 6 hours can be used for streptococcal disease, while cephalexin (12.5 mg per kilogram every 6 hours) or dicloxacillin (12.5 mg per kilogram every 6 hours) is suitable for staphylococcal infection.

Complications

Pulmonary involvement in the form of segmental atelectasis or pneumonia occurs in about 25 percent of patients. Other extraepiglottic foci of infection are uncommon, seemingly a result of the brief and low-density bacteremia observed in this disease. These include pericarditis, suppurative arthritis, cervical adenitis, tonsillitis, and otitis media. Concurrent epiglottitis and meningitis is rare. However, a lumbar puncture should be performed in patients with suspicious neurologic findings and in young infants with *H. influenzae* bacteremia in whom meningeal signs may be difficult to assess.

Other potential complications include shock, hypoxic brain injury, and cardiorespiratory arrest. The latter may occur spontaneously or as a result of inappropriate management. Pulmonary edema occurs in an estimated 10 percent of patients, usually after relief of airway obstruction. The abrupt reduction in airway pressure that accompanies relief of the upper airway obstruction produces a sudden increase in right-sided venous return and intravascular hydrostatic pressure. This mechanism, along with hypoxic damage to the integrity of the capillary walls, favors the formation of pulmonary edema. The use of 4 cm of water of CPAP, instead of the 2 cm usually needed to maintain a normal functional residual capacity, may be helpful in preventing the development of pulmonary edema. Once this complication occurs, treatment consists of oxygen, fluid restriction, diuretics such as furosemide (1 mg per kilogram, administered intravenously), and mechanical ventilation, if needed.

Endotracheal intubation is associated with a number of complications including obstruction by inspissated secretions, pneumothorax, bleeding, and accidental extubation. Subglottic stenosis is unlikely following brief periods of intubation. In addition to these complications, tracheostomy may also be associated with subcutaneous emphysema, fistula formation, and tracheal granuloma.

Extubation

It is generally safe to extubate patients once significant regression of supraglottic edema has been demonstrated. This assessment is best made by visualizing the epiglottis using direct or flexible fiberoptic laryngoscopy. For most patients, 24 to 48 hours of endotracheal intubation is adequate, and some children can be safely extubated as early as 12 hours after intubation. In contrast, children with group A streptococcal disease usually require longer durations of tracheal intubation. It is preferrable to extubate patients during the morning hours when the maximal number of medical and nursing personnel is available. Sedation should be discontinued several hours before the child is taken to the operating room for extubation and complete endoscopy. The patient should be carefully observed for recurrence of obstructive symptoms following extubation. If subglottic edema is detected during endoscopy, nebulized racemic epinephrine may be helpful. Reintubation is rarely needed.

There is no correlation between the duration of fever in epiglottitis and the rate of resolution of supraglottic edema. The presence of fever should therefore not be used as a reason to prolong intubation.

Patients can usually be discharged 24 hours after extubation if there are no respiratory symptoms and oral intake is adequate.

Prognosis

The outcome for children electively intubated early in the course of epiglottitis is excellent. The few deaths that continue to occur may be due to the rapid progression to complete upper airway obstruction before medical care can be sought or to secondary complications such as severe pulmonary edema or septic shock. Unfortunately, some deaths are due to delayed diagnosis and others are a direct result of inappropriate management. Brief periods of nasotracheal intubation are only rarely associated with long-term sequelae.

Prevention

The incidence of epiglottitis is expected to decrease with the recent licensing of the *Haemophilus* b polysaccharide vaccine. This vaccine should be given to all children 2 to 5 years of age. Epiglottitis has already been described in children immunized with this vaccine. Therefore, a history of vaccination should not preclude consideration of this diagnosis in the appropriate clinical setting.

Rifampin prophylaxis is recommended for all household contacts of children with *H. influenzae* type b epiglottitis, including the index case, if other children 4 years old or younger live in that household. The dosage of rifampin is 20 mg per kilogram (maximum, 600 mg per day) once daily for 4 consecutive days.

UVULITIS

Uvulitis may occur either as an isolated infection or in association with pharyngitis or epiglottitis. Both *H. influenzae* type b and group A beta-hemolytic *Streptococcus* have been incriminated as etiologic agents. An elderly patient with concurrent uvulitis and epiglottitis caused by *Streptococcus pneumoniae* has recently been reported. Finding uvular edema and erythema should warn the physician that epiglottitis may be present. Lateral neck roentgenograms should be obtained in all patients with uvulitis, including those without apparent airway obstruction, to rule out a concurrent epiglottic infection unless its presence is clinically obvious.

Management of uvulitis depends on its clinical presentation. When it is associated with pharyngitis in an older child (older than 5 years) with no signs of airway obstruction, the etiologic agent is usually group A *Streptococcus*. The organism can be isolated from throat or uvular surface cultures. These patients can be treated as outpatients with oral penicillin V at a dosage of 25 to 50 mg per kilogram per day in three or four divided doses for a total of 10 days. Erythromycin, in a dosage of 40 mg per kilogram per day in four divided doses, is a suitable alternative for the penicillin-allergic patient. Afebrile adolescents with pharyngitis and uvulitis from whom an infectious agent cannot be isolated should be suspected of using hashish and approached accordingly.

Children with concurrent uvulitis and epiglottitis usually have findings consistent with the latter condition and should be managed accordingly.

Febrile children whose only focus of infection appears to be the uvula should be considered to have *H. influenzae* bacteremia. They should be hospitalized and treated with parenteral antibiotics. The regimens and dosage schedules are similar to those I outlined for the treatment of epiglottitis.

SUGGESTED READING

Bass JW, Fajardo JE, Brien JH, et al. Sudden death due to acute epiglottitis. Pediatr Infect Dis 1985; 4:447–449.
Battaglia JD. Severe croup: the child with fever and upper airway obstruction. Pediatr Rev 1986; 7:227–233.
Daum RS, Smith AL. Epiglottitis (supraglottitis). In: Feigin RD, Cherry JD, eds. Textbook of pediatric infectious diseases, 2nd ed. Philadelphia: WB Saunders, 1987; 224–237.
Lacroix J, Ahronheim G, Arcand P, et al. Group A streptococcal supraglottitis. J Pediatr 1986; 109:20–24.
Wald ER. Uvulitis. In: Feigin RD, Cherry JD, eds. Textbook of pediatric infectious diseases, 2nd ed. Philadelphia: WB Saunders, 1987; 222–223.

BRONCHIOLITIS AND BRONCHITIS

W. PAUL GLEZEN, M.D.

BRONCHIOLITIS

Bronchiolitis is a common cause of hospitalization of infants. Respiratory syncytial (RS) virus is the most common etiology of bronchiolitis, but other viruses such as parainfluenza virus type 3 also cause this illness. The risk of hospitalization for infants during the annual RS virus epidemic is about 1 in 100. Mortality for hospitalized infants is less than 5 percent, overall, but may range up to 30 to 40 percent for infants with congenital heart disease or bronchopulmonary dysplasia. The risk appears to be higher for infants born prematurely and for those infected during the first 3 months of life.

Virtually all children are infected with RS virus at least one time by their second birthday, and many have experienced two infections. The severity of infection in the first months of life may be modified by high concentrations of maternally derived antibody. Older children (9 months of age or older) may have less severe infections as the diameter of their airways increases. Infants younger than 4 months of age, who were born with relatively small amounts of maternal antibody, have the most severe illnesses.

Infants admitted to the hospital with bronchiolitis usually have low-grade fever, dyspnea, retractions, and expiratory wheezes. The chest roentgenogram usually reveals evidence of air trapping and patchy infiltrates involving multiple lobes. Atelectasis ranging from subsegmental to lobar (usually involving the right middle or right upper lobe) is common. Hypoxemia is the rule, and apnea may be an alarming feature of the illness.

Treatment

Consideration should be given to aerosol administration of ribavirin to any infant admitted to the hospital with bronchiolitis during the RS virus season. Ribavirin aerosol treatment has been shown to hasten resolution of signs and symptoms, improve hypoxemia, and reduce virus excretion. No side effects have been noted when the drug is administered properly. Because criteria for admission to hospital vary considerably, some guidelines for use of the drug have been developed. Under these guidelines, any infant with congenital heart disease, bronchopulmonary dysplasia, severe immunodeficiency, or other debilitating illness should be treated immediately at the onset of an acute respiratory illness during RS virus prevalence. Also recommended for therapy are infants younger than 6 weeks of age and hypoxic infants with PO_2 at 65 mm Hg or less.

Ribavirin is usually administered for 3 to 5 days by oxyhood or small croup tent with oxygen or room air. For desperately ill infants, it may be administered through a ventilator if care is taken to prevent clogging of valves and airways. Filters must be inserted in the lines, and the machine must be monitored closely by trained respiratory therapists. Therapy has been continued for as long as 30 days without ill effect. The drug is placed in the reservoir of the aerosol generator at a concentration of 20 mg per milliliter. The therapy is maintained for 18 to 20 hours per day. The dose is determined by the minute volume of the respirations of the patient. High concentrations of the drug—100 times those required to inhibit the virus in culture—have been measured in respiratory secretions during aerosol administration, but the drug is cleared rapidly when the aerosol is stopped.

Wheezing illness similar to bronchiolitis may occur in older children with *Mycoplasma pneumoniae* infection. When *M. pneumoniae* is known to be prevalent, this etiology should be suspected and appropriate diagnostic studies performed. When this etiology is suspected, the child is treated with erythromycin, 50 mg per kilogram of body weight per day, in four divided doses.

Of nonspecific therapies, oxygen is the most important. Infants with bronchiolitis requiring hospitalization should have blood gas determinations, and hypoxic infants should receive oxygen by hood or small tent. Infants with severe apnea or a rising PCO_2 may require mechanical ventilation. Oxygen concentrations should be monitored by pulse oximetry.

Bronchodilators should be used cautiously in small infants with severe bronchiolitis. Studies have shown that some virus infections alter metabolism of theophylline, resulting in toxic serum concentrations if large dosages are used. Blood concentrations should be monitored carefully—especially in infants who are on chronic theophylline therapy for bronchopulmonary dysplasia. Studies have shown that only about 30 percent of infants with bronchiolitis improve with bronchodilators. This form of therapy should not be continued if no definite beneficial response is seen with initial efforts.

Infants with severe bronchiolitis may have difficulty taking oral nourishment. Intravenous fluids may be required to maintain hydration and nutrition, but precautions must be taken to avoid overhydration because heart failure and pulmonary edema may be precipitated by overhydration of hypoxic infants.

BRONCHITIS

Bronchitis or tracheobronchitis in children is usually caused by a respiratory virus or *M. pneumoniae* infection. Hospitalization is usually not required, and most children can be cared for at home. When *M. pneumoniae* infection is suspected on clinical and epidemiologic grounds, erythromycin should be prescribed. Amantadine can be prescribed for children during influenza A prevalence (see chapter on *Influenza*). Humidification of sleep rooms of infants is important, and cough suppressants can be used for older children.

In addition to *M. pneumoniae* and influenza A virus, two other less common causes of tracheobronchitis also have specific therapy available. Afebrile infants younger than 3 months of age with a progressively worsening cough of at least 2 weeks' duration may be infected with *Chlamydia trachomatis*. The index of suspicion is increased if the infant had conjunctivitis during the first 2 weeks of life. Erythromycin is also the treatment of choice for this infection. Bacterial tracheitis may develop in slightly older children, particularly during croup epidemics. The condition appears to be a bacterial superinfection following infection with viruses such as parainfluenza type 1. The most common etiologies of bacterial tracheitis are *Staphylococcus aureus* and *Streptococcus pneumoniae*. Children with bacterial tracheitis usually require hospitalization because they may need emergency intubation to secure the airway. Nafcillin or a related drug is the recommended treatment until the results of bacterial cultures are available.

Children with recurrent acute bronchitis may require special diagnostic studies to rule out anatomic distortions of the major airways or the presence of acquired conditions such as bronchiectasis. Some atopic children present with recurrent bronchitis without much evidence of bronchospasm. In rare instances abnormalities of the immune system, such as a deficiency of a component of the complement system, have been reported.

SUGGESTED READING

AAP Committee on Infectious Diseases. Ribavirin therapy of respiratory syncytial virus. Pediatrics 1987; 79:475–478.

Chapman RS, Henderson FW, Clyde WA Jr, et al. The epidemiology of tracheobronchitis in pediatric practice. Am J Epidemiol 1981; 114:786–797.

Glezen WP, Paredes A, Allison JE, et al. Risk of respiratory syncytial virus infection for infants from low-income families in relationship to age, sex, ethnic group and maternal antibody level. J Pediatr 1981; 98:708–715.

Glezen WP, Taber LH, Frank AL, Kasel JA. Risk of primary infection and reinfection with respiratory syncytial virus. Am J Dis Child 1986; 140:543–546.

Hall CB, McBride JT, Gala CL, et al. Ribavirin treatment of respiratory syncytial virus infection in infants with underlying cardiopulmonary disease. JAMA 1985; 254:3047–3051.

PERTUSSIS

MOSES GROSSMAN, M.D.

Pertussis (whooping cough) is a respiratory disease characterized by a long catarrhal stage followed by the paroxysmal stage, which features episodes of paroxysmal cough with or without an inspiratory whoop. Episodes of apnea are common in young infants. The infection is caused by *Bordetella pertussis,* a gram-negative bacterium. A slightly milder but almost identical illness, parapertussis, is caused by *B. parapertussis.* Pertussis is often, but not universally, characterized by profound lymphocytosis, a feature that is often helpful diagnostically. The disease is highly contagious—more than 90 percent of susceptibles in the household acquire the infection. The diagnosis is clinical and confirmed by culture of the organism from nasopharyngeal swabs or by examination of nasopharyngeal smears with fluorescent antibody microscopy.

The disease is serious in the first 6 months of life, a period accounting for some 30 percent of cases in the United States. Mortality in the first year of life is a little under 1 percent, a significant reduction from past years; this represents improvement in intensive care and life support measures.

The infants and children at highest risk should be hospitalized for monitoring, administration of oxygen, and intravenous fluids. This includes most infants younger than 6 months, as well as older infants with very severe symptoms, apneic or cyanotic spells, or vomiting to the point of needing intravenous nutritional support, as well as infants with underlying pulmonary or cardiac disease. Older infants and children can usually be managed as ambulatory patients. Protection of susceptibles, those already exposed and not yet exposed, needs to be addressed.

GENERAL SUPPORTIVE MEASURES

Nursing care is of paramount importance. Giving attention to feeding and handling of secretions, and most of all avoiding anoxia and dealing with episodes of apnea are the essentials of management.

Hospitalized infants should be handled with respiratory isolation precautions. They should have their cardiorespiratory function and their state of oxygenation monitored. This is best done with a percutaneous oxymeter, if available, because arterial punctures often provoke a paroxysm. Infants should be protected from invasive procedures that are not absolutely necessary, as well as from tobacco smoke, because these tend to trigger paroxysm. Attention must be paid to caloric intake. Small, frequent feedings in a quiet setting are often retained, but prolonged periods of vomiting with paroxysms may necessitate parenteral alimental supplements. Cough medicines and suppressives are of no value. Nasopharyngeal suctioning may be required, and chest physiotherapy may be helpful.

The same principles apply to the care of *ambulatory children.* They need not stay in bed or at home, but obviously should not be placed in an environment that permits them to infect others.

Five days after antimicrobial therapy is initiated the children may be considered noninfectious and can return to day care or school. Parents should be appraised of possible complications, and the children should be examined if they become febrile.

ANTIMICROBIAL THERAPY

Several antimicrobial agents are effective in achieving an early microbiologic cure, but none affects the clinical course of the disease when administered during the paroxysmal stage of the disease. The best of these antimicrobial drugs is erythromycin. There is some evidence that erythromycin (and other drugs) can alter the clinical course of the disease when given during the catarrhal stage (the diagnosis is seldom made at this point except in a second family case), and that it may abort the disease if it is given during the incubation period. Despite the lack of proof of its clinical effectiveness, erythromycin should be administered whenever the disease is diagnosed, because it limits the period of infectivity and thus limits the spread of infection. The recommended dosage of erythromycin is 40 to 50 mg per kilogram per day divided into four doses, with a maximal dose of 1 g per day, given over a period of 14 days. A recent review article (Bass, 1986) suggests that erythromycin estolate produces somewhat higher serum concentrations and is also more effective in eradicating the organism than other formulations of this drug. If the patient is not able to tolerate erythromycin, trimethoprim–sulfamethoxazole or ampicillin might be used instead.

OTHER MEDICATIONS

Two controlled studies in the literature show that administration of glucocorticoids resulted in reduction of the number, severity, and duration of paroxysms. There is little published information beyond those two studies and not much accumulated clinical experience. Based on those studies one might consider adding glucocorticoids to the management of a severely ill child with exceptionally severe paroxysms.

Another drug that has been used to treat this disease is albuterol (or salbutamol), a beta$_2$-agonist. There are several studies of the drug in the literature—some showing effectiveness, some showing lack of it. Because the drug has not been tried in infants younger than a year, and it is not licensed for that age group, and because older children are seldom very ill with pertussis, the role of this agent in therapy remains to be determined.

TREATMENT OF COMPLICATIONS

The most common complications of pertussis are pneumonia, hypoxia, convulsive seizures, and otitis media. The convulsive seizures are best treated with phenytoin; the loading dose is 15 to 20 mg per kilogram per day divided into three doses and followed by a daily dose of 5 to 7 mg per kilogram, given once daily to older children and divided into two doses for infants. The management of the other complications is straightforward (see relevant chapters).

MANAGEMENT OF CONTACTS

Pertussis is a very communicable infection, and household contacts should be treated to prevent further spread of the organism. All household and very close contacts, adults and children alike, should receive erythromycin 40 to 50 mg per kilogram per day in four divided doses for a period of 14 days (maximum dosage 1 g per day). In addition children who are younger than 7 years and who have been immunized with diphtheria–pertussis–tetanus (DTP and have not received a DTP booster during the preceding 3 years should be given a DTP booster. Those who are still in the midst of their basic DTP immunization should continue with the series, in addition to receiving erythromycin prophylaxis.

Day care center contacts should be treated like household contacts with a view to preventing an outbreak. This includes erythromycin prophylaxis, as outlined earlier, and the necessary DTP booster. Secondary cases may be expected up to 14 days after exposure (incubation period is 7 to 10 days) and should be watched for. The primary case may return to the classroom after 5 days of erythromycin therapy if his clinical condition permits.

SUGGESTED READING

Bass JW. Pertussis: current status of prevention and treatment. Pediatr Infect Dis 1985; 4:614–619.
Bass JW. Erythromycin for treatment and prevention of pertussis. Pediatr Infect Dis 1986; 5:154–157.
Cherry JD. The epidemiology of pertussis and pertussis immunization in the United Kingdom and the United States: a comparative study. Curr Probl Pediatr 1984; 14:1–78.
Hinman AR, Koplan JP. Pertussis and pertussis vaccine. JAMA 1984; 251:3109–3113.
Report of the Committee on Infectious Diseases (Red Book). Elk Grove Village, IL: American Academy of Pediatrics, 1986.

DIPHTHERIA

PISESPONG PATAMASUCON, B.Sc.(Med), M.D.

Diphtheria is a vaccine-preventable disease caused by *Corynebacterium diphtheriae.* The disease is characterized by membranous inflammation of the tonsils, pharynx, and larynx. The clinical onset is generally insidious with low-grade fever, cough, hoarseness, and mild sore throat. Complications such as myocarditis, neuritis, nephritis, and hepatitis are the results of toxin from *C. diphtheriae,* which interrupts protein synthesis and causes cell death.

The disease is transmitted by direct contact with infected materials from a patient or carrier. These materials include discharge from the nose, throat, and lesions on the skin, eyes, and even the vagina.

The incidence of diphtheria has decreased dramatically with immunization programs, and is now rare in developed countries like the United States, but with the influx of immigrants from South East Asia, plus a small incompletely or nonimmunized population, clinical diphtheria may not be so rare in the United States in the future. In addition, the cases may be imported from endemic areas. Hence, travelers with fever, sore throat, and white patches or membrane in the faucial area, should be suspected of having diphtheria until proved otherwise. Empiric treatment is advised in such a patient, especially one who presents with a bull neck or who is severely ill.

SPECIFIC THERAPY

Prompt treatment with diphtheria antitoxin (DAT) from horse serum is mandatory following conjunctival or skin tests for hypersensitivity.

Of the three forms of diphtheria toxin (circulating or unbound, bound, and internalized in the cytoplasm), only the circulating form can be neutralized by DAT.

Skin testing is done by using 0.1 ml of a 1:100 dilution of DAT injected intradermally and read in 20 minutes. Formation of a wheal greater than 1 cm in diameter is a positive reaction. The conjunctival test is done by placing 1 drop of DAT, diluted 1 to 10 in physiologic saline, on the conjunctiva of a lower lid. The control eye has a drop of physiologic saline. A positive reaction is seen in 20 minutes with conjunctivitis and lacrimation. This can be alleviated by 1 drop of 1:100 epinephrine. Epinephrine 1:1,000 should be ready to be given in case of anaphylaxis. The doses are about 0.01 ml of epinephrine per kilogram and can be repeated every 15 to 30 minutes. To desensitize, DAT should be given slowly in small increments every 20 minutes. The following schedule is suggested:

1. 0.5 ml of 1:20 dilution subcutaneously.
2. 0.1 ml of 1:10 dilution subcutaneously.
3. 0.3 ml of 1:10 dilution subcutaneously.
4. 0.1 ml of undiluted antitoxin subcutaneously.
5. 0.2 ml of undiluted antitoxin subcutaneously.
6. 0.5 ml of undiluted antitoxin subcutaneously; if there is no reaction, the rest of DAT is given intramuscularly.

There is no definite dosage for the DAT, but I usually give 20,000 to 40,000 U for pharyngeal or laryngeal involvement of < 48 hours' duration, 40,000 to 60,000 U for nasopharyngeal disease, and 80,000 to 100,000 U for disease of 3 or more days or "bull neck" diphtheria. For cutaneous diphtheria, the dose of DAT is 20,000 U. Antitoxin should be diluted 1:20 in isotonic saline given in a single injection intravenously at a rate not exceeding 1 ml per minute.

In order to eradicate the microorganism and to decrease the number of carriers, penicillin should be given in addition to the antitoxin. The dosage is 50,000 to 100,000 U per kilogram per day, intravenously in divided doses every 4 to 6 hours, for 10 to 14 days. However, if the patient can be fed, intravenous penicillin can be stopped after 5 days and continued orally. Erythromycin is the alternative to penicillin, for the same duration of treatment. The dosage for the estolate form is 30 mg per kilogram per day orally, in three divided doses, and 50 mg per kilogram per day orally, in four divided doses for the other forms of erythromycin.

Three negative pharyngeal and nasal cultures should be documented before the patient is discharged.

GENERAL SUPPORTIVE CARE

All patients with diphtheria should rest in bed because of the danger of cardiac complications. They should be under strict isolation until three nose and throat cultures, taken at least 24 hours apart, are negative. Those with cutaneous diphtheria should be handled by contact isolation until two cultures from the cutaneous lesions are negative. In laryngeal diphtheria I prefer to do early and elective tracheostomy rather than intubation because of the ease of toilet care. The cardiac rhythm should be monitored. Dysrhythmia can occur as early as the second day or as late as 6 weeks after onset. The question of whether steroid therapy should be used in diphtheria myocarditis is unsettled. Some reports have suggested that steroids given in those with bundle branch block will decrease mortality, but steroids have no beneficial effect in mild to moderate cases. I prefer to give steroids in bull neck diphtheria, in the severely ill, and in those with electrocardiographic (ECG) changes typical of myocarditis. The dosage of corticosteroid is 2 mg per kilogram per day of prednisolone or equivalent, given intramuscularly. Digitalis is probably more harmful than beneficial.

Neurologic complications such as paralysis of the palate, extraocular muscles, the pharynx, the diaphragm, and the muscles of the extremities may occur. Palatal paralysis is characterized by a nasal voice and regurgitation of fluids through the nose. This usually develops by around the fifth to the sixth day of the disease, or maybe as late as the sixth week. Management of the neurologic complications is purely symptomatic.

I usually keep the patient with diphtheria in the hospital for at least 10 days to allow detection of early complications. The patient should be educated, as well, to the signs and symptoms of late complications.

If the patient is too ill to be fed, nutritionally balanced intravenous therapy should be provided. Liquid diet can be started later if the patient has no swallowing problem.

A patient with diphtheria does not develop immunity to the causative microorganism; thus, for future protection, active immunization with diphtheria toxoid is recommended. Diphtheria toxoid can be given alone or in combination with pertussis and tetanus toxoid (DTP) to patients under the age of 7 years old and adult-type diphtheria toxoid to those over the age of 7.

PROTECTION OF EXPOSED INDIVIDUALS

All close contacts, irrespective of their immunization status, should have throat swab cultures and be kept under surveillance for 7 days. If the culture is positive for *C. diphtheriae,* treatment with a single dose of benzathine penicillin (600,000 to 1,200,000 U intramuscularly, the smaller dosage being for patients weighing less than 30 kg) or oral erythromycin in the same dosage as previously suggested, but not exceeding 2 g, should be given for 7 days. I prefer to use benzathine penicillin rather than erythromycin because of the compliance problem. Throat cultures should be taken for *C. diphtheriae* after completion of antimicrobial therapy. Close contacts who were previously fully immunized should receive a booster dose of diphtherial toxoid (D, DTP, DT) if they have not received a booster dose within 5 years.

DAT should not be given routinely to nonimmunized or incompletely immunized individuals, because of the risk of hypersensitivity to the horse serum.

ACTIVE IMMUNIZATION

Universal immunization for diphtheria is the only effective control measure. We like to start immunization at age 2 months. This consists of three doses of diphtheria, pertussis, and tetanus combination intramuscularly at bimonthly intervals. The fourth reinforcing dose is given a year after the third dose, i.e., at age 18 months, and a booster at 5 years. For children older than 7 years immunization is done with the adult-type diphtheria toxoid and tetanus (DT). Two doses are given 1 to 2 months apart, and a third dose 6 to 12 months after the second. Booster doses should be given every 10 years.

SUGGESTED READING

Committee on Infectious Diseases Report, 20th ed. Elk Grove Village, IL: American Academy of Pediatrics, 1986.
Dobie RA, Tobey DN. Clinical features of diphtheria in the respiratory tract. JAMA 1979; 242:2197–2201.
Krugman S, Ward R. Infectious diseases of children, 8th ed. St Louis: CV Mosby, 1986.
Munford RS, Ory HW, Brooks GG, Feldman RA. Diphtheria deaths in the U.S.A. 1959–1970. JAMA 1974; 229:1890–1893.
Naiditch MJ, Bower AG. Diptheria: a study of 1433 cases observed during a ten-year period at the Los Angeles county hospital. Am J Med 1945; 17:229–245.
Zalma VM, Older JJ, Brooks GF. The Austin, Texas, diphtheria outbreak. Clinical and epidemiological aspects. JAMA 1970; 211:2125–2129.

INFLUENZA

W. PAUL GLEZEN, M.D.

Influenza virus infections are the most important etiologies of acute respiratory illnesses that cause children to be brought for medical care. The rate of visits to health care facilities for preschool children with acute respiratory disease (ARD) during influenza epidemics ranges from 25 to 30 per 100 and from 8 to 20 per 100 for school children. ARD hospitalizations for school children peak annually during influenza epidemics, with rates ranging from 2 to 8 per 10,000. Rates of hospitalization with ARD are higher for preschool children, varying between 20 and 40 per 10,000.

Influenza epidemics occur annually; the earliest warning of influenza virus activity is provided by systematic culturing of children with febrile or flulike illnesses as they present for health care. If systematic surveillance is not available in your community, you can rely on bulletins from the Centers for Disease Control and from state and local health departments for information about the occurrence of influenza virus infections in your area. A strong clue to the presence of influenza is the sudden appearance of many school children with febrile or flulike illnesses; school children are usually the first group in the community to become infected. Only about one-half of children presenting for care have atypical flulike illness; about 15 percent have pharyngitis or upper respiratory infection (URI). Otitis media is common in young children, and tracheobronchitis is common for all ages. Croup and primary viral pneumonia constitute less than 5 percent of illnesses of children seen in the ambulatory setting.

TREATMENT

Ideally, diagnosis should be based on rapid detection of viral antigen in upper respiratory tract secretions by a technique such as immunofluorescence or ELISA. Unfortunately, these methods are not generally available, so that the clinician must rely on evaluation of the clinical and epidemiologic features described previously and prevalence data published by national, state, and local virus laboratories. This information should be sufficient to make a presumptive diagnosis and decisions about management and therapy.

Uncomplicated influenza virus infections of children without underlying conditions or household contacts who have high-risk conditions may not require specific therapy. Rest and administration of acetaminophen for fever, glycerol guaiacolate for cough, and fluids may be sufficient. Aspirin should *not* be given to children suspected of having an influenza virus infection because of the reported association of influenza and aspirin therapy in the development of Reye's syndrome. Cough suppressants are not recommended for children younger than 2 years of age, but older children with a persistent nonproductive cough may be treated with an antitussive such as dextromethorphan.

When influenza A viruses are known to be prevalent, an antiviral drug, amantadine, may be used for treatment. Amantadine is *not* effective for influenza B virus infections. When started early after the onset of an influenza A illness, amantadine shortens the course of fever and other symptoms and reduces the amount of virus in respiratory secretions. The dosage is 5 mg per kilogram of body weight, administered in two divided doses per day for 7 days or until symptoms have subsided. The total daily dosage for children younger than 10 years of age should not exceed 150 mg; for children 10 years of age or older, the total daily dosage is 200 mg. The usual course recommended for adults is only 5 days, but because children commonly excrete virus for 7 or more days, a longer course of therapy is warranted. The drug should be administered cautiously to children with seizure disorders because the therapy may trigger seizures. Amantadine is excreted unaltered by the kidneys; children with chronic renal insufficiency require reduced dosages.

Children with chronic underlying conditions that put them at special risk for developing serious illness or complications should be treated as soon as possible if they develop a flulike illness during influenza A prevalence. This recommendation should be followed even if the child has received influenza vaccine for that year, because the epidemic virus may drift antigenically from that included in the vaccine, reducing the protective effect. Early treatment is also indicated for children who live in a household including a high-risk person; this should reduce the risk that the child will spread the infection to the high-risk contact.

Severe pneumonitis or laryngotracheobronchitis may require hospitalization. Treatment with amantadine is indicated for influenza A infection. For life-threatening infections with influenza B virus, ribavirin aerosol therapy should be considered. This form of therapy is licensed for treatment of infants with bronchiolitis or pneumonia caused by respiratory syncytial virus, and studies have shown that it shortens the course of influenza A or B infections in college students.

In addition to the specific therapies, children with severe pneumonias may require ventilatory assistance. Ampicillin therapy should be started initially and bacterial flora should be monitored to guide specific antibiotic therapy for superinfection. Children with severe croup may need to have their airway secured by intubation or tracheostomy.

COMPLICATIONS

If fever persists after about 3 days, children should be reevaluated for the emergence of a suppurative complication such as otitis media, sinusitis, tracheobronchitis, or pneumonia. If a secondary infection is suspected, appropriate bacterial cultures should be obtained and antibiotics initiated. The most likely pathogens are *Streptococcus pneumoniae* or *pyogenes, Haemophilus influenzae,* and *Staphylococcus aureus.*

Reye's syndrome is a rare but serious complication of influenza in children that usually occurs when aspirin has been administered early in the course of the prodromal illness. The first sign is persistent vomiting, which may be followed by lethargy, coma, and convulsions. Children suspected of having Reye's syndrome should be managed in a pediatric intensive care unit where complete supportive care is available. Vital functions must be supported while efforts are made to reduce the elevated intracranial pressure that is usually present.

Acute myositis is another rare complication of influenza and is usually seen with influenza B virus infection. About 5 days after onset of a typical flulike illness, affected children complain of bilateral lower leg pain and may refuse to bear weight. Marked tenderness and some swelling may involve the calf muscles symmetrically. The serum creatine phosphokinase value may be markedly elevated. The myositis is usually self-limited and recovery uneventful, but renal shutdown has been reported because of excessive myoglobinuria.

PROPHYLAXIS

Influenza virus infections may be prevented by immunization with inactivated vaccine. The currently available vaccine contains antigens for the three prevalent viruses. The antigen content is reviewed each year and altered to reflect emergence of new variants considered to have epidemic potential for the United States. Influenza vaccine is especially recommended for children 6 months of age and older who have underlying conditions that place them at risk for development of complications of influenza virus infection. Highest priority for immunization is given to children with impairment of heart or lung function, including congenital heart disease, bronchopulmonary dysplasia, asthma, and cystic fibrosis. Annual vaccinations are also recommended for children with sickle cell disease, diabetes, and chronic renal disease. Children with malignancies and immune suppression of any type need protection, but their response to the vaccine may not be optimal. Amantadine should be prescribed for them at time of exposure to persons infected with influenza A virus. Children taking chronic aspirin therapy for diseases such as rheumatoid arthritis or Kawasaki syndrome should also receive vaccine because of their risk of developing Reye's syndrome with influenza virus infection.

Infants with chronic conditions may be too young for vaccination or, if more than 6 months of age, may not have an adequate antibody response to vaccine. Their household contacts, including older siblings, should be vaccinated to reduce the risk of infection of the high-risk child. Household contact vaccination is also indicated for families of children who are immunosuppressed. In fact, this measure has been logically extended to all household contacts of any high-risk person as well as to the health care team.

Amantadine can be a useful adjunct to vaccine for prevention of influenza A infection in many settings. Studies have shown that it can be used as both the primary preventive and reinforcement of vaccine in reducing nosocomial infections. It should similarly be prescribed for high-risk persons when a household contact develops a flulike illness during influenza A epidemics. Since the epidemic virus often has drifted antigenically from that included in the vaccine, the added protection of the antiviral drug can avert vaccine failures.

SUGGESTED READING

Glezen WP, Decker M, Joseph SW, Mercready RG Jr. Acute respiratory disease associated with influenza epidemics in Houston, 1981–1983. J Infect Dis 1987; 155:1119–1126.

Glezen WP. Serious morbidity and mortality associated with influenza epidemics. Epidemiol Rev 1982; 4:25–44.

McClung HW, Knight V, Gilbert BE, ct al. Ribavirin aerosol treatment of influenza B virus infection. JAMA 1983; 249:2671–2674.

Peter G, ed. AAP report of the Committee on Infectious Diseases: influenza. Elk Grove Village, IL: American Academy of Pediatrices, 1986; 204–212.

ASPIRATION PNEUMONIA AND LUNG ABSCESS

GEORGE H. McCRACKEN Jr., M.D.

Infants and children with aspiration pneumonia or secondary lung abscess usually have an underlying condition that predisposes them to inhalation of microorganisms. Such conditions include altered consciousness (e.g., coma, seizure, or anesthesia), dysphagia, anatomic defects (e.g., tracheoesophageal fistula, cleft larynx, or gastroesophageal reflux), periodontal disease, alteration in host immunity (e.g., chronic granulomatous disease, alpha$_1$-antitrypsin deficiency, or the immotile cilia syndrome), and a foreign body in the trachea or bronchus.

Anatomic defects should be sought in patients with unexplained or repeated aspiration pneumonia or in young infants with lung abscess. Surgical correction of such defects is curative, as is removal of a foreign body. Disease caused by rarely encountered microorganisms or in patients with repeated respiratory infections should prompt an investigation for impairment of host immunity.

The microorganisms associated with aspiration pneumonia are varied, frequently multiple, and often represent members of the oropharyngeal bacterial flora. Among the putative pathogens are aerobic and anaerobic streptococci, *Bacteroides* species, especially *B. melaninogenicus* or *B. oralis,* and less commonly aerobic and anaerobic gram-negative bacilli. Depending on the underlying condition, lung abscesses can be caused by the same organisms associated with aspiration pneumonia, by *Staphylococcus aureus,* or by unusual organisms in patients with defects in host immunity. In the chronically hospitalized patient, nosocomial infection by enteric gram-negative bacilli with multiple resistance should be considered.

Whenever possible, the physician should attempt to establish the etiologic diagnosis before initiating antimicrobial therapy. Culture of sputum or oropharyngeal secretions is unreliable and often misleading. In the older child or adolescent, transtracheal aspiration is satisfactory and safe if performed by an experienced physician. The preferred procedure is bronchoscopy, which permits one to visualize directly the airway for anatomic defects or a foreign body to culture purulent material from the lesion, and to provide drainage, if necessary. A putrid odor to the secretion suggests anaerobic infection. If a pleural effusion is noted on chest roentgenogram, a diagnostic thoracentesis should be performed. Material obtained at bronchoscopy, at thoracentesis, or by transtracheal aspiration should be examined for cell morphology and number and for microorganisms by Gram and acid-fast stains, and cultured by both aerobic and anaerobic techniques.

ANTIMICROBIAL THERAPY

While awaiting results of cultures, one can guide initial empiric therapy of aspiration pneumonia or lung abscess by examination of purulent material. The drugs should be effective against aerobic and anaerobic microorganisms that compose the oropharyngeal flora. Although penicillin G is effective against most mouth organisms, some *Bacteroides* species and staphylococci are resistant. I prefer clindamycin (20 to 30 mg per kilogram daily in four divided doses, intravenously or orally) for initial therapy. This regimen can be combined with gentamicin (5 to 7.5 mg per kilogram daily in two or three divided doses, depending on age, intravenously or intramuscularly) in patients with gastroesophageal reflux, neonates, and chronically hospitalized individuals in whom gram-negative enteric bacilli could be causative agents.

Once results of cultures and susceptibility testing are available, more specific antimicrobial therapy can be used, if appropriate. For aerobic and anaerobic gram-positive cocci, penicillin G (75,000 to 100,000 units per kilogram daily in four or six divided doses, intravenously) is preferred. For *Bacteroides* species, either clindamycin or metronidazole (15 to 35 mg per kilogram daily in four divided doses, intravenously or orally) can be prescribed. Gram-negative enteric bacillary pneumonia is best treated with an aminoglycoside or with a third-generation cephalosporin such as ccfotaxime (100 mg per kilogram daily in four divided doses, intravenously) or ceftriaxone (50 to 80 mg per kilogram once or in two divided doses daily, intravenously or intramuscularly), especially for aminoglycoside-resistant strains. Disease caused by *Staphylococcus aureus* is treated with either nafcillin (150 mg per kilogram daily in four divided doses, intravenously) or vancomycin (40 mg per kilogram daily in four divided doses, intravenously).

DRAINAGE

Aspiration pneumonia often involves the posterior segment of the right upper lobe or basilar portions of the lower lobes and can be a necrotizing process. In some patients, clinical improvement is hastened by positional drainage under the guidance of a trained pulmonary therapist. For lung abscess, drainage is essential and is best accomplished by bronchoscopy and subsequent positional drainage. Although empyema is uncommonly associated with aspiration pneumonia, when present, it is best managed by placement of one or two catheters for drainage as soon as possible. A foreign body should be removed by bronchoscopy.

Duration of antimicrobial therapy is guided by the patient's clinical and roentgenologic responses. In uncomplicated aspiration pneumonia, 7 to 10 days of antimicrobial therapy usually suffices. In those with necrotizing pneumonitis, therapy for 2 or 3 weeks, or longer, is usually necessary. For patients with lung abscesses, serially performed roentgenography, sonography, or computed tomography is the best guide to determine duration of therapy. Purulent material should be completely evacuated by drainage procedures and the lesion considerably smaller or no longer visualized before therapy is stopped. This can take 3 weeks or longer, but during this time, treatment with orally administered antibiotics is recommended if the susceptibility of the pathogen has been defined, serum bactericidal titers against the pathogen can be determined to achieve optimal effect, and ingestion and retention of the drug can be ensured.

SUGGESTED READING

Asher MI, Spier S, Beland M, et al. Primary lung abscess in childhood. Am J Dis Child 1982; 136:491–494.
Berquist WE, Rachelefsky GS, Kadder M, et al. Gastroesophageal reflux-associated recurrent pneumonia and chronic asthma in children. Pediatrics 1981; 68:29–33.
Brook I, Finegold SM. Bacteriology and therapy of lung abscess in children. J Pediatr 1979; 94:10–12.

ACUTE PULMONARY EXACERBATIONS IN CYSTIC FIBROSIS

JAMES C. CUNNINGHAM, M.D.
LYNN M. TAUSSIG, M.D.

Cystic fibrosis (CF) is an autosomal recessive disorder that primarily involves exocrine glands. It is the most common lethal genetic disease in Caucasians and the most common cause of bronchiectasis in childhood. CF is a multisystem disease but the pulmonary involvement remains the major cause of morbidity and mortality in these patients. During the past 20 years, increased physician and public awareness, early diagnosis by sweat electrolyte quantitative iontophoresis, improved nutrition, improved antibiotics against *Pseudomonas aeruginosa,* and aggressive management of chest complications have resulted in significant improvement in both the quality and the length of life for these patients.

Although the basic defect in CF remains unclear, the generalized exocrine dysfunction results in the production of secretions that inherently have, or develop, altered rheologic properties, resulting in inspissation of secretions in ducts and passageways. In the lungs this results in airway obstruction and altered mucociliary clearance.

The lower respiratory tract of CF patients becomes chronically colonized with bacteria. The common infecting microorganisms in CF include *Staphylococcus aureus, Haemophilus influenzae,* and *Pseudomonas aeruginosa. Staphylococcus aureus* is often the first bacterial pathogen to colonize the airways, with *H. influenza* and *P. aeruginosa* frequently appearing later. In recent years, *S. aureus* appears to have decreased in frequency, even as an initial pathogen. The presence of *H. influenzae* may be overlooked because of more rapid growth in vitro of the other two pathogens. Virtually all CF patients eventually become colonized with mucoid strains of *P. aeruginosa.* Recently, *Pseudomonas cepacia* has emerged as a serious pathogen in some CF centers.

Acute pulmonary exacerbations in cystic fibrosis are usually characterized by increased cough, tachypnea, dyspnea, an increase in sputum production, a decrease in appetite, malaise, and an increase in pulmonary findings on physical examination. Although the exact cause of the acute pulmonary exacerbation is often unclear, it may result from proliferation of the bacteria colonizing the airways. This may occur with or after a viral infection, or other intercurrent acute pulmonary infections caused by *Mycoplasma pneumoniae,* fungi, mycobacteria, *Legionella pneumophila,* or other agents. Although total eradication of *Pseudomonas* from the airways is usually impossible, the goal of treatment is to restore a new stable state of airway colonization patterns and regain and/or preserve pulmonary function.

SPECIFIC THERAPY

Antibiotics

The patient with a mild pulmonary exacerbation who has mild or minimal chronic pulmonary disease may respond to oral antibiotics. We routinely do sputum cultures and susceptibility tests to help guide our therapy. In the young or recently diagnosed patient, we generally begin with antistaphyloccocal drugs such as dicloxicillin, 100 mg per kilogram per day in divided doses every 6 hours, or cefaclor, 40 mg per kilogram per day in divided doses every 8 hours, pending sputum culture results. In the older child, or those known to be colonized with *Pseudomonas,* we begin trimethoprim–sulfamethoxazole, 8 to 12 mg (of trimethoprim) per kilogram per day in divided doses every 12 hours, or tetracycline, 20 to 50 mg per kilogram per day in divided doses every 6 hours (for patients older than 7 years), until culture results are available. Some alternative oral antibiotics used in the treatment of CF are listed in Table 1.

Although *Pseudomonas* usually shows in vitro resistance to most oral antibiotics, many patients appear to show an in vivo response to these agents. Failure to see improvement in 3 to 5 days, however, or worsening of symptoms at any time after oral therapy is instituted, necessitates intravenous antibiotics for more adequate coverage against *Pseudomonas.*

Most patients with an acute pulmonary exacerbation require intravenous antibiotics. Initially, in infants with minimal or no chronic pulmonary disease and no history of *Pseudomonas* colonization, we begin nafcillin, 150 mg per kilogram per day in divided doses every 6 hours, and tobramycin, 8 to 10 mg per kilogram per day in divided doses every 6 hours. For older children, or those patients known to be colonized with *Pseudomonas,* we initially begin ticarcillin, 300 to 400 mg per kilogram per day in divided doses every 6 hours, and tobramycin, 8 to 10 mg per kilogram per day in divided doses every 6 hours. Initial antibiotic choices may be altered in both cases, as indicated by sputum culture results. Although one may debate the usefulness of two agents versus one in treating *Pseudomonas,* we still favor the simultaneous use of two antibiotics because of their potential synergistic activity and the possible delayed emergence of resistance. Some alternative intravenous antibiotics used in the treatment of the acute pulmonary exacerbations in CF are listed in Table 2.

The use of aminoglycosides in cystic fibrosis deserves special mention. *Pseudomonas aeruginosa* is frequently more susceptible to tobramycin than to gentamicin. Regardless of which aminoglycoside is used, however, it is important to measure peak and trough serum concentrations. In many CF patients there is increased clearance of semisynthetic penicillins and of aminoglycosides, requiring increased dosages. Additionally, many CF patients have a shortened serum half-life of aminoglycosides necessitating dosing every 6 hours. We try to keep peak tobramycin concentrations in the 8 to 10-μg per milliliter range to ensure adequate sputum penetration of the drug. Trough tobramycin concentrations should be less than 2 μg per milliliter. Fortunately, for reasons that are not entirely clear, nephrotoxicity and ototoxicity in CF patients are rare. Nonetheless, serum creatinine tests should be done weekly and audiologic evaluations should be done on patients who require frequent or prolonged administration of aminoglycosides.

We also routinely screen each week for adverse reactions to the semisynthetic penicillins. This includes a complete blood count with differential and platelet count to look for eosinophilia and platelet abnormalities as well as an AST or ALT to look for evidence of hepatotoxicity.

The use of aerosolized aminoglycosides in CF is controversial. It seems to offer some benefit in certain patients, but it may be irritating to the airways. We therefore reserve its use for the moderate-to-severely ill patient who has not responded to more conventional therapy. In the adolescent or adult, we use 40 to 80 mg of tobramycin in 2 ml of normal saline three times a day. The dosage for younger children has not been clearly established.

TABLE 1 Oral Antibiotics Used in Cystic Fibrosis

Antibiotic	Dosage (mg/kg/day)	Frequency (hourly)	Comments
Dicloxacillin	25–100	6	Absorbed best with food; occasionally diarrhea
Erythromycin	30–50	6–8	GI side effects; take with meals
Cephalexin	50–100	6–8	GI side effects
Cefaclor	20–40	8	Occasionally diarrhea or rash; do not use <1 month of age
Trimethoprim–sulfamethoxazole	8–12 (tri)	12	Occasionally rashes or blood dyscrasias; take with meals, do not use <2 months of age
Tetracycline–oxytetracycline	25–50	6	Do not use <8 years; take 1 hr before meals
Doxycycline	4–5	12	Do not use <8 years; similar to tetracycline
Chloramphenicol	50–100	6	Blood dyscrasias; monitor CBC

TABLE 2 Intravenous Antibiotics Used in Cystic Fibrosis

Antibiotic	Dosage (mg/kg/day)	Frequency (hourly)	Comments
Nafcillin/ oxacillin/ methicillin	150–200	4–6	Phlebitis, nephritis
Ticarcillin	200–400	4–6	5.2 mEq Na/g; occasionally hypersensitivity, liver and platelet abnormal
Azlocillin/ mezlocillin	300–400	4–6	1.8 mEq Na/g; toxicity similar to ticarcillin
Piperacillin	300–450	4–6	1.8 mEq Na/g; platelet abnormal
Carbenicillin	600	4–6	4.7 mEq Na/g; liver and hematocrit abnormal
Tobramycin/ gentamicin/ netilmycin	7–10	6–8	Nephro- and ototoxicity; monitor serum concentrations (peak 7–10, trough <2 μg/ml)
Cefoperazone	100	12	Hematocrit abnormal
Cefotaxime	50–180	6	75% of *Pseudomonas* susceptible
Ceftazidime	300	6	Best *Pseudomonas* coverage of cephalosporins

Bronchodilators

Bronchodilators may be useful in some CF patients to treat heightened bronchial reactivity, as well as for potential positive effects on mucociliary clearance. However, they also have the potential actually to worsen airway obstruction because of relaxation of bronchial smooth muscle, leading to greater airway collapse in bronchiectatic areas. Therefore, we do not routinely use bronchodilators, but reserve their use for patients with demonstrable clinical response to them by clinical examination and/or by pulmonary function studies.

Most commonly, we aerosolize a beta-agonist (metaproterenol, 0.01 cc per kilogram to a maximum of 0.4 to 0.5 cc, or terbutaline, 0.03 mg per kilogram, diluted in 2 ml of normal saline) four times a day. When further bronchodilation is needed, we begin theophylline, 10 to 20 mg per kilogram per day in three divided doses. It is important to monitor serum concentrations when using theophylline, attempting to keep the level between 10 and 20 μg per milliliter.

Chest Physiotherapy

Chest percussion and postural drainage are important adjuncts to therapy as they help to clear secretions and relieve airway obstruction. We routinely do this four times a day during an acute exacerbation. Chest physiotherapy should be done just after aerosol therapy for maximal benefit.

Oxygen

Each CF patient with an acute pulmonary exacerbation should undergo oxygen saturation determination by pulse oximetry or arterial blood gas determination. If oxygen saturation is 90 to 92 percent or the PO_2 is 55 to 60 mm Hg, the patient is given low-flow (2 liters per minute) O_2 during sleep to prevent periods of desaturation. If the oxygen saturation is less than 90 percent or the PO_2 is less than 55 mm Hg, the patient is given continuous oxygen sufficient to raise the PO_2 above 60 mm Hg. This allows for increased pulmonary healing, improved weight gain (because of decreased caloric expenditure for work of breathing), and decreases the risk of and progression of pulmonary hypertension.

Mucolytics

As mucus inspissation in the airways and resultant airway obstruction appear to play a key role in the pathophysiology of cystic fibrosis, an effective mycolytic agent would obviously be of great potential benefit to these patients. Unfortunately, these agents are of questionable efficacy and have adverse effects. *N*-acetylcysteine's efficacy has not been well-documented and it has the capacity to damage ciliated respiratory epithelial cells, as well as to cause wheezing and airway irritation. However, we occasionally use this agent (1 to 2 cc of 20 percent solution added to an inhaled bronchodilator and normal saline) in very sick patients with large volumes of thick sputum. Saturated solution of potassium iodide (SSKI) has been shown to decrease sputum viscosity in vitro, but has not been clearly shown to be effective in vivo. Sodium bicarbonate is also of questionable benefit and has the potential to be very irritating to the airways. Expectorants such as guaifenesin are also of questionable efficacy. We do not routinely use any of these agents.

Cough Suppressants

Cough is an effective mechanism for clearing secretions from large airways and an important host defense mechanism. Cough suppressants play no role in the treatment of the acute pulmonary exacerbation in CF.

Bronchial Lavage

Bronchial lavage to remove obstructing pulmonary secretions is controversial at best. It appears to have no documented long-term benefit, and the procedure itself entails considerable risk. We use it only as a last resort, after failure of all conventional therapies, when significant mucus plugging is preventing adequate ventilation. Even in this setting, it is merely a temporizing measure. Bronchoscopy with endobronchial lavage should play an extremely limited role in the treatment of CF and should be done only by skilled pulmonary or surgical specialists.

Steroids

Cystic fibrosis patients who also have allergic bronchopulmonary aspergillosis (ABPA) or airway reactivity may respond to steroid therapy. Routine alternate-day steroids have also been tried in mildly symptomatic CF patients based on the hypothesis that the inflammatory process may contribute to the airway damage. At the present time, however, routine use of steroids in CF patients cannot be advocated until more information is available. Their use may be associated with significant side effects, including the onset of diabetes mellitus for which CF patients are already at an increased risk.

Diuretics

Diuretic therapy is needed occasionally during acute pulmonary exacerbations, especially for patients with advanced disease. Diagnosis of congestive heart failure is not always easy in the CF patient but often can be made based on physical findings (especially liver tenderness) and echocardiographic demonstration of right ventricular dilatation. Digitalis preparations appear to have a limited role in the management of CF patients, and we rarely use them. Salt restriction is occasionally required for severely ill patients.

Assisted Ventilation

Intubation and use of artificial ventilation are not indicated for the progressively deteriorating CF patient with advanced lung disease who suffers from frequent pulmonary exacerbations. However, such support may be of benefit to the patient with mild or more advanced disease, who has been relatively stable but suddenly suffers an episode of acute deterioration. Improvements in ventilator care, nutrition, and a better understanding of the disease over the past one to two decades appears to have improved the prognosis from some CF patients who are managed with ventilators.

SUPPORTIVE THERAPY

It is important to ensure adequate hydration and normal electrolyte concentrations as there may be excessive sweat electrolyte losses. Additionally, water soluble forms of multivitamins and vitamins A, E,

and K should be supplemented. The prothrombin time should be measured. Adequate nutrition with a high-calorie, high-protein diet should be maintained and pancreatic enzymes should be replaced as indicated. Dietary fat intake should *not* be restricted. We routinely do nutritional assessments and calorie counts when the patient is hospitalized, because CF patients often have decreased intake during an acute pulmonary exacerbation. Additionally, they have increased caloric expenditures from their work of breathing. Fasting blood glucose values should be measured to ensure early detection of diabetes.

ASSESSMENT OF THERAPEUTIC RESPONSE

There is frequently a 3- to 5-day lag after therapy is instituted before significant respiratory improvement is noted. Often, the first thing noted is the patient's subjective impression of feeling better and breathing easier, followed by improved appetite, a decrease in sleeping respiratory rate, improvement in oxygen saturation, and a decrease in the amount and the purulence of the sputum. We routinely perform pulmonary function tests on admission and weekly thereafter. Length of therapy is generally 2 to 3 weeks and is defined by a plateau in the improvement of pulmonary function or a return of pulmonary function tests to the patient's previous baseline.

In the event that the patient does not respond to therapy, sputum cultures should be repeated, looking specifically for multiply resistant strains of *Pseudomonas aeruginosa,* as well as for *Pseudomonas cepacia,* or other bacterial agents. Other confounding conditions that would hinder improvement should also be evaluated, such as allergic bronchopulmonary aspergillosis, heightened bronchial reactivity, or worsening pulmonary hypertension. Last, a search for other pulmonary infections should be considered, including respiratory viruses, *Mycoplasma pneumoniae,* fungi, mycobacteria, *Legionella pneumophilia,* and Ebstein-Barr virus.

SUGGESTED READING

Davis PB, di Sant'Agnese PA. Diagnosis and treatment of cystic fibrosis-an update. Chest 1984; 85:802–809.

MacLusky I, McLaughlin FJ, Levison H. Cystic fibrosis: Part 1. Curr Probl Pediatr 1985; 15:1–49.

MacLusky I, McLaughlin FJ, Levison H. Cystic fibrosis: Part 2. Curr Probl Pediatr 1985; 15:1–39.

Nelson JD. Management of acute pulmonary exacerbations in cystic fibrosis: a critical appraisal. J Pediatr 1985; 106:1030–1034.

Taussig LM. Cystic fibrosis. New York: Thieme-Stratton, 1984.

Taussig LM, Landau LI. Cystic fibrosis. Semin Respir Med 1979; I:167–182.

Wagener JS, Taussig LM. Cystic fibrosis. In: Cherniack RM, ed. Current therapy of respiratory disease. Toronto: BC Decker, 1984/1985.

Wood RE, Boat TF, Doershuk CF. Cystic fibrosis. Am Rev Respir Dis 1976; 113:833–878.

ACUTE PNEUMONIA OF UNKNOWN ETIOLOGY

ELLEN R. WALD, M.D.

A reasonable approach to the treatment of pneumonia depends on the suspected etiology of the lower respiratory tract infection. This, in turn, is best categorized according to the age of the child, associated symptoms, and radiographic findings. Although some may dispute the need for a roentgenogram in all cases of suspected pneumonia, pneumonia in childhood is sufficiently uncommon that radiographic documentation, if available, should be sought.

Specific microbiologic diagnosis of lower respiratory tract infection caused by bacterial agents is difficult because readily available culture material (from nose, throat, nasopharynx, or blood) is either not predictive or is infrequently positive, and more diagnostic sources (lung aspirate) cannot be easily justified in the otherwise normal host with only mild to moderate illness. We have just begun to enjoy the availability of rapid diagnostic testing for selected viral agents including, most notably, respiratory syncytial virus.

THE NEWBORN

Acute lower respiratory tract disease immediately after birth is caused by the same agents that cause neonatal sepsis. Group B streptococcus and *Escherichia coli* are the most likely pathogens; other enteric organisms or, rarely, staphylococci (in the setting of skin disease, conjunctivitis, or an infected circumcision site) may cause pneumonia. A standard combination of choice would be a penicillin, usually ampicillin at 75 to 100 mg per kilogram per day in three or four divided doses, and an aminoglycoside such as gentamicin, at 5.0 to 7.5 mg per kilogram per day given in two or three divided doses. Therapy is generally maintained for 7 to 10 days. If staphylococcal disease is seriously suspected, a semisynthetic penicillin such as methicillin at 75 to 100 mg per kilogram per day, divided into three or four doses should be prescribed. In areas where methicillin-resistant staphylococci have been a clinical problem, vancomycin can be prescribed in a dosage of 30 to 45 mg per kilogram per day divided three or four times per day. For each of the recommended dosages, the lower dose and less frequent interval should be used in the first week of life. In older neonates, the larger dosage, given more often, is prescribed.

In cases of severe neonatal pneumonia that do not respond to antimicrobials within 24 hours, serious consideration should be given to the addition of acyclovir in a dosage of 30 mg per kilogram per day as a 1- to 2-hour infusion in three divided doses to provide antiviral activity for herpes simplex. Viral cultures of throat, conjunctiva, blood, and cerebrospinal fluid should be done; liver function tests should likewise be obtained.

CHILDREN 1 TO 3 MONTHS OF AGE

Management of pneumonia in this age group is perhaps the most challenging of the therapeutic questions because it is a crossover time for various bacterial agents (a decreasing prevalence of conventional neonatal pathogens—group B streptococcus and *E. coli*—and an increasing prevalence for the usual bacterial pathogens acquired in childhood—*Haemophilus influenzae* type b and *Streptococcus pneumoniae*). In addition, an interesting set of infectious agents can cause the so-called afebrile pneumonitis syndrome (*Chlamydia trachomatis, Ureaplasma urealyticum, Pneumocystis carinii,* and cytomegalovirus). Furthermore, the usual respiratory viruses, respiratory syncytial, and parainfluenzae viruses are common causes of lower respiratory tract disease in this age group as well.

In the febrile and ill-appearing infant whose clinical state calls for hospitalization, cefotaxime (150 mg per kilogram per day in three to four divided doses) is appropriate therapy. In the mild to moderately ill infant, ampicillin (200 mg per kilogram per day in four divided doses) would suffice since ampicillin-resistant *E. coli* or *H. influenzae* type b account for very few cases of pneumonia.

In afebrile infants with wheezing or stridor and pneumonia who have been ill only a few days, no treatment is necessary, because these babies almost certainly have mild viral infection. (For management of more severe cases, see the next section.) In afebrile infants with protracted cough (at least 7 days) and tachypnea, erythromycin, administered at 40 mg per kilogram per day in four divided doses for 14 days, provides coverage for *C. trachomatis*.

CHILDREN 3 MONTHS TO 5 YEARS OF AGE

Most cases of pneumonia in this age group (75 percent) are caused by ordinary respiratory viruses. The two most common agents are respiratory syncytial virus (RSV) and parainfluenzae virus. Influenza viruses and adenovirus may also be important. Most often the nonbacterial nature of the illness is apparent because of low-grade fever, wheezing or stridor, and interstitial infiltrates on chest radiograph. In addition to supportive therapy, ribavirin aerosol is available for infants with RSV who are deemed to be high risk (i.e., those with congenital heart disease, bronchopulmonary dysplasia, and either congenital or acquired immunodeficiency) or to have severe disease. However, the ability of ribavirin to (1) prevent the need for mechanical ventilation, (2) shorten time on mechanical ventilators, (3) lower the requirement for supplemental oxygen, or (4) shorten hospitalization has not been demonstrated at this time. The routine use of ribavirin in all infants hospitalized with RSV is not indicated. Ribavirin is administered by aerosol within a hood for 18 to 22 hours of each 24-hour period.

Bacterial pneumonia in this age group is suggested by the acute onset of high fever, cough (without wheeze or stridor), and lobar infiltrates in the chest roentgenogram. The common agents responsible for bacterial infection are *S. pneumoniae* and *H. influenzae* type b. The relative frequencies of these two bacterial agents are uncertain but they are probably nearly equal. Fifteen to 30 percent of *H. influenzae* type b isolates are beta-lactamase-positive and thereby amoxicillin-resistant.

Assuming that no more than 25 percent of pneumonias in this age group are bacterial, that 50 percent of these are caused by *H. influenzae,* and that 30 percent of these are beta-lactamase producing, approximately 5 percent of all pneumonias would be caused by a beta-lactamase–producing bacterial species. For this reason, amoxicillin at 40 to 50 mg per kilogram per day in three divided doses for 7 to 10 days is appropriate treatment for most children. In a particularly sick youngster, Augmentin (amoxicillin plus potassium clavulanate) may be preferred (40 to 50 mg per kilogram per day in three divided doses for 7 to 10 days). An additional alternative is erythromycin–sulfisoxazole (Pediazole) in a dosage 50 mg per kilogram per day of the erythromycin component in three to four divided doses for 7 to 10 days. For the child who requires parenteral therapy, cefuroxime (150 mg per kilogram per day in three divided doses) is appropriate for the initiation of treatment in the hospitalized child. Once the patient becomes afebrile or a specific etiology has been defined, an alternative orally administered antimicrobial can be prescribed.

6 YEARS OF AGE TO ADULT

Pneumonia is considerably less common in children older than 5 years of age than in younger children. The single most prevalent agent in this age group, and the one that remains an important etiologic agent in adolescents and young adults, is *Mycoplasma pneumoniae*. Bacterial agents become less common, with *H. influenzae* virtually disappearing in children older than 6 or 7 years of age. *S. pneumoniae* remains a prominent cause of acute bacterial pneumonia, but is less prevalent than in the preschool years. Respiratory viruses, influenza virus, and adenovirus are important causes of lower respiratory tract disease; respiratory syncytial virus and parain-

fluenzae viruses are less common causes of pneumonia because repeated infections result in milder respiratory events.

If the patient has a mild to moderate illness for which bacterial agents or mycoplasma are suspect, erythromycin (40 to 50 mg per kilogram per day given orally in three to four divided doses) is a good selection. The regimen can be continued for 10 to 14 days. This provides coverage for *S. pneumoniae* and *M. pneumoniae*. In the case of severe illness with lobar infiltrates and/or empyema, it might be best to provide antibacterial coverage for *H. influenzae* and *S. aureus* as well, until culture results are available, unless the Gram stain of the pleural fluid is easily interpreted. Accordingly, it may be advisable to use cefuroxime (150 mg per kilogram per day in three to four divided doses) plus erythromycin in the previously noted dosage. If laboratory tests yield an etiology, oral treatment with an appropriate agent can be substituted to complete a 10-day course of treatment. If there is no help from the laboratory, erythromycin–sulfisoxazole can be used.

GENERAL ADVICE

In the outpatient management of pneumonia at any age, a follow-up phone call or clinic visit is recommended at 48 hours to ensure that the patient is doing well. It is always advisable to encourage parents to contact the physician if the child becomes increasingly febrile, tachypneic, or distressed at any time. An episode of pneumonia provides a good opportunity to apply a 5 TU PPD to eliminate the possibility of tuberculosis.

The child should be reexamined at 10 days. If the history ensures a complete return to normal of appetite and activity, and the auscultation and respiratory rate are normal, no further evaluation is necessary. Repeat radiographs are not essential after the first episode of pneumonia if the clinical course is uncomplicated and clinical recovery is complete. On the other hand, persistent abnormalities call for an additional evaluation at 4 to 6 weeks. If there is a failure to return to normal by 6 weeks, a repeat radiograph is appropriate to guide further evaluation.

SUGGESTED READING

Denny FW, Clyde WA Jr. Acute lower respiratory tract infections in non-hospitalized children. J Pediatr 1986; 108:635–646.

Long SS. Treatment of acute pneumonia in infants and children. Pediatr Clin North Am 1983; 30:297–321.

Paisley JW, Lauer BA, McIntosh K, et al. Pathogens associated with acute lower respiratory tract infection in young children. Pediatr Infect Dis 1984; 3:14–19.

Stagno S, Brasfield DM, Brown MB, et al. Infant pneumonitis associated with cytomegalovirus, chlamydia, pneumocystis, and ureplasma: a prospective study. Pediatrics 1981; 68:322–329.

PNEUMONIA OF KNOWN ETIOLOGY

BISHARA J. FREIJ, M.D.

Pneumonia in infants and children can be caused by numerous bacteria, viruses, fungi, or parasites. The probability of infection being due to a specific pathogen depends on the clinical syndrome, the patient's age, and the presence of predisposing conditions. Initial therapy is empiric (see chapters on *Acute Pneumonia of Unknown Etiology* and *Nosocomial Pneumonia*), but every effort should be made to identify the causative agents, especially in severely ill patients. An etiologic diagnosis allows the selection of appropriate, narrow-spectrum antimicrobials, thereby reducing the potential adverse effects of antibiotic combinations. It also defines the likelihood of infection at other body sites, the risk for various complications, and the total duration of therapy.

Pneumonias caused by *Actinomyces israelii, Bacillus anthracis, Bordetella pertussis, Coxiella burnetti, Francisella tularensis, Listeria monocytogenes,* mycobacteria, *Nocardia* species, *Pseudomonas pseudomallei, Yersinia pestis,* cytomegalovirus, herpes simplex virus, influenza virus, respiratory syncytial virus, varicella-zoster virus, fungi, helminths, and protozoa are discussed in other sections of the book and are not covered in this chapter.

Optimal management of pneumonia requires the selection of effective antibiotics and the judicious use of supportive measures. The total daily dosage, frequency, and route of administration of individual antibiotics for neonates (Table 1) differ from those for infants and older children (Table 2).

SUPPORTIVE THERAPY

Careful attention to fluid and electrolyte balance is essential. Increased insensible water losses from fever and tachypnea and reduced oral intake result in dehydration and difficulty in clearing pulmonary secretions. Intravenous or oral fluid replacement and, when necessary, administration of humidified oxygen are helpful. Fluid restriction may be required because of the inappropriate secretion of antidiuretic hormone that occasionally accompanies pulmonary infections caused by *Streptococcus pneumoniae* or *Legionella,* or if a concomitant meningitis is present, as in *Haemophilus influenzae* type b disease.

Mechanical ventilation may be required in severe cases. These children require frequent monitoring of arterial blood gases, chest physiotherapy, and suctioning of excess pulmonary secretions.

If a pleural effusion is present, drainage may be required to relieve dyspnea and allow lung reexpansion. If an empyema is found, closed chest tube drainage using large-caliber tubes should be instituted promptly. Inadequate drainage prolongs morbidity and sometimes results in the formation of a restrictive pleural "peel." The chest tubes should be removed when drainage becomes minimal, to avoid additional complications such as pleural fluid superinfection.

ANTIMICROBIAL THERAPY

Aerobic Gram-Positive Bacteria

Staphylococcus aureus

A definitive diagnosis of staphylococcal pneumonia is established by recovering the organism from cultures of blood, pleural fluid, lung parenchyma, or aspirates of other simultaneously infected sites such as joints. Because *S. aureus* is frequently present in the throat and nasopharynx of normal children, its isolation from these sites is not diagnostic, although a pure culture in a patient with a compatible clinical picture is highly suggestive. Measurement of serum teichoic acid antibody titers is rarely diagnostic, except in children with concomitant endocarditis whose levels are markedly elevated.

Staphylococcal pneumonia should be treated initially with a parenteral beta-lactamase-resistant antibiotic such as nafcillin or methicillin, since about 90 percent of *S. aureus* strains are resistant to penicillin. Nafcillin has more in vitro activity than methicillin against *S. aureus,* but both drugs are effective clinically. Nafcillin is predominantly metabolized by the liver and is preferred to methicillin for children with impaired renal function. In contrast, I prefer to use methicillin in children with liver dysfunction. If *S. aureus* is found to be susceptible in vitro to penicillin G, this drug should be used because of its greater safety and lower cost.

Patients with immediate-type hypersensitivity reactions (anaphylaxis, urticaria) to penicillin should be treated with intravenous vancomycin or clindamycin. Vancomycin should be infused over 1 hour because more rapid administration can cause a histaminelike reaction with flushing, pruritus, and a rash involving the face, neck, upper arms, and upper trunk. Serum concentrations of vancomycin should be monitored, and levels of 15 to 30 μg per milliliter are desirable. Some staphylococcal strains are resistant to clindamycin, and this antibiotic should not be used before in vitro susceptibility is demonstrated. Clindamycin should be avoided in the presence of a central nervous system infection because of its poor penetration into the cerebrospinal fluid. If penicillin hypersensitivity is of the delayed type, cephalosporins may be used cautiously because cross-reactions occur in 5 to 15 percent of patients. First-generation cephalosporins such as cephalothin or cefazolin are more active against *S. aureus* than the second- or third-generation agents.

TABLE 1 Neonatal Pneumonia: Recommended Dosage Schedule for Selected Antibiotics

Antibiotic	Route of Administration	Individual Dose (mg/kg) and Frequency	
		Age < 1 Week	Age 1–4 Weeks
Amikacin	IV, IM	7.5–10 q12h*	7.5–10 q8h
Ampicillin†	IV, IM	25 q8h or q12h‡	25 q6h or q8h
Carbenicillin	IV	100 q8h or q12h	100 q6h or q8h
Cefotaxime	IV, IM	50 q12h	50 q8h
Ceftazidime	IV, IM	50 q12h	50 q8h
Ceftriaxone	IV, IM	50 q24h	50–75 q24h
Chloramphenicol	IV, PO	25 q24h	25 q12h or q24h
Erythromycin	PO	10 q12h	10–15 q8h
Gentamicin	IV, IM	2.5 q12h	2.5 q8h
Kanamycin	IV, IM	7.5–10 q12h	7.5–10 q8h
Methicillin†	IV, IM	25 q8h or q12h	25 q6h or q8h
Mezlocillin	IV, IM	75 q12h	75 q8h
Moxalactam	IV, IM	50 q12h	50 q8h
Nafcillin†	IV	25 q12h	25 q6h or q8h
Penicillin G†	IV	25,000 U q12h	25,000 U q6h or q8h
Ticarcillin	IV, IM	75 q8h or q12h	75 q6h or q8h
Tobramycin	IV, IM	2 q12h	2 q8h
Vancomycin	IV	15 q12h	15 q8h

* Lower dose for neonates with body weight less than 2,000 g.
† Dosage is doubled if meningitis is present.
‡ Less frequent administration for neonates with body weight less than 2,000 g.

Pneumonias caused by methicillin-resistant strains of *S. aureus* are uncommon and hospital-acquired in most instances. These staphylococci are often resistant to cephalosporins, erythromycin, tetracycline, and aminoglycosides, but susceptible to vancomycin. Because of frequent treatment failures, cephalosporins should not be used even if these strains are susceptible in vitro. Penicillin-tolerant staphylococci have also been described, but their role in pneumonia is not known. These strains are inhibited but not killed by normally achievable penicillin concentrations, but the tolerance can be overcome by the addition of an aminoglycoside.

The response to therapy in staphylococcal pneumonia is generally slow. Fever commonly persists for 1 to 2 weeks. Parenteral antibiotic therapy should be continued for 1 to 3 weeks. When a patient's condition has improved sufficiently, treatment may be continued with a large-dosage regimen of an oral antistaphylococcal agent such as cloxacillin, dicloxacillin, cephalexin, or clindamycin. The total duration of therapy depends on the rate of improvement and the presence of pulmonary or extrapulmonary complications, but should not be shorter than 3 weeks.

If pleural empyema is present, closed chest-tube drainage should be instituted promptly. Repeated thoracenteses do not provide adequate drainage in most patients and should not be attempted. Acute respiratory deterioration in a child who was otherwise improving is usually secondary to tension pneumothorax from a ruptured pneumatocele, and closed chest-tube drainage is also required for this complication. Bronchopleural fistula is an uncommon complication and requires surgical correction after the infection is cured. Decortication for removal of the pleural "peel" is rarely necessary because most resolve spontaneously within several months.

Wound precautions are recommended for children with draining empyema, but respiratory isolation is sufficient for those with uncomplicated pneumonia. Isolation precautions are continued for the duration of the illness or until staphylococci can no longer be recovered.

In spite of effective antimicrobial agents and the availability of intensive care, mortality remains high, and most of the deaths occur in infants younger than 1 year of age. For the surviving children, roentgenographic abnormalities may persist for weeks or months, but the prognosis for pulmonary function is excellent.

Streptococcus pneumoniae

The diagnosis of pneumococcal pneumonia is confirmed by isolating *S. pneumoniae* from blood, pleural fluid, lung aspirate, or cerebrospinal fluid cultures. Nasopharyngeal or throat cultures are of no value in establishing or excluding a pneumococcal etiology for the pulmonary infection. The detection of pneumococcal polysaccharide antigens in urine, blood, or pleural fluid by counterimmunoelectrophoresis (CIE), latex particle agglutination (LPA), or coagglutination methods provides a presumptive etiologic diagnosis. Antigen detection is particularly helpful in patients who had received antibiotics before cultures from relevant sites were obtained.

Penicillin is the antibiotic of choice for pneumococcal pneumonia except in children allergic to this medication. The route of antibiotic administration depends on the severity of the illness and the presence

TABLE 2   Pneumonia in Infants and Children: Recommended Dosage Schedule for Selected Antibiotics

Antibiotic	Route of Administration	Individual Dose (mg/kg) and Frequency
Amikacin	IV, IM	7.5–10 q8h
Amoxicillin	PO	10–15 q8h
Amoxicillin + potassium clavulanate (amoxicillin component)	PO	15 q8h
Ampicillin*	IM, IV	25–50 q6h
	PO	25 q6h
Azlocillin	IV	75 q4h
Bacampicillin	PO	12.5–25 q12h
Carbenicillin	IV	100 q4h or q6h
Cefaclor	PO	20 q8h
Cefazolin	IV, IM	25 q6h or q8h
Cefoperazone	IV, IM	50 q8h or q12h
Cefotaxime†	IV, IM	25–50 q6h
Cefoxitin	IV, IM	25 q4h or q6h
Ceftazidime	IV	50 q8h
Ceftizoxime	IV, IM	50 q6h
Ceftriaxone†	IV	25–50 q12h
Cefuroxime‡	IV, IM	25–50 q8h
Cephalexin	PO	12.5 q6h
Cephalothin	IV, IM	25 q4h or q6h
Chloramphenicol	IV, PO	20–25 q6h
Clindamycin	IV	7.5–10 q6h
	PO	5–7.5 q6h
Cloxacillin	PO	12.5–25 q6h
Dicloxacillin	PO	7.5–12.5 q6h
Erythromycin	PO	10 q6h
	IV	7.5–12.5 q6h
Gentamicin	IV, IM	1.5–2.5 q8h
Imipenem–cilastatin	IV, IM	15–25 q6h
Kanamycin	IV, IM	7.5 q8h
Methicillin	IV, IM	37.5–50 q6h
Metronidazole	IV, PO	7.5 q6h
Mezlocillin	IV	75 q6h
Moxalactam†	IV	40–50 q6h
Nafcillin	IV, IM	37.5 q6h
Oxacillin	IV, PO	25 q6h
Penicillin G†	PO	12.5 q6h
	IV, IM	20,000–40,000 U q4h
Penicillin G, procaine	IM	25,000 U q12h or q24h
Penicillin V	PO	12.5–25 q6h
Piperacillin	IV	50 q4h or q6h
Rifampin	PO	10 q12h or q24h
Sulfisoxazole	PO	30 q6h
Tetracycline	PO	6–12.5 q6h
Ticarcillin	IV	50 q4h or q6h
Tobramycin	IV, IM	1–2 q8h
Trimethoprim–sulfamethoxazole (trimethoprim component)	PO, IV	6 q12h
Vancomycin§	IV	10 q6h

* Double the dosage if meningitis is present.
† Larger dosage is used if meningitis is present.
‡ Doses are increased to 75 every 8 hours if meningitis is present.
§ Doses are increased to 15 every 6 hours if a central nervous system infection is present.

of underlying disorders. Children with extensive pneumonia, empyema, or associated extrapulmonary infections such as meningitis or endocarditis, and patients with underlying disorders such as sickle cell anemia, cirrhosis, asplenia, or hypogammaglobulinemia should be treated with intravenous penicillin G. In otherwise healthy children with mild or moderate pneumonia, an oral penicillin preparation is adequate in most instances. Penicillin V achieves a sig-nificantly higher serum concentration than an equivalent dosage of oral penicillin G and is the preferred oral penicillin preparation. Intramuscular penicillin preparations may be useful in certain clinical situations. Intramuscular aqueous penicillin G is well absorbed from injection sites and can be used in patients in whom venous access is difficult and who cannot be treated reliably with an oral penicillin. This preparation, however, is painful and should not be used for an extended period of time. Intramuscular procaine penicillin G is less painful, but does not attain peak serum levels comparable to the aqueous preparation; however, penicillin activity persists for several hours. This preparation is particularly useful for children who cannot tolerate oral penicillin preparations because of vomiting. These children may be treated initially with daily intramuscular injections of procaine penicillin G followed by penicillin V 2 to 3 days later. Benzathine penicillin G should not be used for pneumococcal pneumonia because of its high failure rate.

Erythromycin is the drug of choice in the penicillin-allergic patient, but in rare instances, pneumococci are resistant to erythromycin. The oral form is commonly associated with gastrointestinal disturbances, and this limits its usefulness in some children. The intravenous erythromycin preparations (lactobionate, gluceptate) are associated with pain during the infusion and thrombophlebitis. Both of these side effects may be minimized by slowly infusing erythromycin over 30 to 60 minutes. Erythromycin should never be administered intramuscularly. Erythromycin also causes elevated concentrations of theophylline in children receiving the drugs concomitantly. The theophylline dosage should be reduced in these patients to avoid toxicity.

Chloramphenicol is another effective alternative in the penicillin-allergic patient, but its use should be avoided in neonates because of its erratic serum concentrations and the potential for myocardial and central nervous system toxicity, and in children with sickle cell anemia because of its adverse effects on the bone marrow. Other effective alternatives include vancomycin and clindamycin. Cephalosporins should not be used in children with immediate hypersensitivity reactions to penicillin, but may be used cautiously in those with delayed hypersensitivity reactions.

Pneumococcal isolates can no longer be assumed to be uniformly susceptible to penicillin, and screening with oxacillin disks is essential. Penicillin resistance may be relative or absolute. Relatively resistant (tolerant) strains have a minimum inhibitory concentration of 0.1 to 1.0 μg per milliliter and account for about 10 percent of pneumococcal isolates from pediatric patients. Penicillin tolerance can be overcome by using large dosages of penicillin or adding an aminoglycoside. Absolute resistance is rare, but should it be encountered, alternative antibiotics include vancomycin and, possibly, trimethoprim–sulfamethoxazole and rifampin.

The response of fever and symptoms to therapy may be dramatic or gradual. Patients who fail to respond to antibiotics should be carefully examined for previously unsuspected extrapulmonary infections such as meningitis or endocarditis, and their pneumococcal isolates evaluated for penicillin tolerance or resistance. The duration of treatment is usually 7 to 10 days, but may be prolonged if empyema or extrapulmonary infections are present. A minimum of 3 days of therapy following defervescence is recommended. Roentgenographic abnormalities usually require longer periods for complete resolution, but antimicrobial therapy need not be prolonged for that purpose.

Respiratory isolation is recommended for a period of 24 hours after initiation of effective antimicrobial therapy.

Streptococcus pyogenes (Group A Beta-Hemolytic Streptococcus)

A definitive diagnosis of Group A streptococcal pneumonia is difficult to establish. It is uncommon in the absence of viral infections such as chickenpox, measles, or influenza and can complicate certain bacterial infections such as pertussis, pneumococcal pneumonia, or *Mycoplasma pneumoniae* pneumonia. Although parapneumonic effusions or empyema are found in 90 percent of patients, pleural fluid cultures grow the organism in only 30 to 55 percent of cases. Bacteremia is present in only 2 to 15 percent of patients. Recovery of the organism from throat cultures is not sufficient for an etiologic diagnosis. Serologic studies documenting a fourfold or greater rise in antistreptolysin-O titer may help to establish the etiologic diagnosis retrospectively.

Parenteral penicillin G is the drug of choice for streptococcal pneumonia. Cephalosporins, clindamycin, and chloramphenicol are effective alternatives. Erythromycin is the antibiotic of choice in penicillin-allergic children who do not require further parenteral therapy.

The response to antimicrobial therapy is generally slow, and fever may persist for 1 week or longer. This may be related to the concomitant illnesses rather than the streptococcal pneumonia per se. Empyema is a frequent complication and requires early, effective closed chest-tube drainage. The duration of therapy is 10 days in uncomplicated cases, but may be as long as 3 weeks in patients with pleural empyema.

Respiratory isolation is recommended for a period of 24 hours following the start of antibiotic therapy.

Streptococcus agalactiae (Group B Beta-Hemolytic Streptococcus

Group B streptococcal (GBS) pneumonia is seen exclusively in neonates as part of a septicemic illness. A definitive diagnosis is made by recovering the organism from blood, cerebrospinal fluid, pleural fluid, or urine cultures. The isolation of GBS from surface cultures represents colonization and not necessarily disease. A presumptive etiologic diagnosis can be made by detecting GBS polysaccharide antigens in blood, urine, or cerebrospinal fluid by means of CIE, LPA, or staphylococcal coagglutination methods.

Neonates with GBS sepsis and pneumonia can

be treated with parenteral ampicillin or penicillin alone. The addition of an aminoglycoside to ampicillin enhances bacterial killing and prolongs survival of laboratory animals with experimentally induced GBS sepsis. No clinical trials demonstrate a similar benefit for neonates. Susceptibility studies should be performed to detect tolerant strains of GBS. These strains are best killed with a penicillin-aminoglycoside regimen.

The total duration of antibiotic therapy is 10 to 14 days in uncomplicated cases. The presence of extrapulmonary sites of infection may prolong therapy. Early-onset GBS sepsis and pneumonia is a severe disease requiring aggressive therapy (see chapter on *Neonatal Sepsis*). Overall mortality is about 50 percent, with the majority of deaths occurring in premature infants. Late-onset GBS disease is less severe, having a case fatality rate of 15 to 20 percent.

Aerobic Gram-Negative Bacteria

Haemophilus influenzae

The majority of invasive *H. influenzae* infections are due to the type b encapsulated strains and, occasionally, type f. Nonencapsulated strains rarely cause pulmonary infections. A definitive etiologic diagnosis is established by isolating the organism from blood, pleural fluid, or lung aspirate cultures. Extrapulmonary sites of infection are common, and *Haemophilus* may be recovered from cerebrospinal fluid, joint fluid, or pericardial fluid cultures in affected children. Throat and nasopharyngeal cultures are of no value because the majority of children harbor this organism at these sites, and more than 95 percent of the isolates are nonencapsulated forms. The detection of capsular antigens using CIE or LPA in blood, cerebrospinal fluid, urine, or pleural fluid provides presumptive evidence for *H. influenzae* type b invasive disease. The occurrence of false-positive reactions with these antigen detection tests, especially when serum is being tested, appears to be related to either nonspecific agglutination or cross-reactivity with certain pneumococcal, meningococcal, staphylococcal, or *Escherichia coli* strains.

About 25 percent of *H. influenzae* type b strains in the United States are beta-lactamase producers, but this may be as high as 50 percent in certain geographic areas. Standard initial therapy therefore consists of intravenous ampicillin and chloramphenicol. Cefuroxime, cefotaxime, or ceftriaxone are suitable alternatives. Cefamandole should not be used because of its relatively poor stability to the beta-lactamase. Ampicillin is the drug of choice for susceptible strains. Chloramphenicol should not be used in neonates or those with sickle cell disease. Sporadic cases of disease caused by ampicillin- *and* chloramphenicol-resistant *H. influenzae* strains have been described. These strains are susceptible to cefuroxime, cefotaxime, and ceftriaxone. If the prevalence of these strains increases, as predicted by some authorities, the standard initial ampicillin-chloramphenicol regimen will no longer be adequate and will probably be replaced by third-generation cephalosporins.

Oral antibiotics may be used in children with milder infections and in those with severe illness after a period of parenteral therapy. Pneumonias resulting from beta-lactamase-negative strains are adequately treated with amoxicillin, bacampicillin, or ampicillin, whereas those caused by beta-lactamase–producing strains can be treated orally with chloramphenicol, cefaclor, or the combination of amoxicillin and potassium clavulanate (Augmentin).

The duration of therapy in uncomplicated cases is 7 to 10 days. More than half the cases are complicated by pulmonary empyema, and about 15 to 30 percent of patients may have a concomitant meningitis, which may prolong therapy.

Respiratory isolation is recommended during the first 24 hours of antimicrobial therapy. All household contacts of children with *H. influenzae* pneumonia, including the index case, should receive rifampin prophylaxis if there are other children aged 4 years or younger in that household. The dose of rifampin is 20 mg per kilogram (maximum, 600 mg per day) once daily for 4 days. Patients younger than 2 years of age should be immunized with the recently licensed *Haemophilus* b vaccine at the age of 24 months. Vaccination is not indicated for those who develop invasive disease after their second birthday.

Neisseria meningitidis

Primary meningococcal pneumonia is uncommon and usually affects adolescents and young adults. The clinical picture is not distinctive enough to suggest the etiology, and microbiologic confirmation is difficult. Bacteremia occurs in about 15 percent of patients, and pleural effusions are usually small and detected in one-fifth of all cases. Isolating the organism from throat cultures is not helpful because up to 15 percent of healthy individuals may be carriers. Antigen detection using CIE and LPA in blood, urine, and pleural fluid is helpful, but cross-reactions with certain *E. coli* and *Bacillus* strains may occur. Meningococcal pneumonia may also be part of a generalized illness such as meningococcemia or meningococcal meningitis, or may develop as a complication of a preceding viral illness such as influenza.

The drug of choice for primary meningococcal pneumonia is parenteral penicillin G. Chloramphenicol is recommended for penicillin-allergic children. After a minimum of 3 days, oral penicillin or erythromycin can be used. The total duration of therapy is 10 to 14 days.

Respiratory isolation is required during the first 24 hours of antibiotic therapy. Rifampin prophylaxis is recommended for all household and nursery school contacts. The dosage is 10 mg per kilogram every 12 hours for 2 days, not to exceed 1,200 mg per day. The dose for neonates is 5 mg per kilogram every 12 hours for 2 days.

Branhamella catarrhalis

Pneumonias caused by *B. catarrhalis,* formerly known as *Neisseria catarrhalis,* are rare. Most affected patients are adults with chronic lung disease or immunosuppression. The few pediatric cases have involved premature newborns and at least one otherwise healthy child. The diagnosis is made by recovering the organism from tracheal secretions in pure culture or as the predominant isolate. Nasopharyngeal or throat cultures are not helpful because a third of all children are colonized with this organism. Bacteremia is extremely rare.

About 75 percent of *B. catarrhalis* strains are beta-lactamase producers. Initial therapy should consist of a beta-lactamase–resistant antibiotic until the results of susceptibility tests are available. Cefotaxime can be used for parenteral therapy, while erythromycin, trimethoprim–sulfamethoxazole, or the combination of amoxicillin and clavulanic acid are suitable for oral therapy. The optimal duration of therapy is not known but should not be shorter than 5 days.

Coliforms

Pneumonias caused by *Escherichia coli, Klebsiella-Enterobacter* species, *Proteus,* and *Serratia* are mostly nosocomial in origin and affect newborns, children requiring ventilatory support or inhalation therapy, and immunocompromised patients. The diagnosis is established by isolating the pathogens from blood, pleural fluid, lung aspirate, or a concurrently infected site such as the central nervous system.

Treatment of specific coliform pneumonias should be guided by the results of antibiotic susceptibility tests. In general, the most useful classes of drugs are third-generation cephalosporins, such as cefotaxime or cefoperazone, and the aminoglycosides. Some coliform bacilli are resistant to gentamicin and tobramycin. Ampicillin is active against *Proteus mirabilis* and about half of the *E. coli* strains. Antipseudomonal penicillins such as ticarcillin or mezlocillin are active against *E. coli, Enterobacter,* and *Proteus,* but are not suitable for *Klebsiella. Serratia* is usually susceptible to trimethoprim–sulfamethoxazole.

When aminoglycosides are used, careful monitoring of serum concentrations is essential because of their low therapeutic index. The recommended serum concentrations measured 30 to 60 minutes after intravenous or intramuscular doses are 5 to 8 μg per milliliter for gentamicin or tobramycin and 15 to 25 μg per milliliter for amikacin or kanamycin. Trough levels measured just before the following dose is administered should be less than 2 μg per milliliter for gentamicin or tobramycin and less than 10 μg per milliliter for amikacin or kanamycin. Children with impaired renal function require dosage adjustment.

The total duration of therapy is usually 3 weeks, but it may be prolonged in patients with pulmonary abscesses or empyema. Care should be taken to prevent transmission of multiply resistant organisms. Effective measures include careful handwashing and disinfection of respiratory therapy equipment.

Acinetobacter

Although pneumonias caused by *Acinetobacter calcoaceticus* have been reported in otherwise healthy children, the majority of cases are nosocomial and occur in premature infants and patients in intensive care units; in those with tracheostomies, endotracheal tubes, or severe underlying disorders; and in those who received prior antibiotic therapy. A definitive diagnosis can be based on the isolation of *Acinetobacter* from blood, pleural fluid, or lung parenchyma cultures.

Acinetobacter pneumonia is best treated with an antipseudomonal penicillin such as carbenicillin or ticarcillin in combination with an aminoglycoside. Amikacin appears to be the most active aminoglycoside. The incidence of resistance to gentamicin and tobramycin is variable, but may be as high as 30 and 15 percent, respectively. This organism is also susceptible to trimethoprim–sulfamethoxazole, but resistant to penicillin, ampicillin, cephalosporins, erythromycin, and chloramphenicol. In bacteremic patients, removal of intravenous catheters present before onset of the illness is recommended.

The duration of therapy is 2 to 3 weeks in uncomplicated cases. More than one-third of these patients die in the first few days of the illness, mostly from inappropriate antibiotic therapy or development of empyema.

The occurrence of more than one case of *Acinetobacter* infection should prompt a careful search for the environmental sources of contamination such as the hands of hospital personnel or contaminated nebulizers.

Pseudomonas aeruginosa

The majority of these pneumonias are nosocomial and occur in children with burns, cystic fibrosis, or granulocytopenia. A definitive diagnosis is reached by isolating the organism from blood, pleural fluid, or lung parenchyma. Oropharyngeal and rectal isolates may reflect colonization rather than disease.

A number of antipseudomonal penicillins are currently available including carbenicillin, ticarcillin, mezlocillin, azlocillin, and piperacillin. Of these drugs, piperacillin is the most active in vitro; carbenicillin is the least active. However, the clinical efficacies of these five drugs are comparable. Some properties of individual antibiotics may render them more desirable in certain clinical settings. Mezlocillin and piperacillin penetrate inflamed meninges well and may be advantageous in patients with concomitant meningitis. Platelet dysfunction is least pronounced with mezlocillin, and this is desirable for thrombocytopenic patients. The sodium content of mezlocillin, azlocillin, or piperacillin is 40 to 50 percent that of carbenicillin or ticarcillin, and this may be an important consideration for patients with cardiac or renal failure.

The regimen of choice for *P. aeruginosa* pneumonia consists of an antipseudomonal penicillin such as ticarcillin in combination with an aminoglycoside. The combination provides a synergistic effect against *Pseudomonas*. Third-generation cephalosporins such as cefotaxime or cefoperazone are active in vitro, but resistance may develop during therapy. Ceftazidime has in vitro activity exceeding that of antipseudomonal penicillins. Penicillin-allergic patients are treated with aminoglycosides alone. These patients should have the peak serum bactericidal activity against *Pseudomonas* measured to ensure adequate therapy. A titer of at least 1:8 is desirable.

The duration of therapy is usually 3 weeks. The illness is very severe, with a case fatality rate of 50 to 80 percent. Many potential sources of infection exist in the hospital, including sinks, incubators, nebulizers, and resuscitation equipment. Extreme care should be taken to prevent spread to other patients. Careful handwashing and identification of reservoirs of *Pseudomonas* are helpful in reducing this risk.

Pseudomonas cepacia

Pseudomonas cepacia, an opportunistic pathogen, is being increasingly recognized as a cause of nosocomial respiratory infections, especially in patients with altered host defenses such as those with cystic fibrosis, burns, and chronic granulomatous disease. In contrast to *P. aeruginosa,* it is resistant to the aminoglycosides, antipseudomonal penicillins, and most cephalosporins. The drug of first choice is trimethoprim–sulfamethoxazole. Ceftazidime and chloramphenicol are often active against *P. cepacia.* The duration of therapy is 3 weeks or longer.

The isolation of *P. cepacia* should prompt a careful search for an environmental source, which is frequently a contaminated water supply, including such items as detergents or chlorhexidine solutions.

Legionella

Legionellosis is difficult to diagnose with certainty. The organism does not grow on the routine media used in diagnostic laboratories. Special media, such as the commercially available buffered charcoal yeast extract, are necessary for primary isolation. *Legionella* has been recovered from cultures of blood, sputum, pleural fluid, and lung aspirates. Growth may require 3 or more days. Staining of lung tissue or respiratory secretions with direct fluorescent antibody techniques is helpful in half the cases. This test remains positive for at least 3 days, even with antibiotic therapy. Measurement of indirect fluorescent antibody titers helps in making a retrospective diagnosis by documenting a fourfold or greater rise in titer to 1:128 or higher. A single titer of 1:256 or greater is presumptive evidence of a current or past *Legionella* infection. Because about a fourth of all patients with culture-proven disease do not seroconvert, the sensitivity of serologic methods is reduced.

Erythromycin is the drug of choice for legionellosis. The gluceptate form of erythromycin is administered intravenously for about 1 week, after which oral erythromycin is given. Patients usually respond to therapy within 2 days, but others may remain febrile for 1 week. Rifampin is added if a patient fails to respond to erythromycin. Rifampin should not be used alone because of the potential for emergence of resistance. *Legionella* is susceptible in vitro to the penicillins, cephalosporins, chloramphenicol, aminoglycosides, and tetracycline, but these antibiotics are not effective clinically. *Legionella* multiplies within the alveolar macrophages in pulmonary infections. The superiority of erythromycin and rifampin derives from the fact that both of these antibiotics are concentrated in these macrophages. Chronically ill children receiving steroids or other immunosuppressive agents should discontinue their use whenever possible until the infection subsides. Patients who do not respond to therapy should be suspected of having a dual infection. Second pathogens may include *H. influenzae, Mycobacterium tuberculosis, Pneumocystis carinii,* and other organisms.

The total duration of therapy is usually 3 weeks. Relapses are rare, and patients generally respond to a second course of erythromycin.

A number of complications can occur. These include cerebellar ataxia, confusion, seizures, cranial nerve palsies, hemoptysis, empyema, renal failure, severe abdominal or back pain, and several other complications.

Respiratory isolation is recommended. In the event of an outbreak, potential environmental sources of *Legionella* contamination such as water systems and air-conditioning cooling towers should be investigated and properly disinfected.

Anaerobic Bacteria

Anaerobic pulmonary infections in children are uncommon and usually result from aspiration of oropharyngeal secretions. Patients with altered states of consciousness and those with gingivitis or periodontal disease are at greatest risk. The diagnosis is confirmed by recovering the organisms from lung parenchyma or pleural fluid. The material to be cultured should be collected and transported to microbiology laboratories in special anaerobic transport media. Most of the pulmonary infections are polymicrobial.

Penicillin G is the drug of choice for most isolates except *Bacteroides fragilis* and *Bacteroides melaninogenicus.* These two species are susceptible to clindamycin, chloramphenicol, and metronidazole. These three drugs are also useful for penicillin-allergic patients or those who fail to respond to penicillin.

Uncomplicated anaerobic pneumonia is usually treated for 7 to 10 days. Therapy is prolonged if empyema, lung abscess, or necrotizing pneumonia develops. A minimum of 4 weeks of antimicrobial therapy is recommended for patients with necrotizing pneumonia to prevent relapses.

Chlamydiae

Chlamydia trachomatis

Chlamydial pneumonia is confirmed when the organism is recovered from nasopharyngeal aspirates, tracheobronchial secretions, or lung parenchyma by means of tissue culture techniques. *C. trachomatis* may be recovered from the nasopharynx of infants with chlamydial conjunctivitis who do not have pneumonia. Rapid diagnosis of *C. trachomatis* infections is now possible by direct fluorescent antibody staining of nasopharyngeal secretions. Serologic diagnosis is based on the detection of IgM antibodies to *C. trachomatis* by means of the microimmunofluorescence method. A titer of 1:64 or greater is considered diagnostic.

The drug of first choice is erythromycin, but sulfisoxazole is effective as well. Limited experience suggests that ampicillin or amoxicillin may also be beneficial. Antimicrobial therapy provides significant clinical improvement within 7 days and reduces the duration of nasopharyngeal shedding of *C. trachomatis*. The total duration of therapy is 2 to 3 weeks. Respiratory isolation of these infants is recommended for the duration of their hospitalization. However, many infants are managed as outpatients, and complications are rare.

C. trachomatis can cause severe pneumonia in premature infants and recovery can be very protracted. Recent studies also suggest that chlamydial pneumonia in infancy may be associated with long-term pulmonary abnormalities.

Chlamydia psittaci

Psittacosis is rare in children. Microbiologic confirmation is difficult and requires that the organism be grown in the yolk sac of embryonated chicken eggs or in tissue cultures. *C. psittaci* can be isolated from sputum, blood, or lung tissue specimens. The diagnosis is more commonly based on a fourfold or greater rise in complement fixation antibody titers. These antibodies are usually first detected during the second week of illness. A single titer of 1:64 or greater is suggestive of a current or recent infection. Serologic data should be interpreted cautiously because the complement-fixation antibody titer may be elevated in *C. trachomatis* infections.

The drug of choice is tetracycline. This antibiotic should not be used in children younger than 8 years of age. Chloramphenicol and erythromycin have been effective in some patients, but experience with these two agents is limited.

The response to therapy is prompt in some children, with defervescence within 24 to 48 hours; others have a more protracted course. Psittacosis should be treated for 3 weeks, even in patients who improve rapidly. Shorter durations of therapy are associated with relapses. Patients should be observed carefully for extrapulmonary complications such as myocarditis, endocarditis, and liver dysfunction.

Respiratory isolation is required during the acute phase of the illness, especially in patients with severe coughing. Bed linens and other articles contaminated by secretions should be disinfected. The source of infection is most frequently a bird that may or may not appear ill. The suspected pet should be sacrificed. No intervention is necessary for individuals exposed to the same potential sources of infection, but they should be observed for signs and symptoms of psittacosis and treated early if they develop the illness.

Mycoplasma

Pneumonia caused by *Mycoplasma pneumoniae* is usually confirmed serologically and, in rare instances, by recovering the organism from sputum or throat washings. Microbiologic diagnosis requires the use of special media. Furthermore, excretion of the organism persists for a long time, and its isolation may indicate a recent rather than a current infection. A fourfold or greater rise in complement-fixation antibody titer is considered diagnostic. A single titer of 1:256 or greater is suggestive of *Mycoplasma* infection.

The drug of choice is erythromycin. For children older than 8 years of age, tetracycline is a suitable alternative. The benefits of antimicrobial therapy have not been systematically evaluated, but treatment does appear to shorten the duration of fever and cough and hasten resolution of the roentgenographic abnormalities. The total duration of therapy is 14 to 21 days. Shorter periods may be associated with relapses.

A number of complications can occur. These include myocarditis, meningoencephalitis, peripheral neuropathy, Stevens-Johnson syndrome, and cold agglutinin-induced hemolytic anemia.

Children with *Mycoplasma* pneumonia are usually managed as outpatients. Patients with sickle cell disease usually have more severe pulmonary disease when infected. Respiratory isolation is recommended for hospitalized children. No antibiotic prophylaxis is needed for contacts, but they should be cautioned about the possibility of familial spread.

Viruses

Adenovirus

The isolation of the virus from the pharynx, eyes, or feces provides a presumptive etiologic diagnosis. Demonstrating a fourfold or greater increase in antibody titers by complement fixation or enzyme-linked immunosorbent assay (ELISA) is essential for confirmation. Detection of adenovirus-specific IgM is diagnostic of acute infection.

Adenoviral pneumonia is a severe and sometimes fatal infection. Hepatitis, nephritis, encephalopathy, and other extrapulmonary complications are common. Therapy is supportive and recovery is gradual. Anecodotal reports suggest that aerosolized ribavirin may be of therapeutic benefit. Respiratory isolation is required for the duration of the illness in hospitalized children.

Long-term sequelae are common and include bronchiectasis, bronchiolitis obliterans, and unilateral hyperlucent lung.

Measles Virus

The diagnosis of measles is usually made clinically, and laboratory confirmation is seldom needed. Viral isolation from throat, blood, or urine specimens is difficult. The detection of measles-specific IgM antibodies in a single serum sample or the demonstration of a fourfold or greater rise in ELISA, hemagglutination-inhibition, or complement-fixation antibody titers is diagnostic.

Pneumonia complicates measles in 3 to 7 percent of patients and is the most common cause of death in this condition. Therapy is supportive. Secondary bacterial infection often complicates measles pneumonitis and is suspected in patients who develop respiratory deterioration or have persistent high fever. The most common secondary invaders are *Staphylococcus aureus, Streptococcus pneumoniae,* and *Haemophilus influenzae,* and these should be treated with appropriate antibiotics.

Rhinoviruses

An etiologic diagnosis can be established by isolating the virus from respiratory secretions, but this is usually difficult. Serodiagnosis is also difficult because of the large numbers of antigenic types.

No specific antiviral therapy is currently available, and management is strictly supportive. Interferon, interferon inducers, and compounds such as enviroxime have been shown to reduce the incidence of rhinovirus infections when administered prophylactically to human volunteers.

For hospitalized children, respiratory isolation for the duration of symptoms is recommended.

SUGGESTED READING

Doern GV. *Branhamella catarrhalis*—an emerging human pathogen. Diagn Microbiol Infect Dis 1986; 4:191–201.

Edelstein PH. Legionnaires disease, Pontiac fever, and related illnesses. In: RD Feigin, JD Cherry, eds. Textbook of pediatric infectious diseases, 2nd ed. Philadelphia: WB Saunders, 1987; 1163–1172.

Klein JO. Bacterial pneumonias. In: RD Feigin, JD Cherry, eds. Textbook of pediatric infectious diseases, 2nd ed. Philadelphia: WB Saunders, 1987; 329–339.

Knight V, Gilbert BE. Chemotherapy of respiratory viruses. Adv Intern Med 1986; 31:95–118.

Weiss SG, Newcomb RW, Beem MO. Pulmonary assessment of children after chlamydial pneumonia of infancy. J Pediatr 1986; 108:659–664.

DISEASES RELATED TO THE GASTROINTESTINAL TRACT

MEDIASTINITIS

THEODORE P. VOTTELER, M.D.

Mediastinitis is usually a devastating infection requiring prompt aggressive therapy to achieve a successful outcome. These infections may be caused by esophageal perforation, median sternotomy contamination, penetrating injury, retropharyngeal or dental abscess, pleural and pulmonary extension, lymphadenitis, subphrenic extensions, vertebral osteomyelitis, and hematogenous seeding from distant infection. The bacterial flora responsible should be anticipated by consideration of the underlying etiology. Therapy is directed to control the source of infection and provide appropriate antibiotics with effective drainage.

DRUG THERAPY

Antibiotic administration must be prompt, preferably by the intravenous route, and appropriate to the source of infection. Pure cultures of responsible bacteria occur, usually beta-hemolytic streptococcus, *Staphylococcus aureus,* or *S. epidermidis.* However, because of the severity of infections in the mediastinum, broad-spectrum coverage should be used initially. Anaerobic organisms should be expected in dental, retropharyngeal, and esophageal sources. Nafcillin, 150 mg per kilogram per day, given intravenously in divided doses, every 6 hours, with amikacin, 15 to 30 mg per kilogram per day in divided doses every 8 hours, are my initial choices. Anaerobic coverage, when anticipated, should be clindamycin, 40 mg per kilogram per day, given in divided doses every 6 hours, or metronidazole, 30 mg per kilogram per day given in divided doses every 8 hours. Drug therapy should be continued for a minimum of 7 to 10 days, switching drugs in response to culture results or failure of the patient to show satisfactory response within 48 hours.

SURGICAL THERAPY

Surgical drainage is mandatory when fluid collections are present. A vigorous search for abscess should be made by standard radiographs, with or without soluble contrast media, sonography, computed tomography (CT), or magnetic resonance imaging. Prompt response of signs such as fever is to be anticipated if adequate drainage and bacterial control has been established. Absence of such response indicates the need for aggressive search for loculations of pus or sources of continued mediastinal contamination.

Esophageal Perforation Mediastinitis

Minor perforations of the esophagus can be managed by administration of antibiotics alone. This approach should be taken only after water-soluble esophagograms have shown no leakage of contrast material. Mediastinitis after variceal obliteration injections by esophagoscopy is an example. Contrast studies revealing passage of dye into the mediastinum or pleural spaces after instrumentation, vomiting, swallowing of a foreign body, penetrating injury, or leakage of an esophageal suture line indicate the need for prompt thoracotomy with debridement and closure of the esophagus. Wrapping the closure site with muscle flaps and pleura increases the rates of success. Drainage by chest tube is mandatory after saline lavage of all contaminated areas. Antibiotic solutions may be used if desired for lavage. Triple antibiotic solution consisting of neomycin, 200 mg, polymyxin B, 1,000,000 U, and bacitracin, 100,000 U, mixed in 1,000 cc normal saline is appropriate. If the perforation is retropleural, preservation of an intact pleura should be the objective. Massive contamination with necrosis of the esophagus, preventing closure, requires consideration of exclusion procedures to prevent continuing mediastinal–pleural soilage by saliva or gastric juices. Daily assessment of the adequacy of mediastinal drainage is necessary. Cervical perforation may be drained by neck incision, which also prevents infection descending into the thorax. Foreign bodies, if present, should be removed. Rib segment resection to accomplish direct open drainage may be necessary in chronic infection.

Median Sternotomy Wound Mediastinitis

Mediastinitis results in 1 to 2 percent of cardiac procedures using this approach. Some infections are superficial, but most involve the anterior mediastinum, with sternal dehiscence and instability. *S. aureus* and *S. epidermidis* predominate, but gram-negative rods should be suspected. Resistant organisms may be responsible as a consequence of the intensive care environment. Anaerobic infections are rare. Successful management requires adequate debridement, drainage, and removal of foreign material if this is feasible. The sternum is left open after debridement and loculation control are accomplished and cultures are obtained. The open wound is packed loosely and soft catheters are placed to irrigate the mediastinum. Triple antibiotic solutions are used with gauze packing changes done every 12 hours, and catheter irrigations every 6 hours. Very dilute, 0.5 percent povidone–iodine may be substituted, but a more concentrated solution can result in toxic serum concentrations of iodine. After infection control and granulation formation, secondary sternal closure is attempted. Rarely, pectoral muscle flaps are required to obliterate dead space, leaving the sternum open.

Orodental Descending Mediastinitis

Suppurative mediastinal infection may be a result of extension from dental or deep cervical fascial space abscess. The majority occur within 48 hours of onset of the primary infection, but a delay of up to 3 weeks may be seen. Prompt recognition of this potentially lethal complication is necessary for survival. The usual oral flora of bacteria, including anaerobes, should be anticipated. Extension is usually to the posterior mediastinum, with pleural involvement as well as pericardium. CT scans may be required to establish mediastinal involvement. Thoracotomy is needed for adequate drainage, in addition to wide cervical fascial space exposure.

Miscellaneous Sources of Mediastinitis

Extension of infection to the mediastinum from the lung or pleural spaces should be treated by controlling the primary infection. Lung cysts, sequestrations, bronchial stricture abscesses, and foreign bodies require appropriate resections of tissue. Mediastinal lymphadenitis usually responds to drug therapy, but biopsy and drainage by either cervical or thoracic incision may be required to establish the correct pathology and bacteriology. Laparotomy is preferable to thoracotomy if a subphrenic source is suspected, e.g., liver abscess, pancreatitis, or peritonitis. Mediastinitis secondary to infected central venous catheters indicates the need to remove the catheter and administer appropriate antibiotics. Fungal infections may be present after long periods of catheter placement, but drainage of fluid collections is rarely required.

SUGGESTED READING

Brewer LA III, Carter R, Mulder GA, et al. Options in the management of perforations of the esophagus. Am J Surg 1986; 152:62–69.

Estrera AS, Landay MJ, Grisham JM, et al. Descending necrotizing mediastinitis. Surg Gynecol Obstet 1983; 157:545–552.

Glick PL, Guglielmo BJ, Tranbaugh RF, et al. Iodine toxicity in a patient treated by continuous povidone-iodine mediastinal irrigation. Ann Thorac Surg 1985; 39:478–481.

Levine TM, Wurster CF, Yosef PK. Mediastinitis occurring as a complication of odontogenic infections. Laryngoscope 1986; 96:747–750.

Saks BJ, Alan EK, Peter AD, et al. Pleural and mediastinal changes following endoscopic injection sclerotherapy of esophageal varices. Radiology 1983; 149:639–642.

Sarr MG, Vincent LG, Timothy RT. Mediastinal infection after cardiac surgery. Ann Thorac Surg 1984; 38:415–426.

Scully HE, Yves L, Raymond DM, et al. Comparison between antibiotic irrigation and mobilization of pectoral muscle flaps in treatment of deep sternal infections. J Thorac Cardiovasc Surg 1985; 90:523–531.

CHOLANGITIS AND BACTERIAL HEPATITIS

THOMAS L. KUHLS, M.D.

Bacteria in the biliary tract are able to proliferate when normal flow is obstructed. This can lead to inflammation of the bile ducts (cholangitis), with occasional extension to liver parenchyma (hepatitis). Bacterial cholangitis is most commonly observed in infants and children who have received a surgical procedure that uses an intestinal conduit for bile drainage from the liver hilum. Patients who have had a portoenterostomy (Kasai procedure) or orthotopic liver transplant fall into this category. Rarely, cholangitis resulting from other etiologies of biliary tract obstruction are observed, including gallstones in the common bile duct, tumors, cysts, parasitic infections, and previous biliary tract instrumentation.

Cholangitis should be suspected when a child develops fever, obstructive jaundice, and right upper quadrant abdominal pain. More often, patients with intestinal biliary conduits present with fever and leukocytosis. Abdominal findings are often absent or of variable intensity. Treatment strategies of cholangitis and bacterial hepatitis should include hemodynamic support if necessary, antimicrobials, attempts to relieve the biliary obstruction if possible, and measures to prevent recurrent illness following therapy.

HEMODYNAMIC SUPPORT

Pediatric patients with bacterial cholangitis occasionally develop or present in septic shock. Each infant or child should be assessed for early signs of hemodynamic instability and treated accordingly.

ANTIMICROBIAL THERAPY

Gram-negative enteric bacilli, particularly *Escherichia coli* and *Klebsiella* sp can commonly be isolated from the blood of pediatric patients with cholangitis. Other normal intestinal flora as well as *Pseudomonas* sp have been associated with this illness. The role of anaerobes in the pathogenesis of cholangitis has been debated and remains unresolved.

I start prompt empiric therapy with cefoperazone, 150 mg per kilogram per day in divided doses every 8 hours, given intravenously, and tobramycin, 6 mg per kilogram per day in divided doses every 8 hours, also given intravenously. An alternative regimen I have used is ticarcillin, 300 mg per kilogram per day administered intravenously in divided doses every 6 hours, in addition to tobramycin.

The advantage of cefoperazone over other antipseudomonal agents is its ability to achieve extremely high concentrations in the bile even in the presence of biliary obstruction. Patients with intestinal biliary conduits, however, often have evidence of chronic liver disease, poor nutritional status, and occasional varices; thus, the risk of increasing the child's bleeding time from hypoprothrombinemia associated with cefoperazone use must be assessed in each patient. Also, cefoperazone is not approved by the FDA for use in children younger than 12 years of age.

When these regimens are used, fever resolves within 5 days in more than 90 percent of patients with intestinal biliary conduits. When prolonged fever occurs, I assess the possibility of hepatic abscess formation and consider other possible sites of inflammation. If I still suspect cholangitis, I either add metronidazole (30 mg per kilogram per day, intravenously, in divided doses every 6 hours) to my empiric regimen for improved *Bacteroides fragilis* coverage or suggest a percutaneous liver biopsy with appropriate aerobic, anaerobic, and fungal cultures for a specific microbiologic diagnosis. I treat uncomplicated cholangitis with intravenous therapy for a minimum of 10 days.

METHODS TO RELIEVE BILIARY OBSTRUCTION

Surgical intervention to relieve biliary tract pressure and stasis of flow should be completed as soon as the patient is clinically stable and has received antimicrobials. Removal of intrinsic (gallstones) or extrinsic (tumors, cysts, etc.) obstructions of the biliary system is necessary, because antimicrobial therapy alone rarely causes total resolution of disease. Pediatric patients with intestinal conduits, however, have small bile ducts, chronic liver disease, and scarring at the liver hilum; thus, the biliary tract obstruction is not amenable to surgery. In these patients, recurrent cholangitis following antimicrobial therapy is common.

PREVENTION OF RECURRENCES

Since cholangitis and bacterial hepatitis are common in the first year following surgery in patients with intestinal conduits, I begin prophylactic oral therapy with trimethoprim–sulfamethoxazole (6 mg per kilogram per day of trimethoprim component) as soon following surgery as the infant or child is tolerating feeding. Prophylaxis is continued for 1 to 2 years. Trimethoprim–sulfamethoxazole is usually well tolerated, and high concentrations of antimicrobial activity are achieved in the bile. Adverse reactions, including hematologic abnormalities, are infrequent but need to be monitored.

Occasionally, recurrent cholangitis occurs shortly after the discontinuation of intravenous antimicrobials despite oral trimethoprim–sulfamethoxazole prophylaxis. Reinstitution of intravenous antimicrobials usually brings prompt resolution of symptoms, although they reappear shortly following another full course of therapy. In this situation, I pursue a definitive diagnosis by percutaneous liver biopsy. Often trimethoprim–sulfamethoxazole-resistant microorganisms are isolated. I have successfully treated such patients with prolonged intravenously administered cefoperazone and tobramycin at home. Surgical revision of the portoenterostomy anastomosis occasionally brings increased biliary flow and resolution of the recurrent bouts of cholangitis.

SUGGESTED READING

Chaudhary S, Turner RB. Trimethoprim-sulfamethoxazole for cholangitis following hepatic portoenterostomy for biliary atresia. J Pediatr 1981; 99:656–658.

Hays DM, Kimura K. Biliary atresia: new concepts of management. Curr Probl Surg 1981; 18:541–608.

Kuhls TL, Jackson MA. Diagnosis and treatment of the febrile child following hepatic portoenterostomy. Pediatr Infect Dis 1985; 4:487–490.

LIVER ABSCESS

SHELDON L. KAPLAN, M.D.

Pyogenic liver abscesses occur rarely in normal children, but children with underlying illnesses associated with altered host defense are at greater risk for developing a liver abscess. *Staphylococcus aureus* is commonly recovered from solitary liver abscesses of children with chronic granulomatous disease. Gram-negative enteric bacilli and anaerobic organisms are frequently isolated when multiple liver abscesses occur. Such cases are usually associated with underlying biliary tract disease (e.g., cholelithiasis or a complication of a portoenterostomy procedure for biliary atresia) or secondary to inflammation of a contiguous organ. Neutropenic immunosuppressed children are at risk for fungal liver abscesses.

SPECIFIC THERAPY

Antibiotics and surgical drainage are the basic treatment for hepatic abscesses in children. When it is possible, antimicrobial therapy is based on information gained from Gram stain and culture of the purulent material from the liver abscess.

A penicillinase-resistant penicillin plus an aminoglycoside or a third-generation cephalosporin is a suitable combination for initial therapy in a patient with a suspected liver abscess. Therapy may need to be changed when culture results are known. Nafcillin or methicillin is preferred when a susceptible *S. aureus* is isolated. An aminoglycoside or third-generation cephalosporin, or both in combination, is selected on the basis of in vitro susceptibility testing of gram-negative enteric isolates. Cefoperazone enters the biliary tract in very large concentrations and is particularly useful for treatment of liver abscesses associated with inflammation or infection of the biliary tree.

When anaerobic bacteria are encountered, the physician has several antibiotics from which to select, depending on the anaerobe isolated and its antimicrobial susceptibility. Penicillin is usually adequate for gram-positive anaerobic or microaerophilic streptococci. Clindamycin, metronidazole, and chloramphenicol are effective against most gram-negative anaerobes.

When multiple microorganisms are isolated, the optimal combination of antibiotics is determined by susceptibility test results.

The optimal duration of antimicrobial therapy for liver abscesses has not been established in children or adults, but most authorities recommend a minimum course of 6 weeks: 2 to 4 weeks of parenterally administered drugs followed by orally administered drugs for the remaining weeks when appropriate agents are available. Recommended dosages of antibiotics are given in Table 1. Some antibiotics require alteration of dosage in hepatic dysfunction.

Amphotericin B is the principal antifungal agent for treatment of fungal liver abscesses in children. The optimal duration of treatment and total amount of amphotericin B for therapy have not been established, and the antifungal management must be tailored for each patient. In general, amphotericin B is administered in doses of 1.0 mg per kilogram per day for 3 weeks, after which time the doses can be given every other day, depending on the clinical response and tolerance of the drug by the patient. The addition of flucytosine, 150 mg per kilogram per day, to amphotericin B might be useful. The role of other oral antifungal agents, such as ketoconazole, in the treatment of fungal liver abscesses is unknown. (See the chapter on *Aspergillosis* and the chapter on *Sporotrichosis* for treatment of specific fungal infections.)

Drainage of a solitary liver abscess is usually best accomplished by a transperitoneal abdominal exploration, although the surgical approach depends on the size and location of the abscess. A surgical approach, besides establishing adequate drainage, allows the surgeon to explore the abdominal cavity for other foci of infection. An abdominal computed tomographic (CT) scan can define the anatomic relationships between the liver abscess and contiguous structures in order to plan the optimal surgical approach. Drains are placed and advanced under the direction of the surgeon. Multiple liver abscesses usually cannot be adequately drained surgically, and prolonged medical therapy is required. In this situation, the duration of antibiotic administration can be guided by the size and number of liver abscesses on follow-up CT scans or by ultrasonography.

Percutaneous transhepatic drainage of the liver can be performed successfully in children. With this technique, a catheter is placed into the abscess cavity under CT scan guidance. The abscess cavity is irrigated with normal saline and the catheter left in place. This approach should be attempted only by experienced physicians who have adequate surgical and radiologic backup, in case immediate surgery is required. This approach is an alternative to surgical drainage of liver abscesses in the child who is a poor operative risk. Complications of either surgical or percutaneous drainage include peritoneal spillage, hemorrhage, and inadvertent spread of infection to other organs or the development of septicemia. Percutaneous drainage should not be considered if there is another indication for surgery, if there are more than two liver abscesses, and if the location of the abscesses precludes a safe performance of the procedure. Possible complications of pyogenic liver abscesses include pleural pulmonary involvement, peritonitis, suphrenic or subhepatic abscess and hemobilia.

"

TABLE 1 Antimicrobial Agents for the Treatment of Liver Abscesses in Children

Organism	Antibiotic	Dosage (mg/kg/day)	Frequency	Route
Staphylococcus aureus	Nafcillin or methicillin	150–200	q4h or q6h	IV
	Dicloxacillin	75–100	q6h	PO
Gram-negative enteric bacilli	Aminoglycoside	standard dosages		IV
	Cefotaxime	150	q6h–q8h	IV
	Cefoperazone*	150	q8h	IV
Anaerobes	Clindamycin*	40	q6h	IV
		30	q8h	PO
	Penicillin	150,000 units	q4h–q6h	IV
	Metronidazole	15 mg/kg loading then 30 mg/kg/day	q6h	IV or PO
	Chloramphenicol*	50–75	q6h	IV or PO
Candida	Amphotericin B	1.0	q24h	IV

* Requires dosage modification in severe hepatic dysfunction.

SUGGESTED READING

Bartley DL, Hughes WT, Pawey LS, Parham D. Computed tomography of hepatic and splenic fungal abscesses in leukemic children. Pediatr Infect Dis 1982; 1:317–321.

Chusid MJ. Pyogenic hepatic abscess in infancy and childhood. Pediatrics 1978; 62:554–559.

Diament MJ, Stanley P, Kangarlos H, Donaldson JJ. Percutaneous aspiration and catheter drainage of abscesses. J Pediatr 1986; 108:204–208.

Kaplan SL. Pyogenic liver abscess. In: Feigin RD, Cherry JD, eds. Textbook of pediatric infectious diseases. 2nd ed. Philadelphia: WB Saunders, 1987.

Lebel MH. Pharmacology of antimicrobial agents in children with hepatic dysfunction. Pediatr Infect Dis 1986; 5:686–690.

INTRA-ABDOMINAL SEPSIS

JANE D. SIEGEL, M.D.

Intra-abdominal sepsis is encountered less frequently by the pediatrician than by the internist and the surgeon. However, when it does occur, it is usually associated with substantial morbidity. The most common preceding events are appendicitis, necrotizing enterocolitis, biliary tract disease, amebic colitis, pseudomembranous colitis associated with *Clostridium difficile,* trauma, and, in the compromised host, typhlitis. The usual course of events is perforation of intra-abdominal viscera, spillage of fecal material within the peritoneal cavity, and the development of acute peritonitis. Bacteria readily pass through small intercellular openings in the mesothelium of the inferior diaphragmatic surface and enter the lymphatic and vascular systems, causing sepsis and bacteremia. Localized intra-abdominal abscess, liver abscess, pleural empyema, and, in rare instances, brain abscess and endocarditis occur as late complications. Treatment with appropriate antibiotics combined with surgical debridement of necrotic tissue and drainage of localized abscesses has been life-saving.

The etiology of intra-abdominal sepsis is usually polymicrobial. The synergistic effect of aerobic gram-negative rods, including *Pseudomonas* species in as many as 20 to 30 percent of patients, combined with anaerobes produces the characteristic clinical picture. *Bacteroides* species, especially *Bacteroides fragilis,* are frequently beta-lactamase producers and are resistant to most of the routinely used beta-lactam drugs. Although it has been popularly believed that antimicrobial treatment directed against aerobic gram-negative rods are sufficient to achieve clinical cure, studies in both animals and humans, including children, have demonstrated a lower incidence of infectious complications when specific antimicrobial agents with activity against beta-lactamase-producing *Bacteroides* species are used. The role of the enterococcus in the pathogenesis of intra-abdominal sepsis has not been clearly defined. Specific antibiotic coverage for the enterococcus does not appear to be necessary in the early phases. *Entamoeba histolytica* and *Clostridium difficile* should be considered when the etiology of an intestinal perforation is not apparent, because routinely used antibiotic regimens are not active against those pathogens.

The diagnosis of intra-abdominal sepsis is based on such clinical findings as anorexia, nausea, vomiting, fever, and abdominal tenderness, supported by an elevated white blood cell count (WBC) with a left shift. Acute urinary retention is an unusual presentation of appendiceal abscess in children. Endotoxic shock with hypotension and disseminated intravascular coagulation (DIC) may be seen in the most severely affected patients. Urinalysis, Gram stain, and culture of urine are useful because patients with pyelonephritis may present with the physical findings of an acute abdomen. Diagnoses of amebiasis and of *C. difficile* colitis are discussed in the chapters on *Specific Diarrheal Diseases* and *Antibiotic-Associated Diarrheal Syndrome,* respectively. Localized abscesses, especially subphrenic and pelvic, must be identified because surgical drainage is usually required. Ultrasonography, computerized tomography (CT), magnetic resonance imaging (MRI), and radionuclide scintigraphy using gallium citrate or indium III-labeled leukocytes have been used for the diagnosis of intra-abdominal abscess. Of these techniques, the most accurate method is the CT scan, with sensitivity and specificity of 95 to 98 percent. The CT scan is especially useful in the postoperative patient when other techniques yield results that are often difficult to interpret. MRI has been useful for identification of abscesses located within an organ (i.e., liver, spleen). This technique has been disappointing for localizing abscesses within the abdominal cavity, however, because of the inability to distinguish abscess from loops of bowel. Gallium and indium-labeled leukocyte studies have proved to be too nonspecific. I recommend that a Gram stain be obtained as well as culture for aerobes and anaerobes of infected peritoneal fluid and of purulent material obtained from localized abscesses. The information obtained may prove to be especially useful in the case of the patient who does not respond to the initial surgical procedure and antibiotic therapy.

TREATMENT

Successful treatment consists of surgical repair of the underlying condition and resection of necrotic bowel with drainage of localized abscess when it is present. If an abscess is readily accessible, percutaneous needle aspiration and catheter drainage under radiographic guidance may be successful in 85 to 90 percent of selected patients. (See the chapter on *Surgical Infections.*)

The choice of antibiotics for intra-abdominal sepsis has varied considerably. It is now clear that optimal antibiotic combinations used for treatment of intra-abdominal sepsis following intestinal perforation must include activity against the beta-lactamase-producing strains of *B. fragilis* and aerobic gram-negative rods including *P. aeruginosa.* Dosage regimens of the commonly used drugs are presented in Table 1. My preference for the treatment of early intra-abdominal sepsis in a patient who has not previously received a course of antibiotics is clindamycin and an aminoglycoside. The choice of aminoglycoside is determined primarily by the antibiotic susceptibility pattern in each institution and, secondarily, by cost. Gentamicin or tobramycin is appropriate in most settings. Amikacin is preferred for patients who have had prior prolonged hospitalizations and are likely to have become colonized with resistant aerobic enteric gram-negative rods. Addition of ampicillin to the clindamycin–aminoglycoside regimen is suggested for coverage of the enterococcus in patients who have previously received prolonged courses of

TABLE 1   Antimicrobial Agents Frequently Used for Treatment of Intra-abdominal Sepsis

Drug	Dosage (mg/kg/day)	Comments
Clindamycin*	30, div q8h	Resistant *Bacteroides* species in some areas of the country
Metronidazole*	30, div q6h	Excellent activity against anaerobes; inactive against aerobes
Cefoxitin	160, div q6h	Poor activity against *Clostridial* species
Chloramphenicol*	75, div q6h	Inactivated by anaerobic bacteria; bacteriostatic against aerobic gram-negative rods
Ceftazidime	150, div q8h	Variable activity against anaerobes; very active against aerobic gram-negative rods; little experience
Moxalactam	150, div q8h	Associated bleeding tendency makes this drug less desirable in surgical patients; variable activity against anaerobes; inactive against *Pseudomonas* species
Cefotaxime	150, div q6h	Variable activity against anaerobes; inactive against *Pseudomonas* species
Ceftriaxone	50–75, div q12h	Variable activity against anaerobes; inactive against *Pseudomonas* species; little experience
Ampicillin	100, div q6h	Active against enterococcus
Ticarcillin	200–300, div q6h	Adequate activity against enterococcus when combined with an aminoglycoside; variable activity against anaerobes
Mezlocillin	200–300, div q4h–q6h	Active against enterococcus; variable activity against anaerobes
Gentamicin	5–7.5, div q8h	Reduced activity at acid pH and in anaerobic environment of abscesses and deep tissue infections
Tobramycin	5–7.5, div q8h	
Amikacin	22.5, div q8h	

* Oral route may be considered when gastrointestinal function is normal.

antibiotics. Compatibility and stability of the admixture of clindamycin with gentamicin or tobramycin have been demonstrated, a fact that considerably simplifies administration of these drugs.

Alternative regimens warrant discussion. Metronidazole is preferred over clindamycin in combination with an aminoglycoside for treatment of clindamycin-resistant strains of *B. fragilis* or very extensive persistant infection associated with *B. fragilis*. Ceftazidime, a third-generation cephalosporin that is active against *Pseudomonas* species and multiply resistant aerobic gram-negative rods, is a suitable alternative to an aminoglycoside, especially in patients with renal dysfunction. Ceftazidime should be combined with either clindamycin or metronidazole because of its poor activity against *Bacteroides* species as well as many other anaerobes. Like other third-generation cephalosporins, ceftazidime is more effective than aminoglycosides in the treatment of deep tissue infection or an abscess, because of its relatively increased activity under anaerobic conditions and at an acidic pH. For the reasons listed in Table 1, I do not recommend the routine use of other drugs previously considered. Two antimicrobial agents not yet approved for use in children younger than 12 years of age, aztreonam and imipenem–cilastatin, have exhibited efficacy equivalent to the standard clindamycin-aminoglycoside combination in clinical trials in adults. Aztreonam is a monobactam antibiotic that is active against aerobic gram-negative bacilli only and must therefore be combined with clindamycin. Imipenem–cilastatin is a unique broad spectrum beta-lactam antibiotic that is active against nearly all anaerobes, aerobic gram-positive and aerobic gram-negative microorganisms and can therefore be used as a single-drug regimen. These agents may prove to be particularly useful for treatment of infections associated with multiply-resistant pathogens.

The choice of an appropriate combination of antimicrobial agents for neonates is more difficult. Metabolism of clindamycin by the neonate is highly variable, and there are no high-pressure liquid chromatography (HPLC) methods available for rapid and easy measurement of serum clindamycin concentrations. Metabolism of metronidazole by the liver as well as potential mutagenicity of this drug make it undesirable as a first-line drug in neonates. Therefore, clindamycin in combination with an aminoglycoside is recommended only if there is definite evidence for serious anaerobic infection, e.g., gross fecal contamination of the peritoneal cavity, putrid peritoneal fluid, or abscess contents with Gram stain evidence of *Bacteroides* or *Clostridial* species. For most other cases, I still prefer to use either ticarcillin or mezlocillin in combination with an aminoglycoside. The dosages of the commonly used drugs for neonates are presented in Table 2.

Duration of therapy is variable and is determined by the extent of infection, adequacy of drain-

TABLE 2 Neonatal Dosages for Antimicrobial Agents Frequently Used for Treatment of Intra-abdominal Sepsis

	Dosage (mg/kg/day) and intervals of dosages	
Drug	*0–7 Days of age*	*7–30 Days of age*
Clindamycin*		
Term	15, div q8h	20, div q6h
Preterm	15, div q8h	15, div q8h
Metronidazole* (15 initial dose)		
Term (after 24 h)	15, div q12h	30, div q12h
Preterm (after 48 h)	15, div q12h	15, div q12h
Ampicillin		
Term	75, div q8h	100, div q6h
Preterm	50, div q12h	75, div q8h
Ticarcillin		
Term	225, div q8h	300, div q6h
Preterm	150, div q12h	225, div q8h
Mezlocillin	150, div q12h	225, div q8h
Cefotaxime	100, div q12h	150, div q8h
Ceftazidime	100, div q12h	150, div q8h
Gentamicin	5, div q12h	7.5, div q8h
Tobramycin	5, div q12h	7.5, div q8h
Amikacin		
Term	20, div q12h	30, div q8h
Preterm	15, div q12h	30, div q8h

* Optimal dose not clearly established.

age, and promptness of clinical response. A 7- to 10-day course of broad-spectrum antibiotics is recommended for uncomplicated peritonitis following intestinal perforation. Prolonged courses of antimicrobial therapy are occasionally required for the patient with multiple abscess formation. Antimicrobial susceptibilities should be reviewed to determine the appropriateness of the chosen drug regimen. However, anaerobic susceptibilities are not routinely determined in most clinical microbiology laboratories. Requests for such testing should be made in cases of clinical failure. If the testing is unavailable and if adequate surgical drainage has been performed, resistance of *Bacteroides* species to clindamycin should be assumed. The oral route of administration may be considered for clindamycin and metronidazole if prolonged therapy is required and the gastrointestinal tract is functioning reliably. All other drugs should be administered intravenously.

Occasionally, patients with intra-abdominal sepsis are slow to respond or develop secondary fevers. The most common infectious complications to look for in such patients are wound infection, thrombophlebitis, and development of subphrenic or pelvic abscess. A late complication sometimes seen after discharge is intestinal obstruction secondary to development of adhesions.

SUGGESTED READING

Bartlett JG. Recent developments in the management of anaerobic infection. Rev Infect Dis 1983; 5:235–245.
Bell MJ, Shackleford P, Smith R, Schroeder K. Pharmacokinetics of clindamycin phosphate in the first year of life. J Pediatr 1984; 105:482–486.

Dobrin PB, Gully PH, Greenlee HB, et al. Radiologic diagnosis of an intra-abdominal abscess. Arch Surg 1986; 121:41–46.
King DR, Browne AF, Birken GA, et al. Antibiotic management of complicated appendicitis. J Pediatr Surg 1983; 18:945–950.
Weinstein WM, Onderdok AB, Bartlett JG, et al. Antimicrobial therapy of experimental intraabdominal sepsis. J Infect Dis 1975; 132:282–286.

VIRAL HEPATITIS

WILLIAM BORKOWSKY, M.D.

Acute hepatitis can occur or be mimicked in a variety of infectious diseases (e.g., cytomegalovirus, Epstein-Barr virus, toxoplasmosis, rubella, Q fever, secondary syphilis, salmonellosis, amebic liver abscess, and malaria) in which the liver is not the primary target of infection. This discussion emphasizes primary liver disease caused by hepatitis A virus (HAV), hepatitis B virus (HBV), the delta agent or hepatitis D virus (HDV), and non A, non B hepatitis viruses (NANB agents). The prophylaxis or treatment of hepatitis depends in great part on the identity of the viral etiology.

Shown in Table 1 are initial and confirmatory serologic results that can help one in reaching an appropriate diagnosis. Serum from all patients with hepatitis should be tested initially for the presence of hepatitis B surface antigen (HBsAg), antibody to HBsAg, and antibody to HAV. The results obtained may be diagnostic or may suggest the need for additional testing for antibody to the hepatitis B core antigen (anti-HBc). The differential presence of immunoglobulin G (IgG) or IgM anti-HBc may allow further recognition of the duration of HBV infection. When the etiology of the hepatitis has been determined, appropriate prophylactic and therapeutic strategies can be instituted. However, the treatment of acute infection, regardless of cause, is largely supportive; this is summarized in Table 2. Additional interventions are discussed for each specific virus.

HEPATITIS A VIRUS (HAV)

This virus, classified as enterovirus type 72, accounts for 20 to 40 percent of the cases of sporadic hepatitis in the United States. It can be detected in the liver, bile, blood, and stools within 2 weeks of exposure to the virus. Clinical symptoms appear about 4 weeks (range, 15 to 40 days) after exposure, and the presence of virus (i.e., infectivity) usually diminishes rapidly after jaundice appears. Transmission of HAV by blood transfusion is rare. No chronic carrier state has been seen.

Numerous studies have documented the efficacy of immunoglobulin (Ig) therapy given before exposure or during the early part of the incubation period.

Preexposure Prophylaxis

Because more than half of American adults are HAV antibody negative and presumably at risk for infection, preexposure prophylaxis is recommended for international travelers to areas where hepatitis is endemic. A single dose of Ig (0.02 ml per kilogram of body weight) is adequate for travel terminating within 2 months. A larger dosage of Ig (0.06 ml per kilogram every 4 to 6 months) is suggested for prolonged travel. Avoidance of potentially contaminated foods (i.e., uncooked shellfish or fruits and unprepared vegetables) and water is suggested.

Postexposure Prophylaxis

Prophylaxis with Ig is recommended when potential contact with infectious material is less than 2 weeks or when prolonged contact is anticipated. These situations include all household and sexual contacts of HAV-infected individuals. In situations in which group activity may spread the virus (i.e., in day care centers, where members and staff are involved in diapering, in institutions for custodial care, etc.), postexposure prophylaxis may reduce the potential for an epidemic. The occurrence of a case of hepatitis in elementary and secondary schools, hospitals, offices, and factories is usually not followed by an outbreak. However, Ig prophylaxis may be indicated because of special epidemiologic circumstances. For postexposure Ig prophylaxis, a single intramuscular dose of 0.02 ml per kilogram is recommended. The development of safe and effective hepatitis A vaccines will change prophylactic strategies in the future from passive to a combination of passive and active immunization.

HEPATITIS B VIRUS (HBV)

This virus belongs in the hepadna class of viruses. These agents have produced acute and chronic hepatitis in humans, primates, squirrels, woodchucks, and ducks. HBV infection has an incubation period of 45 to 120 days after exposure. This range is related to (1) inoculum size, (2) route of infection, (3)

TABLE 1　Acute Hepatitis Infection: Interpretation of Serologic Results*

Initial serologic results

HBsAg	Anti-HBs	Anti-HAV	Possible Diagnosis	Confirmatory Tests and Probable Final Diagnosis
+	−	−	Acute hepatitis B or Chronic HBV carrier or Simultaneous hepatitis D	Anti-HBc 　Negative = early acute hepatitis (before onset of symptoms) 　Positive = either acute or chronic hepatitis B Anti-HBc IgM 　Negative = chronic hepatitis B 　Positive = acute hepatitis B Anti-HD antibody
−	+	−	Acute hepatitis B or Past hepatitis B	Anti-HBc 　Negative = past hepatitis B infection + possible non-A, non-B hepatitis 　Positive = acute or past hepatitis B infection or non-A, non-B hepatitis Anti-HBc IgM 　Negative = past hepatitis B infection + possible non-A, non-B hepatitis 　Positive = late acute hepatitis B
−	−	+	Acute hepatitis A or Past hepatitis A or Non-A, non-B hepatitis	Anti-HAV IgM 　Negative = possible non-A, non-B hepatitis and past hepatitis A 　Positive = acute hepatitis A
−	+	+	Acute or past hepatitis A and/or Acute or past hepatitis B and/or Non-A, non-B hepatitis	Anti-HAV IgM 　Negative = past hepatitis A 　Positive = acute hepatitis A Anti-HBc IgM 　Negative = past hepatitis B infection 　Positive = acute hepatitis B infection
+	−	+	Acute hepatitis A or Acute or chronic hepatitis B or Simultaneous hepatitis D	Anti-HAV 　Negative = past hepatitis A infection 　Positive = acute hepatitis A Anti-HBc IgM 　Negative = chronic hepatitis B or non-A, non-B hepatitis 　Positive = acute hepatitis B Anti-HD antibody
−	−	−	Non-A, non-B hepatitis	Exclusion of other etiologies

* Key: anti-HAV—hepatitis A antibody; anti-HAV IgM—IgM-specific anti-HAV; HBsAg—hepatitis B surface antigen; anti-HBs—hepatitis B surface antibody; HBcAg—hepatitis B core antigen; anti-HBc—hepatitis B core antibody; anti-HBc IgM—IgM-specific anti-HBc; anti-HD—hepatitis delta antibody.

possible inactivation of some virus particles by physicochemical means, and (4) specific viral host interactions.

Persons infected with the virus may have asymptomatic disease, symptomatic self-limited disease, or fulminant disease. About 1 percent of icteric hospitalized individuals develop fulminant disease. Recuperating individuals may continue to have chronic disease with or without an inflammatory component to the disease. Chronic HBV infection may progress to cirrhosis and primary hepatoma.

The management of acute HBV hepatitis is supportive care (see Table 2). Early treatment with steroids may predispose to persistent infection. The administration of hepatitis B immune globulin (HBIG) is of no benefit once the infection is symptomatic.

HBV immune complexes have been associated with other extrahepatic manifestations of hepatitis. These include (1) a transient serum-sickness-like syndrome with fever, polyarthritis, and a rash preceding the onset of jaundice by days or weeks and (2) chronic membranous glomerulonephritis and nephrosis. Only simple supportive measures are indicated, because these manifestations resolve spontaneously. A papulovesicular peripherally located skin rash has been associated with HBV infection in children (Gianotti-Crosti syndrome). The rash is erythematous and nonpruritic. It appears on the face, buttocks, and extremities, and is accompanied by lymphadenopathy, and anicteric hepatitis lasting 2 months. The rash lasts for 2 to 3 weeks and resolves spontaneously. Although the disease (limited to HBV of the ayw subtype) is prevalent in Italy and Japan, it is rarely associated with HBV in North America, where the ayw subtype is uncommon. When it does appear, the syndrome may represent a late exanthematous response to multiple viral or bacterial antigens, with the eruption appearing at the time of the resolution of the infection.

Postexposure Prophylaxis

HBV is transmitted most commonly by (1) percutaneous route through contaminated blood, blood products, or instruments; (2) sexual intimacy; and (3)

**TABLE 2 Supportive Treatment of Acute
and Fulminant Hepatitis**

	Treatment
Acute hepatitis	Bed rest
	Nutrition—adequate calories, high fat, adequate protein (1 g/kg)
	Hydration—IV if necessary
	Antiemetics
	Vitamin K—10 mg IM if prothrombin time is prolonged
Fulminant hepatitis	ICU supportive care for renal failure
	Reduce hyperammonemia—enemas, lactulose PO; limit protein
	Nutrition and hydration—10% IV glucose; check for hypoglycemia
	Correct clotting abnormalities—fresh frozen plasma
	Control seizures—diazepam (Valium)
	Controversial therapies to remove toxin may cause complications (i.e., exchange transfusion, extracorporeal liver perfusion plasmapheresis and exchange, cross-circulation in humans and other primates)

perinatal transmission from an HBsAg positive mother to her infant.

The frequency of HBV infection following a needle-stick exposure is less than 10 to 20 percent when the HBV source is HBeAg positive (indicating the presence of extremely large numbers of HBV particles in the plasma), and considerably less when the source is HBeAg negative.

Although sexual transmission is less efficient than percutaneous means, the frequency of exposure may result in a 25 to 40 percent acquisition rate of HBV infection among sexual contacts of infected individuals.

In the Far East and certain developing countries, perinatal exposure is the primary mode of HBV transmission. Transplacental infection is rare; and infection usually occurs at birth. The transmission rate in children born to mothers who are HBeAg positive exceeds 80 percent; it is about 10 to 15 percent in those born to HBsAg-positive/HBeAg-negative mothers. Acute infection in the infant is usually asymptomatic, but it is followed by a high incidence of chronic disease. Therefore, all pregnant women at high risk for being an HBV carrier should be screened for HBsAg.

Infants born to HBsAg-positive mothers should receive a combination of (1) HBIG, 0.5 ml administered intramuscularly, within the first hours of life and (2) hepatitis B vaccine, 0.5 ml (10 μg of the plasma-derived vaccine or 5 μg of the yeast recombinant DNA–derived vaccine) administered intramuscularly, in the first week of life and repeated at 1 and 6 months of age. The HBIG and vaccine must be injected at separate sites. Blood should be tested at 6 and 15 months for HBsAg and anti-HBsAg. The presence of antibody at 15 months indicates successful protection.

Although breast milk from an HBV carrier may contain HBV, its role in infecting infants is unknown. Infants treated with HBIG and HBV vaccine may be breast fed.

HBIG (0.06 ml per kilogram) has also been shown to interrupt transmission of HBV that might result from a needle stick, swallowing of virus-infected blood or secretions, or sexual contact. The HBIG should be given as soon as possible after exposure and repeated at 1 month in the case of the percutaneous or mucosal exposure. The HBIG should be given within 2 weeks of a sexual exposure to a chronic carrier, although it may be efficacious as late as 30 days after exposure. A second dose can be given 3 months later if the sexual contact remains HBsAg positive. If the chronic infection persists beyond 6 months, hepatitis B vaccine should be given to obviate repeated HBIG injections.

Active Immunoprophylaxis

Individuals at increased risk for HBV infection should receive HBV vaccine. Potential candidates are listed in Table 3. HBV vaccine is available in both plasma-derivative and recombinant DNA–derived forms. Both are equally safe. The dosage of vaccine for children less than 10 years of age is 0.5 ml given intramuscularly three times at 0-, 1-, and 6-month intervals. The dosage for older children, adolescents, and adults is 1 ml, given at the same intervals.

Experimental Therapies

Various antiviral agents and immunologic modifiers have been used to treat chronic active hepatitis. Steroid therapy by itself appears to worsen the disease. However, prednisolone pulses followed by antiviral therapy with adenine arabinoside therapy for 4 weeks appear to accelerate the progression from an HBeAg-positive to an HBeAg-negative state. The spontaneous rate of this occurrence is 5 to 15 percent per year. Alpha- and beta-interferon therapy, alone or in combination with adenine arabinoside or acyclovir, also appears to be of some benefit in suppressing viral replication.

**TABLE 3 High-Risk Individuals Who Represent
Potential Candidates for Hepatitis B Vaccine**

Health care professionals exposed to blood and blood products
Residents and staff of institutions for the developmentally handicapped
Hemodialysis patients
Homosexually active males
Users of illicit injectable drugs
High-risk populations (e.g., Alaskan Eskimos, immigrants from HBV endemic areas such as Southeast Asia, Haiti, and sub-Saharan Africa)
Household and sexual contacts of HBV carriers
Postexposure victims (i.e., through needle sticks, sexual contact, and newborns of carrier mothers)
Recipients of multiple transfusions (e.g., thalassemics, sickle cell homozygotes, and hemophiliacs)

HEPATITIS D VIRUS (HDV)— THE DELTA AGENT

HDV was originally described in 1977 and is now recognized as a defective RNA virus that exists as a hybrid composed of an HDV core encapsidated by an HBsAg coat. The RNA may be related to plant virioids. The virus can infect only HBsAg-positive individuals and appears to compete with HBV DNA for the HBsAg coat. HDV hepatitis may exist (1) simultaneously with acute HBV, (2) as an acute infection superimposed on chronic HBV, and (3) as a chronic infection superimposed on chronic HBV hepatitis. Most persons infected with HDV have evidence of liver damage. In fact, the coinfection of HDV and HBV is more often associated with fulminant hepatitis than is HBV alone.

Serologic diagnosis is made by radioimmune assay. However, diagnosis of acute infection is often difficult because the anti-HDV titers are short-lived. Chronic hepatitis D can be diagnosed by the presence of either IgM or IgG anti-HDV antibody. Epidemiologic studies in the United States have found HDV in 24 percent of HBsAg-positive Los Angeles drug addicts and in 50 percent of HBsAg-positive hemophiliacs. Although perinatal transmission of HDV from HBeAg-positive mothers has been seen, it is an infrequent event.

The best prevention of hepatitis D is immunization of susceptible persons with hepatitis B vaccine.

NON A, NON B (NANB) HEPATITIS

NANB hepatitis was first recognized in 1974 and, since the introduction of HBV screening of blood products, has been responsible for 80 to 90 percent of posttransfusion hepatitis and 25 to 50 percent of spontaneous hepatitis. This form of hepatitis is transmitted both parenterally and nonparenterally. Implicated blood product vectors include cells, plasma, factor VIII and factor IX concentrates, and even intravenous Ig. The most common incubation period ranges from 40 to 100 days, but periods as short as 2 weeks and as long as 6 months have been reported. Individuals with NANB hepatitis may have a monophasic rise in serum alanine aminotransferase (ALT) levels, a plateaulike response, or a biphasic pattern (seen in 25 percent of cases). Jaundice occurs infrequently (i.e., in 20 percent of those infected), but chronicity is common, with 40 percent of infected individuals maintaining elevated ALT levels for several years. Half of hemophiliacs receiving substantial factor VIII or factor IX concentrates have increased ALT levels for longer than 6 months, in the absence of HBV infection.

The etiologic agents of NANB hepatitis have not been identified. Blood and blood products may induce two episodes of NANB hepatitis in chimpanzees. This suggests the presence of at least two different NANB agents in human plasma. Diagnosis of NANB infection is made by exclusion of other potential causes of hepatitis. Most blood bank facilities are now employing two surrogate tests for the prevention of NANB posttransfusion hepatitis: serum ALT and anti-HBc. These nonspecific tests may identify donors who are carriers of NANB hepatitis viruses. In one study, the attack rate in recipients of blood that had an ALT level of greater than 45 IU was five times as great as those who received blood with lower ALT levels.

Standard Ig (0.06 ml per kilogram) has been recommended by some authorities for postneedle-stick prophylaxis, but there is no evidence for its efficacy.

Although there is currently no effective therapy for NANB chronic hepatitis, a recent report suggests that prolonged therapy with recombinant alpha-interferon may be effective in controlling activity of the disease in some patients. Steroid therapy has been tried and is of no benefit.

SUGGESTED READING

Dienstag JL. Non A, non B hepatitis. Part 1. Recognition, epidemiology and clinical features. Gastroenterology 1983; 85:439–462.

Dienstag JL. Non A, non B hepatitis. Part 2. Experimental transmission, putative virus agents and markers, and prevention. Gastroenterology 1983; 85:743–768.

Friedman LS, Dienstag JL. Recent developments in viral hepatitis. DM1986; 32:314–385.

Krugman S. Viral hepatitis: 1985 update. Pediatr Rev 1985; 7:3–11.

Seeff LB, Hoofnagle JH. Immunoprophylaxis of viral hepatitis. Gastroenterology 1979; 77:161–182.

ACUTE DIARRHEAL DISEASE OF UNKNOWN ETIOLOGY

JOSEPH F. FITZGERALD, M.D.

When one considers that the gastrointestinal mucosa is a two-way barrier between body fluids and the outside world, the fragile balance between absorption and secretion can be better appreciated. Any process that disturbs this delicate balance leads to diarrhea. Approximately 9 L of fluid enter the adult gastrointestinal tract each day; two are consumed in the diet and seven result from gastrointestinal secretions. All but 100 to 200 ml are absorbed.

Most episodes of acute-onset diarrhea in infants and children have an infectious etiology. The diarrheal illness is typically accompanied by other signs and symptoms of infection, such as fever, vomiting, rash, and, perhaps, headache and myalgia in the older child. Other family members are often similarly affected. Occasionally, parents relate the onset of diarrhea to the introduction of a food or the administration of a medication, most commonly an antibiotic.

I am often as surprised as the parent(s) when I find an abundance of rock-hard stool in the rectal vault of an infant or child with fecal "overflow." In general, the history of recurrent diarrhea with intervening periods of decreased stool frequency should suggest that constipation, not diarrhea, is the problem.

I often provide consultation on well-hydrated infants with persistent diarrhea, thought to be infectious at the outset, who are continuing to pass diarrheal stools. These infants are receiving excessive amounts of "clear liquids," which are undoubtedly contributing to their persistent diarrhea. The reinstitution of an age-appropriate diet is curative.

True diarrhea results from impaired fluid absorption or excessive secretion. Secretory diarrhea is characteristically high-volume (greater than 10 ml per kilogram per hour), high in fecal sodium (greater than 85 mEq per liter), and unaffected by bowel rest.

EVALUATION

Physical examination includes determination of the blood pressure, heart rate, respiratory rate, temperature, length, weight, and head circumference. The growth measurements, including weight/length ratio, must be plotted on an anthropometric chart. Examination also includes an assessment of the hydration status, and careful abdominal and anorectal examinations.

A fluid deficit of 5 percent (weight [kg] $\times$ 0.05 = deficit [ml]) is suggested by dry mucous membranes. A deficit of 7 percent is accompanied by very dry mucous membranes, sunken eyes, and a depressed fontanel. These findings plus a loss of skin turgor (evidenced by a capillary filling time greater than 2 seconds), a weak rapid pulse, and cold extremities indicate a deficit of 10 percent or greater.

Abdominal examination may detect distention, asymmetry, a fluid wave, organ enlargement, or a mass. Anorectal examination rules out obstruction and impaction and provides a ready stool sample that can be tested for the presence of blood.

Microscopic examination of a fresh stool for fecal leukocytes is very helpful. Abundant polymorphonuclear leukocytes are found in the stool of the infant with a bacterial enteritis or enterocolitis; fewer than 5 per high-power field (HPF) suggests a nonbacterial etiology. I obtain a complete blood count (CBC) and determine the serum electrolyte, urea nitrogen, and creatinine values of patients whose estimated fluid deficit is 5 percent or greater. The urea nitrogen/creatinine ratio (normal is less than 25) can be calculated and the urine specific gravity measured to further assess the hydration deficit. If the patient is malnourished, manifested by a weight/length ratio

below the fifth percentile after correction for the calculated fluid deficit, the carotene, albumin, transferrin, prealbumin, and retinol binding protein blood concentrations should be measured. Fecal electrolytes should be determined in patients with *persistent* high-volume diarrhea, as discussed earlier.

MANAGEMENT

Severely dehydrated infants (greater than 7 percent fluid loss) should be hospitalized and their deficits corrected with parenteral fluid therapy. There is little doubt, however, that infants with fluid deficits of 7 percent or less can be corrected by the oral route with careful monitoring. The Committee on Nutrition of the American Academy of Pediatrics recognizes three stages in the management of the dehydrated infant: rehydration stage, maintenance fluid stage, and early refeeding stage. The recommended therapeutic volume for the rehydration stage is the estimated deficit (see preceding). This volume is provided over 4 hours. The oral rehydration solution (ORS) should contain 60 to 90 mEq per liter of sodium and 100 to 120 mMol per liter (2 percent) of glucose. I prescribe Rehydralyte (Ross), formerly Pedialyte RS, because of its convenience (dispensed in 8-oz bottles) and availability.

Even severe dehydration in infants can be corrected with an ORS after the signs of shock have been alleviated with the infusion of intravenous fluid, e.g., Ringer's lactate at a rate of 40 ml per kilogram per hour. The ORS can be administered by mouth or continuously through a nasogastric tube. Vomiting is *not* a contraindication for oral rehydration therapy. More than 90 percent of infants tolerate ORS if it is given slowly. A decrease in stool volume is usually noted during the rehydration stage.

The maintenance stage follows the 4-hour rehydration stage. The administration of sodium must be reduced during this stage because of high insensible water losses in infancy. This is most readily accomplished by alternating the ORS with breast milk or water, or by substituting an oral solution containing 45 to 50 mEq per liter of sodium, e.g., Resol (Wyeth), Pedialyte (Ross), Lytren (Mead-Johnson), or Infalyte (Penwalt), in a volume of 150 ml per kilogram every 24 hours. There is a growing body of opinion that human milk or a lactose-free formula can be offered immediately after the rehydration stage, as long as ongoing stool losses are replaced milliliter for milliliter with the ORS. Common sense dictates that the milk/formula be discontinued if the stool volume increases after it is restarted.

Infants with a deficit less than 5 percent can be managed with a solution containing 45 to 50 mEq per liter of sodium (see earlier) in a volume of 150 ml per kilogram every 24 hours. Some would alternate this solution with human milk or lactose-free formula, limiting the total fluid volume to 150 ml per kilogram every 24 hours. I question the need to substitute a lactose-free formula in the management of these mildly affected infants.

There is now general agreement that early refeeding is desirable. I consider the duration of diarrhea and the infant's response to my initial management strategy in the planning of the refeeding stage. For example, an infant with acute-onset diarrhea of 6 to 12 hours' duration before the rehydration stage, and who passes one to two stools during the maintenance stage, can be advanced to his or her usual diet after 24 hours. On the other hand, an infant with a 2- to 3-day history of diarrhea and a fluid deficit greater than 7 percent when initially seen should not be advanced as rapidly. Dietary increases should be made over a period of 2 to 3 days in this patient. Neither prolonged nor repeated protein-calorie deprivation can be permitted. Parenteral nutrition should be initiated if optimal nutrition is not attained in 5 days.

The older infant and child, who was accepting a mixed diet previously, can be offered familiar solids before undiluted milk or formula is reintroduced. I usually avoid high-fat solids on the first day of refeeding, but this practice is without scientific basis.

Antidiarrheal preparations such as kaolin, pectin, paregoric, diphenoxylate, loperamide, and bismuth subsalicylate should not be prescribed. None, with the possible exception of bismuth subsalicylate, positively affects the pathophysiology of the process. Drugs that decrease intestinal transit prolong the time that the injurious agent is in contact with the intestinal epithelium. Likewise, empirical antibiotic therapy is unwarranted in the management of the nontoxic infant with acute diarrhea.

Most infants and children recover uneventfully. Some demonstrate lactose intolerance for greater than 1 month after recovery, and a rare patient remains lactose-intolerant indefinitely. It is important to provide proper dietary instructions to the family to prevent conscious or unconscious adverse alterations of the infant's or child's diet.

SUGGESTED READING

Brown KH, MacLean WC Jr. Nutritional management of acute diarrhea: an appraisal of the alternatives. Pediatrics 1984; 73:119–125.

Finberg L. The role of oral electrolyte-glucose solutions in hydration for children—international and domestic aspects. J Pediatr 1980; 96:51–54.

Hirschhorn N. The treatment of acute diarrhea in children. An historical and physiological perspective. Am J Clin Nutr 1980; 33:637–663.

Santosham M, Brown KH, Sack RB. Oral rehydration therapy and dietary therapy for acute childhood diarrhea. Pediatr Rev 1987; 8:273–278.

SPECIFIC DIARRHEAL DISEASES

LARRY K. PICKERING, M.D.

Gastrointestinal tract infections include a wide range of symptom complexes that can be produced by a variety of enteropathogens. A presumptive etiologic diagnosis can be established on the basis of a medical history, including epidemiologic clues, clinical manifestations, physical examination, and knowledge of the pathophysiologic mechanisms of enteropathogens. Laboratory studies are often performed to establish the definitive diagnosis and to guide therapy. All patients with diarrhea require some degree of fluid and electrolyte therapy, a few need other nonspecific support, and some may benefit from specific antimicrobial therapy.

BACTERIAL ENTEROPATHOGENS

Many bacterial species have been shown to be important causes of gastroenteritis in various parts of the world. In selected patients with diarrhea, antimicrobial agents decrease symptoms and/or reduce fecal shedding of the organism.

Aeromonas

Species of *Aeromonas*, including *A. caviae*, *A. hydrophila*, and *A. sobria*, have been shown in some studies to be causes of acute gastroenteritis; other studies do not support this observation. The illness associated with *Aeromonas* appears to be seasonal with a midsummer peak. It is more common in children younger than 2 years of age, and often presents with relatively nonspecific clinical symptoms. Watery diarrhea with mild fever of brief duration is most common, but both prolonged diarrhea and dysentery-like illness have been reported. The true frequency of *Aeromonas* in stool cultures is probably underestimated because the organism resembles normal enteric flora. Treatment is not indicated for patients with mild self-limited illness, although for those with an illness that persists for weeks or presents in a dysentery-like fashion, trimethoprim–sulfamethoxazole (TMP/SMZ) is recommended (Table 1).

Campylobacter

C. fetus subspecies *jejuni* is an enteric pathogen that has been shown by DNA homology studies to be

TABLE 1   Antimicrobial Therapy for Patients with Diarrhea Caused by Bacterial Enteropathogens

Enteropathogens	Antimicrobial Agent	Dosage for Children
Aeromonas hydrophila	None for most patients; TMP/SMZ for severe or prolonged illness	TMP 10 mg/kg/day plus SMZ 50 mg/kg/day orally, in 2 divided doses for 5 days
Campylobacter jejuni	None	
	or	
	Erythromycin	40 mg/kg/day orally, divided 4 times daily for 5–7 days
E. coli		
Enterotoxigenic	None or TMP/SMZ	See above
Enteropathogenic	None or TMP/SMZ	See above
Enteroinvasive	TMP/SMZ	See above
Enterohemorrhagic	TMP/SMZ	See above
Shigella species	TMP/SMZ	See above
	or	
	Ampicillin	50–75 mg/kg/day orally, divided 4 times daily for 5 days
Salmonella		
Carrier state	None	None
Acute gastroenteritis	None	None
Bacteremia and/or		
enteric fever	Ampicillin	200 mg/kg/day IV, divided every 4 hours for 2 weeks
	or	
	Chloramphenicol	75 mg/kg/day orally or IV, divided every 6 hours for 2 weeks
	or	
	TMP/SMZ	TMP 10 mg/kg/day plus SMZ 50 mg/kg/day divided every 12 hours for 2 weeks
V. cholerae	TMP/SMZ	Dosage as above, treat for 2 days
Vibrio parahemolyticus	None (?)	None
Y. enterocolitica	None (?)	None

two organisms, *C. jejuni* and *C. coli*. These organisms are generally not distinguished in most clinical microbiology laboratories and are reported as *C. jejuni*. Clinically, *C. jejuni* frequently resembles bacillary dysentery with bloody diarrhea containing fecal leukocytes or it may cause watery diarrhea. In North America *Campylobacter* is increasingly being recognized as the most commonly documented bacterial cause of diarrhea. Selective techniques are required to culture *Campylobacter* in the laboratory. Erythromycin therapy (see Table 1) has been shown to alter clinical findings only if provided early in the course of disease. Therapy reduces fecal shedding of the organism. Resistance to erythromycin has not been reported in the United States, but has been reported in Thailand. The quinolone antibiotics have been shown to be effective, but are not yet approved for therapy of gastrointestinal tract infections.

Escherichia coli

E. coli that cause disease can be divided into several categories based on their mechanism of disease production and clinical manifestations: (1) enterotoxigenic, (2) enteropathogenic, (3) enteroinvasive, and (4) enterohemorrhagic.

Enterotoxigenic

Illness caused by enterotoxigenic strains results from heat-stable and/or heat-labile enterotoxins that cause small bowel derangement in absorption of electrolytes and water. The heat-labile enterotoxin is similar to that of *V. cholerae*. Gastrointestinal tract symptoms include nausea, vomiting, cramps, and frequent watery stools. There are no fecal leukocytes in the stool. This syndrome is usually self-limited and lasts about 5 days (rarely as long as 10 days). The preferred treatment is symptomatic, although some antimicrobial agents such as TMP/SMZ have been shown effective in shortening the course of disease. TMP/SMZ also has been used for prophylaxis for persons traveling from developed to developing countries, but prophylactic antimicrobial therapy is not currently recommended.

Enteropathogenic

The mechanism of disease production by enteropathogenic *E. coli* (EPEC) is not fully understood. These strains do not produce enterotoxin and are not invasive. Among these strains are some that destroy the microvilli, lower the disaccharidases, and cause inflammation of the small bowel and malabsorption. Diarrhea is usually self-limited in older children and adults. Nausea, vomiting, cramps, and voluminous diarrhea without blood or mucus are common. No fecal leukocytes are present in stool. These strains, in rare instances, cause protracted diarrhea in infants. Thus, EPEC should be considered in infants who have had diarrhea lasting 2 weeks or longer. In patients with protracted diarrhea, diagnosis can be made by examination of small intestinal contents by biopsy, microscopic evaluation, and culture. Treatment of these protracted episodes in infants includes the use of TMP/SMZ if the strains are susceptible.

Enteroinvasive

Enteroinvasive strains are associated with a clinical picture and pathogenesis comparable to those observed with *Shigella*. The strains, which belong to restricted serotypes, colonize the colon and distal part of the small intestine and cause damage to the epithelium. Nausea and vomiting frequently accompany abdominal pain. The diarrhea is less in volume than that seen with ETEC strains and contains mucus and blood. Fever, headache, and myalgia are common. Treatment with TMP/SMZ is recommended for susceptible strains (see Table 1). Ampicillin can be used against susceptible strains in a dosage of 75 mg per kilogram per day orally in divided doses every 6 hours for 5 days.

Enterohemorrhagic

E. coli 0157H7 has been shown to produce diarrhea and hemorrhagic colitis. This organism is associated with severe abdominal cramps, low-grade fever, grossly bloody diarrhea, nausea, and vomiting. Symptoms are usually self-limited and last about 5 days. This organism also has been found in association with hemolytic uremic syndrome (HUS). If one suspects this etiology as a cause of hemorrhagic colitis or HUS, stool samples for culture should be obtained early in the illness. If the microbiology laboratory identifies *E. coli* that are sorbitol negative, the organism should be sent to a reference laboratory that can identify the serotype. Treatment with TMP/SMZ in dosages used to treat shigellosis is recommended (see Table 1).

Salmonella

Currently, three species of *Salmonella* are differentiated on the basis of biochemical characteristics: *S. cholerae-suis, S. typhi,* and *S. enteritidis.* Nearly all of the over 1,700 serotypes of *Salmonella* are now grouped under the single species name *S. enteritidis.* Determining serotypes remains a useful epidemiologic tool for outbreak situations, although definition of one of the three species is still adequate for the vast majority of patients. *S. typhi,* the cause of typhoid fever, is considered the most virulent *Salmonella* serotype.

Although it is still considered inappropriate to give antibiotic therapy to the vast majority of patients with *Salmonella* gastroenteritis, several groups of patients should receive therapy, including those with marked toxicity, infants younger than 6 months of age, patients with malignancies, and patients with hemoglobinopathies such as sickle cell anemia. Many *Salmonella* strains are now resistant to multiple antibiotics. Ampicillin, chloramphenicol, and TMP/SMZ are appropriate agents for patients with *Salmonella* who require therapy and should be provided for all patients with typhoid fever, bacteremia caused by nontyphoidal strains, and dissemination with localized suppuration (see Table 1). Patients with resistant strains may benefit from a third-generation cephalosporin. (See chapter on *Typhoid Fever*).

Patients with hemoglobinopathies and children younger than 6 months of age who have *Salmonella* infection and fever are treated with antimicrobial agents as if they had blood invasion until proved otherwise. Patients with chronic or debilitating disease, or those receiving immunosuppressive therapy, should be treated the same as the group with hemoglobinopathies. These special groups are often hospitalized and treated with parenteral therapy. Therapy can be modified once blood, CSF and other culture results become available.

Shigella

There are four serogroups of *Shigella* containing more than 40 serotypes. *S. sonnei* is currently the most common cause of bacillary dysentery in the United States and Europe, whereas *S. flexneri* serotypes account for a majority of the remaining cases. The fecal leukocyte examination has been found to be helpful in evaluating patients thought to have shigellosis; however, this evaluation may also be positive in patients who have other invasive enteropathogens. About half of the strains of *S. sonnei* are resistant to ampicillin, therefore TMP/SMZ has become the treatment of choice for shigellosis. Ampicillin is still acceptable therapy for those patients known to be infected with *S. sonnei* that is susceptible to ampicillin and for patients infected with *S. flexneri,* which have remained relatively susceptible to ampicillin (see Table 1). Amoxicillin is not as effective as ampicillin in the treatment of patients with susceptible strains and should not be used. The quinolone antibiotics have been shown to be effective but are not currently approved for this use. Any antidiarrheal compound that decreases intestinal motility should be avoided because of the likelihood of prolonging the infection.

Vibrio cholerae

A focus of cholera is present in the Gulf Coast of the United States. Epidemic cholera is caused by O group 1 strains of *V. cholerae.* However, non-O1 or nonagglutinating *V. cholerae* also cause disease. All clinical isolates of *V. cholerae* O1 from the United States have been hemolytic, biotype El Tor, serotype Inaba, and have had the same unique phage type and toxin gene sequence. The major mechanism by which this organism causes fluid loss is the production of a heat-labile enterotoxin. The isolation of *V. cholerae* from stools requires a special culture medium, thio-sulfate-citrate-bile salt-sucrose agar (TCBS), which is not routinely used by most laboratories for evaluation of stool specimens. Therapy for this disease calls for the administration of large volumes of electrolytes to replace the almost isotonic fluid loss in stools. It is useful to keep a record of the volume of stools as well as the volume of fluid administered because the goal is a one-to-one replacement. The electrolytes of these children should be followed closely for development of hyperkalemia, a common complication in children with cholera. Monitoring blood glucose concentrations is important because hypoglycemia occurs in about 10 percent of children. The vaccine currently available provides fair but short-lived protection. Treatment with antimicrobial agents results in a reduction of fluid loss and duration of diarrhea. TMP/SMZ is an appropriate choice for treatment of children too young to receive tetracycline, which is the drug of choice for adults (see Table 1).

Vibrio parahemolyticus

V. parahemolyticus is a common marine isolate that has been found in water, shellfish, fish, and plankton. The illness associated with *V. parahemolyticus* may be either dysentery-like or, more commonly, a nonspecific diarrheal illness. Illness is uncommon in most of the world except in areas such as Japan, where seafood is consumed uncooked. In the United States, children develop diarrhea caused by *V. parahemolyticus* infrequently because their diets seldom include raw seafood. The mechanism of disease caused by this pathogen is not clear, although at least some strains are capable of producing a cytotoxin. Like *V. cholerae,* this organism requires TCBS agar to be isolated; routine stool cultures therefore do not identify it. Currently it is unclear whether antibiotics have any role in therapy of *V. parahemolyticus* gastroenteritis.

Yersinia enterocolitica

Gastroenteritis caused by *Y. enterocolitica* is uncommon in the United States, although it is a common cause of gastroenteritis among children in Canada and Europe. Illness is much more common in children during the first 4 years of life than in older children or adults, and it may resemble shigellosis or acute appendicitis, although endemic infection usually results in diarrhea, vomiting, abdominal pain, and fever. Although *Y. enterocolitica* is occasionally identified on routine stool cultures, cold enrichment increases the yield of positive cultures. Because cold enrichment requires subculturing in a nutrient broth over a 3-week period of time, diagnosis is delayed. When illness has already resolved in the setting of late laboratory diagnosis, no therapy is given. For those patients who are still symptomatic when cultures become positive, appropriate therapy for *Y. enterocolitica* gastroenteritis has not been established. Because the illness is usually self-limited, most patients probably require no therapy. If a decision is made to treat, TMP/SMZ or chloramphenicol are the agents to be cosidered.

PARASITIC ENTEROPATHOGENS

The four most frequent causes of parasitic diarrhea in persons in the United States are *Giardia lamblia, Entamoeba histolytica, Cryptosporidium,* and *Strongyloides steracoralis.* (See the related chapters for detailed information about these parasites.)

Giardia lamblia

G. lamblia is a flagellated protozoan that exists in trophozoite and cyst forms. Disease caused by this organism is common in certain high-risk populations and in persons who travel to hyperendemic areas. Infection with *Giardia* ranges from asymptomatic excretion to acute explosive, watery, foul-smelling diarrhea with abdominal distention, flatulence, nausea, and anorexia. Chronic diarrhea with malabsorption and significant weight loss over many months may also occur. Studies in day care centers have shown that *Giardia* cysts, and even trophozoites, are common in children manifesting no symptoms. Stool examination is less reliable than examination of upper intestinal secretions. Quinacrine, metronidazole, and furazolidone are the drugs used for treatment of patients with giardiasis (Table 2). Side effects occur in 23 percent of patients treated with quinacrine, in 10 percent with furzaolidone, and in 7 percent with metronidazole. Quinacrine is significantly less expensive than metronidazole and furazolidone. Because furazolidone is the only drug available in a liquid preparation, this is generally the one used in pediatric patients. Asymptomatic excretors of *Giardia* are not generally treated.

Entamoeba histolytica

Amebiasis is a major health problem in Asia, Latin America, and Africa. The influx of refugees into the United States over the past 10 years has increased the likelihood that physicians will see children with amebiasis. Childhood intestinal amebiasis generally presents with diarrhea containing blood and mucus and no fever. Diarrhea without blood, fulminating colitis, appendicitis, and ameboma occur infrequently in children. A diagnosis of *E. histolytica* is made by examination of fresh stool specimens or bowel wall scrapings for cysts or trophozoites. Serologic tests for amebas are almost always positive in acute amebic dysentery and hepatic amebiasis. A

TABLE 2 Parasites that Produce Gastroenteritis

Enteropathogens	Therapy	Dosage for Children
Giardia lamblia	Quinacrine	6 mg/kg/day orally divided 3 times daily for 7 days (maximum 300 mg/day)
	or	
	Metronidazole	15 mg/kg/day orally divided 3 times daily for 7–10 days (maximum 750 mg/day)
	or	
	Furazolidone	9 mg/kg/day orally divided 3 times daily for 10 days (maximum 400 mg/day)
Entamoeba histolytica		
Asymptomatic cyst excretor	Iodoquinol	30 mg/kg/day divided 3 times daily for 20 days (not to exceed 2 g per day)
	or	
	Paromomycin	25–30 mg/kg/day divided 3 times daily for 7 days
	or	
	Diloxanide furoate*	20 mg/kg/day divided 3 times daily for 10 days (not to exceed 1.5 g per day)
Intestinal amebiasis	Metronidazole	30–50 mg/kg/day divided 3 times daily for 10 days (maximum 2,250 mg/day)
	plus	
	Iodoquinol	See above
	or	
	Dehydroemetine*	1 to 1.5 mg/kg/day (maximum 90 mg/day) IM in 2 doses for up to 5 days
	plus	
	Iodoquinol	See above
Cryptosporidium	None	
Strongyloides stercoralis	Thiabendazole	25 mg/kg/dose every 12 hours for 4 doses (alternative 25 mg/kg once daily for 5 days)

* Available from the CDC Drug Service, Centers for Disease Control in Atlanta, Georgia [(404) 329-3670 or (404) 329-3311].

liver scan or computerized tomography scan may detect a liver abscess. In treating patients with amebiasis, iodoquinol is the best luminal amebicide presently available in the United States. It is effective against cysts and trophozoites in the intestine but is not effective against tissue forms of disease. Invasive amebiasis of the intestine, liver, or other organs necessitates the additional use of tissue amebicides such as metronidazole (see Table 2).

Cryptosporidium

In 1976 the first human infections caused by *Cryptosporidium* were reported. With the onset of the AIDS epidemic, many patients with chronic malabsorption syndrome and severe protracted, watery diarrhea were recognized as having cryptosporidiosis. Other reports have demonstrated that *Cryptosporidium* is a common intestinal parasite of immunocompetent humans, particularly of children in the first 4 years of life. The illness is generally self-limited, although watery diarrhea persists in some patients for more than a month (median 15 days). Weight loss, vomiting, abdominal discomfort, anorexia, and occasionally fever also occur. This pathogen probably accounts for less than 5 percent of diarrheal illness in most populations. For reasons that are not yet clear, illness is more common in late summer and early fall than in winter or spring. Diagnosis is made by modified Kinyoun acid-fast stain of stool with demonstration of oocysts. Supportive therapy should be provided; no effective antimicrobial therapy is available.

Strongyloides stercoralis

Although other nematodes (*Capillaria philippinensis*), and trematodes (*Schistosoma japonicum, Fasciolopsis buski*) cause diarrhea and eosinophilia, only *S. stercoralis* is a common cause of this syndrome in the United States. Characteristically, children with this pathogen have diarrhea that lasts many weeks with epigastric pain, steatorrhea, weight loss, and eosinophilia. This organism can produce a devastating illness in certain immunosuppressed hosts. Because diagnosis of this pathogen by stool examination is difficult, examination of duodenal fluid is frequently required. The optimal method of obtaining duodenal fluid for this purpose appears to be a string test, although duodenal aspirates and biopsies are sometimes positive. Thiabendazole remains the treatment of choice (see Table 2).

VIRAL ENTEROPATHOGENS

Rotavirus, Norwalk-like virus, and enteric adenovirus are recognized causes of acute infectious gastroenteritis. Other viruses that may cause infectious gastroenteritis include astroviruses, calicivirus, coronavirus, and minirotavirus. These viruses exhibit different epidemiologic and clinical features, although most episodes are self-limited and characterized by various combinations of diarrhea, nausea, vomiting and abdominal cramps, headache, myalgia, and low-grade fever. Bowel movements are watery and generally do not contain blood or mucus. Rotavirus is the only one of these agents for which commercial kits are available for diagnosis.

Rotavirus

Rotavirus is one of the most important enteric pathogens throughout the world, particularly in infants. Illness is prevalent in temperate climates in winter months and may account for as much as 50 to 60 percent of diarrhea in infants and young children. The precise significance of asymptomatic shedding of rotavirus is unclear at present, although it is a common event. Because of increased insensible fluid losses with fever, intestinal losses of diarrhea, and emesis interfering with rehydration, rotavirus is commonly associated with significant dehydration. Careful attention to fluid and electrolyte balance is required to care for a child with rotavirus infection adequately. Because there are multiple serotypes, reinfection can occur. Rotavirus causes minimal or no symptoms among neonates. Commercially available rapid diagnostic tests using enzyme immunoassays or latex agglutination are available to detect rotavirus in stools. Testing of various rotavirus vaccines using several sources of antigen is underway.

Norwalk Virus

Norwalk-like virus agents are much smaller than rotavirus (27 nm versus 70 nm), and therefore diagnosis is made by immune electron microscopy (IEM) of stools or by serology. Commercial assays are not available. These viruses have been shown to affect children in elementary school outbreaks in which 50 percent primary and 35 percent secondary attack rates have been described. Upper gastrointestinal tract symptoms such as nausea and vomiting occur; diarrhea is not as common as with rotavirus and, when it occurs, has no mucus or blood, is not foul smelling, and usually does not contain fecal leukocytes. An illness usually lasts for 24 to 48 hours. There is no specific treatment, and fluid replacement is dictated by the patient's condition. There are no preventive measures such as immunization.

Enteric Adenoviruses

At least two distinct subgroups of enteric adenovirus, F (type 40) and G (type 41), have been described. These agents primarily affect children younger than 2 years of age. They cause increased morbidity in infants who undergo surgical procedures. Diagnosis can be made by electron microscopy or by ELISA, but commercial assays are not available. These agents cause a febrile gastrointestinal tract illness that may be associated with respiratory findings. The symptoms include frequent vomiting and diarrhea, but no blood or mucus in stool. Treatment is nonspecific, and fluid replacement is dictated by the patient's condition. Nosocomial spread is common. No immunization methods are available.

SUGGESTED READING

Cleary TG, Pickering LK. Update on infectious diarrhea. Adv Pediatr Infect Dis 1986; 1:117–143.
Pickering LK, Cleary TG. Approach to patients with gastrointestinal infections and food poisoning. In: Feigin RD, Cherry JD, ed. Textbook of pediatric infectious diseases. Philadelphia: WB Saunders, 1987; 622–651.

NECROTIZING ENTEROCOLITIS

MORVEN S. EDWARDS, M.D.

Necrotizing enterocolitis (NEC) is a disease of multifactorial origin that is estimated to occur in 0.2 percent of live births, or approximately 4,000 neonates annually in the United States. Predominantly a disease of the premature, it affects 1 to 5 percent of infants admitted to neonatal intensive care units (NICUs). In the very low birth weight infant, the incidence may be as high as 12 percent. Although no consensus as to its pathogenesis has been reached, risk factors associated with NEC are established. These include low or very low birth weight, enteric feeding or feeding of hyperosmolar solutions, the occurrence of bacterial sepsis, patent ductus arteriosus, respiratory distress syndrome, umbilical vessel catheterization, and perinatal asphyxia. Each of these may predispose to the development of selective bowel ischemia, characteristically involving the "watershed" (cecum, distal ileum, and proximal colon) of splanchnic blood flow. Bowel ischemia promotes the invasion of gut by intestinal flora. The radiographic finding of pneumatosis intestinalis is thought to be caused by gas-producing intestinal bacteria. Unimpeded, the process may progress to peritonitis with or without abscess formation, intestinal perforation, gangrenous bowel, septicemia, and death.

MEDICAL MANAGEMENT

Treatment of NEC varies depending on the severity of disease at the time of presentation. Designation of clinical staging according to the criteria of Bell and associates, as modified by Walsh and Kliegman, provides a basis for the extent of therapeutic intervention. Infants with stage I infection are those with suspected or "rule-out" NEC, in whom common features include feeding intolerance, abdominal distension, microscopic evidence of blood in stools, and abdominal radiographs that *lack* diagnostic evidence of NEC. For infants with stage IIA disease, the radiographic finding of pneumatosis intestinalis confirms the diagnosis of NEC, but infants are not clinically toxic. Stage IIB disease is distinguished by moderate systemic toxicity manifested as mild acidosis or thrombocytopenia and by focal abdominal findings consistent with early peritonitis such as cellulitis of the abdominal wall, right lower quadrant mass, rebound tenderness, or hepatic portal vein gas. Infants with stage III disease are critically ill and have impending (stage IIIA) or overt (stage IIIB) evidence of intestinal perforation.

A direct role for bacteria and their toxins in the development of NEC is now undisputed. In most instances the organisms causing bacteremia or peritonitis are secondary invaders of damaged mucosa rather than the primary cause of ischemic damage. The epidemic clusters of cases reported from some nurseries probably reflect invasion in susceptible hosts by the prevalent nosocomial agents endemic to particular NICUs. Thus, all patients suspected of having NEC should be evaluated for possible sepsis. Culture of blood should be obtained peripherally and through umbilical, central venous, and/or arterial access catheters, if applicable. If feasible (i.e., the infant is not in shock), cerebrospinal fluid should be obtained for total cell count, glucose and protein, Gram stain, and culture. Urine should be collected sterilely for culture, and, if the infant requires ventilatory support, tracheal aspirate secretions should be examined microscopically and sent for culture.

Antibiotic therapy should be initiated, after appropriate cultures are performed, in all infants with suspected or proven NEC. Initially, antimicrobial therapy should be directed toward the microorganisms that most commonly cause peritonitis or bacteremia in these young hosts, especially within a particular NICU, *and* based on knowledge of the relative virulence of potential infecting organisms (Table 1). For infants with rule-out NEC or who are mildly ill with NEC (with a low risk of perforation), treatment is directed primarily toward the Enterobacteriaceae likely to be associated with bacteremia. Among infants with suspected microscopic or gross leakage

TABLE 1 Microorganisms Frequently (F), Less Commonly (L), Occasionally (O), or Rarely (R) Isolated from Blood and/or Peritoneal Fluid of Neonates with Sporadic (S) or Epidemic (E)* NEC

Microorganism	Frequency and Occurrence	Relative Virulence†
Escherichia coli	F,S,E	+++
Klebsiella pneumoniae	F,S,E	++
Staphylococcus epidermidis	F,S	+
Enterobacter cloacae	L,S,E	++
Pseudomonas aeruginosa	L,S,E	+++
Clostridium perfringens	L,S,E	+++
Other *Clostridia*	O,S,E	++
Streptococcus faecalis	O,S	++
Bacteroides fragilis	L,S,E	++
Other *Bacteroides*	O,S	++
Staphylococcus aureus	R,S	++
Listeria monocytogenes	R,S	+
Group B *Streptococcus*	R,S	++
Salmonella	O,E	++
Candida albicans	O,S	+

* Coronavirus, rotavirus, and enteroviruses have also been implicated in NEC outbreaks.

† Extremely virulent and often associated with fatal infection (+++); moderately virulent (++); less virulent and unlikely to cause bacteremia or fungemia-associated death (+).

from the bowel, treatment is broadened to include bowel anaerobes.

Guidelines for *initial* antimicrobial therapy in NEC are shown in Table 2. The aminoglycoside employed initially will depend on the resident microflora in an individual nursery. In our nurseries, for example, resistance patterns dictate the use of amikacin routinely for late-onset infections. If resistance is not prevalent, gentamicin may be employed for possible or proven NEC. Similarly, the decision to employ an antipseudomonal penicillin, such as ticarcillin or piperacillin, for initial treatment of NEC should be based on the risk of *Pseudomonas* in the NICU. (Piperacillin is not approved for use in children under 12 years of age.) Serum concentrations should be measured and dosage adjusted to maintain peak and trough gentamicin concentrations of 5 to 10 μg per milliliter and less than 2 μg per milliliter, respectively, or peak and trough amikacin concentrations of 25 to 40 μg per milliliter and less than 10 μg per milliliter, respectively.

For stages IIB and III NEC, I use clindamycin to provide broad anaerobic coverage. If thrombocytopenia is present or platelet adherence is a concern, piperacillin may be substituted for ticarcillin, and obviates the use of clindamycin. I often withhold vancomycin initially. However, if staphylococcal infection is a consideration in the differential diagnosis (and *Pseudomonas* is *not* of concern), it may be substituted for the penicillin. Although vancomycin has no gram-negative spectrum of activity, it has activity against enterococci and the gram-positive anaerobes, including most strains of *Clostridia*. If vancomycin is employed, serum concentrations should be moni-

TABLE 2 Guidelines for Initial Antimicrobial Therapy in Necrotizing Enterocolitis (NEC)

NEC Stage	Antibiotic	Dosage (mg/kg) and Interval (hr) of Doses by Infant's Age and Weight			
		<7 Days/<1 kg	<7 Days/>1 kg	>7 Days/<1 kg	>7 Days/>1 kg
I*, IIA	Ampicillin or	50q8	50q6	50q6	50q4–6
	ticarcillin and	50q12	50q6	50q6	50q4–6
	Amikacin or	7.5q18	7.5–10q12	10q12	10q8–12
	gentamicin	2.5q18	2.5q12	2.5q18	2.5q8–12
IIB	As for stages I/ IIA and				
	clindamycin	7.5q12	7.5q8	10q8	10q6
IIIA, IIIB	Aminoglycoside, ticarcillin, and clindamycin as above or aminoglycoside and				
	piperacillin†	50q8	50q6	50q6	50q4–6
Any-*S. epidermidis* isolated	Vancomycin	7.5q12	10q12	10q12	10q8

* If staphylococcal infection is suspected independently of NEC, methicillin or vancomycin should be added.
† If thrombocytopenia is present or platelet adherence is considered abnormal.

tored to maintain a peak of 25 to 40 μg per milliliter and a trough of less than 15 μg per milliliter. Antimicrobial therapy should be altered, if necessary, based on the results of cultures. Antimicrobial agents employed as adjunctive therapy for the treatment of NEC at our hospitals are shown in Table 3.

The duration of therapy varies depending on stage and culture results. For stage I NEC in which cultures are sterile, antibiotics usually can be discontinued in 3 days. For stage IIA with lack of clinical progression and sterile cultures, a 7- to 10-day course usually suffices. Among infants with stages IIB or III, the usual duration of therapy ranges from 2 to 3 weeks, depending on culture results and clinical progress. I usually continue clindamycin for about 7 days unless a specific anaerobe resistant to penicillin is isolated. Treatment should be provided for a minimum of 10 days after sterilization of the bloodstream is documented in patients with bacteremia. Usually, the clinical progress of intestinal and peritoneal disease is the feature on which ultimate duration is based. Orally administered antibiotics have no role in the treatment of NEC.

Particular mention should be made of therapy in fungal peritonitis, with or without documented fungemia. If *Candida albicans* (or another *Candida* species) is isolated from peritoneal fluid, treatment with amphotericin B should be initiated. I consider fungal peritonitis in the premature infant to be a systemic infection and provide a full course of therapy (30 mg per kilogram) for these infants.

Supportive measures should be undertaken at the first clinical suspicion of NEC. These include cessation of enteral feeding and provision of gastric decompression by nasogastric tube. Fluids, electrolytes, and parenteral nutrients are provided intravenously. Serial radiographs, performed initially at 6- to 8-hour intervals are a critical adjunct to monitoring the progress of infection. Infants with stage III NEC often require aggressive fluid resuscitation, correction of acidosis, ventilatory support, and pressor therapy for treatment of septic shock. Dopamine should be restricted to a dosage (5 to 15 μg per kilogram per minute) that improves cardiac output without further compromising splanchnic and renal blood flow. For further support, dobutamine may be initiated at 5 to 10 μg per kilogram per minute and increased as needed. Transfusion with platelets is indicated for infants with clinical evidence of bleeding (usually those with fewer than 10,000 per cubic millimeter). In my

TABLE 3 Adjunctive Antibiotics for Treatment of NEC

Antibiotic	Dose (mg/kg) and Interval (hr) by Infant's Age		Indication
	<7 Days	>7 Days	
Metronidazole	7.5q12	15q12	Anaerobe resistant to clindamycin
Cefotaxime	50q12	50q8	Susceptible Enterobacteriaceae
Cefoxitin	50q12	50q8	Susceptible Enterobacteriaceae; also has good anaerobic spectrum
Ceftazidime	50q12	50q8	Alternative to antipseudomonal penicillin

experience, recovery from neutropenia, if present initially, usually occurs within 48 hours after initiation of antimicrobial and supportive therapy. Transfusion of white blood cells should not be employed routinely for the treatment of NEC.

More than half of those infants with NEC respond to medical therapy alone. The duration of the bowel rest period may be as short as 3 to 5 days for suspected NEC with persistently negative radiographs. For infants with stage IIA NEC, our routine is a 10-day period of bowel rest. A 14-day minimum period of bowel rest is employed for stage IIB or III disease.

SURGICAL THERAPY

NEC is the most common surgical emergency in the newborn. Surgical intervention is mandatory when intestinal perforation has occurred. It should be considered for infants with a persistent right-lower-quadrant mass, a persistent (nonshifting) bowel loop seen by radiography, abdominal wall erythema, or failure to respond to medical therapy. For these infants we perform a diagnostic paracentesis and, if perforation is documented, exploratory laparotomy. If the infant is at high risk for perforation, abdominal radiographs are taken at 6-hour intervals with the infant's right side up. When possible, the infant is placed in this position for 4 or 5 minutes before the roentgenogram is taken, to allow free air to rise.

There are three surgical options for the infant with perforation. If the area of necrotic bowel is contained, resection and primary enteroenterostomy is performed. During the past 5 years our surgeons have shifted toward the option of primary anastomosis, when feasible, as a means by which the enteric stream can be maintained and the risk for stricture reduced. When the affected area of necrotic bowel is more extensive, resection is performed and enterostomy and mucous fistula are established. In these patients, efforts are made to close the enterostomy within 3 to

4 weeks of the primary diversion. This approach is intended to minimize the problems associated with ileostomy care and electrolyte balance in the premature infant, as well as to maintain dilitation of the injured mucosa. For critically ill infants unable to undergo major resection and for those with massive involvement, lavage and drainage are carried out, usually in the nursery, and a "second look" procedure is performed 24 to 48 hours after the infant's condition has stabilized and devitalized bowel can be more positively delineated. The overall survival of infants requiring surgical intervention at our hospitals is approximately 80 percent.

PREVENTION

We observe routine cohorting of infants admitted to the NICU. When NEC activity rises above the baseline, the index infants are placed in contact isolation, involved sections of the unit are closed to new admissions, and surveillance cultures of index and asymptomatic infants in the unit are initiated. Infants colonized with a potential epidemic strain are monitored closely for symptoms of NEC and are maintained in their cohorts until their discharge from the hospital.

SUGGESTED READING

Kliegman RM, Fanaroff AA. Necrotizing enterocolitis. N Engl J Med 1984; 310:1093–1103.
Kosloske AM. Pathogenesis and prevention of necrotizing enterocolitis: a hypothesis based on personal observation and a review of the literature. Pediatrics 1984; 74:1086–1092.
Milner ME, de la Monte SM, Moore GW, Hutchins GM. Risk factors for developing and dying from necrotizing enterocolitis. J Pediatr Gastroenterol Nutr 1986; 5:359–364.
Rotbart HA, Levin MJ. How contagious is necrotizing enterocolitis? Pediatr Infect Dis 1983; 2:406–413.
Walsh MC, Kliegman RM. Necrotizing enterocolitis: treatment based on staging criteria. Pediatr Clin North Am 1986; 33:179–201.

ANTIBIOTIC-ASSOCIATED DIARRHEAL SYNDROMES

THOMAS G. CLEARY, M.D.

The spectrum of antibiotic-associated diarrhea varies from severe life-threatening pseudomembranous colitis to mild self-limited diarrhea without inflammatory changes. Pseudomembranous enterocolitis was described before 1900, thus preceding the introduction of antibiotics by many years. Currently, although spontaneous nonantibiotic associated cases still occur, the vast majority of pseudomembranous colitis occurs in the setting of antibiotic therapy. It has become clear, in the 10 years since pseudomembranous colitis was first associated with the toxins of *C. difficile,* that its usual cause is *C. difficile.* Antibiotics upset the balance of intestinal microflora, with resulting proliferation of *C. difficile* and production of toxin. Although many antibiotics have been associated with this syndrome (Table 1), it most often occurs in the setting of oral therapy with clindamycin, a penicillin, or a cephalosporin. Paradoxically,

TABLE 1 Antibiotics Associated with Diarrhea or Pseudomembranous Colitis

Amoxicillin	Clindamycin	Miconazole
Ampicillin	Cloxacillin	Nafcillin
Amphotericin B	Erythromycin	Neomycin
Carbenicillin	Ethambutol	Penicillin G
Cefazolin	Flucloxacillin	Penicillin V
Cefoxitin	Flucytosine	Rifampin
Cefuroxine	Gentamicin	Sulfasalzine
Cephalexin	Isoniazid	Sulfamethoxazole
Cephaloridine	Kanamycin	Tetracycline
Cephalothin	Lincomycin	Tobramycin
Chloramphenicol	Metronidazole	Trimethoprim

even antibiotics that kill *C. difficile* are occasionally associated with colitis. A milder syndrome without pseudomembranes occurs commonly. Although diarrhea developing in the patient who is taking antibiotics is sometimes clearly associated with *C. difficile,* for the majority of cases of antibiotic-associated diarrhea without pseudomembranous colitis, the etiology remains obscure. In the past, this syndrome was thought to be caused by *S. aureus.* It is now doubtful that staphylococci have any role in this syndrome.

Although illness typically occurs between the fourth and ninth day of antibiotic therapy, onset can be delayed up to several weeks after its completion. Diarrhea is typically watery without gross blood, although occult blood is commonly present. Low-grade fever, hypogastric pain, nausea, and vomiting may also occur. The diagnosis of pseudomembranous colitis is generally made by demonstration of characteristic changes on colonoscopy (discreet elevated yellow or white plaques of fibrinous exudate) as well as the demonstration of *C. difficile* and its toxins in feces. The diagnosis of antibiotic-associated diarrhea without pseudomembranous colitis is usually made on the basis of the clinical setting. In about 25 to 30 percent of cases of antibiotic-associated diarrhea, *C. difficile* and its toxins are demonstrated in stool.

THERAPEUTIC ALTERNATIVES

Since antibiotic-associated diarrhea is often related to *C. difficile* and pseudomembranous colitis is nearly always caused by *C. difficile,* most authorities consider these illnesses to be on a continuum. The treatment literature thus far has focused on patients who have well-documented *C. difficile* infection. It remains unclear what ought to be done for those in whom *C. difficile* cannot be documented. In the current state of ignorance, I have managed these patients in a fashion identical to those with well-documented *C. difficile* disease.

The treatment options currently available for *C. difficile* are aimed at either killing the offending microorganism (vancomycin, metronidazole, bacitracin) or preventing adsorption of the toxin (cholestyramine). Several other possible alternatives that theoretically might be of interest either are of un-

proved benefit (lactobacillus preparations, corticosteroids, serum immunoglobulin) or may actually be dangerous (antimotility agents).

PREFERRED APPROACH

The most important therapeutic maneuver for the child ill with *C. difficile,* is the discontinuation of the offending antibiotic. In many children, no other treatment is required. However, there are several settings in which specific therapy is indicated. One should treat the child who has life-threatening fluid and electrolyte losses without delay as described herein rather than wait for a response to withdrawal of the offending drug. In addition, it is sometimes impossible to discontinue the drug presumed to be offending. In other children, diarrhea continues unabated several days after the antibiotic has been stopped. For each of these situations, therapy aimed at eradication of *C. difficile* is indicated. The usual patient is able to take oral therapy. In general, vancomycin is the drug of choice. For the uncommon child who is unable to tolerate vancomycin or other oral medications, or for whom cost is a major consideration, metronidazole is the usual choice. Bacitracin, although shown to be efficacious in adults, has not been well studied in children and should probably not be used. Cholestyramine has been reserved primarily for mild cases although some data in adults indicate that it may be useful to give cholestyramine for 2 to 3 weeks after a course of vancomycin to prevent relapse. Management of fluid and electrolyte status will not be discussed here though obviously, as with all children who have diarrhea, metabolic balance is the first issue to be addressed.

PATIENT SELECTION

A difficult issue regarding *C. difficile* in the pediatric patient is deciding who really has illness caused by the organism. Because *C. difficile* and its toxins are commonly demonstrable in the stools of normal infants up to about 8 months of age, interpretation of "positive" laboratory studies is difficult. As a practical approach to this dilemma, all children with positive laboratory studies and a clinical picture consistent with severe *C. difficile*-associated diarrhea, ought to receive vancomycin. Obviously, since there is no way to make the diagnosis with certainty in the young child, response to treatment must often be part of the criteria for diagnosis. The physician must keep an open mind to other possible diagnoses. Thus, in the infant a course characterized by failure to respond to vancomycin should be interpreted as suggesting that the positive stool studies for *C. difficile* do not explain the illness.

MEDICAL THERAPY

Oral vancomycin is effective therapy because the concentrations of drug achieved in the gut lumen far exceed those required to kill *C. difficile*. In adults, a dose of 500 mg given four times daily achieves a stool concentration of about 2,000 μg per milliliter, and a dose of 125 mg four times daily has been shown to achieve concentrations of 500 to 1,000 μg per milliliter. These concentrations are vastly in excess of those required to inhibit the organism (median minimum inhibitory concentration [MIC] 0.2 μg per milliliter). Metronidazole and bacitracin are presumably effective because they also achieve large concentrations in stool.

Cholestyramine has been thought to be effective because of its ability to bind toxin and thereby prevent its adsorption.

Dosage

Vancomycin has been used in children and adults in dosages of 500 to 2,000 mg per day in four divided doses, given for 7 to 14 days. In infants, a dosage of 500 mg per 1.73 m^2 every 6 hours is appropriate. Metronidazole has been used in adults in dosages of 250 to 500 mg given three to four times daily. An optimal pediatric dosage for *C. difficile* has not been established. Bacitracin has been used in adults in dosages of 25,000 U given orally four times daily for 7 to 10 days. It appears to be nearly as effective as vancomycin. The usual dosage of cholestyramine in older children or adults is 4 g given three to four times daily. For infants, dosages of 500 mg given every 6 hours have been suggested.

Route

Usually vancomycin is given by mouth or by nasogastric tube. In the rare patient who cannot take vancomycin, intravenous metronidazole is an option. Metronidazole can also be given orally as an alternative to oral vancomycin.

The most important practical consideration in choosing between the possible therapeutic options is cost. Vancomycin is the best studied of the available options. It clearly works well. The only reason not to use vancomycin in all patients requiring therapy is its high cost, which is 30 to 50 times that of metronidazole. In some patients, this consideration may prompt use of either metronidazole or cholestyramine. For example, the patient who is not ill enough to be hospitalized could be given either metronidazole or cholestyramine.

Side Effects

The major side effect of vancomycin is its foul taste. Because systemic absorption is minimal even in the face of severe mucosal inflammation, toxicity is rare. The major risk associated with metronidazole is the theoretical risk of malignancy. Although the true risk may be nil, most authorities still prefer vancomycin to metronidazole because of this potential risk.

With cholestyramine, the major side effect is constipation. Complications of treatment with these agents are extremely uncommon. Before adequate therapy existed, children occasionally died of pseudomembranous colitis. A literature review suggests a mortality of 28 percent in the prevancomycin treatment era. Currently, children rarely die of this illness.

THERAPEUTIC RESPONSE

Ideally, the assessment of therapeutic response should include determination of presence or absence of toxin in the stool near the end of vancomycin therapy as well as follow-up of the patient for several weeks. Both children and adults respond clinically within a few days of initiation of vancomycin, metronidazole, or bacitracin therapy. However, the determination of the presence or absence of fecal cytotoxin at about day 7 of therapy may be useful even when clinical response has been good. Patients who still have cytotoxin in the stool appear to be more likely to relapse than those who do not. Thus, fecal toxin determination to determine whether to discontinue treatment at 10 or 14 days is probably useful. Unfortunately, regardless of the drug regimen (vancomycin, metronidazole, or bacitracin), a significant number of patients relapse after treatment. In most studies, about 15 percent (range of 10 to 40 percent) of patients require a second or sometimes a third course of vancomycin. Those who relapse respond well to the same therapy given initially because the failures do not reflect drug-resistant *C. difficile*. Follow-up evaluations during the several weeks after vancomycin therapy is completed are required because of this risk of relapse.

ROLE OF SURGERY

Currently the role for surgery in the management of *C. difficile*-related diarrhea or colitis is limited. Rarely, development of toxic megacolon requires surgical intervention.

PROS AND CONS OF TREATMENT

The major advantage of treatment is that significant morbidity and occasional mortality can be avoided by therapy. The major disadvantage of treatment is that the best-studied drug is very expensive.

SUGGESTED READING

Borriello SP. Antibiotic-associated diarrhea in colitis: the role of *C. difficile* in gastrointestinal disorders. Boston: Martinus, Nijhoff, 1984.

Feigin RD. Antimicrobial agent induced pseudomembranous colitis. Pediatr Rev 1981; 3:147–152.

Teasley DG, Gerding DN, Olson MM, et al. Prospective randomized trial of metronidazole vs vancomycin for *C. difficile* associated diarrhea and colitis. Lancet 1983; 1043–1046.

Young GP, Ward PB, Bayley N, et al. Antibiotic associated colitis due to *Clostridium difficile:* double blind comparison of vancomycin with vasotracin. Gastroenterology 1985; 89:1038–1045.

TRAVELERS' DIARRHEA

WILLIAM J. RODRIGUEZ, M.D., Ph.D.

Travelers' diarrhea is a term used to describe a gastrointestinal syndrome, usually acute and self-limited, caused by multiple enteric infectious agents. The patient experiences an increase in frequency of unformed bowel movements (twofold or more over the patient's baseline). Besides diarrhea, other symptoms include cramps, nausea, fever, and malaise. One estimate is that each year at least 100 million out of 250 million people who travel from one country to another develop travelers' diarrhea. Most of the world literature deals with the experience of adults without regard for the children who accompany them; thus, most of our data are derived from the observation in these adults.

ETIOLOGY

Bacterial Agents

Enterotoxigenic *Escherichia coli* are implicated in approximately 50 percent of cases in which a cause is detected. *Campylobacter* species may account for approximately 10 percent of cases. *Salmonella* species and *Vibrio cholerae,* although rare, are more common in certain geographical areas such as Asia. *Shigella* species are recovered from about 15 percent of patients with travelers' diarrhea, mostly in Mexico. *Vibrio parahemolyticus* is reported among certain traveling groups. Other bacterial agents are also recovered. One recent report suggests that enteroadherent *Escherichia coli* may very well be responsible for one-third of travelers' diarrhea cases in which heretofore no agents have been detected.

Viral Agents

Rotaviruses and Norwalk-like viruses have been known to cause approximately 10 percent of illness among American adults traveling to Mexico. Because certain viral infections are more prevalent in children, it follows that viruses probably constitute an even higher percentage of the causative agents for travelers' diarrhea in the pediatric age group.

Parasitic Agents

Parasites vary in their importance. *Giardia lamblia* causes between 0 and 9 percent of the disease, and presence of *Entamoeba histolytica* has been proved in a few cases. Still other parasites such as *Cryptosporidium* may be involved.

Unfortunately, in 20 to 50 percent of cases, the cause of the syndrome is unknown. It has been noted, however, that even patients with travelers' diarrhea of unknown etiology are likely to respond to antimicrobial therapy. This applies even to severe cases with symptomatology in which no enteric bacterial agent has been recovered.

MANAGEMENT

Prevention

Because travelers' diarrhea is a multifactorial syndrome, the best way to manage it is by prevention. The well-informed traveler certainly has a decided advantage.

Diet and Food Preparation

Cooked meals, hot or steaming, are less likely to cause disease than leafy, cool, or rewarmed food. Raw vegetables, meat and seafood, unpasteurized milk, and fruits that cannot be peeled should be avoided. Water by itself does not appear to be as important as food in travelers' diarrhea, but ice used in alcoholic mixed drinks and soft drinks or melted (hidden) in them, can be the means of transmission to the unsuspecting victim. Bottled beverages, both carbonated and flavored, hot and boiled drinks, boiled water, and drinks pretreated with iodine or chlorine are generally considered safe.

Immunization

There is no prospect for immunization in the near future.

Nonspecific Agents

Kaolin and pectin and, more recently, Diasorb give symptomatic relief; however, their effect on total loss of body water is negligible.

Nonantimicrobial Agents

Imodium and Pepto-Bismol have had some prophylactic effectiveness in adult travelers who have been studied.

Prophylactic Antibiotics

Some antimicrobial agents have been able to prevent illness in certain adult groups. Disease in adults has been prevented by the use of trimethoprim-sulfamethoxazole, one double-strength tablet once a day for 14 days. A rash has been the only side effect with this agent. Trimethoprim, 200 mg per day for 14 days, has also been effective; however, the possibility exists of a higher incidence of microbial resistance when trimethoprim is used alone.

Doxycycline in a dosage of either 100 or 200 mg once daily for 21 days has been successful in prophylaxis compared with control subjects, but this antimicrobial agent has no role in the management of infants and young children.

Bismuth subsalicylate (60 mg orally four times a day for 21 days) has resulted in a 62-percent protection rate in young adults. No solid guidelines exist for the use of this preparation in children. One caveat, when doxycycline and bismuth subsalicylate are used together in treating adults or adolescents, is that if bismuth subsalicylate is given 2 hours before doxycycline, peak serum concentrations of the latter can be significantly decreased. This interference has not been noted when Pepto-Bismol is given 2 hours after doxycycline.

Bicozamycin, a nonabsorbable antimicrobial agent not available in the United States, has been used with success in dosages of 400 mg four times a day for 21 days. More recently, norfloxacin has also been used successfully (400 mg per day orally for 14 days); however, this antimicrobial agent is not approved for use in children and young adolescents.

Prophylaxis with any of these antimicrobial agents or bismuth subsalicylate, is not currently indicated in pediatric patients. Adolescents could follow the advice given to adults, with the necessary adjustment of dosage. The overall rationale regarding prophylaxis in children is that the agents used have potential toxicities (which may be even more likely in children), and generally the disease is self-limited. Thus, in prevention, our main recommendation is attention to diet and safe food preparation.

Therapeutics

The treatment of travelers' diarrhea could be approached from various directions: (1) hydration; (2) use of nonspecific agents such as Kaopectate and Pepto-Bismol; (3) other non-specific methods with potential for higher toxicity such as administration of Lomotil and Loperamide; and (4) use of antimicrobial agents.

Hydration

Oral rehydration is the superior method and involves no discomfort other than waiting for the disease to run its course. The World Health Organization's (WHO) oral rehydration preparation is generally available worldwide. It contains 90 mEq of sodium per liter, 20 mEq of potassium per liter, and 2 g of carbohydrate per deciliter. The 90 mEq of sodium is more than ample to handle acute dehydration caused not only by choleralike agents but by other enteric pathogens.

Another preparation, Rehydralyte (formerly Pedialyte RS), has about 75 mEq of sodium per liter and concentrations of potassium and carbohydrate similar to those of the WHO preparation. Both preparations are adequate to handle the initial phase of rehydration. Theoretically, a child who is mildly or moderately dehydrated could be rehydrated with the WHO preparation in the first 4 hours. After the first 4 hours of hydration, a solution containing less sodium (45 to 50 mEq per liter), such as Pedialyte or Lytren, should be started. In acute dehydration, lactose feeding should not be reintroduced soon after initial oral hydration.

It is postulated that hydrating solutions containing starch or cereal actually improve the rate of absorption of sodium and water: when digested, long-chain glucose polymers provide an excess of glucose molecules and, simultaneously, overall low osmolar concentrations. Homemade salt preparations are not to be used in children because they may contain too much sodium, which could lead to hypernatremia. Commercially available beverages or sodas contain rather small amounts of sodium and potassium and also have too much carbohydrate, which could lead to even more diarrhea. In children, careful attention should be paid to such signs as tearing, urinary output, and moistness of mucous membranes. Parents should be cautioned to call a physician if they have questions.

In planning a trip, travelers could contact an organization such as the International Association for Medical Assistance to Travelers (IAMAT), 736 Center Street, Lewistown, NY 14902 (telephone: 716-754-4883), to obtain information about physicians in the areas on their itinerary.

Nonspecific Agents

A variety of absorbants have been used traditionally to stem the outflow of fluid from the gastrointestinal tract. Agents such as Kaopectate or Kaolin promote the formation of stool with greater consistency; however, there has been no indication that they decrease water loss. Diasorb, a nonfibrous activated attapulgite, is a new over-the-counter liquid antidiarrheal preparation, whose manufacturer claims it is superior to Kaopectate in reducing the number of bowel movements, cramping, and abdominal distention. The manufacturer also claims that Diasorb absorbs the toxins, bacteria, and viruses associated with diarrhea. The validity and significance of these claims await clarification and further experience.

Pepto-Bismol, in dosages of 1 oz every 30 minutes for eight doses, has been known to decrease stool frequency in adult travelers with diarrhea compared with placebo; however, this preparation is not generally recommended for children. If used at all, it should be used with caution and only in children older than 2 years of age. The salicylate load could conceivably lead to intoxication. This preparation should also not be consumed by patients with allergy to aspirin or bleeding problem. Prophylaxis with the new bismuth subsalicylate tablet preparation is effective and may ultimately provide a more convenient way to medicate both symptomatic adults and children. The protection rate against diarrhea in adults who have taken the tablet was recently reported to be 65 percent for a large-dosage regimen (2 tablets, 524 mg of bismuth subsalicylate, four times daily). This regimen was used for 3 weeks and well tolerated, the most common side effect being black stools and tongue and a small incidence of tinnitus.

Other Nonspecific Methods

Antimotility agents such as the natural opiates (paregoric) should not be used in children. Diphenoxylate (Loperamide) should not be used in children younger than 3 years of age. In a study conducted in Egypt, Loperamide in a dosage of 0.24 mg per kilogram of body weight per day, in three divided doses, was given to children younger than 2 years of age with diarrhea. The beneficial result did not differ significantly from that in children receiving placebo.

Antimicrobial Agents

Generally, afebrile children can be managed conservatively with oral fluids to ensure hydration. Those with fever and/or blood or mucus in the stool could be treated with a short course of trimethoprim–sulfamethoxazole (TMP/SMZ), particularly if they have a rectal temperature of 38.5°C or higher and abdominal discomfort. Dosage of TMP/SMZ should be calculated at about 50 mg of the sulfamethoxazole component per kilogram per day in divided doses twice daily for 5 days. *Shigella,* or another potentially invasive agent as yet not defined, could be postulated as the causative agent.

Furazolidone can be prescribed in a dosage of 5 mg per kilogram per day in 4 divided doses for approximately 7 days. This antimicrobial agent may be useful in patients who are allergic to TMP/SMZ or when patients do not respond to the first course of treatment with TMP/SMZ. In these situations, furazolidone could be used with the hope of exploiting its activity against other suspected agents such as *Giardia lamblia* or *Campylobacter jejuni.* Furazolidone should not be used in patients with presumed or proved severe shigellosis and/or those who need to be hospitalized.

Finally, because travelers' diarrhea can manifest itself several days after a person has been infected, it is very important for the physician to ask the family about travel whenever treating a child with diarrhea. About 10 percent of travelers develop chronic diarrhea. In these patients, a concerted clinical evaluation is needed to explore the possibility of parasitic infection or other conditions such as tropical sprue, small bowel bacterial overgrowth, and inflammatory bowel disease, in relation to the acute episode.

SUGGESTED READING

Committee on Nutrition. Use of oral fluid therapy and post-treatment feeding following enteritis in children in a developed country. Am Acad Pediatr 1985; 75:358–360.

DuPont HL. Non-fluid therapy and selected chemoprophylaxis of acute diarrhea. Am J Med 1985; 78(Supp 6B):81–90.

Johnson PC, DuPont HL, Ericsson CD. Chemoprophylaxis of travelers' diarrhea in children. Pediatr Infect Dis 1985; 4:620–621.

Listernick R, Zieserl E, Davis T. Outpatient oral rehydration in the United States. Am J Dis Child 1986; 140:211–220.

Steffen R, van der Linde F, Gyr K, et al. Epidemiology of diarrhea in travelers. JAMA 1983; 249:1176–1180.

Travelers Diarrhea Consensus Conference, Office of Medical Applications of Research, NIH, Bethesda, MD JAMA, 1985; 253:2700–2704.

DISEASES OF THE MUSCULOSKELETAL SYSTEM

SUPPURATIVE ARTHRITIS AND OSTEOMYELITIS

SHELDON L. KAPLAN, M.D.

SUPPURATIVE ARTHRITIS

The initial approach to management of the child with suppurative arthritis is based on several factors. The age of the child provides some clue as to etiology. *Haemophilus influenzae* type b is the most common organism isolated from children with suppurative arthritis between 6 and 24 months of age, although it should be considered for children up to 10 years old. *Staphylococcus aureus,* which is recovered from all age groups, is the next most common organism overall in children. *Streptococcus pneumoniae* and group A *Streptococcus* should also be considered in all age groups. *Neisseria gonorrhoeae* may be responsible for arthritis at any age, but particularly so during adolescence. Group B *Streptococcus, S. aureus,* and Enterobacteriaceae account for most cases in neonates, although *Candida* sp are isolated increasingly frequently in association with central hyperalimentation. *Fungi* and Enterobacteriaceae are major causes of joint infection in children who are immunocompromised. Infections caused by *Salmonella* sp and *S. pneumoniae* occur more commonly in young children with hemoglobinopathies.

Gram stain of synovial fluid may help guide initial antibiotic therapy. If definite gram-positive cocci are noted, treatment can be directed against *S. aureus* and streptococci. When gram-negative pleomorphic rods are identified, antibiotics that are active against *H. influenzae* type b (including β-lactamase–producing strains) are administered. Occasionally, bacterial polysaccharide antigen in synovial fluid, blood, or urine can be detected. When suppurative arthritis is associated with other systemic infections such as meningitis, the causative agent is likely to be responsible for both sites of infection.

The parenteral administration of antibiotics achieves antibiotic concentrations in synovial fluid exceeding in vitro minimal inhibitory concentration (MIC). Therefore, antibiotics do not need to be injected directly into the joint space, a procedure that may actually lead to greater damage of the joint. Furthermore, in my experience, continuous irrigation of the joint space is even more hazardous and has been associated with serious secondary bacterial infections.

Once an organism has been recovered, the most active, specific, and safe antibiotic is administered as established by in vitro susceptibility tests. In some patients, particularly those with abnormalities in host defense, determining the MIC and the minimal bactericidal concentration (MBC) for selected antibiotics is helpful for choosing the most appropriate antimicrobial therapy. Unfortunately, even when adequate cultures of synovial fluid and blood are obtained, the etiology of the suppurative arthritis is frequently not determined.

In the neonate, a combination of methicillin (100 to 150 mg per kilogram per day) and an aminoglycoside provides adequate initial antibiotic coverage. Alternatively, cefotaxime could be substituted for the aminoglycoside, if *Pseudomonas* sp is not a concern. Knowledge of the antimicrobial susceptibility of the organisms colonizing the infant, as well as the nursery flora in general, is invaluable for selecting appropriate initial therapy. In addition, it is necessary to evaluate the infant for concomitant osteomyelitis, which frequently precedes neonatal suppurative arthritis.

Initial Antibiotic Therapy

Cefuroxime therapy adequately covers the most common organisms causing septic arthritis in normal children between 2 months and 10 years of age. I usually recommend that cefuroxime be administered in a dosage of 100 to 150 mg per kilogram per day, in three divided doses, as initial therapy until an organism is isolated. When *S. aureus* is recovered, nafcillin or oxacillin (150 to 200 mg per kilogram per day IV in four to six divided doses) is continued if the organism is susceptible to methicillin. During therapy with nafcillin, the white blood cell and differential count should be determined twice weekly to detect the development of neutropenia, which generally occurs during the second to third week of treatment. Cefazolin (100 mg per kilogram per day) and clindamycin (30 to 40 mg per kilogram per day in three divided doses) are alternative agents for the penicillin-allergic patient. Vancomycin (40 to 60 mg per kilogram per day in four divided doses) is the drug of choice for treating infection caused by methicillin-resistant *S. aureus* or *S. epidermidis,* predominantly nosocomial pathogens. Ampicillin (150 to 200 mg per kilogram per day in four to six divided doses) is administered if ampicillin-susceptible *H. influenzae* type b is recovered. Cefuroxime can be continued if ampicillin-resistant *H. influenzae* type b is isolated, although chloramphenicol (50 to 75 mg per kilogram per day in four divided doses) remains the gold standard for the treatment of infections caused by *H. influenzae* type b that is resistant to ampicillin. Ampicillin- and chloramphenicol-resistant strains of *H. influenzae* type b currently are not common in the United States; however, either cefotaxime (100 to 200 mg per kilogram per day in four divided doses) or ceftriaxone (50 to 75 mg per kilogram per day in two divided doses) is probably the drug of choice. Susceptible strains of *S. pneumoniae, S. pyogenes, N. meningitidis,* and *N. gonorrhoeae* are best treated with aqueous penicillin G (100,000 to 200,000 U per kilogram per day in four to six divided doses). Penicillin G should be adequate therapy for arthritis caused by strains of *S. pneumoniae* relatively resistant to penicillin; however, if there is any question that the patient is not responding to penicillin therapy as expected, chloramphenicol or vancomycin is the most established alternative antibiotic.

For normal children older than 10 years of age, nafcillin or oxacillin (not to exceed 12 g per day) alone is adequate initial coverage. For immunocompromised older children, nafcillin or oxacillin plus an aminoglycoside or cefotaxime is reasonable. Fungal arthritis requires therapy with amphotericin B.

Surgical Therapy

In addition to antimicrobial therapy, the infected joint should be drained either by needle aspiration or by surgical incision and drainage. Orthopaedic colleagues should be consulted to help determine the optimal approach to drainage. Except for the hip joint, in many instances, repeat needle aspiration is all that is required to obtain adequate drainage. If the erythema, swelling, and tenderness surrounding the joint do not respond to repeated aspirations or are clearly increasing, open surgical drainage should be undertaken. Open surgical management is also required for removal of foreign bodies secondary to penetrating injuries.

Suppurative arthritis of the hip can compromise blood supplied to the femoral head through the acetabular branch of the medial femoral circumflex artery, which courses into the acetabular fossa and reaches the femur by means of the ligamentum teres; therefore, surgical incision and drainage of the hip is considered mandatory by most authorities. Immobilization of the affected joint may help relieve pain. As the infection is clearly responding, some physical therapy to promote joint mobility and strengthen unused muscles generally is desirable.

Duration of Therapy

The duration and route of administration for the antibiotics is somewhat dependent on the circumstances. In general, *H. influenzae* type b disease requires at least 2 weeks of total therapy. Arthritis caused by *S. aureus* or Enterobacteriaceae should be treated for a minimum of 3 weeks. Suppurative arthritis secondary to *N. gonorrhoeae* should be treated for at least 7 days. Immunocompromised hosts and neonates should be treated longer than normal patients. Most children are afebrile after 5 to 7 days of therapy. I recommend that antibiotics should be administered for the minimum duration already stated, or until the erythrocyte sedimentation rate is less than 20 mm per hour, whichever is longer.

Alternative Modes of Therapy

Several studies have demonstrated that oral administration is as effective as parenteral administration of antibiotics once the patient has responded satisfactorily to initial treatment. However, the decision to switch from parenteral to oral antibiotics requires several prerequisites. First, an oral antibiotic exists with adequate antimicrobial activity against the patient's isolate, assuming that an organism has been recovered. Second, there is a responsible adult who can assure the physician that the child will get the desired antibiotic at the correct intervals. Third, the child can take and tolerate the oral agent. Finally, the physician must be able to monitor the patient frequently to ensure compliance and continued improvement.

If oral antibiotics have been initiated, I like to obtain peak (1 to 1½ hours after a dose) and trough (immediately before administration of a dose) serum bactericidal titers (SBT) while the child is still in the hospital. Optimally, the peak SBT is equal to or greater than 1:8, and the trough level is measurable (equal to or greater than 1:2). After discharge, the child is seen weekly, at which time I continue to monitor the SBT as a means of assessing compliance. Oral therapy is continued while the criteria, stated earlier, are met. In some children, oral antibiotics are continued in the hospital because no one at home can reliably administer the drug. Dicloxacillin (75 to 100 mg per kilogram per day in four divided doses) is my initial choice for an oral agent to complete therapy of *S. aureus* infection. Unfortunately, many children cannot tolerate this dosage of dicloxacillin, and an alternative agent such a cephalexin or clindamycin is required. Chloramphenicol is the best-studied agent for oral therapy of arthritis caused by ampicillin-resistant *H. influenzae* type b. Although ampicillin–clavulanate potassium is adequate for ampicillin-resistant *H. influenzae,* I have found that many children have excessive diarrhea with the large dosage of ampicillin (75 mg per kilogram per day) I employ. (Interpreting the SBT during oral therapy for *H. influenzae* type b arthritis is tricky; I prefer to measure the serum concentration of the antibiotic in this instance.)

Another alternative to parenteral therapy in the hospital is home intravenous therapy under the supervision of a home therapy team. In this situation, ceftriaxone is particularly convenient to use because of its prolonged half-life in serum. Ceftriaxone can be administered either twice (50 to 75 mg per kilogram per day in two divided doses) or once (50 mg per kilogram) daily for serious infections caused by *H. influenzae* type b. I do not use this agent for disease caused by *S. aureus.*

Although the joint infection may be adequately controlled by antibiotic therapy and the drainage procedures, some children continue to have synovial inflammation for several weeks. This seems to respond to aspirin.

Young age (less than 6 months), prolonged duration of symptoms prior to treatment, infection of the hip and infection caused by *S. aureus* are risk factors for orthopaedic sequelae such as irreversible cartilage damage, stiff joint with poor mobility, abnormal bone growth, unstable joint, and chronic dislocation. Fortunately the majority of children have no permanent sequelae following septic arthritis.

OSTEOMYELITIS

Staphylococcus aureus is the most common organism causing hematogenously acquired osteomyelitis in children. Puncture wounds of the foot through soft-soled shoes are associated with osteochondritis caused by *Pseudomonas aeruginosa* or organisms recovered from soil. Osteomyelitis contiguous to a wound usually is related to the organism causing the wound infection. Group B streptococcus, *Staphylococcus aureus,* and the Enterobacteriaceae are the most likely causes of neonatal osteomyelitis. As with suppurative arthritis, an underlying host-defense deficiency may lead to infection with unusual organisms such as Enterobacteraciae or fungi. *Salmonella* is a major pathogen causing osteomyelitis in children with sickle cell hemoglobinopathies. Anaerobic bacteria are infrequent causes of childhood osteomyelitis, but are usually associated with an indolent course. Unlike suppurative arthritis, *H. influenzae* type b is not commonly isolated from children with osteomyelitis.

Antibiotic Therapy

Optimal therapy of osteomyelitis requires the isolation of a pathogen or pathogens and determining the antimicrobial susceptibility pattern of the isolate.

Thus, every effort should be expended to recover a pathogen from blood cultures, bone aspiration, and/or surgical specimens. After adequate cultures have been obtained, initial antibiotic therapy may be guided by the findings on Gram stain. If osteomyelitis is thought to have occurred by the hematogenous route in an otherwise normal child and the Gram stain shows either gram-positive cocci or no organisms, I recommend starting therapy with nafcillin or oxacillin (200 mg per kilogram per day in four to six divided doses). For patients with osteomyelitis of the foot secondary to puncture wounds, ticarcillin plus an aminoglycoside is a reasonable combination to start until the culture results are known. Vancomycin is included in initial empiric therapy if methicillin-resistant staphylococci are a known nosocomial pathogen and the child is at risk for a hospital-acquired infection (e.g., osteomyelitis secondary to a surgical procedure). If gram-negative bacilli are seen in specimens from infection associated with open fracture, penetrating or puncture wound, or postoperative infection, a combination of an extended-spectrum penicillin (ticarcillin, piperacillin, etc.) plus an aminoglycoside is recommended. Methicillin plus an aminoglycoside or cefotaxime is a reasonable empiric combination for the neonate. Once an organism is isolated, the most specific therapy should be continued intravenously (Table 1).

In vitro MIC and MBC determinations are useful to confirm antibiotic susceptibilities by disk testing. I also obtain peak and trough serum bactericidal titers (SBT). Antibiotics should be administered intravenously until the child is afebrile for several days and has demonstrated definite clinical evidence of response. At this time, depending on the experience of the physician and available resources, therapy is completed by the intravenous route, or oral administration is considered. Several studies have shown that osteomyelitis, particularly that caused by *S. aureus,* can be treated successfully with an oral antibiotic when the proper precautions are understood. Clindamycin may not be bactericidal for some strains of *S. aureus* and, for this reason, should be avoided for the child with a host-defense abnormality. As with suppurative arthritis, optimal oral treatment is undertaken when a pathogen has been isolated and adequate SBT can be documented while the child remains under hospital care. The same careful approach to follow-up and monitoring of compliance is required for oral therapy of osteomyelitis as was outlined for suppurative arthritis. Home intravenous therapy is another alternative to complete therapy.

Unfortunately, it is common not to recover a pathogen even when appropriate cultures are obtained. In this instance, if the patient has responded to initial antibiotic therapy, which in most cases is nafcillin or oxacillin, the same antibiotic is continued to complete the course of therapy. I am reluctant to recommend oral therapy when a pathogen has not been isolated.

TABLE 1 Antibiotic Therapy for Osteomyelitis

Pathogen	Antibiotic	Dosage (mg/kg/day except as noted)
Staphylococcus aureus	Nafcillin or oxacillin	200
	Dicloxacillin	75–100
	Clindamycin	30–40
Methicillin-resistant *S. aureus*	Vancomycin	40
Group A or B *Streptococcus*	Aq penicillin G	200,000–250,000 U
Pseudomonas	Ticarcillin or piperacillin plus appropriate aminoglycoside	300
	Alternative—ceftazidime	100–150
Salmonella	Ampicillin	200
	Chloramphenicol	50–75
	Trimethoprim–sulfamethoxazole	10-15 (trimethoprim component)
Enterobacteriaceae	Appropriate aminoglycoside	
	or	
	Cefotaxime	100–150
	or	
	Ceftriaxone	50–75
H. influenzae type b		
Ampicillin susceptible	Ampicillin	150–200
Ampicillin resistant	Chloramphenicol	50–75
	or	
	Cefuroxime	100–150
	or	
	Cefotaxime	100–150
	or	
	Ceftriaxone	50–75

Surgical Therapy

Surgical intervention for osteomyelitis is indicated to obtain adequate specimens for culture, especially in unusual cases, and is probably also indicated to drain suppurative collections identified by aspiration of bone. The timing and extent of the surgical procedure is individualized for each child, in consultation with an orthopaedic surgeon. Some authorities recommend that surgical intervention for osteomyelitis be restricted to drainage of pus in the subperiosteal space or other tissue planes. Surgical debridement is crucial for successful therapy of *Pseudomonas* osteochondritis following a puncture wound of the foot. In the neonate, other sites of osteomyelitis not clinically evident should be sought initially by skeletal survey; bone scan may be positive when the plain radiographs are equivocal for osteomyelitis. Infection of a contiguous joint is common in neonates.

Duration of Therapy

For most children with osteomyelitis, the minimum duration of antibiotic therapy is 3 weeks. I prefer to treat children for at least 3 weeks, or until the erythrocyte sedimentation rate (ESR) is 20 mm per hour or less, whichever takes longer. Roentgenograms of the involved extremity are also followed until healing is complete. If thorough surgical debridement has been performed for *Pseudomonas* infection of the foot, 2 weeks of antibiotic therapy appears to be adequate.

Affected extremities should be immobilized initially to help reduce pain and possible further injury resulting from trauma. Weight bearing should be avoided for affected lower extremities until some healing has occurred, because of the risk of pathologic fracture.

Most children have no skeletal sequelae from osteomyelitis. Inadequate or delayed therapy may lead to chronic osteomyelitis, growth disturbance (or total destruction) of bone, pathologic fracture, and joint deformities. These complications are more likely to occur in the neonate.

SUGGESTED READING

Dich VQ, Nelson JD, Haltalin KC. Osteomyelitis in infants and children. A review of 163 cases. Am J Dis Child 1975; 129:1273–1278.

Edwards MS, Baker CJ, Wagner ML, et al. An etiologic shift in infantile osteomyelitis: the emergence of the Group B streptococcus. J Pediatr 1978; 93:578–583.

Goldenberg DL, Reed JI. Bacterial arthritis. N Engl J Med 1985; 312:764–771.

Jacobs RF, Adelman L, Sack CM, Wilson CB. Management of pseudomonas osteochondritis complicating puncture wounds of the foot. Pediatrics 1982; 69:432–435.

Nelson JD. The bacterial etiology and antibiotic management of septic arthritis in infants and children. Pediatrics 1972; 50:437–440.

Prober CG, Yeager AS. Use of the bactericidal titer to assess the adequacy of oral antibiotic therapy in the treatment of acute hematogenous osteomyelitis. J Pediatr 1979; 95:131–135.

Rotbart HA, Glode MP. *Haemophilus influenzae* type b septic arthritis in children: report of 23 cases. Pediatrics 1985; 75:254–259.

Tetzlaff TR, McCracken GH Jr, Nelson JD. Oral antibiotic therapy for skeletal infections of children. II. Therapy of osteomyelitis and septic arthritis. J Pediatr 1978; 92:485–490.

Waldvogel FA, Medoff G, Swartz MN. Osteomyelitis: a review of clinical features, therapeutic considerations and unusual aspects. N Engl J Med 1970; 282:198–206, 260–266, 316–322.

Welkon CJ, Long SS, Fisher MC, Alburger PD. Pyogenic arthritis in infants and children: a review of 95 cases. Pediatr Infect Dis 1986; 5:669–676.

SUPPURATIVE BURSITIS

KEVIN M. SHANNON, M.D.

The bursae are fluid-filled spaces lined with synovial membranes that function as physiologic cushions in skeletal movements. Bacterial infections of the bursae are uncommon in infants and children. A history of antecedent trauma is often elicited; physical findings include fever and erythema, swelling, and tenderness of the affected bursa. The prepatellar bursa is most often involved. *Staphylococcus aureus* is isolated from the bursal fluid of 90 percent of patients with suppurative bursitis.

Management of suppurative bursitis involves surgical drainage and specific antimicrobial therapy. Early percutaneous aspiration of the involved bursa is essential for accurate diagnosis and may provide adequate initial drainage unless the fluid is thick and tenacious. In suppurative bursitis, bursal aspirates are exudative with white blood cell counts in excess of 1,000 per mm^3 (predominantly polymorphonuclear cells). The fluid should be Gram stained and cultured. Additional studies include a complete blood count, blood cultures (in febrile children), and an erythrocyte sedimentation rate (ESR). Technitium pyrophosphate imaging should be performed to rule out other sites of involvement, particularly in contiguous bones and joints.

I believe that all children with suppurative bursitis should be admitted to the hospital and treated with intravenous antibiotics. The choice of antimicrobial therapy should be guided by the results of the Gram stain and by the data showing that *Staphylococcus* sp. and *Streptococcus* sp. cause more than 95 percent of cases. In most patients, single-agent therapy with either nafcillin (100 to 150 mg per kilogram per day in divided doses given every 6 hours) or cefazolin (75 to 100 mg per kilogram per day in divided doses given every 8 hours) is appropriate. In the infant or young child who is febrile and "looks sick," I favor an initial antimicrobial regimen that provides broad-spectrum coverage. The first dose of antibiotics should be deferred until the bursa has been aspirated.

Most patients are considerably improved after one day of therapy. Serial examinations of the involved bursa are essential to assess the adequacy of initial drainage. Patients not originally treated by incision and drainage are at risk for residual or recurrent bursal exudates that should be drained. Clinical improvement is characterized by improvement of acute inflammatory findings in the affected bursa and by resolution of fever and other systemic signs. Studies in adults have shown that bursal fluids are sterile after 2 to 3 days of antimicrobial therapy. In one series, all bursal infections were cured in patients who received antibiotics for an additional 5 days.

Excellent antibiotic concentrations can be achieved in bursal fluid after oral administration of large dosages of antibiotics. I therefore feel that parenteral therapy can be safely discontinued after 48 to 72 hours in children who show a good clinical response and in whom there is no evidence of concurrent osteomyelitis or septic arthritis. In these patients, oral antibiotics are continued for an additional 5 to 7 days on an outpatient basis. At the completion of antibiotic therapy, the patient should be carefully reassessed. I repeat the ESR if it was elevated at diagnosis. It should be normal or near-normal; persistent elevation suggests inadequate drainage or an undiagnosed site of infection. Complete recovery is universal in childhood suppurative bursitis managed with drainage and antibiotics. Long-term local complications and recurrent infections have not been reported.

SUGGESTED READING

Ho G, Su EY. Antibiotic therapy of septic bursitis. Arthritis Rheum 1981; 24:905–911.

Ho G, Tice AD. Comparison of septic and nonseptic bursitis. Arch Intern Med 1979; 139:1269–1273.

Ho G, Tice AD, Kaplan SD. Septic bursitis in the prepatellar and olecranon bursae. Ann Intern Med 1978; 89:21–27.

Meyers S, Lonon W, Shannon K. Suppurative bursitis in early childhood. Pediatr Infect Dis 1984; 3:156–158.

Paisley JW. Septic bursitis in childhood. J Pediatr Orthop 1982; 2:57–61.

PYOMYOSITIS

PISESPONG PATAMASUCON, B.Sc.(Med), M.D.

Pyomyositis is a suppurative infection of large skeletal muscles formerly called tropical pyomyositis because of the prevalence in tropical areas of Asia and Africa. Although unusual in areas with a temperate climate, pyomyositis has been reported in the United States since 1971. The disease is more common among males, with a male:female ratio of 1.4–4.0:1.0.

In Asia the disease is commonly seen among those under 10 years old, but in Africa, it is common around age 20 to 40. A single skeletal muscle is involved more often than multiple sites. It is more common in a large skeletal muscle such as the thigh, followed by the buttock, shoulder, back, abdominal wall, and leg. The psoas and iliacus are obscure sites of pyomyositis that I have encountered in the last 5 years.

The pathogenesis of pyomyositis is still not agreed on, but various predisposing factors have been identified, such as trauma, parasites, viruses, malnutrition, and anemia. Because the site of entry is rarely apparent and multiple, distant sites are involved in some cases, one cannot exclude hematogenous spread. If this occurs, it must be transient and early in the course of the disease, because blood cultures are generally negative. *Staphylococcus aureus* is the most common etiologic agent, accounting for more than 95 percent of cases. Streptococci, *Escherichia coli, Staphylococcus epidermidis,* and *Pasteurella* make up the rest.

The diagnosis of pyomyositis should be considered in a child returning from tropical countries, having more than 10 percent eosinophiles, and presenting with fever plus edema and tenderness of a specific skeletal muscle. The definitive diagnosis can be obtained by needle aspirate of the involved muscle or from surgical exploration. However, the disease need not be excluded because the child has not been abroad. The disease can occur in obscure sites such as pelvic muscles, mimicking appendicitis or arthritis of the hip joint. Radionuclide imaging, ultrasonography, and computerized tomography can help in making the correct diagnosis even in obscure sites.

Pyomyositis can be divided into three stages:

1. *The invasive stage* occurs within 1 week of the disease, and there is no pus in the infected muscle.
2. *The suppurative stage* occurs about 10 to 21 days after onset. The patient is usually febrile, with definite signs of inflammation and tenderness of the muscle. Aspiration usually yields pus.
3. *The late stage* occurs after 21 days, when the patient may look very sick, with definite sign of abscess and occasionally septicemia.

Blood cultures and needle aspirate should be followed by use of intravenous antibiotic. Nafcillin, cloxacillin, or methicillin (100 to 150 mg per kilogram per day) should be given intravenously in four divided doses. (Cloxacillin for intravenous use is not available in the United States.) If pus is obtained, surgical drainage must be done. Aside from the Gram stain and culture of the pus, susceptibilies of the causative microorganism must be done to identify methicillin-resistant staphylococci. If pus cannot be obtained, I empirically give the preceding antibiotic for 2 days and reaspirate. The antibiotic is given intravenously for 7 to 10 days in the hospital and then orally (dicloxacillin 50 to 75 mg per kilogram per day in three divided doses) at home for 7 more days. If satellite involvement occurs, such as osteomyelitis or pericarditis, the duration of antibiotic administration should be longer and the necessary surgical support should be given. In the case of methicillin-resistant *Staphylococcus aureus* infection vancomycin, 40 mg per kilogram per day, should be given intravenously, in divided doses every 6 hours, for 7 to 10 days.

SUGGESTED READING

Chacha PB. Muscle abscesses in children. Clin Orthop 1970; 70:174–180.

Chiedozi LC. Pyomyositis: review of 205 cases in 112 patients. Am J Surg 1979; 137:255–259.

Firor HV. Acute psoas abscess in children. Clin Pediatr 1972; 11:228–231.

Joseph SC. Pyomyositis a "tropical" disease? Am J Dis Child 1975; 129:775–776.

Sirinavin S, McCracken GH. Primary suppurative myositis in children. Am J Dis Child 1979; 133:263–265.

DISEASES OF THE SKIN AND SKIN STRUCTURES

CELLULITIS

CHARLES G. PROBER, M.D.

Cellulitis, an infection of the skin and subcutaneous tissues, is a common infection in children. The etiology is best predicted from a carefully performed history and physical examination. When tissue aspiration is performed, bacteria can be recovered from culture approximately 50 percent of the time. In general, blood cultures have a low diagnostic yield except in very young, systemically ill children. Empiric antibiotic therapy is based on a prediction of the most likely pathogen(s), and definitive therapy is based on a positive culture, when available. Assessing the response to therapy is primarily based on frequent examination of the involved area and monitoring for evidence of spread to deeper tissues (e.g., muscle, fascia, or bone) or dissemination. Unless a complication ensues, surgical intervention is unnecessary.

For the sake of ease of presentation, I discuss cellulitis under the following headings: cellulitis in the neonate, cellulitis in infants and children, cellulitis following trauma, and blistering dactylitis.

CELLULITIS IN THE NEONATE

Cellulitis is not a common infection in neonates. When it does occur, streptococci (especially group B) and staphylococci are the most likely causitive agents. Enteric pathogens, an otherwise common cause of neonatal sepsis, are rarely implicated. I recommend empiric therapy with parenteral nafcillin, 50 to 100 mg per kilogram of body weight per day in two to three divided doses. If group A or B streptococci are isolated, parenteral penicillin G, 50,000 to 100,000 units per kilogram per day in two to four divided doses, is recommended. For both nafcillin and penicillin, the lower dosage and less frequent dosing intervals are used in low-birth weight (under 2,000 g) and/or young (less than 7 days) neonates. In the unusual event that a gram-negative bacillus is isolated, therapy with parenteral gentamicin, 5 to 7.5 mg per kilogram per day in two to three divided doses, is appropriate unless susceptibility testing identifies a gentamicin-resistant pathogen. Five to 7 days of treatment is usually sufficient. I usually recommend that the total course of therapy be given by the parenteral route.

CELLULITIS IN INFANTS AND CHILDREN

The most common etiologies of cellulitis in infants and children are *Haemophilus influenzae* type b, group A *Streptococcus,* and *Staphylococcus aureus.* The specific etiology often can be predicted by the clinical circumstances. For example, cellulitis involving the face (buccal or preseptal periorbital areas) of children younger than 3 years of age is most often caused by *H. influenzae* type b, unless the cellulitis was preceded by trauma (see later). *Streptococcus pneumoniae* has been identified as a less frequent cause of this form of cellulitis. Before initiating therapy in these young, often systemically ill children, one should perform a blood culture. In those children younger than 12 to 18 months of age, a lumbar puncture should also be performed even if undue irritability or signs of meningeal irritation are absent. Meningitis may be silently present in these young children. Because many isolates of *H. influenzae* type b are resistant to ampicillin, I favor treatment with parenteral cefuroxime, 100 mg per kilogram per day in three divided doses. The third-generation cephalosporins, cefotaxime (100 mg per kilogram per day in three divided doses), and ceftriaxone (75 mg per kilogram per day in two divided doses), are suitable alternatives. I recommend 7 days of therapy. Parenteral therapy is continued until clinical resolution is almost complete (usually 2 to 3 days), at which time oral therapy can be substituted. Cefaclor, 40 mg per kilogram per day in three divided doses, is my preference for the oral phase of therapy.

Two other causes of cellulitis, often predictable from clinical presentation, are cellulitis caused by group A streptococci (erysipelas) and cellulitis caused by *Erysipelothrix rhusiopathiae* (erysipeloid). Erysipelas can occur in a child of any age. A history of preceding trauma (including surgery) may or may not be obtained. Typically, the spread of brilliant erythema is rapid and the leading edge is elevated. It may present anywhere on the body. I initiate therapy intravenously with penicillin G, 150,000 units per kilogram per day in four divided doses. After nearly complete clinical resolution, I change therapy to oral penicillin V, 50 mg per kilogram per day in four divided doses, and complete a total course of therapy of 7 days. Erythromycin, 40 mg per kilogram per day in four divided doses, is my alternative choice for the penicillin-allergic patient. It is common for the skin lesion to continue to spread during the first 12 hours or so of therapy.

The cause of erysipeloid, *E. rhusiopathiae,* is a gram-positive microaerophilic bacillus. Patients with this infection usually present with cellulitis, typically evolving 1 to 7 days after exposure to raw fish, crab, poultry, or pork products. Fishermen and butchers are therefore most at risk for this infection, although it has occurred in settings without a recognized environmental exposure. Progression after inoculation is usually by centrifugal spread with central clearing, from a red maculopapular lesion to a target-shaped lesion with a clear center and a red or blue peripheral ring. When the cellulitis is on the hands, the typical clinical lesions are violet or purple, warm, tender plaques. The patient is usually afebrile, and even without treatment, the disease tends to regress spontaneously over a 2- to 3-week period. However, because this organism can cause septicemia with or without focal complications, antibiotic treatment is indicated. The choice and duration of treatment are precisely the same as was described for erysipelas.

CELLULITIS FOLLOWING TRAUMA

Cellulitis following trauma, even if the trauma is only a superficial scratch, is almost always caused by group A streptococci and *S. aureus.* If a foreign body has complicated the trauma, it must be removed for therapy to be successful. Also, cellulitis unresponsive to antibiotic therapy should always raise the consideration of a foreign body.

Regarding antibiotic therapy; if the cellulitis is localized and the patient is not systemically ill, outpatient therapy is often sufficient. Under this circumstance, I recommend dicloxacillin, 25 to 50 mg per kilogram per day in four divided doses. Erythromycin, 40 mg per kilogram per day in four divided doses, is my alternative choice for the penicillin-allergic patient. If the cellulitis is not localized, or the patient is systemically ill, I would hospitalize the patient and initiate parenteral therapy with both nafcillin, 100 mg per kilogram per day in four divided doses, and

penicillin G, 150,000 units per kilogram per day also in four divided doses. Although nafcillin alone may be adequate, I have seen clinical progression on this therapy, presumably because of insufficient activity against group A streptococci. Duration of therapy depends on the extent of the cellulitis and response to treatment. In general, however, a 7-day course of antibiotics is sufficient.

An unusual form of cellulitis of the foot occurs after puncture-wound injuries. This cellulitis is often secondary to *Pseudomonas aeruginosa* and it may be complicated by osteomyelitis of the bones of the foot. An aggressive diagnostic workup is indicated, including a soft-tissue aspirate for bacterial culture, a radiographic assessment of the contiguous bones, and a bone aspirate for bacterial cultures if there is any question of osteomyelitis. Therapy with parenteral ticarcillin, 200 mg per kilogram per day in four divided doses, and tobramycin, 5 mg per kilogram per day in three divided doses, is recommended. After surgical debridement of any infected tissue, therapy is continued for approximately 2 weeks.

BLISTERING DACTYLITIS

Blistering dactylitis, an infection that involves the distal portion of a digit, is caused by group A streptococci and results in a painful, superficial blistering lesion over the fat pad of the digit. Treatment consists of antistreptococcal antibiotics. Oral penicillin V, 50 mg per kilogram per day in four divided doses, or erythromycin, 40 to 50 mg per kilogram per day in three divided doses, is the antibiotic of choice. Therapy should be continued for 7 to 10 days.

SUGGESTED READING

Carter S, Feldman WE. Etiology and treatment of facial cellulitis in pediatric patients. Pediatr Infect Dis 1983; 2:222–224.
Fleisher G, Ludwig S, Campos J. Cellulitis; bacterial etiology, clinical features, and laboratory findings. J Pediatr 1980; 97:590–593. 97:590–593.
Lacroix J, Delage G, Mitchell G. Erysipeloid in an infant. J Pediatr 1981; 99:745–746.
Uman SJ, Kunin CM. Needle aspiration in the diagnosis of soft tissue infections. Arch Intern Med 1975; 135:959–961.

IMPETIGO AND PYODERMA

HUGH C. DILLON JR., M.D.

Pyoderma and impetigo are common terms for superficial skin infection. Group A streptococci and *Staphylococcus aureus* are the causative organisms. Distinct forms of impetigo can be related to the spe-

cific infectious agent. Streptococcal lesions are purulent, tend to form shallow craters, and become covered with honey-colored or brown crusts. Pyoderma is an accurate term to describe them. Such lesions often become secondarily colonized with staphylococci. Cultures usually reveal either pure growth of group A streptococci or streptococci plus a variable number of staphylococcal colonies. Bullous lesions, large fluid-filled lesions that contain very few leukocytes, are *not* purulent, and are uniformly caused by certain toxin-producing strains of *S. aureus* that are closely related to those causing the scalded skin syndrome in young infants. Bullous impetigo is rarely secondarily colonized by group A streptococci.

Bullous impetigo usually occurs during hot weather. Minor skin trauma is not a predisposing condition. The infection is most common in infants and young children. Lesions typically occur on the buttocks, trunk, axillae, and face. Crops of lesions occur and may coalesce; when they rupture, a thin, varnishlike crust develops. Neither bacteremia nor suppurative complications are associated with this disease. Nasal carriage of the staphylococcus is common and likely contributes to reinfection as well as spread to close contacts.

Streptococcal impetigo occurs most often during hot and humid months and during rainy seasons in tropical and semitropical climates. Minor skin trauma, especially mosquito bites, plays an important role in the pathogenesis of the infection. Lesions occur on exposed extremities and the face. Blisters, minor burns, puncture wounds, and other breaks in the skin commonly become infected. Acute lymphadenitis is common early, and regional lymphadenopathy is a hallmark of persistent, untreated infection. Cellulitis or acute lymphangitis may occur, usually early in the infection. Bacteremia is uncommon. The disease is most common in lower socioeconomic groups, in young children. Children with streptococcal pharyngitis occasionally develop skin lesions around the nose or mouth.

Acute poststreptococcal glomerulonephritis may occur following skin infection with "nephritogenic" serotypes of streptococci. It has not been demonstrated that treatment regularly prevents acute glomerulonephritis (AGN). This is partly because patients delay seeking treatment. It is important to evaluate and treat infected contacts of patients with AGN, to minimize spread of nephritogenic streptococci and prevent further cases.

THERAPY

Systemic antibiotic therapy for impetigo (Table 1) or pyoderma is based on providing a regimen of proved value for the specific form of infection being treated. Several effective regimens are listed in the table for the two common forms of impetigo. Benzathine penicillin G (BPG), although effective for streptococcal impetigo, can cause painful local reactions, and there is also a slightly higher risk of acute allergic reactions with intramuscular than with oral penicillin. I prefer to limit the use of BPG for patients unable or unwilling to comply with oral treatment. BPG should *not* be given to infants and children with bullous impetigo. Staphylococci causing this infection are uniformly resistant to penicillin G.

Penicillin, either the oral or the intramuscular preparation, is effective therapy for streptococcal impetigo, including cases in which lesions yield both group A streptococci and *S. aureus.* More than 85 percent of the latter strains are now resistant to penicillin. However, the staphylococci are of secondary importance and are usually eradicated as the streptococcal infection clears. Thus, penicillin remains an inexpensive and effective agent and can be chosen as initial treatment for nonbullous cases of impetigo. Treatment for a minimum of 7 days is required; I prefer 10 days of treatment to reduce the risk of reinfection. Erythromycin is a very good alternative oral antibiotic regimen, and is effective against both streptococcal impetigo (with or without staphylococci in lesions) and staphylococcal bullous impetigo. If erythromycin estolate is used, a lower dosage (20 mg per kilogram) can be prescribed. At this dosage, the estolate preparation compares favorably in cost and efficacy with a 40-mg-per-kilogram dosage regimen of the ethyl succinate preparation. Currently, approximately 90 to 95 percent of group A streptococci and *S. aureus* in this country are susceptible to erythromycin.

Clindamycin is effective for both streptococcal and staphylococcal forms of skin infection. Although I have not encountered significant adverse reactions, I reserve this drug for patients allergic to other agents, or for those who experience treatment failure with one or more normally effective drugs. Clindamycin is

TABLE 1 Recommended Antibiotic Therapy for Impetigo

Antibiotics	For Streptococcal Impetigo (±S. aureus in Lesions)	For Staphylococcal Impetigo
Benzathine penicillin G*	600,000 U IM < 60 lb 1.2 million U IM > 60 lb	Not recommended
Penicillin V	500 mg/day < 40 lb 1 g/day > 40 lb (bid, tid, or qid)	Not recommended
Erythromycin (estolate or ethyl succinate)	20–40 mg/kg/day (bid, tid, or qid)	30–50 mg/kg/day (tid or qid)
Cephalosporins (cephalexin, cephradine, or cefaclor)	25–50 mg/kg/day (tid or qid)	Same
Penicillinase-resistant penicillins, e.g., dicloxacillin	20 mg/kg/day (max. 750; tid) 12.5 mg/kg/day (qid; max. 500)	Same Same
Clindamycin palmitate	8–12 mg/kg/day (bid, tid, or qid)	12–15 mg/kg/day (tid or qid)

* Mixtures containing BPG plus procaine penicillin may be substituted; a minimum dosage of 600,000 U of BPG is needed to ensure an adequate duration of therapy (7–10 days).

particularly effective in eradicating nasal carriage of staphylococci.

Oral cephalosporins are also very effective against either common form of skin infection. In recently completed, unpublished studies, I found cephalexin, given for either 7 or 10 days, to be somewhat more effective than penicillin for patients with streptococcal and mixed streptococcal–staphylococcal impetigo. The drug is well-tolerated, palatable, and safe.

Patients with staphylococcal bullous impetigo should be treated with an appropriate oral antibiotic. Treatment for 7 days is usually sufficient, but it may be continued for 10 days if the case is severe or if healing is delayed. The primary reasons for therapy are to hasten clearing of lesions, abort the infection, and reduce the risk of spread to others. Several regimens, as noted, have proved to be effective. Most recently, I have compared cephalexin and dicloxacillin therapy, using the former on a twice-daily schedule. Both drugs are quite effective, but cephalexin is better tolerated and more palatable for young children.

Summing up my current recommendation for streptococcal and staphylococcal impetigo, I prefer oral penicillin V for streptococcal infection because it is both effective and inexpensive. I use erythromycin or cephalexin for bullous impetigo; erythromycin is somewhat less expensive and most strains are susceptible. Both the latter drugs are acceptable alternatives for penicillin in the treatment of streptococcal skin infection. If one is uncertain of etiology, and cultures are not available, erythromycin is a good empirical "first choice" for patients with superficial skin infection.

Topical antibiotic therapy (bacitracin or combinations of bacitracin, neomycin, and polysporin) has a limited place in the treatment of impetigo. It is seldom useful in bullous impetigo; new crops of lesions tend to occur and the infection is difficult to bring under control without systemic antibiotic therapy. Topical therapy is occasionally useful in patients with a few streptococcal lesions, provided the antibiotic is applied regularly and diligently. I do not recommend decrusting lesions after healing begins and crusts become adherent. When using *systemic* therapy, it is *not* advisable to scrub lesions or remove crusts. In fact, this may delay healing by interfering with development of normal granulation tissue.

Recently, we have reported on the use of topical antibiotic therapy for prevention of streptococcal skin infection. This was demonstrated to be effective in a high-risk population in a day care center, where impetigo was an annual problem. It may be useful to use this approach, which involves application of the antibiotic ointment to minor forms of skin trauma, such as scratches, abrasions, and inflamed mosquito bites, in children known to be in contact with others with impetigo.

SKIN INFECTIONS ASSOCIATED WITH WHIRLPOOLS AND HOT TUBS

In recent years there have been reports associating skin infections with the use of whirlpool baths or hot tubs. The infection is usually caused by *Pseudomonas aeruginosa*. Epidemics have been described with a specific serotype of the latter organism being traced to the whirlpool. The typical infection includes folliculitis, a pruritic skin rash and, in some cases, otitis externa. Serious eye infections have also occurred. The skin infection is usually self-limited, but cases of invasive disease have required systemic therapy with antipseudomonal drugs. This is an infection that is best prevented by efforts to eliminate *Pseudomonas* from public facilities, and by acquainting users with potential risk. Showering after use has been suggested as one means of reducing risk of infection.

SUGGESTED READING

Dillon HC Jr. Impetigo contagiosa: suppurative and non-suppurative complications. I. Clinical, bacteriologic and epidemiologic characteristics of impetigo. Am J Dis Child 1968; 115:530–541.

Dillon HC, Jr. Topical and systemic therapy for pyodermas. Int J Dermatol 1980; 19:443–451.

Dillon HC Jr. Treatment of staphylococcal skin infections: a comparison of cephalexin and dicloxacillin. J Am Acad Dermatol 1983; 8:177–181.

Maddox JS, Ware JC, Dillon HC Jr. An investigation of the natural history of streptococcal skin infection and prevention with topical antibiotics. J Am Acad Dermatol 1985; 13:207–212.

Ratnam S, Hogan K, March SB, Butler RW. Whirlpool-associated folliculitis caused by *Pseudomonas aeruginosa:* report of an outbreak and review. J Clin Microbiol 1986; 23:655–659.

ACNE

LYNNE J. ROBERTS, M.D.

Acne vulgaris is an important disease because of its nearly universal occurrence as well as its considerable emotional impact. Acne is the most common skin disorder, affecting more than 85 percent of the American population at some time during their lives. Although mild in some, acne vulgaris is a devastating disease for many. Fortunately, recent advances have vastly improved the management of this disorder.

Acne is a multifactorial disease with three absolute requirements for clinical expression: (1) normal concentrations of circulating androgens, (2) sebaceous gland function and/or production of sebum, and (3) abnormal keratinization of follicular epithelium. Androgens are responsible for stimulating and maintaining sebaceous gland activity. Secondary factors modulate the expression of acne, including familial susceptibility, environmental insults, and bacterial flora. Bacteria are felt to play an indirect role in the pathogenesis of acne by releasing free fatty acids from triglycerides in sebum. Free fatty acids are irritants and are comedogenic (promote the formation of comedones). Bacteria also may release proteases capable of injuring the follicular epithelium and may produce chemotactic factors that attract polymorphonuclear cells.

The most important factor in the development of acne is abnormal maturation and differentiation (keratinization) of the follicular epithelium. The initial lesion to develop in acne, a microcomedone, is a keratin plug impacted within the follicle. The earliest detectable change is a hyperplastic follicular epithelium that sheds increased numbers of adherent cells, producing a solid mass rather than loose debris. This mass expands steadily and distends the follicle to produce a closed comedone ("whitehead"), clinically apparent as a noninflammatory white or flesh-colored papule 1 to 2 mm in diameter. The follicular orifice is tiny and generally cannot be seen. There is a common misconception that acne begins with an obstruction at the surface or follicular orifice, causing retention of follicular contents behind it. The obstruction actually occurs in a lower portion of the follicle, well below the skin surface. Closed comedones may rupture or transform into open comedones. Open comedones ("blackheads") are 5 mm or more in diameter and have a darkly pigmented central plug. These are fairly stable structures because their follicular contents are slowly extruded through the dilated orifice. When a closed comedone ruptures sebum, free fatty acids, hair fragments, and keratin are released into the dermis, provoking a foreign-body type of inflammatory reaction that leads to the development of erythematous papules, pustules, and cysts.

Acne is classified as follows, according to the predominate type of lesion present:

1. Noninflammatory acne
   a. Comedonal acne
2. Inflammatory acne
   a. Papulopustular acne
   b. Nodulocystic/conglobate acne

The ultimate prognosis and the approach to treatment depend on the type of acne.

THERAPY

It is important to explain the natural history of acne to patients and their parents. With the possible exception of isotretinoin, there is no cure for acne.

Patience is crucial, as improvement occurs slowly over weeks to months. Maximum therapy should be used to obtain control, after which treatment modalities are reduced to the fewest necessary to maintain control until natural remission of the disease occurs.

Comedonal Acne

Comedonal acne can usually be controlled with the use of topical preparations alone; systemic antibiotic therapy is rarely required (Table 1). Benzoyl peroxide gels have been a mainstay in the treatment of acne. Benzoyl peroxide is a potent antimicrobial agent that also has a comedolytic effect, i.e., it promotes the dissolution of existing comedones, and inhibits the formation of new ones. Benzoyl peroxide gels are available in 2½, 5, and 10 percent concentrations and the vehicle may be either water, acetone, or alcohol. Water-based products are less drying and are particularly helpful in patients with relatively dry or sensitive skin. Alcohol- or acetone-based gels are more useful in patients with excessively oily skin. Most patients tolerate a 2½ or 5 percent benzoyl peroxide on the face and a 10 percent gel on the trunk. Initial dryness or chapping of the skin frequently resolves despite ongoing therapy. When used alone benzoyl peroxide may be applied once or twice daily in the smallest amount needed to cover the affected area lightly. Spot treating lesions is not as effective as treating the entire affected area, as benzoyl peroxide will both speed resolution of existing lesions and help prevent the formation of new ones. Allergic contact dermatitis from benzoyl peroxide occurs in a small percentage of patients, and the drug may bleach colored fabrics.

Tretinoin (Retin-A) is the most effective topical drug in the treatment of acne, but it may be more difficult to use because of a greater incidence of drying and irritation. Tretinoin is a more potent comedolytic agent than benzoyl peroxide and also interferes with comedone formation by reversing

TABLE 1   Treatment Guidelines

Comedonal acne
   Tretinoin
   Benzoyl peroxide
Mild papulopustular acne
   Tretinoin
   Benzoyl peroxide
   Topical antibiotics
Moderate papulopustular acne
   Tretinoin
   Benzoyl peroxide
   Systemic antibiotics
   Topical antibiotics
Nodulocystic acne
   Systemic antibiotics
   Intralesional steroids
   Tretinoin
   Benzoyl peroxide
   Isotretinoin

abnormal keratinization of the follicular epithelium. Epithelial turnover is accelerated and the ultimate result is increased production of loose debris, which is expelled rapidly. Tretinoin may produce a considerable amount of redness, irritation, and peeling, but these effects are not necessary or even desirable. Retin-A is available in three bases: 0.01 and 0.025 percent gel, 0.1 and 0.05 percent cream, and 0.05 percent lotion. Although the gels contain lower concentrations of tretinoin, they are more drying and less easily tolerated than the cream base in some patients. I rarely prescribe the lotion because this is the most irritating base.

A thin layer of Retin-A should be applied once daily to all affected areas, avoiding the sensitive skin around the eyes, nasolabial folds, and lips. It is important to wait 20 or 30 minutes after washing the face before applying Retin-A, to minimize irritation. Patients should be warned that Retin-A often worsens the acne during the first few weeks of therapy, and this is to be expected. Retin-A may result in a heightened susceptibility to sunburn. Combined use of Retin-A and benzoyl peroxide may be more effective in those patients who have not responded adequately to single-drug therapy after 2 to 3 months. When both preparations are used, one should be applied in the morning and the other at bedtime. Sulfur, resorcinol, and salicylic acid are less effective topical agents. Acne surgery to remove comedones is occasionally helpful and can be accomplished with a comedo extractor, surgical blade, or blood lancet.

Papulopustular Acne

Mild papulopustular acne usually responds to Retin-A and benzoyl peroxide alone or in combination, as described in the management of comedonal acne. If adequate control has not been obtained, a topical antibiotic may be considered in addition to Retin-A and benzoyl peroxide. Clindamycin, erythromycin, and tetracycline are available as hydroalcoholic solutions. I believe topical clindamycin and erythromycin are more effective than topical tetracycline. Instruct patients to apply the topical antibiotic twice daily, in the morning and evening, before applying benzoyl peroxide or Retin-A. A new topical gel combination of benzoyl peroxide and erythromycin is available under the trade name of Benzamycin.

Patients with moderate to severe papulopustular acne often require the use of systemic antibiotics, in addition to benzoyl peroxide and Retin-A, to obtain control after which topical antibiotic solutions can be substituted as needed. Tetracycline is the most widely used systemic antibiotic in the management of acne, but erythromycin, minocycline, and trimethoprim-sulfasoxazole are also effective, particularly in patients who have become refractory to tetracycline therapy. I usually begin therapy with tetracycline or erythromycin, 500 mg twice daily. A twice-daily dosage appears to be as effective as a three- or four-times-a-day schedule, and compliance is much better.

The question has been raised as to whether or not tetracycline decreases the effectiveness of oral contraceptives. In patients for whom this is an issue, I use erythromycin. Systemic antibiotics are probably effective because they suppress bacterial growth as well as inhibit neutrophil chemotaxis. Ultraviolet light and cryotherapy with liquid nitrogen or carbon dioxide slush produce erythema and desquamation, which may speed resolution of superficial lesions.

Nodulocystic Acne

Nodulocystic acne is more resistant to treatment than other types of acne lesions. Initial treatment includes a systemic antibiotic, usually tetracycline or erythromycin, 1 to 2 g daily, in addition to topical treatment with benzoyl peroxide, Retin-A, and occasionally topical antibiotics. I use topical antibiotics in conjunction with oral antibiotics only when patients have been refractory to therapy. Resolution of cystic lesions also may be promoted by intralesional injection of a low concentration of corticosteroids, such as triamcinolone acetonide in a 2.5-mg-per-milliliter concentration, although atrophy of the skin is a potential complication. In the past, estrogen, usually in the form of estrogen-dominant contraceptives, was used to reduce sebum production. Unfortunately, oral contraceptives with high estrogen levels are also associated with other, potentially more serious, side effects. Patients with severe acne who have elevated plasma concentrations of dehydroepiandrosterone sulfate have responded to small doses of dexamethasone.

Isotretinoin (Accutane), a derivative of vitamin A, may be used for severe cystic acne that has not responded to standard treatment. Accutane reverses the abnormal pattern of keratinization of the follicular canal, thus preventing formation of comedones. In addition, it induces a reduction in sebum production and is anti-inflammatory. Accutane is available in 10-, 20-, and 40-mg capsules. The recommended dosage is 1 mg per kilogram per day for a total duration of 16 to 20 weeks. Complete remission occurs in up to 65 to 80 percent of patients who complete this regimen. A small number of patients may require a second course of therapy, which should be postponed until they have been off therapy for at least 2 months. A third course is rarely indicated.

A significant number of side effects occur during Accutane therapy, including the nearly universal occurrence of cheilitis and dry skin. Other side effects include dryness of the eyes, nose, and mouth, pruritus, peeling of the palms and soles, and increased sensitivity to sunburn. Contact lens wearers may not be able to tolerate their lenses because of dryness of the eyes during therapy. Ten to 15 percent of patients may experience nonspecific pain, tenderness, or stiffness of their muscles or joints. In 10 percent of patients nonscarring diffuse alopecia has been reported, which usually resolves when therapy is discontinued. Less common side effects include headache, which may be a symptom of pseudotumor cerebri, visual disturbances, and emotional instability. Concomitant tetracycline therapy increases the risk of pseudotumor cerebri.

Administration of isotretinoin is teratogenic in animals and congenital malformations, including major central nervous system and cardiac defects, have occurred in newborn infants of mothers who conceived while taking the drug. *All females of childbearing age must employ an effective method of birth control while on isotretinoin therapy.* Skeletal hyperostoses have been reported rarely in patients treated for nodulocystic acne. In general, the severity of the side effects is dosage-related and reversible in most instances, with the exception of teratogenicity and skeletal hyperostoses. Attempts to decrease the dosage or shorten the course of therapy to reduce side effects have resulted in a much higher relapse rate. Elevation of hepatic enzyme values, triglycerides, and, less commonly, cholesterol may occur during therapy. Diabetics may experience hyperglycemia while taking isotretinoin. I obtain liver function studies, triglyceride, and cholesterol studies before beginning therapy and at 1 and 2 months during therapy.

MISCONCEPTIONS

There is no evidence that diet plays a role in the development or perpetuation of acne. Obviously, for general health purposes, patients should be encouraged to eat sensibly. Another misconception is that acne patients are unclean or have poor hygiene. Because acne patients tend to have oily skin, they feel they must wash frequently and scrub with a vengeance. There is no evidence that lack of washing is harmful or that frequent cleansing is helpful; in fact, excessive cleansing may aggravate the problem. Washing simply removes surface lipids. Acne patients should be advised to wash only as often as necessary to eliminate the unpleasant oily feeling; once or twice daily should be sufficient. I prefer the use of unmedicated bath soaps. Scrubbing, including the use of abrasive cleansers, sponges, or washcloths, does not eliminate lesions and often irritates the skin, which can complicate topical treatment. Control of scalp oil or seborrheic dermatitis has no effect on the presence or severity of acne. Hair overlying the forehead is not a factor unless it has been treated with an oily or greasy comedogenic substance. Glycerin is a noncomedogenic alternative for those patients who feel the need for a scalp hair treatment.

ENVIRONMENTAL FACTORS

A discussion of treatment would be incomplete without considering external factors that may complicate the management of acne. Topically applied comedogenic agents include some cosmetics as well as facial creams referred to as night creams, cleansing creams, and moisturizers. Because variation in concentration as well as additive effect of ingredients may significantly alter the final comedogenicity of a given product, it is often difficult to determine the degree of comedogenicity of a preparation from the ingredient list alone. I recommend that patients minimize the use of moisturizers and limit their use to those emollients that have been proven to be noncomedogenic, including Keri Lotion, Keri Light Lotion, Neutrogena Facial Moisturizer, Complex 15, and Dermatology Formula. Water-base makeup should be used ("oil free" is not water base) and powder rather than cream blush is recommended. Astringents should be avoided because they exacerbate dryness resulting from topical acne medications. Sunscreens may also be a problem, and noncomedogenic brands such as Total Eclipse or Coppertone Supershade should be used. Hair grooming pomades come into contact with the skin and are suspect if comedones are clustered over the forehead and temples. Glycerin is noncomedogenic and may be used safely on the hair of acne patients. Trauma in the form of excoriation of lesions should be avoided.

It is important to remind patients that manipulation of lesions retards healing and promotes scarring. Mechanical forces of pressure and friction produced by postures such as resting the chin on the hand or by contact with external agents such as chin straps, shoulder pads, and helmets may aggravate acne. Certain occupations predispose to acne in unusual locations as a result of exposure to comedogenic agents including greases, oils, coal tar, or pitch. Be alert for adolescents with full- or part-time jobs as mechanics, fast-food cooks, or road workers.

COMPLICATIONS

Papulopustular or nodulocystic acne may result in significant scarring of the skin. Attempts at improving the appearance of the skin with collagen injection, chemical peels, dermabrasion, and punch grafting should generally be delayed until the disease process is inactive.

SUGGESTED READING

Dicken CH. Retinoids: a review. J Am Acad Dermatol 1984; 11:541–552.

Gammon WR, Meyer C, Lantis S, et al. Comparative efficacy of oral erythromycin versus oral tetracycline in the treatment of acne vulgaris: a double blind study. J Am Acad Dermatol 1986; 14:183–186.

Leyden JJ, Shalita AR. Rational therapy of acne vulgaris: an update on treatment. J Am Acad Dermatol 1986; 15:907–915.

Plewig G, Kligman AM. Acne: Morphogenesis and Treatment. New York: Springer-Verlag, 1975.

Strauss JS, Rapini RP, Shalita AR, et al. Isotretinoin therapy for acne: results of a multicenter dose-response study. J Am Acad Dermtol 1984; 10:490–496.

FUNISITIS AND OMPHALITIS

KEITHA FARMER, M.B., Ch.B., F.R.C.P.(UK),, F.R.A.C.P., Ph.D.

Funisitis (inflammation of the umbilical cord) and omphalitis (inflammation of the umbilicus and surrounding tissues) are rare in developed countries. Staphylococcal and streptococcal infections are the most common causes, but most pathogenic bacteria have caused umbilical sepsis. Funisitis is infection of devitalized tissue, but extension can occur through the umbilical arteries or vein. There is a need for recognition and prompt treatment of presumed sepsis and continued vigilance in the management of this open wound in the newborn. If the current trends toward home birth continue, I predict an increase in omphalitis. Neonatal tetanus and the other severe complications of primitive rituals that occur in developing countries are not within my experience, and therefore I shall not deal with those problems (see chapter on *Tetanus*).

It is important to exclude other disorders causing discharge from the umbilical stump, varying from granuloma and patent vitellointestinal duct to a patent urachus. Causes of delayed separation of the umbilical cord other than sepsis, such as leukocyte mobility problems, should also be considered.

My management of suspected funisitis or omphalitis is influenced by the presence of constitutional symptoms, definite evidence of inflammation in the form of erythema, induration or pustules, and the gestational age of the infant, which will determine the environment and current surrounding bacterial flora. The physician should be aware of the antimicrobial susceptibilities of local bacteria as a guide to antimicrobial therapy, and may have the benefit of prior bacterial cultures and other laboratory investigations.

THERAPEUTIC ALTERNATIVES

I believe that in the presence of clinical signs of either systemic or local inflammation, the infant should be hospitalized until the inflammation is diminishing or sepsis is excluded. I prefer to administer antibiotics intravenously, but oral antibiotics may be justified in the presence of subsiding or minimal inflammation. The offensive-smelling noninflamed umbilical cord (usually colonized with saprophytes) can be treated with local antiseptics following culture. However, the other extreme of fasciitis, with extensive inflammation and necrosis of the abdominal wall, may require surgical debridement and supportive therapy, including administration of blood products.

SPECIFIC ANTIMICROBIAL THERAPY
Asymptomatic Infant With Colonized Umbilicus

When cultures from a "normal" umbilicus contain Group A or B beta-hemolytic streptococci, I prescribe a single intramuscular injection of benzathine penicillin (50,000 U per kilogram of body weight), although I am aware that the probability of invasion by Group B streptococci is low compared with that of Group A, and colonization by either group is not erradicated. In the presence of an epidemic of Group A streptococcal infection in a nursery, babies who have had contact should be treated. In general, other organisms such as staphylococci are regarded as normal flora, in the absence of symptoms and signs, but colonization may be reduced by antiseptics. Multiresistant organisms call for isolation of the infant and cohorting of contacts.

Prolonged Serous Discharge From "Uninflamed" Umbilical Cord

If there is prolonged discharge, once anatomic abnormalities are excluded, the possibility of streptococcal infection must be considered. Cultures are taken from the discharge and a single injection of benzathine penicillin (50,000 U per kilogram), given while you are awaiting further progress and cultures. Local application of antiseptic every four hours is also indicated to reduce superficial bacteria.

Omphalitis With Surrounding Erythema and Induration in a Term Infant

When erythema extends more than a centimeter from the umbilical stump and there is edema or induration, I obtain bacterial cultures (including anaerobic) from the site, blood cultures, and a white blood cell count. The infant is usually being nursed in a general or postnatal ward with the mother, i.e., *in a nonantibiotic intensive care environment*. I would treat the infant in the hospital with ampicillin and cefoxitin in appropriate dosages (Table 1), pending the results of culture, to cover streptococci with the ampicillin and staphylococci and gram-negative bacteria with the cefoxitin. Ampicillin is effective against the improbable *Clostridium tetani* and cefoxitin provides coverage for anaerobic organisms. However, alternative regimens such as ampicillin and aminoglycoside or cefuroxime alone are effective. I hesitate to use oral antibiotics, particularly at home, because of absorption variability and lack of opportunity for observation. Local antiseptics are also indicated.

Omphalitis in an Infant Born Outside the Hospital

If the infant is born outside the hospital in the presence of doubtful hygiene, I obtain bacterial cultures

TABLE 1 Dosage and Administration of Antimicrobial Agents for Funisitis and Omphalitis

Clinical Signs		Treatment		
Local	*Systemic*	*<1 Week of Age*	*>1 Week of Age*	*Precautions*
Offensive odor—not inflamed	Nil	Local antiseptic	Local antiseptic	Culture for both aerobes and anaerobes
Colonized with Group A or B streptococcus or prolonged serous discharge	Nil	Benzathine penicillin 50,000 U/kg IM as 1 dose	Benzathine penicillin 50,000 U/kg IM as 1 dose	
Erythema, induration > 1 cm abdominal wall >37 weeks gestation	Nil	Ampicillin 100 mg/kg/day IV* divided q12h †cefoxitin 100 mg/kg/day IV* divided q12h	Ampicillin 150 mg/kg/day IV* divided q8h †Cefoxitin IV 150 mg/kg/day divided q8h	Local culture plus blood culture prior to therapy
Erythema, induration < 37 weeks gestation hospital-acquired infection	Nil	Ampicillin 100 mg/kg/day IV* divided q12h plus ‡Netilmicin 5 mg/kg/day IV* divided q12h or <1,250 g divided q18–24h	Ampicillin 150 mg/kg/day IV* divided 8qh ‡Netilmicin 7.5 mg/kg/day IV* divided q8h	Local culture plus blood culture prior to therapy Modification of dosage may be necessary with very immature infants and impaired renal function; serum levels monitored
Erythema, induration	Fever, etc.			
Erythema, induration, pustules or proven *Staphylococcus aureus*	Plus or minus	Methicillin 100 mg/kg/day IV divided q12h	Methicillin 150 g/kg/day IV divided q8h	Check urine RBCs

* IV infusion over 20 to 30 minutes.
† Alternative cover staphylococcus, community-acquired gram-negative organisms and anaerobes.
‡ Routine aminoglycoside of nursery to which local organisms are susceptible, suitable—e.g., gentamicin, same dosage of netilmicin.

and observe carefully for local sepsis, systemic infection, and the very unlikely neonatal tetanus following contamination of the cord. If *Clostridium tetani* is isolated, or symptoms compatible with tetanus are present, management includes use of antiserum, penicillin, and appropriate supportive measures (see chapter on *Tetanus*).

Omphalitis With Pustules or Proven Staphylococcal Colonization

If *Staphylococcus aureus* is a probable pathogen, I use methicillin in appropriate dosages (see Table 1). Other antistaphylococcal penicillins are effective, and intramuscular administration is possible. Cloxicillin, given orally, or erythromycin may be used for susceptible organisms when there is limited inflammation, but the infant must be seen daily by a reliable observer.

Omphalitis Causing Constitutional Symptoms (Fever, Lethargy, Etc.) and Arising in a Low Birthweight Infant in a Special Care Unit

If the infant is symptomatic and may have acquired organisms from the hospital environment, I use netilmicin and ampicillin therapy for 7 to 10 days, depending on whether blood cultures are positive. The aminoglycoside known to be effective against gram-negative organisms occurring in the nursery are a suitable alternative. In a sick low-birthweight infant with an umbilical catheter who is presumed to be infected with *Staphylococcus epidermidis,* the catheter should be removed. If the organism is resistant to methicillin, vancomycin, 30 mg per kilogram per day in two doses infused over an hour, should be prescribed for infants weighing more than 1,200 g. Very low-birth-weight infants require a dosage of 20 mg per kilogram per day at intervals of 24 to 36 hours.

MONITORING FOR COMPLICATIONS OF THERAPY

Aminoglycoside therapy must be modified if renal function is impaired. The serum creatinine should be measured as an index of renal function, and serum concentrations of aminoglycoside should be monitored. Audiologic evaluation is necessary for those neonates with abnormally large serum concentrations. A complete blood count and renal function tests are indicated with the use of methicillin.

PROPHYLACTIC TREATMENT

In our hospital the umbilical cord is occluded with a rubber band, and the base of the cord is treated with iodophor in surgical spirit (1,600 parts per million of iodine [0.16 percent]). In normal term infants, the iodophor is applied with a cotton wool bud by the mother every time she changes the infant's diapers, usually about every 4 hours at feeding time, until the cord has separated and the umbilical stump is dry. No dressing is applied.

We have not had clinical problems with iodine absorption with 0.16 percent iodophor, as has been reported with 1 percent povidone iodine. Alternative therapies such as Triple dye are undoubtedly successful, the rationale being to keep the cord dry with minimal bacterial colonization, leading to early separation and healing of the umbilical stump. In the case of a term infant discharged before the cord separates, the mother is given iodophor in spirit and advised to continue the treatment at home. A district nurse visits the home to inspect the umbilicus. In the case of low-birth-weight infants, the treatment is carried out by the nurses until the cord separates. In the presence of an umbilical catheter, mycostatin powder is applied to the umbilicus and the infant is given oral mycostatin to avoid colonization and invasion by *Candida*. When a catheter is placed in the umbilical vein, it should be removed immediately after a procedure such as exchange transfusion, because unrecognized sepsis may lead to portal vein thrombosis.

EVALUATION OF RESPONSE TO THERAPY

In the case of the colonized umbilicus and the persistent serous discharge, one dose of benzathine penicillin given intravenously is adequate, assuming that the cord separates and no symptoms arise. For the clinically infected umbilicus with negative blood culture, if the induration and erythema begin to subside within 48 hours, 5 days of treatment with parenteral antibiotics is sufficient. Progress can be assessed by measuring the distance of the erythema from the umbilicus. However, if the blood cultures are positive and/or signs of infection are still present after 5 days, treatment should be continued for at least 5 more days. If inflammation, constitutional symptoms, and signs of inflammation remain or increase after 48 hours, it may be necessary to change the antibiotic therapy according to the antibiotic susceptibility tests. With the development of fluntuation or creptitus extension in the abdominal wall, a surgical opinion should be sought, particularly as extending inflammation of the abdominal wall may signify underlying peritonitis.

FOLLOW-UP

Infants who have had significant inflammation of the umbilical area should be observed for complications such as portal vein thrombosis.

SUGGESTED READING

Cushing AH. Omphalitis—a review. Pediatr Infect Dis 1985; 4:282–285.

McKenna H, Johnson D. Bacteria in neonatal omphalitis. Pathology 1977; 9:111–113.

Nelson JD, Dillon HC, Howard JB. A prolonged nursery epidemic associated with a newly recognized type of group A streptococcus. J Pediatr 1976; 89:792–796.

Pyati SP, Ramamurthy RS, Krauss MT, Pildes RS. Absorption of iodine in the neonate following topical use of povidone iodine. J Pediatr 1977; 91:825–828.

Thompson EN, Sherlock S. The aetiology of portal vein thrombosis with particular reference to the role of infection and exchange transfusion. Q J Med 1964; 132:465–479.

NEONATAL BREAST ABSCESS

KEITHA FARMER, M.B., Ch.B., F.R.C.P.(UK), F.R.A.C.P., Ph.D.

Neonatal breast abscess is a rare disorder of term infants that occurs from the end of the first week to the second month of life. The diagnosis is a localized fluctuant or indurated area in one breast, rarely in both breasts, in contrast with physiologic hypertrophy. The disease is often caused by *Staphylococcus aureus* and was more common in past decades. Streptococci and gram-negative organisms may also be the etiological agent.

If there is a fluctuant area, surgical drainage peripheral to the nipple to avoid damage to the breast tissue is indicated. If only erythema and induration are present, however, antibiotic therapy alone may be justified following Gram stain and culture of a needle aspirate or purulent expressed colostrum. Blood culture is also indicated, but rarely positive. The infant should be hospitalized. I use methicillin (150 mg per kilogram per day in three divided doses) plus netilmicin (7.5 mg per kilogram per day in three divided doses). A suitable alternative is an aminoglycoside, used routinely in the nursery, to which most gram-negative organisms are susceptible. Alternative therapy would be a third-generation cephalosporin and another beta-lactamase–resistant penicillin. If the inflammation is minimal and the infant has not been in contact with relatively resistant gram-negative bacilli, a second-generation cephalosporin, which is effective against staphylococci, and gram-negative organisms such as cefoxitin, is justified. Usually the Gram stain of the pus or culture is a guide as to whether gram-positive cocci or other organisms should be covered. If staphylococci are identified, methicillin alone is adequate.

If the inflammation subsides within 1 to 2 days, with or without surgical drainage, and blood cultures are negative, a 5-day course of antibiotic therapy is adequate. However, if the blood culture is positive, 7 to 10 days of intravenous therapy is indicated. An alternative is intramuscularly administered antibiotics. If the lesion is exacerbated in the absence of surgical drainage, a surgical opinion should be sought, and if organisms are resistant to the therapy being used, the antibiotics should be changed appropriately.

If aminoglycosides are used, the peak and trough serum concentrations should be estimated twice weekly. In the case of netilmicin, a peak level should be 5 to 10 mg/L and the trough less than 2 mg/L.

Infants who have received aminoglycosides should have a hearing test performed if abnormally large serum concentrations have been documented or if the monitoring was not adequate. Because there have been a few reports of impairment of breast development, all cases should be followed up to assess

any atrophy of the breast as a consequence of either extension of the pus or the surgical drainage.

Prevention is to avoid expressing colostrum from the infant's breast with physiological hypertrophy in the first month of life. If the organism is a staphylococcus, general measures, such as isolation of infected infants, are indicated.

If a breast abscess caused by staphylococci or group A streptococci occurs in a nursery, the contacts as well as the patient should be isolated; in general, however, breast abscesses arise in healthy term infants at home. The mother's breasts should be assessed for staphylococcal infection and treated appropriately. The infant should be admitted to hospital and, ideally, isolated with the mother.

SUGGESTED READING

McCracken GH, Nelson JD. Antimicrobial therapy for newborns, 2nd ed. New York: Grune & Stratton, 1983.
Rudoy PR, Nelson JD. Breast abscess during the neonatal period. Am J Dis Child 1975; 129:1031–1034.
Walsh M, McIntosh K. Neonatal mastitis. Clin Pediatr 1986; 25:395–399.

INFECTION FOLLOWING A BITE

MORVEN S. EDWARDS, M.D.

Approximately 90 percent of the one million to 2 million animal bites that occur annually are caused by dogs and almost 10 percent by cats. School-aged children are the most frequent victims of animal bite wounds, but some of the most severe injuries are inflicted on toddlers by large dogs. Children from 2 to 5 years of age are the most likely to sustain human bites, and children are victims of approximately 4,000 snake bites yearly.

The incidence of infection following a bite is 10 to 30 percent for dog and human bites. As many as 20 to 50 percent of cat bites for which medical attention is sought develop infection. The risk for infection after a snake bite is unknown.

ANTIMICROBIAL THERAPY

Each of the hundreds of microbial species composing the biting animal's or human's normal oral flora has the potential to cause bite wound infection. Although a myriad of organisms have been occasionally associated with wound infection, empiric therapy

can be directed toward a relatively restricted group (Table 1). Among the aerobic gram-positives, staphylococci (especially *Staphylococcus aureus*) and streptococci are frequently implicated in infected dog, cat, and human bites. Of the gram-negative aerobes and facultative species, *Pasteurella multocida* is a major animal bite pathogen, causing up to 50 percent of dog bite–associated and 80 percent of cat bite–associated infections. *Eikenella corrodens* is almost exclusively a human bite–associated pathogen, but it has, on occasion, been isolated from the canine mouth. Species of *Proteus, Pseudomonas,* and the Enterobacteriaceae are restricted primarily to snake bite–associated wounds, probably because of defecation by reptile-ingested prey. Anaerobes are frequently isolated, alone or in combination, from all types of bite wounds.

Antimicrobial therapy is indicated for suspected bite wound infection and may be provided orally or parenterally, depending on the severity of the bite wound or infection. In addition, parenteral therapy is indicated for children with signs of systemic toxicity, involvement of tendon, bone, or joint, poor response to oral therapy, or impaired immunity, particularly due to splenectomy. All children with poisonous snake bites, except those suspected to have very mild envenomation, should be admitted to the hospital. Before therapy is initiated, a wound culture should be obtained and processed for the isolation of both aerobes and anaerobes. If applicable, a similarly pro-

TABLE 1 Organisms Frequently Associated with Bite Wound Infection

Microorganism	Suspect in Dog (D), Cat (C), Human (H), or Snake (S) Bite
Gram-positive aerobes	
Corynebacterium spp	D,C,H
Staphylococcus aureus	D,C,H
Staphylococcus epidermidis	D,C,H,S
Streptococcus spp*	D,C,H
Gram-negative aerobes and facultative spp	
Acinetobacter spp	D
Eikenella corrodens	H
Neisseria spp	H
Pasteurella multocida	D,C
Proteus spp	S
Pseudomonas spp	S
Anaerobes	
Bacteroides spp	D,C,H,S
Clostridium spp	S
Fusobacterium spp	D,C,H
Peptococcus spp	D,C,H
Peptostreptococcus spp	H
Propionobacterium spp	D

* Includes alpha, beta, and nonhemolytic isolates.

cessed culture should be performed of surrounding areas of cellulitis or purulence. I believe a blood culture is appropriate when signs of systemic toxicity, including temperature exceeding 102°F, are evident.

Guidelines for initial oral and parenteral antimicrobial regimens are shown in Table 2. The availability of agents that broaden the spectrum of penicillins to include antistaphylococcal activity has greatly simplified the approach to treatment of animal and human bites. Ticarcillin-clavulanate (Timentin), administered parenterally, and amoxicillin-clavulanate (Augmentin) given orally are ideal antimicrobials for empiric treatment of dog, cat, and human bites. (Ticarcillin-clavulanate is not approved for use in children less than 12 years of age.) A penicillin is the preferred antibiotic for streptococci, *P. multocida, E. corrodens,* and most anaerobes that cause bite-associated infection, and irreversible beta-lactamase inhibition by clavulanic acid restores the potency of the ampicillin or amoxicillin for *S. aureus.* The formerly employed "standard" regimen of penicillin G or V *plus* a penicillinase-resistant penicillin is equally acceptable but more cumbersome.

In all but mild cases, it is difficult to distinguish signs of infection from those of envenomation in snake bites. When envenomation is sufficiently severe to warrant hospital admission, I provide antibiotic therapy. The use of ampicillin or ticarcillin plus gentamicin is directed toward the most common species—*Clostridia, Bacteroides, Proteus,* and *Pseudomonas*—isolated from infected snake bite wounds.

There is no entirely satisfactory regimen for the treatment of bite wound infection in penicillin-allergic individuals. For serious infections, I would initiate treatment with the regimen suggested in Table 2 and,

TABLE 2 Guidelines for Initial Antibiotic Therapy of Infected Mammal, Reptile, or Human Bites

Indication	Antibiotic Regimen (dosage/kg per 24 hr)	
	Inpatient—Intravenous Regimens	Outpatient—Oral Regimens
Suspected infection—mammal or human bite	Ticarcillin-clavulanate (200–300 mg of ticarcillin component in 4–6 doses)* or Aqueous penicillin G (200,000 U in 4–6 doses)* plus Oxacillin (150 mg in 4 doses)	Amoxicillin-clavulanate (40 mg of amoxicillin component in 3 doses) or Penicillin V (50,000 U in 4 doses) plus Dicloxacillin (50 mg in 4 doses)
Suspected infection—snake bite†	Ampicillin (200 mg in 4–6 doses) or ticarcillin (300 mg in 4–6 doses)* plus Gentamicin (5 mg in 3 doses)‡	Not indicated
Suspected infection—penicillin-allergic patient	Vancomycin (40 mg in 4 doses)§ and Cefotaxime (150–200 mg in 4 doses)* or Chloramphenicol (75 mg in 4 doses)**	Erythromycin (30–50 mg in 4 doses)
Prophylaxis—human bite of hand or face; deep animal wound of hand, face; puncture wound	As above, for suspected infection—mammal or human bite	As above, for suspected infection—mammal or human bite

* Employ the larger dosage and/or more frequent interval for severe infections.
† Infection should be suspected in all cases of moderate or severe envenomation.
‡ Monitor serum concentrations to maintain a peak of 5–10 μg per milliliter and trough less than 2 μg per milliliter.
§ Monitor serum concentrations to maintain a peak of 25–40 μg per milliliter and trough less than 12 μg per milliliter.
** Monitor serum concentrations to maintain a peak of 20–30 μg per milliliter and trough less than the peak.

as soon as is feasible, perform penicillin skin testing, desensitize the patient to penicillin, and switch to the penicillin-containing regimen outlined. In the initial regimen suggested for penicillin-allergic individuals, vancomycin is provided for the treatment of *S. aureus,* streptococci, and gram-positive anaerobes; cefotaxime is an alternative antibiotic for *P. multocida* and *E. corrodens,* and it has a good spectrum of anaerobic activity. Chloramphenicol provides a similar spectrum for patients in whom allergic reaction to a cephalosporin is a concern. *P. multocida* isolates are susceptible, and *E. corrodens* is usually susceptible to chloramphenicol. Clindamycin is omitted from the "alternative-to-penicillin" regimen because it has poor activity against *P. multodica* and *E. corrodens.* Erythromycin is the most reasonable alternative to penicillins for the oral treatment of animal or human bites, providing treatment for staphylococci and streptococci. Since *P. multocida* is only moderately susceptible and *E. corrodens* is relatively resistant to erythromycin, children receiving this regimen should be monitored frequently for signs of progressive infection. Antibiotics should be adjusted in all patients, if necessary, when susceptibility testing is available.

When gentamicin, vancomycin, or chloramphenicol are employed for treatment of infection following a bite, serum concentrations should be monitored and maintained in the range indicated in Table 2. In hospitalized patients I perform a complete blood count, BUN, creatinine, and urinalysis, at biweekly intervals, to assess possible antibiotic-associated toxicity.

The usual duration of parenteral antimicrobial therapy is 5 to 10 days for wound infection with cellulitis or localized (and drained) abscess. For patients treated initially by the intravenous route, a 10- to 14-day total treatment course can often be completed orally, after improvement is evident. Antibiotics should be continued until signs of inflammation have resolved.

Infectious complications of human and animal bites include arthritis, osteomyelitis, and tenosynovitis. Assuming appropriate drainage, 2 to 3 weeks of treatment are usually required for patients with arthritis or tenosynovitis, and 3 or 4 weeks for those with osteomyelitis. Systemic infections such as leptospirosis, cat-scratch disease, brucellosis, and tularemia can be transmitted by means of a bite. The bite serves as the means of inoculation, and the clinical manifestations, discussed in the appropriate chapters, are not unique when a bite has been the source of infection.

In every child sustaining a bite wound, the immunization status should be determined, and tetanus prophylaxis (see chapter on *Tetanus*) should be administered when indicated. The need for rabies prophylaxis (Table 3) should be assessed. With human bites, particularly among children in institutions for the mentally retarded, administration of postexposure prophylaxis for hepatitis B should be considered (see chapter on *Viral Hepatitis*).

SUPPORTIVE AND SURGICAL THERAPY

Visible dirt should be sponged away gently and the wound cleansed using a 1 percent solution of povidone iodine. Subsequently, high-pressure irrigation

---

TABLE 3   Rabies Postexposure Prophylaxis Guide

Animal Species	*Condition of Animal at Time of Attack*	*Treatment of Exposed Person**
Domestic		
Dog and cat	Healthy and available for 10 days of observation	None, unless animal develops rabies†
	Rabid or suspected rabid	HRIG and HDCV
	Unknown (escaped)	Consult public health officials. If treatment is indicated, give HRIG and HDCV
Wild		
Skunk, bat, fox, coyote, raccoon, bobcat, and other carnivores	Regard as rabid unless proved negative by laboratory tests‡	HRIG and HDCV
Other		
Livestock, rodents, and lagomorphs (rabbits and hares)	Consider individually. Local and state public health officials should be consulted on questions about the need for rabies prophylaxis. Bites of squirrels, hamsters, guinea pigs, gerbils, chipmunks, rats, mice, other rodents, rabbits, and hares almost never call for antirabies prophylaxis.	

* *All bites and wounds should immediately be thoroughly cleansed with soap and water.* If antirabies treatment is indicated, both human rabies immune globulin (HRIG) and human diploid cell rabies vaccine (HDCV) should be given as soon as possible, *regardless* of the interval from exposure. Local reactions to vaccines are common and do not contraindicate continuing treatment. Discontinue vaccine if fluorescent-antibody tests of the animal are negative.

† During the usual holding period of 10 days, begin treatment with HRIG and HDCV at first sign of rabies in a dog or cat that has bitten someone. The symptomatic animal should be killed immediately and tested.

‡ The animal should be killed and tested as soon as possible. Holding for observation is not recommended.

Recommendations of the Advisory Committee on Immunization Practices of the Centers for Disease Control.

Note: The recommendations in this table are only a guide. In applying them, take into account the animal species involved, the circumstances of the bite or other exposure, the vaccination status of the animal, and presence of rabies in the region. Local or state public health officials should be consulted if questions arise about the need for rabies prophylaxis.

of the wound should be performed using a 19-gauge needle and a 20- or 35-ml syringe. Approximately 200 ml of normal saline is an adequate volume for all but the most extensive of wounds. Puncture wounds should be cleansed but not irrigated. If rabies is a concern, 1 percent benzalkonium chloride may be used for cleansing to promote virucidal activity.

Wounds that appear to be infected must be left open initially. Infected wounds that were previously sutured should be opened. Fluctuant wounds should be incised and drained. All devitalized tissue must be debrided, in the operating room if necessary. Surgical debridement and exploration is appropriate for all deep or extensive wounds to the hand and for all wounds involving the metacarpophalangeal joint. Surgical consultation should also be obtained for infections possibly extending to bone or joint, extensive infections and those requiring an open drainage procedure, and infections that potentially require skin grafting.

Local therapy includes the application of warm soaks for 30 to 60 minutes, two or three times daily, to promote drainage. Analgesics such as acetaminophen or codeine may be required to relieve pain.

Snake bites with moderate or severe envenomation should be considered infected. At hospital admission, children with Crotalid or pit viper bites (rattlesnake, copperheads, water moccasins) should have a baseline complete blood count, blood typing and crossmatching, assessment of bleeding and clotting times, serum electrolytes, BUN, creatinine, and urinalysis. In cases of severe envenomation, these values should be reassessed serially. Systemic effects of Crotalid envenomation such as the consequences of hemolysis may occur, including hematuria, hematemesis, and shock, with disseminated intravascular coagulopathy. Supportive measures for respiratory insufficiency, cardiac arrhythmias, and renal failure may be required. Coral snake venom is a neurotoxin, and symptoms following a bite may be delayed. These patients are not at high risk for hemolysis but should be observed closely for involvement of cranial nerves and bulbar paralysis. Ventilatory support may be required.

Antivenin is indicated for children with snake bites when, within 30 to 60 minutes after the bite, progressive swelling of the injured area is evident, paresthesias of the mouth or extremities are present, or systemic signs of toxicity occur. All North American antivenins are made from horse serum. Hypersensitivity reactions or anaphylaxis have occurred as the result of antivenin administration. I have administered benadryl (1 mg/kg) intravenously before initiating therapy, and keep epinephrine at the bedside. The specifics of antivenin administration are provided in the package inserts. Both the Crotilidae polyvalent antivenin and antivenin effective against the North American coral snake are available commercially from Wyeth Laboratories.

THERAPEUTIC OUTCOME

With appropriate drainage, response to therapy should be clinically apparent within 48 hours. Patients receiving home therapy should be reassessed at this time to determine the adequacy of their response. For hospitalized patients with more severe infections, systemic toxicity should be less within 2 to 3 days, and wound pain and inflammation should be reduced. With progression or lack of response, the primary concerns are (1) an undrained local or deep focus of infection, (2) retained foreign material, and (3) inadequate antimicrobial therapy. Lack of response thus dictates reassessment of both medical and surgical therapy.

SUGGESTED READING

Edwards MS. Infections due to human and animal bites. In: Feigin RD, Cherry JD, eds. Textbook of pediatric infectious diseases. Philadelphia: WB Saunders, 1987; 2362–2373.
Feder HM Jr, Shanley JD, Barbera JA. Review of 59 patients hospitalized with animal bites. Pediatr Infect Dis J 1987; 6:24–28.
Marcy SM. Infections due to dog and cat bites. Pediatr Infect Dis 1982; 1:351–356.
Russell FE. Snake venom poisoning in the United States. Annu Rev Med 1980; 31:247–259.
Trott A. Care of mammalian bites. Pediatr Infect Dis J 1987; 6:8–10.

DECUBITUS ULCER

JOHN G. BIRCH, M.D., F.R.C.S.(C)

Decubitus ulcers are the product of accident, neglect, or ignorance in an at-risk patient. The offending agent of injury is usually excessive pressure (i.e., tissue pressure that exceeds capillary filling pressure) applied to the soft tissues for a period long enough to cause cell death. Insensitive skin (in the pediatric population most commonly a result of spina bifida, and less frequently a sequela of spinal cord injury) or diminished pain response (acute closed head injury, drug overdose, severe static encephalopathy) are prerequisites. Pressure decubitus are typically located over the ischia or sacrum in sitting patients, or over any bony prominence in a bedridden patient. Decubitus can also be caused by sheer (e.g., over bedsheets, or by crawling), thermal burns, or chemical burns (including urine). Poor nutrition aggravates the situation by increasing the risk of skin breakdown, and prolonging healing time.

PREVENTION OF DECUBITUS ULCER

Prevention of decubitus requires recognition of the at-risk patient, proper acute nursing care, thorough patient education, and application of a fastidious chronic skin care program by the patient. Prevention of a decubitus ulcer is infinitely more satisfying and cost-effective than treatment of established sores.

The acutely at-risk patient (unconscious or acute spinal cord injured) must be turned every 2 hours with padding or support of all bony areas. Pressure distributing pads (I prefer egg crate mattresses) are helpful, but do not replace frequent turning, careful padding of bony prominences, and vigilant skin inspection. Maintenance of maximal nutrition is also very important.

Parents of the mobile child with insensitive (classically spina bifida) skin must be taught that the child can and will hurt the insensitive areas without realizing it. The child should not be left unattended, and the insensitive areas should never be left unprotected. For example, crawling without socks or some clothing over the leg will produce carpet burns on the knees or the dorsum of the feet. These children must be protected from radiators, space heaters, exposed metal components of car seats, and sunlight. Shoes or braces can pinch the skin without complaint from the child. The tip of the great toe is easily ulcerated; when the foot is slipped into a shoe, the toe becomes bunched up in the end, and is left in this position unrecognized. New braces or shoes should be left on only 15 or 20 minutes initially, and then removed and the skin inspected for any area of undue pressure. Patients who are wheelchair bound must be checked for any area of reddening resulting from sitting, specifically over the ischia, trochanters, and sacral region. Any areas of redness must be addressed immediately by being sure that no further excessive pressure is placed there. If the area is inflamed without blanching, tissue damage has occurred. A decubitus is impending, and the area must be made totally pressure-free.

The older child must learn to assume these responsibilities. The sitting child must relieve weight from his bottom by lifting up, rocking side to side, or leaning back in the chair every 15 minutes. There are many excellent seat cushions (ROHO, viscoelastic polymer), but none prevents tissue-killing pressures without weight relief. Furthermore, they must remain clean and dry of urine.

TREATMENT OF ESTABLISHED DECUBITUS

There are four main aspects to proper management of an established pressure sore: (1) assessment of the severity of tissue injury and systemic response; (2) determination as to the cause of the sore; (3) relief of pressure from the injured area; and (4) medical treatment of the injured tissue.

First, I assess the severity of the decubitus. Clean, shallow ulcerations (above the deep fascia) can usually be managed on an outpatient basis. Ulcerations that are deeper than this, particularly those with necrotic tissue present, require initial chemical and/or surgical debridement, so a period of hospitalization is usually necessary. If there is evidence of infection (foul discharge, local erythema, and particularly any systemic symptoms), hospitalization is required not only for appropriate debridement, but also for culture and intravenous antibiotics to control the infection. This is the only circumstance in which I find antibiotics helpful.

The next most important thing is to determine how the ulcer came about. If an ulcer represents one-time direct trauma, simple reeducation may be all that is required. If it is due to increased pressure, its cause must be removed. Ill-fitting shoes or braces are easy to correct. A poor sitting surface (e.g., a hammock-type wheelchair seat) is also readily corrected. Undue moisture present as a result of uncontrolled urinary or fecal incontinence, or poor general hygiene, must be dealt with. If these measures are not undertaken, repeat ulceration is inevitable no matter how good the care of a particular ulcer.

In the case of pressure decubitus, the initial medical management consists of removal of that pressure. Ulcers on the sole of neurogenic feet must be treated by non-weight-bearing. Ulcers caused by sitting must be treated by total weight relief. This involves the prone position, which can be tolerated for up to 8 hours at a time. A reclining wheelchair or stretcher can be used at home, if the ulcer itself permits. Ideally, the child can continue in school, but if not, I arrange homebound teaching for the duration of treatment. Hospitalized patients are managed similarly when the ulcer itself requires more intensive nursing care or antibiotic treatment.

I like to keep the treatment of the ulcer as simple as possible. Clean ulcers that extend to the deep fascia can be managed by a program of cleansing with hydrogen peroxide solution and loose packing of the wound with normal saline-soaked gauze. This should be repeated two or three times daily. The dressing may be covered with some gentle adhesive tape (e.g., Hypafix). I avoid excessive use of adhesive tape because this may sheer the surrounding skin.

Wounds with necrotic tissue require debridement. If there is extensive necrotic tissue, and/or bony involvement, I take the child to the operating room for surgical debridement. Less extensive necrotic tissue can be removed by gentle scrubbing or sharp superficial dissection, using hydrogen peroxide or Betadine diluted with an equal part of saline. Both of these agents are toxic to healthy granulation tissue, as well as any other, and therefore should be carefully cleaned away after debridement. They should be discontinued once only healthy granulation tissue is found in the wound. Commercially available enzyme products (Collagenase ointment, Elase ointment, Carrington gel) can be used during this phase of treatment, but I do not routinely use them in addition to the mechanical debridement and cleansing. After debridement, the wound is dressed with saline-soaked gauze and covered.

Decubitus caused by sitting that extends beyond the deep fascia, particularly one that involves bone, virtually always requires plastic surgical management in addition, to cover the affected area with a flap once the wound is clean. I therefore consult a plastic surgeon early in the course of management. Before reconstructive surgery, the ulcer must be clean and the cause of the ulcer corrected. If this condition is not corrected, the newly rotated flap is just as likely to break down as the original tissue.

The patient's nutritional status, particularly during this stressful period, must be as good as possible. I provide a high-protein, high-calorie diet with the addition of multivitamins and vitamin C (250 mg daily).

The impact from an economic, psychosocial, and physiologic standpoint can be staggering on the patient. Prevention of the decubitus ulcer is infinitely better management than good medical care after it has developed.

SUGGESTED READING

Agris J, Spira M. Pressure ulcers: prevention and treatment. Clin Symp 1979; 31:2–15.

Constantion M. Pressure ulcers: principles and techniques of management. Boston: Little, Brown, 1980.

WARTS

DAVID A. WHITING, M.D.,
M. MED.(DERM.), F.A.C.P., F.R.C.P.

Warts are intraepidermal tumors that affect skin and mucous membranes and are caused by a DNA virus known as the human papilloma virus (HPV). An increasing number of different types of HPV, about three dozen to date, are being identified. They are antigenically distinct, and this feature explains one individual's susceptibility to different types of warts at different sites at different times, despite spontaneous resolution of earlier warts. Warts are transmitted by direct contact, by indirect contact through contamination of objects and immediate environment, and by autoinoculation. All of these means involve direct inoculation of infected material. The incubation period of warts is 1 to 20 months, the average being 4 months. Warts are unusual in infants and young children, increase in frequency during the school years, and peak between the ages of 12 and 16 years.

Because therapy is influenced by the type of wart, a brief review of classification is necessary.

TYPES OF WARTS

Common Warts (Verruca Vulgaris)

These are single or multiple and start as pinhead, flesh-colored or translucent papules and grow within weeks or months into projecting lesions varying from 1 to 12 mm in diameter. They develop a rough horny surface and contain black specks from thrombosed capillaries. In children they are seen commonly on the backs of the hands and fingers and on the knees. Periungual warts, single or multiple, are common and occur especially in nail biters.

Plane Warts (Verruca Plana)

These are multiple small, tan, flattened, round or polygonal lesions 1 to 5 mm in diameter and are found especially on the face, back of the hand, and shins. They are more common in teenagers.

Filiform or Digitate Warts

These occur as single or multiple polypoid projecting lesions and are usually seen on the lips, nose, or eyelids in children.

Plantar Warts (Verruca Plantaris)

These inverted, flattened lesions occur as circumscribed, horny papules of the soles and when shaved show the black specks of thrombosed capillaries. A wart interrupts the natural skin lines, and there is a plane of cleavage between a plantar wart and the surrounding collarette of normal skin, unlike a corn. Lesions are single, multiple, or mosaic. Plantar warts are often painful unless they are of the mosaic variety.

Venereal Warts (Condylomata Acuminata)

These are multiple irregular or pointed papules that are often confluent and found on genital mucosa or adjacent skin. The occurrence of genital warts in small children should arouse suspicion of sexual abuse.

Epidermodysplasia Verruciformis

These multiple lesions resemble plane warts on the face and neck, but they are larger and firmer on the trunk and extremities. They are most numerous on the face and neck, and on the dorsal aspects of the hands and feet.

TYPES OF THERAPY

Warts have a high rate of spontaneous resolution, even while other warts are appearing: 20 to 30 percent of all warts resolve spontaneously within 6 months, 50 percent within 1 year, and 66 percent within 2 years.

Most methods of therapy involve some form of tissue destruction and therefore are often painful and may also lead to scarring. Overtreatment of warts can be a traumatic and mutilating experience, particularly to small children. Therapeutic zeal should be tempered with caution. The natural course of warts and their high spontaneous remission rate should be thoroughly explained and stressed. Warts that remit spontaneously vanish painlessly, often overnight, and leave no scars. Harmless placebos certainly have their place. When it is necessary to treat children, try to find a suitable method that is not too painful and causes minimal scarring (Table 1). The desire to eliminate every wart should be suppressed.

TABLE 1 Specific Recommendations for Treatment of Warts: In Order of Preference

Type of Wart	Treatment
Common warts	
Single or few	Light electrodesiccation and curettage, cryosurgery, keratolytics
Multiple	Cryosurgery, keratolytics, monochloracetic acid
Plantar warts	
Single or few	Keratolytics, light electrodesiccation and curettage with enucleation
Multiple	Keratolytics, formalin soaks, skin paring, and cushion inner soles
Plane warts	Cryosurgery, monochloracetic acid, light electrodesiccation and curettage, topical tretinoin, oral vitamin A
Filiform and digitate warts	Simple excision, light electrodesiccation and curettage, cryosurgery, monochloracetic acid
Venereal warts	Podophyllin, monochloracetic acid, cryosurgery, electrodesiccation and curettage
Periungual warts	Keratolytics, cantharidin, cryosurgery, curettage with enucleation
Epidermodysplasia verruciformis	Cryosurgery, monochloracetic acid, light electrodesiccation and curettage
Recalcitrant warts	Referral for specialized treatment such as carbon dioxide laser therapy, intralesional bleomycin, topical sensitization with a chemical such as diphenylcyclopropenone, topical 5-fluorouracil therapy, or, possibly at some future date, interferon therapy

Cryosurgery

Probably the easiest treatment is to dip a loosely wrapped cotton-tipped applicator into liquid nitrogen and apply it repeatedly to the wart for 10 to 30 seconds until a ring of frosting appears, extending 1 to 3 mm beyond the wart. Choose a swab a little smaller than the wart and apply it intermittently to small lesions and continuously to large lesions. Usually one freeze-thaw cycle is adequate, but for larger and thicker warts, two freeze-thaw cycles are preferable. No anesthesia is necessary. A liquid nitrogen cryospray can also be used with different-sized cones to limit the freezing zone, but for small children I find the swab method easier. Some physicians prefer to use carbon dioxide snow, either compressed into a solid pencil or mixed with acetone to produce a slush. Freezing causes stinging and burning, which peaks about 2 minutes after the treatment, when thawing occurs. It is followed by a wheal and flare reaction and later by blistering. Decompress large blisters with a sterile needle or No. 11 scalpel blade and cleanse them daily with hydrogen peroxide or 70 percent isopropyl alcohol. The blisters later flatten, and the dead wart and blister can be trimmed away. Patients should return for assessment and, if necessary, for retreatment every 2 to 3 weeks.

Electrodesiccation and Curettage

This method is suitable when only a small number of warts are present. Under local anesthesia, the wart is lightly electrodesiccated until it softens and bubbles. It is then removed with a curette (which may be sharp for common warts or blunt for plantar warts), leaving the underlying dermis intact. Hemostasis can be secured by pressure or by the application of a styptic such as ferrous subsulfate (Monsel's) solution. The electrodesiccating current should be kept to a minimum, to minimize scarring. Wounds should be cleansed daily with soap and water and hydrogen peroxide and dressings applied until firm dry scabs form. Many prefer to treat plantar warts with enucleation by blunt curettage alone, to minimize scarring. In this case, in order to obtain a plane of cleavage for the curette, either a light cautery burn or scissors is used to create a shallow trench around the perimeter of the wart.

Keratolytics

Different formulations are available, but I generally find it convenient to use salicylic acid, 5 to 20 percent, and lactic acid, 5 to 20 percent, in flexible collodion or compound tincture of benzoin. A suitable commercially available preparation is Duofilm (Stiefel), which contains 16.7 percent salicylic acid and 16.7 percent lactic acid in flexible collodion. It is best to apply the paint with an applicator when the warts are moist after bathing. Allow to dry, apply a second coat, and when that is dry, cover with an impermeable and occlusive tape such as Blenderm (3M Co.). Leave this in place for 24 hours, then remove it before shower or bath and remove dead skin with an emery board, callus file, pumice stone, or blade. Repeat the process after bathing, and continue until the wart disappears. This regimen removes 70 to 80 percent of common or ordinary plantar warts within 12 weeks, but only about half of mosaic plantar warts. This method is usually painless and free from scarring. Another useful formulation, particularly for plantar warts, is 40 percent salicylic acid plaster, which is available as Mediplast (Beiersdorf, Inc., South Norwalk, CT). This can be cut to the size of the wart, applied after bathing, covered with Blenderm, and left in place for several days at a time.

Acids

Monochlor-, bichlor-, and trichloracetic acids can be applied to warts. Trichloracetic acid causes more superficial destruction and monochloracetic acid causes deeper destruction. All are comparatively painless at the time of application, provided they are carefully applied with wooden applicators trimmed to the size of the wart, to confine the fluid to the warty lesion. I personally prefer a saturated solution of monochloracetic acid, which tends to sink through the wart and cause later blistering. It should be used sparingly at first because there is much individual variation in reaction to it, and severe blistering and ulceration with scarring can ensue. It can be reapplied every 2 to 3 weeks if necessary, and so it is advisable to start with very small amounts and to increase the acid application at follow-up visits as necessary. Severe pain and chemical inflammation can occur within the first few days of treatment. This is most likely to occur on the soles or palms and in the periungual regions; therefore, it is necessary to avoid or carefully control acid usage in these areas. These acids are highly corrosive, and great care must be exercised to protect mucosal surfaces, eyes, or normal skin in general.

Podophyllin

This cytotoxic agent is a metaphase inhibitor, which causes slow cell death and subsequent sloughing of the wart. Irritation during the sloughing process is common. I apply a 20 to 25 percent solution of podophyllin resin (USP) in compound tincture of benzoin, but I sometimes use 95 percent ethanol as the vehicle. Both solutions cause some burning at the time of application, and for small children, podophyllin 25 percent in liquid paraffin is painless, but has to be thoroughly remixed before use. Podophyllin works best in moist or macerated areas and is usually reserved for moist genital warts. Using it for plantar warts commonly results in secondary infection. It should be carefully applied to genital warts with an applicator and then dry dusted with talcum powder such as Zeosorb (Stiefel). It should be washed off within 6 to 8 hours or sooner if irritation occurs. Care should be exercised when using it on penile warts below the foreskin because severe swelling and even paraphimosis could occur. Reapplication every 10 to 14 days may be necessary. Low-potency topical steroid creams may help the irritation during treatment. The warts take 5 to 7 days to slough away. The podophyllin should be freshly prepared because its shelf life is limited. A suitable commercial preparation is Podofin (Syosset Laboratories).

Cantharidin

This preparation, which is a mitochondrial poison and a vesicant, causes dermoepidermal separation. Commercial preparations are Cantharone (Seres Laboratories) or Verrusol (C&M Pharmacal). It needs to be applied precisely to the wart with an applicator and then occluded with a waterproof tape such as Blenderm for 24 hours or until it becomes painful. The tape is then removed and the lesion soaked in warm soapy water. The lesion goes through blister, crust, and scab stages and needs to be trimmed off in 7 to 14 days and then retreated if necessary. No scarring occurs, but ringlike recurrences may be seen, especially if the blister extends well beyond the wart.

Soaks

Soaks are sometimes useful in the treatment of multiple plantar or palmar warts. The affected soles or palms should be soaked for 30 minutes in 3 to 5 percent formaldehyde solution, which should be used as a shallow layer in a flat-bottomed container, such as a large serving plate, to prevent contact with the thinner skin in the webs or on the sides of hands and feet. Formalin is irritating and sensitizing in some cases. Treatment for 2 to 4 weeks is necessary before the warts dry up and fall out. Glutaraldehyde, 10 percent, can be applied in the form of soaks or paints, but is usually less effective than formalin. Note that the glutaraldehyde solution must be freshly made because it deteriorates within a couple of weeks.

Miscellaneous Types of Treatment

Vitamin A Derivatives

Topical retinoic acid (tretinoin) preparations such as Retin-A (Ortho) may be applied to multiple plane warts over the long term. Orally administered vitamin A (such as Aquasol made by USV Pharmaceuticals), in daily doses of 50,000 to 100,000 U, can be tried.

Symptomatic Treatment

In cases of chronic plantar warts in which active intervention is undesirable, regular paring of hyperkeratotic skin and the use of cushion inner soles provides symptomatic relief.

MOLLUSCUM CONTAGIOSUM

CHARLES M. GINSBURG, M.D.

Molluscum contagiosum is caused by *Poxvirus mollusci,* a DNA virus that has a worldwide distribution and affects primates and marsupials as well as humans. The precise incidence of molluscum infection is not known; however, it has been estimated to affect 2 to 5 percent of humans. Although epidemiologic studies indicate that the largest attack rates for disease occur in children who are younger than 5 years old, recent epidemiologic evidence shows that the incidence of the disease is increasing in adolescents and young adults.

Molluscum virus is transmitted by direct contact and, possibly, by fomites. Autoinoculation is common in infants and young children. Although nonsexual transmission of virus among adults has been reported, the recently observed increased incidence of molluscum contagiosum in adolescents and young adults has been attributed to skin contact associated with sexual intercourse.

Following an incubation period of 2 to 7 weeks, the initial lesions of molluscum appear as pinhead-sized, discrete, flesh-colored papules. Over a period of days to weeks the lesions slowly enlarge and the characteristic central umbilication becomes apparent. Individual lesions are generally 3 to 5 mm in diameter and rarely exceed 10 mm in size. The distribution of lesions varies depending on the mode of transmission. In children and in adults with nonsexually transmitted disease, the lesions of molluscum are most common on the trunk, extremities, and, occasionally, the face.

By contrast, the primary lesions of sexually transmitted disease occur on the lower abdomen and in the genital regions. Mucous membrane involvement, uncommon at any age, generally occurs as a result of sexual intercourse or autoinoculation. Five to 10 percent of patients with molluscum contagiosum have a halolike eczematoid dermatitis surrounding the individual lesions. Although the precise explanation for this phenomenon is not known, it has been suggested that the reaction is secondary to delayed hypersensitivity to the viral antigen.

Because of their unique appearance, the lesions of molluscum contagiosum are generally not confused with other dermatologic disorders. In instances when the diagnosis is in question, it is often helpful to express manually material from the center of an umbilicated lesion and to stain it with Wright or Giesma stain to determine whether or not the characteristic inclusion bodies are present.

In most instances, therapy of molluscum contagiosum should be supportive. Parents and patients should be informed that the lesions will generally resolve spontaneously, without scarring, within 2 to 6 months. In instances when secondary infection or an eczematoid dermatitis is present, patients should be treated, respectively, with systemic antimicrobials or a topical corticosteroid. Lesions that do not resolve spontaneously or those that are infected recurrently can be removed by curettage, electrodissection, or cryotherapy, or with topically applied chemicals. No systematic comparative studies demonstrate a superiority of any one of these treatment modalities; therefore, specific therapy should be based on the number, size, and anatomic location of the lesion as well as the age and cooperativeness of the child.

SUGGESTED READING

Becker TM, Blount JH, Douglas J, Judson F. Trends in molluscum contagiosum in the United States, 1966–1983. Sex Trans Dis 1986; 13:88–92.

Felman Y, Nikitis JD. Genital molluscum contagiosum. Cutis 1980; 26:28–32.

Rackoff AS. Molluscum dermatitis. J Pediatr 1978; 92:945–947.

ERYTHRASMA

DAVID A. WHITING, M.D.,
M. MED.(DERM.), F.A.C.P., F.R.C.P.

Erythrasma is a bacterial infection of the skin surface caused by *Corynebacterium minutissimum.* The organism elaborates porphyrins, which produce a characteristic coral-red fluorescence when affected skin is exposed to a Wood's light. This is a reliable diagnostic test for infection, provided the area has not been washed recently. The organism can be cultured on Tissue Culture Medium 199 with 20 percent calf serum and 2 percent agar, provided no antibiotics are added.

C. minutissimum grows best in hot, humid areas, so it favors skin folds and is more common and more likely to cause symptoms in hot climates. It affects toewebs, groins, axillae, and intergluteal and inframammary folds. Patches of erythrasma are well-demarcated and initially red, later turning brownish and sometimes slightly scaly.

Effective topical therapy for erythrasma includes miconazole cream (Monistat-Derm, Ortho), aluminum chloride 20 percent in anhydrous ethyl alcohol (Drysol, Person and Covey), aqueous solution of 2 percent clindamycin hydrochloride, and benzoic and salicylic acid ointment U.S.P. (Whitfield's Ointment, Faugera). These should be applied twice daily for 3 to 4 weeks. Relapses are more likely to occur when agents such as antibacterial soaps, 3 percent sulfur ointment, or 20 percent sodium hyposulfite are used. In resistant or extensive cases, the treatment of choice is oral erythromycin, given four times a day in equally divided doses for 10 days. Children require 30 to 40 mg per kilogram per day, ranging up to an adult dosage of 1 g per day.

SUGGESTED READING

Roberts SOB, Highet AS. Erythrasma. In: Rook A, Wilkinson DS, Ebling FJG, Champion RH, Burton JL, eds. Textbook of dermatology, 4th ed, Vol. 1. Oxford: Blackwell Scientific, 1986; 759–761.

Sindhuphak W, MacDonald E, Smith EB. Erythrasma. Overlooked or misdiagnosed? Int J Dermatol 1985; 24:95–96.

STAPHYLOCOCCAL SCALDED SKIN SYNDROME

JAMES K. TODD, M.D.

The staphylococcal scalded skin syndrome (SSSS) is actually a spectrum of clinical illnesses that presents with different manifestations, depending on patient age and immune status. All disease manifestations are caused by a single epidermolytic toxin (exfoliation) produced by a few strains of *Staphylococcus aureus*. This toxin causes erythema and separation of the epidermis at the granular cell layer.

The various manifestations of toxin exposure depend on the age of the patient as well as preexisting humoral immunity. Newborns develop an extreme variant of SSSS called Ritter's disease, consisting of a generalized, painful erythematous eruption with positive Nikolsky sign. In infants these same manifestations resemble those of an acutely burned child—the classic scalded skin syndrome. The same clinical findings can also be seen in patients with drug eruptions, but a deeper level of epidermal involvement at the basal cell layer with some dermal inflammation is noted on skin biopsy. In older children, the same toxin may cause an erythematous, scarletinaform eruption—staphylococcal scarlet fever—which resembles streptococcal scarlet fever, with the notable absence of a strawberry tongue.

The milder clinical manifestations in older children seem to reflect a more rapid and effective excretion of the toxin. Patients who have preexisting humoral immunity (either transplacental or acquired) may have small areas of skin injury colonized with the same toxin-producing staphylococci, which produce enough toxin at the site of local infection to give large infected bullous lesions (e.g., bullous impetigo, bullous varicella). These lesions represent both the effect of the local infection and its toxin production, whereas the generalized forms represent toxin absorption from a focus of infection with systemic distribution to all areas of the skin in the absence of neutralizing humoral immunity.

Thus, the manifestations of this single staphylococcal toxin range from the severity of Ritter's disease in the newborn to the much milder forms of staphylococcal scarlet fever and isolated bullous lesions, with therapy dependent on the diagnosis and severity of illness in the patient.

RITTER'S DISEASE

Ritter's disease (generalized scalded skin syndrome in a newborn) can be severe. These patients have no preexisting transplacental antitoxin and therefore experience the toxin's maximum effect. The organism producing the toxin usually grows in the nasopharynx, with subsequent systemic absorption resulting in generalized skin injury. Other potential foci of infection (e.g., septic arthritis, osteomyelitis, pneumonia) should be investigated and blood cultures should be performed because some infants may also have staphylococcal bacteremia. Parenteral fluids should be given because these infants may experience significant fluid losses. Parenteral antistaphylococcal antibiotics (e.g., oxacillin, vancomycin) should be administered in appropriate dosages for newborns. The selection of antibiotics depends on the known antimicrobial susceptibility patterns of staphylococci isolated in that particular nursery. If methicillin-resistant *Staphylococcus aureus* strains have previously been identified, vancomycin would be more appropriate initial therapy until the organism is cultured and specific antimicrobial susceptibilities are performed. Although the skin in infants with Ritter's syndrome looks severely affected, the cleavage plane is superficial and full recovery can be expected. Ambitious local skin treatment (e.g., burn wound-type care) is, therefore, ordinarily not indicated. Precautions to accommodate for fluid and heat loss should be taken in small infants. With appropriate therapy (including drainage of any focus of infection) the skin lesions cease to progress within several days and gradually heal after desquamation. If no clear focus of infection that requires more prolonged therapy was established (e.g., osteomyelitis, septic arthritis, abscess, endocarditis), an appropriate oral antistaphylococcal antibiotic (e.g., cephalexin, erythromycin) can be selected to complete 2 weeks of therapy once the patient is afebrile and feeding well. The selection of antimicrobial agent depends on clear identification of the causative organism and appropriate antimicrobial susceptibilities. It should be remembered that some young infants do not absorb oral beta-lactam antibiotics well, and any change from parenteral antistaphylococcal therapy to oral therapy should include the measurement of serum bactericidal power to ensure appropriate absorption. Ordinarily a peak bactericidal titer of 1:8 or more is considered adequate therapy.

SCALDED SKIN SYNDROME

Although known by many names, this is the classical presentation of the epidermolytic toxin produced by *Staphylococcus aureus.* These patients are usually infants who present with painful erythroderma and positive Nikolsky sign. As was previously mentioned, it is important to be sure that the patient is not taking drugs (e.g., antibiotics, anticonvulsants) that might predispose to the same signs and symptoms but can be distinguished by the level of skin separation on a skin biopsy. Usually patients with staphylococcal scalded skin syndrome are irritable because of painful skin, but have normal oral mucous membranes and can take fluids (and antibiotics) orally. Appropriate diagnostic cultures should be considered in patients who have additional evidence of a focal staphylococcal infection. Otherwise, oral treatment with an appropriate antistaphylococcal antibiotic is usually sufficient. Cephalexin or dicloxacillin given orally (50 mg per kilogram per day), in four divided doses, is usually well tolerated and sufficient therapy. It should be emphasized that antimicrobial treatment (except in early cases) probably does little to alter the course of disease, which is self-limited. Parents are usually quite distressed, both at the apparent rejection they sense from their child whenever they attempt to pick him or her up (because of the painful skin) and also by their fear that the skin lesions may persist as permanent scars. With time and patience, both problems completely resolve. With appropriate hydration, the disease usually runs its course within 3 to 5 days, progressing to generalized desquamation with normal skin underneath. Unless there is a clearly identified focus of staphylococcal infection, long-term (more than 10 days) antimicrobial treatment is not indicated.

STAPHYLOCOCCAL SCARLET FEVER

Milder forms of rash associated with the same epidermolytic toxin may be seen, especially in older patients, which may look similar to streptococcal scarlet fever with a scarletinaform eruption, circumoral pallor, and Pastia's lines. Although the rash is similar, patients with staphylococcal scarlet fever have normal oral mucous membranes, which serve as a useful discriminating feature. Most patients are only mildly ill and can be treated as previously indicated with oral antistaphylococcal therapy.

BULLOUS LESIONS

Patients with isolated bullous lesions caused by *S. aureus* (e.g., bullous impetigo, bullous varicella) usually have high levels of humoral antibody against the scalded skin syndrome epidermolytic toxin; however, if the organism initiates a local skin infection (usually at the site of a break in skin or trauma) enough toxin can be formed locally to cause bullous separation of the superficial epidermal layer. These bullous lesions actually contain *S. aureus* and respond readily to oral antistaphylococcal therapy and local skin care consisting of rupture of the lesion, thorough washing, and then allowing the skin to dry.

Outbreaks of bullous impetigo and other diseases associated with the expanded scalded skin syndrome can occur in nurseries heavily colonized with a toxin-producing strain. Such outbreaks may be difficult to contain, however, efforts at cohorting patients and staff with careful skin and umbilical cord care and meticulous handwashing are often of benefit.

THE CARRIER STATE

Most antistaphylococcal therapy does not eradicate the carrier state but rather only treats an infected site. Thus, patients who have had scalded skin syndrome, Ritter's disease, or bullous impetigo may have recurrent bullous lesions because of the continued carrier state and reinfection of traumatized skin. These recurrences are usually milder than the initial episode because of the progressive development of antibody to the epidermolytic toxin. It is likely that other family members also carry the same strain of staphylococcus, so that eradication of the carrier state may be difficult. In the rare circumstance that frequent recurrences warrant an attempt to eradicate the carrier state, all family members carrying the organism (except pregnant women) should be treated with an appropriate oral antistaphylococcal agent (e.g., cephalexin or dicloxacillin, 30 mg per kilogram per day in divided doses four times a day) in combination with rifampin (10 to 20 mg per kilogram per day, twice a day) for 5 days. This combination may be effective in eradicating the carrier state, although recolonization can occur if the patient is reexposed to the same organism.

SUGGESTED READING

Melish ME, Glasgow LA. The staphylococcal scalded skin syndrome: the expanded clinical syndrome. J Pediatr 1971; 78:958–967.

Todd JK. Staphylococcal toxin syndromes. Annu Rev Med 1985; 36:337–347.

GAS GANGRENE

JAMES W. BASS, M.D., M.P.H.

The term *gas gangrene* has been used to refer to a variety of necrotizing soft tissue infections produced by *Clostridium perfringens* and other clostridial species resulting in free gas in the tissues. *Gaseous cellulitis* refers to infection confined to the skin and subcutaneous tissue and *gaseous fasciitis* refers to extension of the infection into fascia and along fascial planes without involvement of muscle. Classic gas gangrene, however, usually refers to fulminant life-threatening clostridial infection involving invasion and necrosis of muscle (clostridial myonecrosis). Other problems in terminology occur when infection is caused by other gas-producing bacteria, including anaerobic bacteroids, peptococci, peptostreptococci, and facultative aerobic coliforms. These variations in the definition of gas gangrene in terms of cause, site, and extent of involvement of infection may be responsible for the discrepancies in morbidity and mortality in response to treatment reported from different medical centers.

Clostridial myonecrosis in children most often occurs as a result of trauma, especially vehicular or agricultural accidents involving open fractures and massive tissue destruction and, as postoperative complications after surgery, usually involving the gastrointestinal tract. Factors favoring clostridial infection in these circumstances include contamination of the wound by foreign material (i.e., soil in open traumatic wounds, fecal material in wounds complicating gastrointestinal surgery), inadequate debridement of devitalized tissues, hemorrhage into the wound and surrounding tissues, and the presence of other proliferating bacteria in the wound. This may be accompanied by tissue ischemia caused by vascular injury, edema-causing compartment syndromes, or constrictive sutures or casts. All of these factors contribute to reduction of the local redox potential in the area, which is essential for clostridium organisms (obligate anaerobes) to thrive. The redox potential of most normal healthy tissues is too high to favor growth of these organisms.

After an incubation period of from 6 to 48 hours following traumatic injury or operative procedure, clostridial myonecrosis usually first manifests with elevation of body temperature, tachycardia, hypotension, and changes in mental status associated with typical skin changes. Early examination of the involved area reveals a characteristic pale yellow to bronze discoloration of the skin, with marked pain and tenderness without palpable subcutaneous emphysema, although radiographs of the affected area reveal soft tissue gas that is not yet palpable. At this stage the patient is usually mentally clear but may be apprehensive or anxious. As infection progresses, the skin becomes more edematous and tense and takes on an erythematous-bronze hue. Bullae filled with dark serosanguinous, foul-smelling fluid appear rapidly, and palpable subcutaneous emphysema becomes evident. All of these changes spread as the infection extends into adjacent tissues. Gram stain of wound exudates or of fluid from bullae usually reveals many gram-positive bacilli without spores and a striking scarcity of leukocytes. With further progression of the disease, severe systemic toxicity develops with high fever, hemolysis, jaundice, hypotension, severe metabolic acidosis, disseminated intravascular coagulation, multiple organ failure, and, without treatment, death in all cases within 48 hours after onset of systemic symptoms.

Clinical differentiation between clostridial cellulitis, fasciitis, myonecrosis, and nonclostridial gas gangrene can be difficult, and delay in treatment results in increased mortality. For these reasons all clinical gas gangrene infections should be treated as clostridial myonecrosis.

MANAGEMENT

General Supportive Treatment

The airway should be secured and high-flow oxygen should be given. Baseline blood studies including cultures, complete blood count (CBC), chemistries, arterial blood gases, and a radiograph of the affected area for soft tissue gas should be obtained. If the infection involves a wound, sutures should be removed and the wound should be opened and cultured. Further surgical treatment should be deferred as an operation room procedure, usually under general anesthesia, which should be scheduled immediately. Vital signs and urinary output should be closely monitored. Intravenous isotonic crystalloids such as saline or Ringer's lactate should be given to maintain blood pressure and visceral perfusion. If shock is present, volume resuscitation should be given. Vasopressors should be avoided, however, because vasoconstriction may further decrease tissue perfusion in the infected area, accelerating spread. Potent hemolysins produced by *C. perfringens* organisms result in severe hemolysis, and marked anemia is frequently seen in patients with advanced infection. Blood should be given sparingly until specific treatment has brought infection and toxemia under control, because transfused blood is also rapidly hemolyzed. Tetanus toxoid should be given if immunization is not current. All of these procedures should be accomplished within the first few minutes as the patient is being evaluated. Survival depends on providing immediate specific treatment, including antimicrobial drugs, surgery, and hyperbaric oxygen therapy. Specific treatment using polyvalent gas gangrene antitoxin has never been proven effective for treatment of gas gangrene, and most recipients experienced serious, occasionally fatal, untoward reactions. It is no longer available.

Antimicrobial Drugs

Based on data from uncontrolled clinical studies during World War II, the Vietnam War, and more recent civilian series, penicillin G is the time-honored recommended antibiotic of choice for treatment of gas gangrene. It should be given in a dosage of 250,000 U per kilogram per day, administered intravenously, in divided doses every 4 hours. More recent controlled studies in experimental animals have shown clindamycin to be the most effective drug, and tetracycline, chloramphenicol, rifampin, and metronidazole all to be superior to penicillin in prevention and treatment of gas gangrene. Pending further more definitive studies, clindamycin, 30 mg per kilogram per day, tetracycline, 25 mg per kilogram per day, or chloramphenicol, 50 mg per kilogram per day, each given in divided intravenous doses at 6-hour intervals, should probably be added as a second drug. Also, since different strains of *C. perfringens* and related clostridium species have varied in their susceptibility to these drugs, it appears appropriate to provide double drug coverage for these organisms. Gentamicin, 5 mg per kilogram per day in three divided doses given intravenously or intramuscularly, should be given as a third drug to cover mixed infection with gram-negative enteric organisms. The first dose of each drug should be given immediately at the initial evaluation.

Surgery

Immediate surgical intervention is necessary to confirm the diagnosis, assess the severity and extent of infection, and permit specific surgical treatment, the single most important determinant in survival. The area should be opened and explored to the full extent of the infection. Foreign material, hematomas, and exudates should be removed and devitalized tissues should be excised. With early intervention, infection may be localized and decompression of the involved fascial compartments, by multiple incisions and fasciotomies and excision of infected muscles alone, may arrest the process and eliminate the need for amputation. Local excision of single muscles or muscle groups may be adequate to conserve a functional extremity. With delay in diagnosis and treatment, irreversible gangrenous changes involving the whole extremity necessitate amputation.

Hyperbaric Oxygen Therapy (HBO)

Hyperbaric oxygen appears to augment antimicrobial and surgical treatment. A Po_2 of 90 mm Hg is lethal to *C. perfringens* organisms, but arterial Po_2 pressures of 800 to 1,000 mm Hg are required to produce tissue oxygen concentrations of this magnitude. Although these concentrations are not practical to achieve, tissue oxygen tensions of 250 mm Hg, a level that inhibits growth and toxin production of *C. perfringens,* are achieved with HBO with 100 percent oxygen at 3 Bar. A treatment schedule using three "dives" of 2 hours at 3 Bar within the first 24 hours, and two "dives" daily thereafter until the infection is under control, is recommended.

SUGGESTED READING

Altemeier WA, Fullen WD. Prevention and treatment of gas gangrene. JAMA 1971; 217:806–813.
Darke SG, King AM, Slack WK. Gas gangrene and related infection: classification, clinical features and aetiology, management and mortality. A report of 88 cases. Br J Surg 1977; 64:104–112.
Freishlag JA, Ajalat G, Busuttil RW. Treatment of necrotizing soft tissue infections: the need for a new approach. Am J Surg 1985; 149:751–755.
Kline KA, Turnbull TL. Clostridial myonecrosis. Ann Emerg Med 1985; 14:459–466.
Myers AM, Schnitsner BA. Hyperbaric oxygen use: update 1984. Postgrad Med 1984; 76:83–95.
Stevens DL, Maier KA, Laine BM, et al. Comparison of clindamycin, rifampin, tetracycline, metronidazole, and penicillin for efficacy in prevention of experimental gas gangrene due to *Clostridium perfringens.* J Infect Dis 1987; 155:220–228.

The opinions or assertions contained herein are the private views of the author and are not to be construed as official or as reflecting the views of the Department of the Army or the Department of Defense.

NECROTIZING FASCIITIS

DALE COLN, M.D.

Necrotizing fasciitis is a rapidly advancing destructive infection along muscle fascia. It is caused by multiple organisms invading the fascial plane, either through a wound in the skin or by outward extension of an intra-abdominal infection. It is seen after puncture wounds of the extremities, colostomy closures, closure of omphaloceles, and intra-abdominal infections. The main feature that distinguishes necrotizing fasciitis from cellulitis is the rapidly advancing painful erythematous wound edge, with accompanying central necrosis of the skin. The necrotic skin is bluish and blistered. The subcutaneous undermining characteristic of necrotizing fasciitis can be confirmed by incising the skin and gently inserting a hemostat below it, along the plane of the fascia. If the hemostat passes unobstructed along the plain of the fascia, a diagnosis of necrotizing fasciitis can be made.

The primary treatment of necrotizing fasciitis is aggressive surgical debridement. Under general anesthesia in the operating room, the wound is opened to all leading edges of erythema. All dead skin is removed, along with any necrotic fascia and muscle. Thorough washing of the wound is done with pulsating application of warm saline. Fine-mesh gauze is then loosely packed into the wound and the wound is dressed in such a manner that it can be inspected in 4 hours to determine whether the infection is spreading or not.

The common offending organisms are *Staphylococcus aureus,* Group A streptococcus, and *Escherichia coli.* The choice of antibiotics is based on the results of Gram stain and culture. Until this information is available, intravenous penicillin, 25,000 U per kilogram of body weight, every 6 hours, and gentamicin, 1.5 to 2 mg per kilogram every 8 hours, is given. These antibiotics are started as soon as the diagnosis is suspected and not withheld until surgical debridement is done. A specimen for culture can be obtained before debridement by aspirating the central area of skin necrosis. A good time to do this is when the incision is made to inspect the fascia to make the diagnosis. Antibiotic therapy is continued for 7 to 10 days after the debridement, pending satisfactory appearance of the wound.

The wound is inspected 4 hours after the initial debridement and then every 4 to 6 hours for the first 24 hours. The patient is returned to the operating room 24 hours after the initial debridement for dressing change and any further debridement. Dressing changes are performed on an every-day to every-other-day basis, under general anesthesia or after the administration of ketamine, 2 mg per kilogram, given intramuscularly or intravenously.

Final reconstruction of the wound is deferred until the life-threatening crisis has passed and the patient is making a good recovery from the metabolic consequences, which can be severe with this serious infection. Complete blood count, platelet count, bleeding and clotting studies, serum electrolytes, and calcium are measured at the time of the initial diagnosis and are monitored on a daily basis for 48 to 72 hours after debridement. Blood transfusions are administered to replace any blood loss at the time of the debridement and to correct the anemia that sometimes accompanies the necrotizing fasciitis. Intravenous calcium may be necessary for infections involving a large surface area, because of saponification of fat. Intravenous nutrition may also be necessary.

Response to therapy is gauged by the disappearance of the signs of toxicity, the halting of the advancing skin erythema and the healthy appearance of the wound when the dressing is changed. Failure of response requires further surgical debridement and assessment of the appropriateness of the antibiotic therapy based on culture and susceptibility testing results.

SUGGESTED READING

Gozal D, Ziser A, Shupak A, et al. Necrotizing fasciitis. Arch Surg 1986; 121:233–235.
Pessa M. Necrotizing fasciitis. Surg Gynecol Obstet 1985; 161:357–361.
Rea JW, Wyrock Jr JW. Necrotizing fasciitis. Ann Surg 1970; 172:957–964.

DISEASES OF THE HEART AND BLOOD VESSELS

INFECTIVE ENDOCARDITIS

STANFORD T. SHULMAN, M.D.

In the preantibiotic era, infective endocarditis was associated with virtually 100 percent mortality. Even though antimicrobial agents clearly revolutionized therapy of this disorder, endocarditis remains a serious medical problem that requires prompt and aggressive therapy.

The accurate diagnosis of endocarditis generally necessitates identification of the infecting microorganism from blood cultures. Except in severely and acutely ill patients, empiric institution of therapy prior to recovery of the causative agent is to be discouraged because failure to isolate the infecting organism complicates management greatly. In patients with the typical subacute presentation, three to four sets of blood cultures should be obtained over the first 24 hours in the hospital (longer if the patient has recently received any antibiotic therapy) to maximize the opportunity to identify the infecting microbe. In those patients with an acute presentation manifested by toxicity or progressive hemodynamic instability, one should obtain three to four sets of blood cultures (by separate venipunctures) over several hours before instituting empiric antibiotic treatment.

PREDISPOSING FACTORS AND ETIOLOGIC AGENTS

Most children with endocarditis have preexisting structural heart disease. In highly developed parts of the world, decreasing proportions of endocarditis patients have preexisting rheumatic heart disease, and increasing proportions have congenital heart disease (with or without previous cardiac surgery) or indwelling intravascular catheters or devices. In developing areas, rheumatic heart disease remains a prominent risk factor for endocarditis. In recent years it has been recognized that children at particularly high risk for endocarditis include those with surgically constructed systemic-pulmonary shunts as well as those with prosthetic valves or other intracardiac prosthetic material. Intravenous drug abuse is a prominent risk factor in adolescents and young adults who develop endocarditis in the absence of preexisting cardiac disease.

Although virtually every microbe ever isolated from humans has been reported at one time or another to have caused infective endocarditis, the majority of such infections are caused by a relatively limited number of pathogens, particularly streptococci and staphylococci. These agents account for approximately 80 percent of pediatric cases of endocarditis on the average. Endocarditis in patients with prosthetic valves, in the early postoperative period, or in drug abusers is more likely to be caused by more unusual agents such as gram-negative bacilli or fungi.

ANTIMICROBIAL THERAPY: GENERAL

Successful treatment of infective endocarditis requires intensive parenteral therapy with bactericidal antibiotic(s). This is not because of antibiotic resistance but because within vegetations the organisms are quite protected from host defenses and also appear to be relatively inactive metabolically. Bacteriostatic drugs have been associated with frequent treatment failures and relapses. Intravenous antibiotics are preferred to intramuscular antibiotics in children because of the lack of muscle mass as well as the psychologic trauma of repeated intramuscular injections. Use of heparin lock devices facilitates ease of therapy and ambulation in older children. Home intravenous therapy can be used in some patients with a particularly stable initial course in hospital. Despite aggressive use of intravenous bactericidal antibiotics, certain patients require surgical intervention in addition to medical therapy to effect a cure (see following).

During therapy, antibiotic concentrations in blood should substantially exceed the minimum bactericidal concentration (MBC), i.e., the minimum drug concentration required to kill the infecting organism in vitro. When combinations of antibiotics are employed, they should be tested in vitro against the patient's isolate for evidence of synergistic activity. Soon after therapy is initiated, documentation of cessation of bacteremia should be sought as a measure of the adequacy of the treatment regimen: this also should be monitored by periodic assessment of the serum bactericidal titer (SBT), i.e., the highest serum dilution that kills the patient's isolate in vitro. Peak SBT titers of 1:32 or greater are associated with a high rate of cure, although lower SBT titers do not necessarily portend failure. Following therapy, several blood cultures should be obtained over the first 1 or 2 months to document that the infection has been cured and to detect the occasional relapse that occurs.

HIGHLY PENICILLIN-SUSCEPTIBLE STREPTOCOCCAL ENDOCARDITIS

Streptococci with minimal inhibitory concentrations (MICs) of penicillin of 0.1 μg per milliliter or less are considered highly penicillin-susceptible and are among the most common organisms that cause endocarditis. In children, the vast majority of these organisms are alpha-hemolytic (viridans) streptococci, and the rest usually either *S. bovis* (a nonenterococcal Group D streptococcus) or Group A streptococci (*S. pyogenes*). For individuals who are not allergic to penicillin, three therapeutic regimens are associated with high cure rates (Table 1): (a) intravenous aqueous crystalline penicillin G for 4 weeks; (b) intravenous penicillin G *or* intramuscular procaine penicillin G for 4 weeks together with a parenteral aminoglycoside such as gentamicin for 2 weeks; and (c) intravenous penicillin G *or* intramuscular procaine penicillin G for 2 weeks in combination with a parenteral aminoglycoside such as gentamicin or streptomycin for 2 weeks. Each of these regimens has certain advantages and disadvantages.

Intravenous aqueous crystalline penicillin G (150,000 U per kilogram per day administered continuously or divided into six doses) for 4 weeks is associated with low relapse rates and avoids exposure to an aminoglycoside. This regimen is preferred for patients with impaired renal or eighth nerve function or at particular risk of aminoglycoside toxicity. Unacceptably high relapse rates have been reported when intravenous penicillin has been administered alone for 2 or 3 weeks.

Because synergy between penicillin G and aminoglycosides (e.g., gentamicin, streptomycin, amikacin) is easily demonstrated for viridans streptococci and for nonenterococcal Group D organisms, and because combinations of penicillin G and an aminoglycoside are superior to penicillin G alone for treatment in the animal model of experimental endocarditis, regimens of 4 weeks of penicillin G combined with an aminoglycoside for the first 2 weeks are widely employed and highly effective. Reported relapse rates are quite low with this therapy, but this regimen has not been established to be superior to penicillin G alone for viridans streptococcal endocarditis. Most published experience with this combination is with twice-daily intramuscular streptomycin (10 mg per kilogram per dose, up to 500 mg), which renders it quite unattractive for treating children. Therapy of 4 weeks of intravenous penicillin G with intravenous gentamicin (2.5 mg per kilogram per dose, up to 100 mg, every 8 hours) or amikacin (7.5 mg per kilogram per dose, up to 240 mg, every 8 hours) is more acceptable for children. Patients with eighth nerve or renal insufficiency should either not receive this regimen or receive smaller dosages of aminoglycoside.

Short-term (2-week) combined penicillin G and aminoglycoside (usually streptomycin) regimens have become increasingly popular in the treatment of highly penicillin-susceptible streptococcal endocarditis in adults because reported relapse rates have been low and because the savings associated with a shortened hospital stay are considerable. Experience

TABLE 1   Treatment of Streptococcal Endocarditis

Drug	Dosage	Duration (Weeks)
Penicillin MIC ≥0.1 μg/ml (also nutritionally variant streptococci)	Penicillin G (150,000 U/kg/day, up to 16 million U/day) IV	4
	+ gentamicin (7.5 mg/kg/day, up to 240 mg/day) IV	4
	or amikacin (22.5 mg/kg/day, up to 720 mg/day) IV	4
	Alternative: vancomycin (40 mg/kg/day, up to 2 g/day) IV	4
	or cephalothin (100 mg/kg/day, up to 12 g/day) IV	4
Penicillin MIC <0.1 μg/ml	Penicillin G (150,000 U/kg/day, up to 16 million U/day) IV	4
	or	
	Penicillin G (150,000 U/kg/day, up to 16 million U/day) IV	4
	+ gentamicin (7.5 mg/kg/day, up to 240 mg/day) IV	2
	or amikacin (22.5 mg/kg/day, up to 720 mg/day) IV	2
	or	
	Penicillin G* (150,000 U/kg/day, up to 16 million U/day) IV	2
	+ gentamicin (7.5 mg/kg/day, up to 240 mg/day) IV	2
	or amikacin (22.5 mg/kg/day, up to 720 mg/day) IV	2
	Alternative: vancomycin (40 mg/kg/day, up to 2 g/day) IV	4
	or cephalothin (100 mg/kg/day, up to 12 g/day) IV	4
Penicillin-resistant (enterococcus)	Penicillin G (150,000 U/kg/day, up to 16 million U/day) IV	4–6
	or ampicillin (200 mg/kg/day, up to 12 g/day) IV	4–6
	+ gentamicin (7.5 mg/kg/day, up to 240 mg/day) IV	4–6
	or streptomycin (15 mg/kg/day in 2 doses, up to 1 g/day) IM	4–6
	Alternative: vancomycin (40 mg/kg/day, up to 2 g/day) IV	4–6
	+ gentamicin (7.5 mg/kg/day, up to 240 mg/day) IV	4–6

* See text for exclusions.

with 2-week regimens in children is limited, but they appear promising. For children, intravenous gentamicin therapy appears to be the preferred aminoglycoside of choice; however, it must be pointed out that the published short-course experience in adults has been with penicillin and streptomycin exclusively. We have used gentamicin with satisfactory results in this way. Consideration of a 2-week treatment regimen for highly penicillin-susceptible streptococcal endocarditis should be limited to those patients in whom the clinical features, as well as the characteristics of the bacterial isolate, strongly suggest a favorable outcome. Short-course therapy clearly should *not* be used for patients infected with "relatively penicillin-resistant" (see following), penicillin-tolerant, or nutritionally deficient strains of viridans streptococci. Furthermore, it should *not* be used for patients who have any of the following clinical features: endocarditis of more than 3 months' duration, prosthetic valve infection, shock or decreased perfusion, extracardiac foci of infection, mycotic aneurysm or cerebritis, renal failure, or ventricular dysfunction. In general, the few relapses that have occurred following short-course therapy have been readily detected and promptly responsive to treatment. The majority of such relapses occur within 2 months.

Penicillin-allergic individuals frequently can be desensitized successfully to allow treatment with the drug of choice, penicillin. An effective alternative regimen when penicillin cannot be employed safely is intravenous vancomycin (10 mg per kilogram per dose, up to 500 mg per kilogram per dose, four times daily) for 4 weeks. Cephalosporins such as cephalothin or cefazolin should be used cautiously in highly penicillin-allergic patients. In vitro susceptibility testing of the patient's organism should be performed with these alternative agents.

RELATIVELY PENICILLIN-RESISTANT STREPTOCOCCAL ENDOCARDITIS

Viridans streptococci with MICs of penicillin 0.1 μg per milliliter or greater are occasionally recovered from pediatric patients with endocarditis and are best treated with 4 weeks each of intravenous aqueous penicillin G and parenteral gentamicin. Four weeks of vancomycin is a reasonable alternative for penicillin-allergic individuals; insufficient clinical data are available at present to determine the advantages of the addition of an aminoglycoside to the latter agent, although we have utilized this for difficult patients with excellent renal function.

PENICILLIN-RESISTANT STREPTOCOCCAL ENDOCARDITIS

Enterococci (*S. fecalis, S. fecium, S. durans*) are fortunately uncommon causes of endocarditis in pediatric patients. Treatment of these infections is diffi-

cult; the mean penicillin MIC for these organisms equals 2 μg per milliliter, which necessitates combination therapy of intravenous penicillin G or ampicillin with a synergistic aminoglycoside, usually streptomycin or gentamicin, for 4 to 6 weeks. Synergy in vitro correlates with the absence of high-level (MIC of 2,000 μg per milliliter or greater) resistance to a given aminoglycoside. In penicillin-allergic patients who cannot be desensitized, 4 to 6 weeks of vancomycin combined with streptomycin or gentamicin is recommended. Patients receiving these regimens should be closely monitored for renal toxicity and ototoxicity.

STAPHYLOCOCCAL ENDOCARDITIS

Because only a small percentage of staphylococcal strains associated with endocarditis are penicillin susceptible, antibiotic therapy must generally include a penicillinase-resistant penicillin (nafcillin or oxacillin, 200 mg per kilogram per day in four to six doses) or cephalosporin (cephalothin or cefazolin 100 mg per kilogram per day in four to six doses) administered intravenously for 4 to 6 weeks (Table 2). Because most staphylococcal endocarditis is serious, the 6-week regimen is more commonly used and is preferable. Although some have recommended oral therapy (with careful monitoring of serum concentrations of antibiotic) during the last several weeks of therapy, this should be undertaken with extreme caution. Patients with endocarditis caused by a penicillin-susceptible strain of *S. aureus* should receive large doses of intravenous penicillin G for 4 to 6 weeks.

Addition of an aminoglycoside or rifampin to a penicillinase-resistant penicillin as adjunctive therapy, to take advantage of frequent synergistic interaction, has been suggested. Although definitive data do not exist, we have used one of these agents in particularly severe or unresponsive instances of staphylococcal endocarditis, with apparent success. The latter category of patient includes, for example, patients with *S. epidermidis* prosthetic valve endocarditis.

Many strains of *S. epidermidis,* as well as a small but increasing number of strains of *S. aureus,* are resistant to the penicillinase-resistant penicillins. These include strains of *S. epidermidis* likely to cause prosthetic valve or postoperative endocarditis. Vancomycin given intravenously for 6 weeks is the mainstay of treatment for these troublesome infections; the possible adjunctive role of other agents such as rifampin and/or an aminoglycoside is still undefined. Both gentamicin and rifampin may be added to vancomycin in the instance of a methicillin-resistant *S. epidermidis* prosthetic valve infection. Cephalosporins should be avoided in the treatment of infections caused by these strains.

Antibiotic tolerance has been reported for some staphylococcal strains, especially with *S. aureus,* although its clinical significance is somewhat unclear. A tolerant organism is one in which a large discrep-

TABLE 2   Staphylococcal Endocarditis

Drug	Dosage	Time (Weeks)
Penicillin-resistant, methicillin-susceptible		
S. aureus		
S. epidermidis (coagulase ⊖)	Nafcillin *or* oxacillin (200 mg/kg/day, up to 12 g/day) IV	4–6
	Alternative:	
	Vancomycin (40 mg/kg/day, up to 2 g/day) IV	4–6
	or cefazolin (100 mg/kg/day, up to 8 g/day) IV	4–6
Penicillin-susceptible (rare)		
S. aureus	Penicillin G (150,000 U/kg/day, up to 16 million U/day) IV	4–6
S. epidermidis (coagulase ⊖)		
	Alternative:	
	Vancomycin (40 mg/kg/day, up to 2 g/day) IV	4–6
	or cefazolin (100 mg/kg/day, up to 8 g/day) IV	4–6
Methicillin-resistant		
S. epidermidis (coagulase ⊖)	Vancomycin (40 mg/kg/day, up to 2 g/day) IV	6
S. aureus		
	Alternative:	
	Select on susceptibility data	

Notes: (*a*) Adjunctive therapy with rifampin and/or an aminoglycoside such as gentamicin may be useful in particularly severe or unresponsive cases and in patients with staphylococcal prosthetic valve infection or infections with tolerant organisms or methicillin-resistant organisms. (*b*) Cephalosporins may elicit cross-allergenicity in penicillin-allergic patients. (*c*) Vancomycin and gentamicin doses must be adjusted for renal insufficiency.

ancy between the MIC and the MBC exists. These organisms may be particularly difficult to eradicate with antibiotics. Successful therapy of tolerant *S. aureus* infections may require the combination of a penicillinase-resistant penicillin and rifampin.

In the penicillin-allergic individual with staphylococcal endocarditis who cannot be desensitized, intravenous vancomycin administered for 6 weeks is the drug of choice.

GRAM-NEGATIVE ENDOCARDITIS

Endocarditis caused by enteric bacilli (*E. coli,* etc.) and *Pseudomonas aeruginosa* requires an individualized antibiotic regimen based on in vitro antibiotic susceptibilities. Most such patients are treated with 4 to 6 weeks (6 weeks is preferable) of intravenous ampicillin or carbenicillin or an expanded-spectrum cephalosporin together with an aminoglycoside (usually gentamicin or amikacin).

More common causes of gram-negative endocarditis are the fastidious gram-negative coccobacilli, including *Haemophilus aphrophilus,* other *Haemophilus* species, *Actinobacillus actinomycetemcomitans, Cardiobacterium hominis, Eikenella corrodens,* and *Kingella kingii.* The most commonly used regimen for these infections is penicillin or ampicillin, frequently in combination with an aminoglycoside. Antibiotic susceptibility data and SBTs are highly useful in managing patients with these infections. Gonococcal endocarditis can be treated with large-dosage intravenous penicillin therapy.

FUNGAL ENDOCARDITIS

Endocarditis caused by *Candida,* or more rarely by other fungi, is seen in the setting of intravenous drug abuse, postcardiac surgery, prolonged antibiotic administration, central hyperalimentation, or immunocompromised states; it is associated with high mortality. Diagnosis is difficult because blood cultures yielding *Candida* do not necessarily indicate the presence of endocarditis; endocarditis caused by other fungi, on the other hand, is rarely associated with positive blood cultures and is frequently diagnosed only at surgery or autopsy. More recently, the echocardiogram has become useful in diagnosing fungal endocarditis.

Treatment of fungal endocarditis with antifungal agents alone is almost always unsuccessful. Surgical excision of the infected tissue with replacement of the infected valve, together with at least 6 postoperative weeks of intravenous amphotericin B therapy, is usually required. The role of adjunctive therapy with other antifungal agents such as flucytosine or ketoconazole has not been clearly defined. Surgery is probably best performed after 1 to 2 weeks of medical therapy if the patient's hemodynamic status permits and earlier if there is evidence of embolic phenomena.

CULTURE-NEGATIVE ENDOCARDITIS

After careful workup, therapy for the rare patient believed to have culture-negative endocarditis should include penicillin G or a penicillinase-resistant penicillin (nafcillin or oxacillin) together with streptomycin or gentamicin. For patients who are allergic to penicillin or for those with prosthetic valves, vancomycin with an aminoglycoside should be used. Discontinuation of the aminoglycoside may be considered after 2 weeks if there has been a substantial response to therapy, although therapy must be individualized. Treatment should be continued for 6 full weeks.

PROSTHETIC VALVE ENDOCARDITIS

Antibiotic therapy for patients with infected prosthetic heart valves must be appropriate for the specific infecting agent and must be administered for at least 4 weeks; 6 weeks of treatment is usually necessary for cure. In general, therapy for endocarditis on a prosthetic valve or other device should be approximately 2 weeks longer than would be appropriate for the same infection on a native valve. For the rare infections with penicillin susceptible (MIC less than 0.1 μg per milliliter) staphylococci, penicillin G is the preferred agent. Penicillin-resistant, nafcillin-susceptible staphylococcal infections are treated with nafcillin or oxacillin, or one of these antibiotics in combination with an aminoglycoside for at least the first 2 weeks. Nafcillin-resistant *S. aureus* or *S. epidermidis* infections, or any staphylococcal infection in a penicillin-allergic individual, should be treated with intravenous vancomycin 10 mg per kilogram every 6 hours (not to exceed 500 mg per dose), probably along with oral rifampin and/or intravenously administered aminoglycoside.

Prosthetic valve infections caused by highly penicillin-sensitive streptococci (MIC 0.1 μg per milliliter or less) should be treated with 6 weeks of intravenous penicillin and gentamicin or amikacin, whereas those caused by "relatively penicillin-resistant" streptococci or enterococci should be treated for up to 8 weeks with the same drugs. For penicillin-allergic individuals who cannot be desensitized, vancomycin in combination with an aminoglycoside is recommended. Prosthetic valve endocarditis caused by diphtheroids is best treated with penicillin and gentamicin, or with vancomycin for penicillin-allergic patients. Therapy for gram-negative bacillary prosthetic valve endocarditis must be prolonged and based on the results of in vitro MIC and MBC tests and in vitro evaluation of synergy between several antibiotics. Common regimens include cephalothin and gentamicin, and carbenicillin and gentamicin, for at least 6 weeks. The role of newer cephalosporins in these infections appears promising but remains to be clarified.

TABLE 3   Antibiotic Regimens for the Prevention of Bacterial Endocarditis

Regimen	Condition	Dosage
Recommended antibiotic regimens for dental/respiratory tract procedures*		
Standard	For dental procedures that cause gingival bleeding and oral/respiratory tract surgery	Penicillin V (2 g orally 1 hour before, then 1 g 6 hours later); for patients unable to take oral medications, 2 million U of aqueous penicillin G IV or IM 30–60 min before a procedure and 1 million U 6 hours later may be substituted
Special	Parenteral regimen for use when maximal protection is desired, e.g., for patients with prosthetic valves	Ampicillin (1–2 g IM or IV) plus gentamicin (2 mg/kg IM or IV), half hour before procedure, followed by 1 g oral penicillin V 6 hours later; alternatively, parenteral regimen may be repeated once 8 hours later
	Oral regimen for penicillin-allergic patients	Erythromycin (1 g orally 1 hour before), then 500 mg 6 hours later
	Parenteral regimen for penicillin-allergic patients	Vancomycin (1 g IV *slowly* over 1 hour starting 1 hour before); no repeat dose necessary
Recommended regimens for gastrointestinal/ genitourinary tract procedures*		
Standard	For genitourinary/gastrointestinal tract procedures	Ampicillin (2 g IM or IV) plus gentamicin (2 mg/kg IM or IV), given 30 min to 1 hour before procedure; 1 follow-up dose may be given 8 hours later
Special	Oral regimen for minor or repetitive procedures in low-risk patients	Amoxicillin (3 g orally 1 hour before procedure and 1.5 g 6 hours later)
	Penicillin-allergic patients	Vancomycin (1 g IV *slowly* over 1 hour), plus gentamicin (2 mg/kg IM or IV given 1 hour before procedure); may be repeated once 8–12 hours later

* Pediatric doses are as follows: ampicillin (50 mg per kilogram per dose); amoxicillin (50 mg per kilogram per dose); erythromycin (20 mg per kilogram for the first dose, then 10 mg per kilogram); gentamicin sulfate (2 mg per kilogram per dose); penicillin V (full adult dose if weight is greater than 27 kg [60 lb]; one-half adult dose if weight is less than 27 kg [60 lb]); aqueous penicillin G sodium (50,000 U per kilogram; 25,000 U per kilogram follow-up); and vancomycin hydrochloride (20 mg per kilogram per dose). The intervals between doses are the same as for adults. Total dosages should not exceed adult dosages.

Adapted from Shulman ST and Committee on Rheumatic Fever and Bacterial Endocarditis, American Heart Association. Circulation 1984; 70:1123.

SURGICAL CONSIDERATIONS

Recent experience in adults with prosthetic valve endocarditis has suggested that early surgical replacement of the infected valve may reduce the excessively high mortality associated with such infections. The timing of surgical removal and replacement of an infected prosthetic valve or other device must be individualized. The clinician must establish that operative intervention is inevitable, but should not delay a decision for surgery in a deteriorating clinical situation until the surgical risk becomes prohibitive. Some have recommended that most or all patients with staphylococcal or early-onset (fewer than 60 days postoperative) prosthetic valve infection should undergo valve replacement. Definite indications for operative intervention include significant valvular obstruction, progressive heart failure secondary to valvular insufficiency or dehiscence, proved or suspected fungal endocarditis, persistently positive blood cultures despite appropriate antibiotics for 10 to 14 days, bacteriologic relapse after an appropriate course of therapy, and recurrent major emboli. Less definite indications for surgery include a single major embolus, echocardiographic demonstration of a large vegetation, and extension of infection to an annular abscess or myocardial abscess.

Surgery for *non*prosthetic valve endocarditis is sometimes necessary as well, and proper timing of surgical intervention is sometimes life-saving. General indications for surgery include (1) intractable congestive failure, usually the result of progressive valvular insufficiency, (2) inability to sterilize the blood despite appropriate medical therapy, (3) valve ring and/or myocardial abscess, (4) embolic event(s) during therapy, and (5) fungal endocarditis.

PREVENTION OF ENDOCARDITIS

The American Heart Association for many years has reviewed data on the efficacy of antibiotic prophylaxis for endocarditis and has recommended specific regimens (Table 3). Prophylaxis is indicated for those patients with prosthetic heart valves, surgically constructed systemic-pulmonary shunts, previous history of endocarditis, most congenital heart conditions, rheumatic and other acquired valvular dysfunction, idiopathic hypertrophic subaortic stenosis, and mitral valve prolapse with regurgitation. Those patients experiencing procedures that are likely to induce bacteremia should receive prophylaxis. The procedures include all dental procedures likely to induce gingival bleeding, tonsillectomy and/or adenoidectomy, surgical procedures involving respiratory mucosa, bronchoscopy, incision and drainage of infected tissue, and genitourinary and gastrointestinal procedures. Patients at particularly high risk for endocarditis (those with prosthetic valves or systemic-pulmonary shunts) should receive parenteral prophylaxis whenever possible.

MYOCARDITIS

NANCY A. AYRES, M.D.

Myocarditis is the infiltration of the myocardium with inflammatory cells. Infectious agents that can result in myocarditis are numerous and varied (Table 1). The signs and symptoms of myocarditis may be difficult to recognize and may present long after the initial phase of infection. In addition, the severity of presenting clinical symptoms ranges from the adolescent with mild chest pain and fatigability to the neonate with tachypnea, cyanosis, and rapidly progressive circulatory collapse. In neonates, coxsackie B virus accounts for more than 50 percent of the cases of acute myocarditis. Viral infections frequently affect other organs, which may result in the primary clinical features. Thus, the diagnosis of myocarditis requires the physician's awareness of the various clinical manifestations and a high degree of suspicion. The diagnosis of myocarditis is sometimes missed and made only at autopsy.

To assist in confirmation of the diagnosis, a gallium scan may be used to monitor the presence and extent of myocardial inflammation. An invasive diagnostic tool, the endomyocardial biopsy is also used to define myocarditis by histologic criteria and to monitor histologic results of therapy. I find two-dimensional echocardiography a helpful noninvasive method to evaluate myocardial contractility, the cardiac chamber dimensions, and the myocardial response to therapeutic interventions.

Some of our therapeutic recommendations originate from studies on the murine model with coxsackie B viral myocarditis. The viral virulence, extent of cardiac necrosis, viral titer, and mortality are accentuated by exercise or poor nutrition in the experimental myocarditis model. Thus, treatment begins with bed rest or at least a marked reduction in physical activity and good nutrition during the acute phase of myocarditis. Corticosteroid therapy administered to the murine model during the first 10 to 14 days of the acute phase of the illness results in accelerated viral replication and myocardial necrosis. However, the treatment of myocarditis with steroids is controversial because several clinical studies contradict the murine studies and document that immunosuppres-

TABLE 1   Infectious Etiologies

Type	Infectious Agent
Viral	Coxsackie A
	Coxsackie B
	Echovirus
	Adenovirus
	Influenza
	Poliomyelitis
	Smallpox
	Hepatitis
	Measles
	Rubella
	Rabies
	Infectious mononucleosis
	Arbovirus
	Cytomegalovirus
	Herpes simplex
	Yellow fever
	Psittacosis
	Coronavirus
	Mumps
Rickettsial	Tsutsugamushi disease (scrub typhus)
	Rocky Mountain spotted fever
	Q fever
Metazoan	Trichinosis
	Schistosomiasis
	Ascariasis
	Filariasis
	Cysticercosis
	Echinococcosis
	Strongyloidiasis
Miscellaneous	*Chlamydia trachomatis*
	Mycoplasma pneumoniae
Bacterial	Diphtheria (toxin)
	Tuberculosis
	Typhoid fever
	Scarlet fever
	Tetanus
	Pertussis
	Brucellosis
	Staphylococcus
	Pneumococcus
	Gonococcus
Spirochetal	Syphilis
	Leptospirosis
	Lyme disease
Protozoan	Chagas' disease (trypanosomiasis)
	Malaria
	Toxoplasmosis
	Leishmaniasis
	Sarcosporidiasis
	Balantidiasis
Fungal	Actinomycosis
	Coccidioidomycosis
	Aspergillosis
	Histoplasmosis
	Blastomycosis
	Sporotrichosis
	Cryptococcosis
	Candidiasis

sive therapy improves cardiac function, decreases myocardial cellular infiltration, and lowers mortality. Presently, most therapy is symptomatic and supportive. If the infectious etiology is known, appropriate specific therapy should be initiated. In most cases, however, the etiology is undetermined. Therefore, therapy is directed toward the complications of myocarditis that account for the 40 to 75 percent mortality, namely, congestive heart failure and arrythmias.

THERAPY IN ACUTE DISEASE

Acute myocarditis most often occurs following a brief prodrome of diarrhea, pyrexia, lethargy, and anorexia. Subsequently, the patient develops tachycardia out of proportion to the fever, irregular or gallop rhythm, tachypnea, and dyspnea, which are signs of the progressing congestive heart failure. However, the first symptom of acute myocarditis may be syncope, secondary to dysrhythmia, or cardiovascular shock. Once the diagnosis of myocarditis is made, I recommend careful observation, preferably in an intensive care unit (ICU) setting, for close monitoring of the hemodynamic status and dysrhythmia.

In myocarditis, the depressed myocardial contractility and resultant congestive heart failure are best managed with inotropic support (Table 2). Inotropic support of the failing myocardium in myocarditis is critical. The selection of the inotropic agent depends on the presenting clinical status.

If the cardiovascular status is stable, I proceed with oral digitalization for inotropic support. However, in the patient with cardiovascular compromise, the intravenous route is preferred. With cardiovascular shock, I initiate inotropic support with dopamine or dobutamine. I prefer dopamine because it has a specific dopaminergic vasodilating effect on the renal and mesenteric vasculature at small dosages (less than 10 μg per kilogram of body weight per minute). Dobutamine is also a potent inotropic agent that acts directly on myocardial receptors. In contrast with dopamine, however, it lacks the peripheral vascular vasodilatory effect. Amrinone, a new inotropic agent, increases cardiac contractility and decreases systemic vascular resistance. In adults, amrinone is effective in treatment of severe congestive heart failure, but presently it is used infrequently in children. I use amrinone in the compromised patient who is unresponsive to other inotropic agents. Caution must be observed with all inotropic drugs because these agents may result in marked tachycardia and precipitate dysrhythmias.

TABLE 2   Inotropic Agents

Drug	Route	Dosage
Digoxin	PO load	20–30 μg/kg over 24 hours* initial dosage = ½ total dosage (10–15 μg/kg), followed by ¼ total dose at 12 and 24 hours
	Maintenance	6 to 10 μg/kg/day divided bid
	IV	⅔ of PO dose
Dopamine	IV	2–20 μg/kg/min
Dobutamine	IV	2–10 μg/kg/min
Amrinone	IV	40 mg/kg/min

* Maximum loading dosage = 1.0 mg.

Cardiac output can also be improved by reducing the myocardial preload or afterload. I restrict fluids at 80 to 120 cc per kilogram per day to reduce the preload. In addition, diuretic therapy is often necessary. In the acutely ill, edematous patient I administe furosemide (Lasix) 1 to 2 mg per kilogram IM or IV. Careful observation of the cardiac output, systemic venous pressure, and systemic arterial pressure guides the clinician in further diuretic therapy. A complication of vigorous diuretic therapy is electrolyte imbalance such as hypokalemia, which may precipitate dysrhythmias. If the patient requires significant diuretic therapy, I use a combination of furosemide and spironolactone to reduce the risk of hypokalemia. Listed in Table 3 are the diuretics I prefer.

Additional pharmacologic intervention with afterload reduction may be indicated. In the acutely ill patient, I frequently use nitroprusside in conjunction with dopamine. Used together these two agents increase cardiac output synergistically. Nitroglycerin is also very effective. A complication of nitroprusside with low cardiac output and poor renal function is cyanide toxicity. Table 4 lists vasodilators and appropriate dosages. If it is apparent that ongoing afterload reduction is necessary, I administer hydralazine to neonates and toddlers. In older children, I prefer to use captopril. Captopril is difficult to administer to small children, and the complication of hypotension may be difficult to detect. I frequently maintain chronic pharmacologic therapy with digitalis, hydralazine or captopril, and alternate-day furosemide for 6 to 12 months after the acute onset of myocarditis.

THERAPY IN CHRONIC MYOCARDITIS

Myocarditis cannot be considered a benign illness because those patients who survive the acute episode frequently progress to chronic dilated cardiomyopathy. These patients experience a protracted downhill course ending in death secondary to congestive heart failure.

Steroid therapy is controversial, as was mentioned previously. However, when standard medical therapy fails, or chronic myocarditis ensues, I recommend an endomyocardial biopsy followed by a therapeutic trial of steroids. As noted previously, steroid therapy is absolutely contraindicated during the acute phase of the illness (initial 10 to 14 days). When treating with steroids, I recommend prednisone in a 40-mg-per-square-meter dosage, with tapering after 6

TABLE 3   Diuretic Agents

Drug	Route	Dosage (mg/kg/day)
Furosemide	IV, IM, or PO	1–4
Spironolactone	PO	1–4
Hydrochlorothiazide	PO	2–4

TABLE 4   Vasodilators

Drug	Route	Dosage
Nitroprusside	IV	0.5–1.5 μg/kg/min
Nitroglycerin	IV	Initial dosage 0.2 μg/kg/min ↑ by 0.2 μg/kg/min q15 min, maximum 5 μg/min
Hydralazine	IV	0.2–3.0 mg/kg/day q6h
	PO	0.75–4.0 mg/kg/day q6h
Captopril	PO	Start at 5 mg/m²/dose q6h, increase slowly, maximum 30 mg/m²/dose

weeks to 25 mg per square meter. A repeat endomyocardial biopsy is necessary to evaluate the therapeutic response. Azathioprine (75 mg per square meter) therapy should be added if little or no improvement is seen with prednisone alone. When all treatment fails, cardiac transplantation is a final option in severe chronic dilated cardiomyopathy.

THERAPY OF DYSRHYTHMIAS

Myocarditis may present as syncope or sudden death. The incidence of histologic myocarditis from autopsy studies of sudden death ranges from 5 to 17 percent. Arrythmias associated with myocarditis are not a rare event, but documentation of a dysrhythmia as a final event is rare. Because of focal inflammation of the cardiac conduction system, various conduction disturbances, including premature atrial or ventricular contractions, transient first- or second-degree atrioventricular block, complete heart block, atrial flutter, atrial fibrillation, and ventricular tachycardia, are seen in acute myocarditis. With complete heart block, mortality is 84 to 100 percent. Thus, careful monitoring of the patient with electrocardiographic (ECG) telemetry or in an ICU setting is mandatory.

Varying degrees of ectopy are seen in myocarditis. Frequently noted are isolated benign unifocal premature ventricular or atrial contractions, which do not require treatment. Multiform premature ventricular contractions, couplets, or brief runs of ventricular tachycardia should be suppressed using one of the drugs listed in Table 5. I prefer to initiate treatment with propranolol. However, serious side effects of propranolol are sinus bradycardia, sinus node arrest, and further depression of myocardial contractility. Thus, before administering propranolol in the compromised myocarditis patient, I have a temporary pacemaker available. If any complications of propranolol therapy occur, I select procainamide or quinidine. Procainamide (intravenous) may be given to predict the ventricular response to quinidine. I prefer quinidine on a chronic basis over procainamide because of the potential induction of lupus along with the frequent-dosing schedule of procainamide.

Atrial flutter, atrial fibrillation, ventricular tachycardia, and complete heart block are medical emergencies. The complete or transient heart block seen in myocarditis often necessitates temporary pacemaker placement. In the hemodynamically compromised patient with atrial tachycardia, electrical synchronized direct-current cardioversion is the fastest method of cardioversion. Low energy usually converts atrial tachycardia (see Table 5). However, if the atria are markedly dilated, 1 to 2 W-sec per kilogram may be necessary for cardioversion. If the patient is hemodynamically uncompromised by the atrial tachycardia, I recommend intravenous digitalization with an initial 10 μg per kilogram administered slowly over 5 minutes. After 8 hours, another 5-μg-per-kilogram dose is given, followed 8 hours later by the final 5-μg-per-kilogram loading digitalis dose. One should not expect immediate cardioversion with the initial dose of digoxin. It may take up to 6 hours for the digitalis to be effective. If pharmacologic cardioversion with digitalis is not successful and electrical conversion is subsequently necessary, lidocaine, 1 mg per kilogram, must be administered before cardioversion. It is also important to note that patients with myocarditis appear to have a lowered threshold for digitalis toxicity. Additional antiarrythmic agents such as quinidine, propranolol, or procainamide may be necessary to control the atrial tachycardia if digitalis alone is not effective. Caution must be observed when beginning quinidine therapy in conjunction with digitalis, because plasma digitalis

concentrations rise and can result in digoxin toxicity. Further depression of myocardial contractility is a complication seen with use of quinidine, procainamide, and propranolol. Because the myocardium is already depressed in the patient with myocarditis, I use digitalis in conjunction with a negative inotropic antiarrythmic agent.

Hemodynamic compromise secondary to ventricular tachycardia also necessitates immediate synchronized direct-current electrical cardioversion. If cardioversion is unsuccessful, the patient may be acidotic, hypoxic, or hypoglycemic. Other treatable etiologies of ventricular tachycardia are the position of an intracardiac catheter, hypokalemia, digitalis, and quinidine toxicity. In the hemodynamically stable patient, lidocaine, 1 mg per kilogram, administered intravenously, is most effective in suppressing acute ventricular tachycardia (see Table 5). However, for chronic control of the ventricular ectopy, I use procainamide or a long-acting beta-blocker. Alternative therapeutic modalities are listed in Table 5. I have used bretylium to convert ventricular tachycardia when standard pharmacologic agents failed. However, there is little experience with bretylium in pediatric patients, and it should be reserved for life-threatening ventricular arrythmias.

To monitor the effectiveness of antiarrhythmic drug therapy, I have found 24-hour electrocardiographic monitoring in conjunction with plasma drug levels to be helpful. I also recommend periodic evaluation of cardiac function with M-mode and two-dimensional echocardiogram, since various antiarrhythmic drugs may further depress the myocardial contractility in the patient with myocarditis.

New antiarrhythmic agents such as flecainide, encainide, mexiletine, and amiodarone have been found to be effective in controlling atrial and ventricular arrythmias in adults. These agents will soon be available for use in pediatrics and may add new alternatives for treatment of arrythmias occurring with myocarditis.

SUGGESTED READING

Adams FH, Emmanouilides GC. Heart diseases in infants, children, and adolescents. Baltimore, MD: Williams & Wilkins, 1983; 37:576–585.

Kaplan MH, Klein SW, McPhee J, Harper RG. Group B coxsackievirus infections in infants younger than three months of age: a serious childhood illness. Rev Infect Dis 1983; 5(6):1019–1032.

Mason JW, Billingham ME, Ricci DR. Treatment of acute inflammatory myocarditis assisted by endomyocardial biopsy. Am J Cardiol 1980; 45:1037–1044.

Reyes MP, Lerner AM. Coxsackievirus myocarditis—with special reference to acute and chronic effects. Prog Cardiovasc Dis 1985; 27(6):373–394.

Woodruff JF. Viral myocarditis. A review. Am J Pathol 1980; 101(2):425–484.

TABLE 5   Management of Dysrhythmias

Ventricular Tachycardia
 Synchronized DC electrical cardioversion 1–2 W-sec/kg
 Lidocaine 1 mg/kg IV-q5 min for 3 doses
  continuous infusion = 10–50 μg/kg/min
 Procainamide 1 mg/kg IV-q5 min for 15 doses*
  continuous infusion = 20–80 μg/kg/min
  PO = 15–50 mg/kg/day q6h
 Phenytoin 10–15 mg/kg IV over 60 min*
  PO = 10–15 mg/kg for 1 day (loading dose)
  2.5–10 mg/kg q12h
 Quinidine sulfate
  PO 7.5–10.0 mg/kg q6h†
 Propranolol
  IV = 0.01–0.1 mg/kg over 10 min‡
  PO = 0.05–1.5 mg/kg q6h
 Bretylium IV = 5 mg/kg q15 min
  maximum 30 mg/kg

Supraventricular Tachycardia
 Synchronized DC electrocardioversion 0.5–1.0 W-sec/kg
 Digoxin§
 Quinidine or procainamide§

---

* May cause hypotension.
† ↑ plasma digoxin concentration.
‡ May result in severe bradycardia requiring a pacemaker.
§ See Table 2.

ACUTE PERICARDITIS

WILLIAM E. FELDMAN, M.D., M.S.

Acute purulent pericarditis should be distinguished from more common etiologies of acute pericarditis, such as viral pericarditis, by obtaining cultures of blood and other infected sites. Pneumonia, meningitis, suppurative arthritis, and skin infections are often associated with acute purulent pericarditis. Rapid diagnostic tests (latex agglutination, coagglutination, etc.) should be done for *Haemophilus influenzae* type b, *Neisseria meningitidis,* and *Streptococcus pneumoniae* antigen in serum and urine (and cerebrospinal fluid [CSF] if indicated). Although *Staphylococcus aureus* is a common cause of acute purulent pericarditis, rapid diagnostic tests for this organism are presently unavailable. Acute purulent pericarditis caused by gram-negative enteric bacilli is rare, but it has been reported in the neonate. Although tuberculosis used to be relatively common, it is now unusual in developed countries.

Echocardiography is a sensitive tool to determine whether or not pericardial fluid is present. If acute purulent pericarditis is suspected, a diagnostic pericardiocentesis should be done to obtain exudate and/or relieve cardiac tamponade, if present. However, pericardiocentesis should not be considered definitive therapy for acute purulent pericarditis.

Treatment consisting of appropriate antibiotics and surgical drainage should be instituted as soon as the diagnosis is established. Initial antibiotic therapy should be guided by Gram stain of aspirated fluid from the pericardial sac. If fluid is unavailable, broad-spectrum coverage for the organisms noted earlier must be provided. A standard regimen for infants and children is nafcillin, 37.5 mg per kilogram every 6 hours intravenously (IV), and chloramphenicol 25 mg per kilogram IV every 6 hours. Newer cephalosporin antibiotics have not been well studied because of the rarity of this disease, although these antibiotics are effective against the major pathogens. Reasonable alternatives to nafcillin and chloramphenicol include cefotaxime, 50 mg per kilogram IV every 6 hours, or cefuroxime, 50 mg per kilogram IV every 8 hours. The latter regimens may also be effective for associated infections (see appropriate chapters).

Surgical drainage of the pericardial sac is indicated on an emergency basis. The optimal surgical approach is unknown at this time, although good results have been reported with an anterior interphrenic or subxiphoid approach and with total pericardiectomy. Patients treated by multiple pericardiocenteses without open drainage do poorly. The lowest mortality has occurred with a combination of appropriate antibiotic therapy and surgical drainage.

Once the antimicrobial susceptibilities are known, broad-spectrum antibiotics should be changed to a more specific antibiotic. The recommended duration of therapy for acute purulent pericarditis caused by *Staphylococcus aureus* is 21 to 28 days, whereas acute purulent pericarditis caused by *H. influenzae* type b, *N. meningitidis,* or *Str. pneumoniae* is treated for 10 to 14 days.

Response may be monitored clinically by resolution of clinical symptoms and signs. Cardiac tamponade must be watched for carefully; it can occur even in a patient in whom the pericardial sac has been partially drained. It is important to correlate serial echocardiograms with clinical response to determine whether or not pus reaccumulates and further surgical intervention is needed. Positive cultures should be repeated to verify in vivo sterilization of the infection. Decreases in white cell count and in sedimentation rate toward normal are useful indicators of response.

Purulent fluid may accumulate in the pericardial sac after antibiotic treatment is started for another illness, so that patients treated for meningitis or other illness should be observed carefully for unsuspected purulent pericarditis. Long-term follow-up of survivors is necessary because of the possibility of constrictive pericarditis developing later. Pericardiectomy may be necessary in a few patients.

Rifampin, in a dosage of 10 mg per kilogram (maximum dosage is 600 mg daily) orally every 12 hours for four doses, should be given to close contacts of patients with *N. meningitidis* infection. The role of rifampin prophylaxis for patients with infection caused by *H. influenzae* type b is unclear at this time, because it has been evaluated only in patients with meningitis.

SUGGESTED READING

Feldman WE. Bacterial etiology and mortality of purulent pericarditis in pediatric patients: a review of 162 cases. Am J Dis Child 1979; 133:641–644.

Morgan RJ, Stephenson LW, Woolf PK, Edie RN, et al. Surgical treatment of purulent pericarditis in children. J Thorac Cardiovasc Surg 1983; 85:527–531.

THROMBOPHLEBITIS

DALE COLN, M.D.

In children, the vast majority of *diagnosed* thrombophlebitis occurs in the subcutaneous veins, as a consequence of venous catheterization. The diagnosis is made when pain, tenderness, and induration along the course of a superficial vein exist. Thrombophlebitis occurring as a result of *central* venous catheters is not usually recognized clinically, unless the catheter becomes occluded. The initial treatment of catheter-induced superficial thrombophlebitis is to remove the catheter. If significant pain and tenderness persist, local heat and analgesia are helpful. Most superficial thrombophlebitis responds to symptomatic treatment and does not require antibiotics, surgery, or anticoagulants.

In children who are immunosuppressed or suffering from third-degree burns, catheter-induced thrombophlebitis can be suppurative. Local signs of inflammation may not be present. If suppurative thrombophlebitis is suspected, it is wise to make an incision over the vein after sedation and local analgesia. The vein is opened and material is taken for culture. *Staphylococcus aureus* is most often the offending organism. Methicillin or nafcillin, 37.5 mg per kilogram every 6 hours, is given until antibiotic susceptibility test results are available. Adequate drainage of the infected vein is obtained by opening the vein the full length of involvement. Excising the involved vein is usually not necessary. Antibiotic therapy is continued for 7 to 10 days.

Deep venous thrombosis is rarely recognized in children. The scenario of silent deep venous thrombosis with subsequent development of pulmonary embolism is a rarity in children. When deep venous thrombosis of the thigh and leg occurs in childhood it is usually the accompaniment of chronic immobolization. It occurs most commonly in children with paraplegia. The diagnosis is suspected when massive swelling of the thigh or leg occurs. Confirmation with venography is done before deep thrombophlebitis is treated with anticoagulation. Heparin is given intravenously with a loading dose of 100 U per kilogram followed by continuous infusion of 20 U per kilogram per hour. The Lee-White clotting time, or activated partial thromboplastin time, is maintained at twice the normal level. Heparin treatment is discontinued by tapering the dosage after 10 days. Elevation is helpful in reducing the swelling, which is slow to disappear in children with neurologic deficit. Oral anticoagulants may be given for 6 weeks, but are not used indefinitely for prophylaxis.

SUGGESTED READING

DeWeese, J. Venous and lymphatic disease. In: Schwartz SI, Shires GT, Spencer FC, Storer EH, eds. Principles of surgery, 3rd ed. New York: McGraw-Hill, 1979; 985–1010.

Matthews DJ, Levin M. Pulmonary thromboembolism in children. Intensive Care Med 1986; 12:404.

DISEASES OF THE CENTRAL NERVOUS SYSTEM

BACTERIAL MENINGITIS

GEORGE H. McCRACKEN Jr., M.D.

Approximately 15,000 cases of bacterial meningitis in infants and children occur yearly. This figure represents age-specific annual attack rates of 100 cases per 100,000 neonates, 57 to 88 cases per 100,000 infants younger than 1 year, 25 cases per 100,000 infants 1 to 2 years, and considerably smaller rates in older children. The case fatality rates for bacterial meningitis in neonates are from 15 to 20 percent, and in infants and children from 5 to 10 percent. As many as 50 percent of survivors have some sequelae of their disease. These include hearing impairment (10 percent), language disorders (15 percent), mental retardation (10 percent), motor abnormalities (3 to 7 percent), and seizures (2 to 8 percent).

The etiology of bacterial meningitis varies with age, involving principally group B streptococci and gram-negative enteric bacilli in neonates and *Haemophilus influenzae* type b (approximately 65 percent of all cases), *Neisseria meningitidis,* and *Streptococcus pneumoniae* in infants and children. Less frequently encountered, but important, pathogens in newborn infants are *Listeria monocytogenes, Citrobacter diversus,* and *Enterobacter sakazaki;* the latter two of these are associated with brain abscesses and a necrotizing cerebritis, respectively, and have a poor prognosis. In the United States, 20 to 25 percent of *H. influenzae* strains are resistant to ampicillin because of beta-lactamase production; a few strains are resistant to ampicillin as a result of diminished diffusion through the cell wall or altered penicillin-binding proteins in the periplasmic space.

Cerebrospinal fluid (CSF) examination and culture are essential to the diagnosis of meningitis. In most patients, CSF examination, protein and glucose concentrations, and a careful evaluation of the gram-stained or acridine orange–stained smear of fluid can distinguish an aseptic process from bacterial meningitis. Identification of antigen in CSF by latex agglutination is a sensitive and specific technique for diagnosing *Haemophilus* meningitis; the technique is less reliable for disease caused by *S. pneumoniae* and *N. meningitidis.* After the meningeal pathogen is identified, the bacteriology laboratory should be instructed to determine the beta-lactamase production and the susceptibility of *H. influenzae* to ampicillin, chloramphenicol, and a cephalosporin, if one is being used for treatment, and that of *S. pneumoniae* to penicillin by use of a 1-μg oxacillin disk (if the zone of inhibition is 19 mm or less, minimal inhibitory concentration [MIC] and minimal bactericidal concentration [MBC] of penicillin should be determined). Ideally, the laboratory should provide MIC and MBC values of penicillin or ampicillin for group B streptococci or of an aminoglycoside or third-generation cephalosporin for gram-negative enteric bacilli, depending on the agent chosen for therapy.

TREATMENT

Initial empiric treatment for bacterial meningitis entails selection of antimicrobial agents that are effective against the likely etiologic agents and use of proper drug dosages and administration schedules to produce adequate bactericidal activity in CSF (Table 1).

Newborn Infants

In neonates the initial empiric regimen used conventionally has been ampicillin (or penicillin G) and an aminoglycoside. Although this combination has been used effectively for more than two decades, it is advisable to monitor serum concentrations of the aminoglycoside, especially in low-birth-weight infants in whom concentrations are unpredictable. Dosages of the aminoglycosides should be tailored to achieve peak serum values in the range considered therapeutic and nontoxic (i.e., 4 to 8 μg per milliliter for gentamicin and tobramycin and 15 to 25 μg per milliliter for kanamycin and amikacin). The aminoglycosides should be avoided in patients with abnormalities in renal function. For these reasons, I prefer ampicillin and cefotaxime for initial treatment, especially if gram-negative enteric bacilli are suspected from stained smears or cultures of CSF and in late-onset (after more than 10 days) meningitis in infants in neonatal intensive care units, if aminoglycoside-resistant nosocomial bacterial infections are present in that unit. Cefotaxime should not be used routinely for initial empiric therapy of suspected neonatal sepsis because cefotaxime-resistant *Enterobacter* strains are likely to develop rapidly in that neonatal unit.

TABLE 1   Daily Dosages* for Antimicrobial Agents for Treatment of Meningitis

| | Neonates | | |
Drugs	0–7 Days	8–28 Days	Infants and Children
Amikacin	15–20 div q12	20–30 div q8	20–30 div q8
Ampicillin	100–150 div q12	150–200 div q8 or 6	200–300 div q6
Cefotaxime	100 div q12	150–200 div q8 or 6	200 div q6
Ceftriaxone	——	——	80–100 div q12 or once daily
Ceftazidime	60 div q12	90 div q8	125–150 div q8
Cefuroxime	——		240 div q8
Chloramphenicol	25 once daily	50 div q12	75–100 div q6
Gentamicin	5 div q12	7.5 div q8	7.5 div q8
Kanamycin	15–20 div q12	20–30 div q8	——
Moxalactam	100 div q12	150–200 div q8 or 6	200 div q6
Penicillin G	100,000–150,000 div q12	150,000–20,000 div q8 or 6	250,000 div q6
Ticarcillin	150–225 div q12 or 8	225–300 div q8 or 6	300 div q6
Tobramycin	4 div q12	6 div q8	6 div q8
Vancomycin	20 div q12	30 div q8	40–60 div q6

* In milligrams per kilogram (units per kilogram for penicillin G) divided every (q) 12, 8, 6, or 4 hours.

Once the pathogen has been identified and the susceptibilities have been defined, the single most appropriate antibiotic or combination of antibiotics should be selected. Penicillin G or ampicillin is preferred for group B streptococci unless the organism is shown to be tolerant in vitro (MBC 32-fold greater than MIC), in which case combined therapy with ampicillin and gentamicin is preferred. Ampicillin is satisfactory for *Listeria* meningitis, and cefotaxime alone or combined with an aminoglycoside is preferred for gram-negative enteric organisms. For *Pseudomonas aeruginosa,* ticarcillin or ceftazidime and an aminoglycoside should be administered.

The duration of antimicrobial therapy for neonatal meningitis depends on the clinical response and duration of positive CSF cultures after therapy is initiated. For disease caused by group B streptococci or *Listeria,* 10 to 14 days of therapy is adequate in most infants. In contrast, a minimum of 2 weeks of therapy after sterilization of CSF cultures or 3 weeks, whichever is longer, is required for gram-negative enteric meningitis, and in some infants, as many as 4 to 6 weeks is necessary. Because of the unpredictable clinical course of illness, and the unreliability of the clinical examination in assessing response to therapy in neonates, we believe that the CSF should be examined and cultured when conventional therapy is completed, to determine whether or not additional treatment is required.

1- To 3-Month-Old Infants

I have designated the 1- to 3-month-old age group as a special category because of the broad array of possible etiologic agents that can cause disease in these infants. I prefer ampicillin and cefotaxime, because this regimen is effective against the commonly encountered pathogens of neonates as well as of older infants and children. If ampicillin and an aminogly-coside are administered and the causative organism is a beta-lactamase–producing strain of *H. influenzae,* only the aminoglycoside is active, and experience with those agents in *Haemophilus* meningitis is inadequate for efficacy to be ensured. Indeed, a few *Haemophilus* strains are resistant to the aminoglycosides. Likewise, use of ampicillin and chloramphenicol in this age group could be problematic if group B streptococci or *Listeria* were the etiologic agent, because antagonism between those two drugs when used against those organisms has been demonstrated in vitro. Under most circumstances cefotaxime could be used singly in infants 1 to 3 months of age because *Listeria* or enterococci rarely causes meningitis beyond the age of 4 to 6 weeks.

The duration of therapy is tailored to the etiologic agent and clinical response to therapy. For the pathogens that are usually encountered in the neonatal period, therapy is administered for the requisite time after sterilization of cultures (see preceding), whereas for the common pathogens of older infants and children, therapy is usually given for 7 to 10 days.

Infants and Children

Conventional therapy for meningitis with ampicillin and chloramphenicol has been effective for many years. Because of the extraordinary in vitro activity of the new cephalosporins against common meningeal pathogens and their apparent excellent safety record, attention has recently focused on them for treatment of meningitis in infants and children. Despite their superior in vitro activity and greater bactericidal activity in CSF, those cephalosporins do not sterilize CSF cultures more rapidly, nor do they improve case fatality rates over the conventional antibiotic regimens in infants and children, providing the pathogens are susceptible to the antibiotic used. Because of the unpredictable metabolism of chloramphenicol in newborn and young infants, and of the pharmacologic interactions of this agent when administered concomitantly with phenobarbital, phenytoin, or rifampin, serum concentrations should be measured and the dosage adjusted accordingly to avoid potentially toxic (more than 40 μg per milliliter) or subtherapeutic (fewer than 10 μg per milliliter) peak concentrations. In those situations it is advisable to use the cephalosporins for therapy to avoid the unnecessary expense and trouble of monitoring serum concentrations; when monitoring is not immediately available, use of chloramphenicol should be avoided.

Presently, I prefer cefuroxime, cefotaxime, or ceftriaxone for initial, empiric treatment of meningitis in older infants and children. Each physician must decide which of these agents is best suited to his or her patients, and the selection process should be based on personal experience, availability of the drug in the hospital formulary, dosing schedules, and cost. Because ceftriaxone can be administered intravenously or intramuscularly on a once-daily basis, its cost of administration is considerably less than that for an agent that must be given three or four times daily. With ceftriaxone therapy I prefer two doses on the first day; thus, the patient receives an 80-mg-per-kilogram dose at diagnosis, at 12 hours, at 24 hours, and then every 24 hours thereafter for 7 to 10 days.

Once the etiologic agent has been identified and the susceptibilities of the organism defined, alteration of therapy may be indicated or the initial cephalosporin could be continued. If ampicillin and chloramphenicol were used initially, one or the other should be continued for *Haemophilus* meningitis, depending on its susceptibility to ampicillin. Either penicillin or ampicillin should be used for pneumococcal or meningococcal disease. Approximately 5 to 15 percent of *S. pneumoniae* strains are relatively resistant to penicillin (MIC, 0.1 to 1.0 μg per milliliter). In this circumstance, vancomycin, cefuroxime, cefotaxime, or ceftriaxone is chosen for therapy. In the rare event that the pneumococcus is resistant to penicillin (MIC greater than 1.0 μg per milliliter), vancomycin, possibly with rifampin, should be used.

On the basis of recently published studies and many years of general experience, we believe 7 days of treatment is satisfactory for most infants and children with uncomplicated meningococcal or *Haemophilus* disease; 10 days is preferred for pneumococcal meningitis. A lumbar puncture performed at completion of therapy in the patient with no complications is unwarranted because the information obtained is not useful in predicting which patient will develop recurrent disease.

SUPPORTIVE CARE

The first 3 or 4 days of treatment are critical because complications of septicemia and meningitis occur most frequently during this time. It is advisable to manage infants and children with meningitis in a hospital that has specialized equipment and staff with expertise in caring for infants and children who are critically ill.

Adequate oxygenation, prompt management of seizures, control of hypoglycemia, and replacement of fluid deficits are important. During the first days of treatment the patient should be evaluated for inappropriate secretion of antidiuretic hormone, and intravenously administered fluids should be restricted to 800 to 1,000 ml per square meter in 24 hours. Fluids should not be restricted in patients with hypotension or hypoglycemia. In patients with clinical evidence of intracranial hypertension, management in an intensive care unit with hyperventilation, mannitol (0.5 to 2.0 g per kilogram), or dexamethasone (0.5 to 0.7 mg per kilogram) should be considered.

COMPUTED TOMOGRAPHY

Computed tomography (CT scan) provides a noninvasive means of diagnosing some intracranial complications of meningitis. These include subdural collection of fluid, ventricular dilatation, ischemic changes secondary to vascular thrombosis, and brain abscess. Simultaneous intravenous administration of contrast material (enhanced CT scan) is often helpful in distinguishing subdural effusion from empyema and abscess from focal cerebritis. A CT scan should be considered in patients with meningitis who have persistent or prolonged fever, clinical evidence of increased intracranial pressure, focal neurologic findings or seizures, enlarging head circumference, prolonged obtundation, or persistently abnormal CSF cell counts, protein concentrations, or cultures. Additionally, all infants with meningitis caused by *Citrobacter diversus* should have a CT scan, because approximately three-quarters of those patients have one or more brain abscesses.

REPEAT CSF EXAMINATION

Although infectious disease consultants disagree on the need for repeat CSF examinations, I prefer to repeat an examination and culture 24 to 36 hours after therapy is initiated to document eradication of the pathogen. This is especially important in newborn and young infants, in whom clinical response to therapy may not accurately reflect the bacteriologic response. In addition, delayed sterilization of CSF cultures in neonates with gram-negative enteric meningitis and in infants and children with *Haemophilus* meningitis is associated with a poorer outcome than in those in whom the pathogen has been promptly eradicated (in less than 24 hours).

When the patient's management and course of illness is uncomplicated, CSF examination and culture when therapy is completed are unnecessary. The information obtained in such patients is not useful in identifying those who will have recurrent disease, and arbitrary rules regarding approximate numbers of white blood cells (WBCs) and protein and sugar concentrations in CSF may unnecessarily prolong treatment. Newborn infants with meningitis, I believe, are an exception; generally they should have a CSF examination and culture before discharge because their clinical course often belies the response to therapy, as reflected by degree of CSF inflammation.

ALTERNATIVE TREATMENT REGIMENS

For some patients with meningitis, alternative treatment regimens might be considered to shorten the duration of hospitalization and complete therapy at home. A shorter period of hospitalization of patients with meningitis could reduce the risk of acquiring nosocomial infections, help to lessen the total course of management, and return the patient to his or her normal environment where family interactions are more complete and meaningful. The physician must individualize each situation in deciding when it is safe for the patient with meningitis to go home. Although I do not condone early discharge from the hospital for home management of infants and children with meningitis, some physicians prefer this alternative to treatment. In such cases, the decision for early discharge must be based on the clinical condition of the patient, the reliability of the parents to assess clinically the child at home and follow instructions, the ability of the child to swallow and retain medication given orally, and the availability of a visiting nurse service or home therapy team to evaluate the patient and administer antibiotics intravenously or intramuscularly. The patient who is alert, stable, and cooperative is a potential candidate for early discharge. If the decision is to provide oral chloramphenicol therapy, it is mandatory for the physician to document adequate absorption of the agent before discharge. Therapeutic serum concentrations of chloramphenicol are from 15 to 25 μg per milliliter. Rifampin should not be administered concomitantly with chloramphenicol because it may reduce serum concentrations of the latter agent below what is observed when the drug is given alone. Experience with using ceftriaxone intramuscularly for treatment of meningitis is limited, and a nurse or physician should administer the drug, preferably intravenously through a heparin lock, rather than attempt to teach a parent the proper technique. The physician or a nurse who is trained to evaluate patients with meningitis should examine the child daily while completing therapy at home and arrangements should be made for a hearing evaluation within several weeks of completing therapy.

FOLLOW-UP EVALUATIONS

Because approximately 10 percent of infants and children develop hearing impairment as a result of meningitis, it is imperative that all patients have an adequate hearing evaluation at the time of discharge from the hospital or within 4 to 6 weeks thereafter. Detection of hearing abnormality should prompt referral of the patient to an audiologist for further evaluation and management. Long-term follow-up of meningitis patients is advised, to identify developmental neurologic, behavioral, or learning communicative abnormalities, some of which may not be detectable until the child reaches school age.

PREVENTION

Vaccines

Immunization is potentially the most effective means of prevention of bacterial meningitis in children. The vaccines currently available are relatively nonimmunogenic in children younger than 18 to 24 months of age, the very age group that is most prone to meningitis. The commercially available *Haemophilus influenzae* type b polysaccharide vaccines are recommended for all children 2 to 6 years of age and for those older than 6 years who have chronic illnesses known to be associated with an increased risk of disease. These conditions include anatomic or functional asplenia, such as patients with sickle-cell disease and Hodgkin's disease, and other malignancies associated with prolonged immunosuppression. The Immunization Practices Advisory Committee of the U.S. Public Health Service advises use of *Haemophilus* vaccine in children 18 to 24 months of age who attend day care. This recommendation is problematic and not supported by the Committee on Infectious Diseases of the American Academy of Pediatrics, because at least 20 to 25 percent of such children do not respond adequately to the vaccine, and efficacy in that age group has not been documented. By early 1988 a conjugated *Haemophilus* vaccine will probably be approved by the Food and Drug Administration. This vaccine is considerably more immunogenic than currently available products and should be effective in infants younger than 12 months of age.

A polyvalent meningococcal vaccine, containing purified polysaccharide capsules from Groups A, C, Y and W135 strains, is available. Monovalent vaccines of each of these components are also available. The vaccine is recommended for children 2 years of age or older who are at high risk, including those with anatomic or functional asplenia or with terminal complement component deficiencies.

The currently manufactured pneumococcal vaccine is composed of purified capsular polysaccharide antigen from 23 pneumococcal serotypes. The vaccine is recommended for children 2 years of age or older who are at increased risk of developing pneumococcal infection. Included in the high-risk category are those with anatomic or functional asplenia, nephrotic syndrome, those undergoing cytoreduction therapy for Hodgkin's disease, and those with recurrent meningitis after head trauma.

CHEMOPROPHYLAXIS

Rifampin prophylaxis is recommended for all household contacts of an index case when at least one contact is younger than 48 months of age and has not received the *Haemophilus* vaccine at 2 years of age or older. The dose is 20 mg per kilogram (maximum, 600 mg) daily, given for 4 days. The index case should also receive rifampin at or near completion of treatment for meningitis. Rifampin should not be administered concomitantly with chloramphenicol because the former reduces the serum concentration of chloramphenicol.

Management of day care and extended home care groups must be individualized. There is disagreement regarding the rate of secondary *H. influenzae* disease in day care attendees. Although secondary cases do occur in this setting, some evidence suggests that the rate of secondary disease is not greater than that of the open population. The efficacy of rifampin prophylaxis in day care attendees is unproved, and the logistics of administering the drug to all day care contacts and personnel can be difficult. Accordingly, prophylaxis is recommended only after two cases of *Haemophilus* disease have occurred in a day care or home care setting, in which case city or county health officials should also be notified. Contacts who have received *Haemophilus* vaccine should also receive rifampin prophylaxis to eradicate the organism from the pharynx.

Household and day care or nursery school contacts of an index case of meningococcal meningitis should be given rifampin prophylaxis. A dosage of 10 mg per kilogram (maximum, 600 mg) is given every 12 hours for five doses. Infants younger than 1 month should receive 5-mg-per-kilogram doses. Contacts are urged to seek medical attention at the first sign of illness.

SUGGESTED READING

Del Rio M, Chrane D, Shelton S, et al. Ceftriaxone versus ampicillin and chloramphenicol for treatment of bacterial meningitis in children. Lancet 1983; 1:1241–1244.

Klein JO, Feigin RD, McCracken GH. Report of the task force on diagnosis and management of meningitis. Pediatrics 1986; 78(Suppl):959–982.

Krasinski K, Kusmiesz H, Nelson JD. Pharmacologic interactions among chloramphenicol, phenytoin and phenobarbital. Pediatr Infect Dis 1982; 1:232–235.

Lin TY, Chrane DF, Nelson JD, et al. Seven days of ceftriaxone therapy is as effective as ten days treatment for bacterial meningitis. JAMA 1985; 253:3559–3563.

McCracken GH, Nelson JD. Antimicrobial therapy for newborns. New York: Grune & Stratton, 1983; 44–65.

McCracken G, Nelson J, Kaplan S, et al. Consensus: current antimicrobial therapy of bacterial meningitis. Pediatr Infect Dis 1987; 6:501–505.

Odio CM, Faingezicht I, Salas JL, et al. Cefotaxime vs. conventional therapy for the treatment of bacterial meningitis of infants and children. Pediatr Infect Dis J 1986; 5:402–407.

Rodriquez WJ, Puig JR, Khan WN, et al. Ceftazidime vs. standard therapy for pediatric meningitis: therapeutic; pharmalogic and epidemiologic observations. Pediatr Infect Dis 1986; 5:408–415.

BRAIN ABSCESS

RALPH D. FEIGIN, M.D.
KATHLEEN A. SHEERIN, M.D.

Brain abscess is uncommon in children. Commonly, infants present with signs and symptoms of vomiting, fever, seizure activity, or hydrocephalus. Older children may present with headache, vomiting, and lethargy. Almost half of the children with brain abscess are afebrile at the time of initial presentation.

Sinusitis, middle ear disease, and mastoiditis are present in 30 to 50 percent of patients who have brain abscesses. Congenital heart disease is an associated or antecedent event in a similar proportion of patients (30 to 50 percent). Additional predisposing factors are pulmonary infection, dental abscesses, furuncles, osteomyelitis, endocarditis, penetrating trauma, and leptomeningitis. Approximately 10 to 25 percent of patients have no identifiable source of infection. Knowledge of the predisposing conditions involved in the pathogenesis of brain abscesses heightens the physician's suspicion of the possibility of an intracranial infection.

A carefully performed history and physical examination are imperative. Diagnostic evaluation should include a total and differential white blood cell count, blood culture, chest and skull radiographs, and computerized tomographic (CT) scan of the head with and without contrast. The CT scan may permit detection of extracerebral intracranial lesions or intracerebral collections of purulent material. Technetium radionuclide scanning also may be helpful in some cases in which the CT scan fails to explain satisfactorily the clinical symptomatology. For many years the pathognomonic finding on CT scan was thought to be a ring enhancing lesion. The thin dense ring surrounding a central lucent area seen with contrast infusion was thought to represent the abscess capsule. Animal studies have shown that ring enhancement occurs in the late stages of cerebritis prior to capsule formation. Ring enhancement also can be seen in patients with infarction of the brain, primary and secondary metastatic tumors, hematoma, and radiation necrosis.

A lumbar puncture should not be performed in someone with a suspected brain abscess prior to the performance of a CT scan. In those patients in whom lumbar puncture is deemed to be appropriate (no evidence of significant increase in intracranial pressure), cerebrospinal fluid may reveal an elevated leukocyte count (10 to 200 cells per cubic millimeter). Lymphocytes generally predominate. Cerebrospinal fluid protein concentrations range from 75 to 400 mg per deciliter. Generally, the cerebrospinal fluid glucose is normal and no organisms are seen on smear, nor are organisms isolated in standard culture media.

THERAPY

Therapy of brain abscess may include operative excision or aspiration coupled with antibiotic therapy or antibiotic therapy alone.

Antibiotic Therapy

There have been more than 40 reports of patients with brain abscesses who have been cured with medical treatment alone.

Antibiotic therapy should be initiated immediately. Empiric therapy requires knowledge of the usual pathogenic organisms involved. When the organisms causing a brain abscess have been identified (following needle aspiration of the abscess), the antibiotic(s) chosen can be adjusted accordingly.

In the past, approximately 25 percent of cultures obtained intraoperatively were sterile. Anaerobes are recovered most frequently. Thus, surgical specimens should be transported and cultured anaerobically. Aerobic bacteria recovered from brain abscesses include streptococci, coagulase positive and negative staphylococci, gram-negative bacilli, and *Haemophilus* species. Many abscesses contain mixed aerobic and anaerobic flora.

Brain abscesses in newborn infants are caused more commonly by gram-negative organisms such as *E. coli.* In immunocompromised patients, opportunistic infection with *Actinomyces, Nocardia, Aspergillus,* and *Rhizopus* should be considered.

Most abscess cavities contain organisms that are susceptible to penicillin. However, anaerobes that are resistant to penicillin, such as certain strains of *Bacteroides* sp., may be recovered.

When brain abscesses occur in a patient who had a paranasal sinus, ear, or mastoid infection, we initiate therapy with penicillin G (300,000 U per kilogram of body weight per day) and chloramphenicol (100 mg per kilogram per day). Consideration must also be given to the use of a penicillinase-resistant penicillin for coverage of penicillin-resistant *S.*

aureus. The concentration of methicillin within brain abscess cavities is sufficient to inhibit penicillin-susceptible strains of *S. aureus* when a dosage of 200 mg per kilogram per day is provided intravenously. Nafcillin, even administered at 200 mg per kilogram per day has not been detected within the cavity of a brain abscess. In patients with brain abscess following trauma or neurosurgery, methicillin should be included in the initial therapeutic regimen; appropriate changes in antibiotic coverage can be made on the basis of culture results.

Metronidazole has been used recently as initial treatment for brain abscesses. It is bactericidal for most anaerobic microorganisms and high concentrations of the drug have been achieved rapidly in both the cerebrospinal fluid and abscess cavities of adults receiving 400 to 600 mg of metronidazole every 8 hours by either the oral or the intravenous route. Metronidazole administration has been associated with vomiting, diarrhea, urticaria, neutropenia, and vaginal and urethral burning. Ataxia, vertigo, and headaches also have been reported in patients receiving the drug. The use of metronidazole in mice has been associated with an increased risk of malignancies.

There are no controlled studies in which metronidazole and penicillin have been compared with penicillin and chloramphenicol for treatment of brain abscess. Metronidazole must be given in combination with penicillin because it is not active against facultative bacteria such as streptococci and is inactive against some anaerobic gram-positive cocci.

The dosage of metronidazole for children with brain abscess is not well established. We have used this drug in some children with brain abscess caused by anaerobic microorganisms in a dosage of 30 mg per kilogram per day (following a loading dose of 15 mg per kilogram). A dosage of 40 to 50 mg per kilogram per day can be given orally. The penetration of antibiotics into brain tissue and brain abscess fluid is recorded in Table 1.

Persistence of viable organisms has been reported in abscess cavities, even with delivery of concentrations of antibiotics 24 to 380 times the minimal inhibitory concentration of the organisms that were recovered. Local factors within the abscess cavity, such as pH, hypoxia, hypertonicity, protein concentration, and divalent cations, may suppress the efficacy of the antibiotics that have been administered.

As a result of recent advances in noninvasive imaging techniques, brain abscesses can be diagnosed early when only cerebritis is present, before a well-defined abscess develops. Currently, there are no definitive guidelines for the physician to follow in deciding whether or not the patient is an appropriate candidate for medical therapy alone. A correlation between successful antibiotic treatment and small lesions (1.7 versus 4.2 cm, mean) in patients with a brief duration of symptoms has been described.

Medical treatment alone should be considered

TABLE 1 Antibiotic Penetration Into Brain Tissue and Abscess Fluid

Antibiotic	No. of Patients	Range of Means of Daily Doses Reported from Various Studies	Serum (1 ml)	Abscess (per ml) or Brain (per g)	Range of Abscess: Serum Ratios
			Range of Mean Concentrations (μg)		
Penicillin	37	1.04–18 MU			0.00–0.95
Methicillin	2	20 g	15.5	4.5	0.29
Ampicillin	12	2–2.5 g	2.8–23	0.39–1.53	0.02–0.53
Nafcillin	1	18 g	8.0	0.0	0.00
Cloxacillin	4	4 g	3.55	1.25	0.35
Cephalothin	7	2 g	13.3	4.2	0.32
Cephaloridine	12	1.9–6 g	2–58	0.9–2.7	0.05–0.79
Moxalactam	4	300 mg–12 g	20–159	10.1–13.2	0.06–0.66
Vancomycin	1	2 g	21.0	16.5	0.79
Chloramphenicol	11	2–4 g	4.2–>7.7	1.0–19.3	0.15–4.60
Gentamicin	4	220 mg	0.95	<0.5	0.53
Fusidic acid	1	1.5 g	6.2	6.2	1.00
Metronidazole	3	1.4 g	38.1	19.7	0.52
Erythromycin	5	1.68 g	3.63	0.15	0.04
Streptomycin	4	3 g	24	0.0	0.00
Tetracycline	8	2.5–3 g	6.5–9.0	0.34–0.56	0.05–0.06

Source: Adapted from Levy RM, Gutin PH, Baskin DS, Pons VG. Vancomycin penetration of a brain abscess: case report and review of the literature. Neurosurgery 1986; 18:634.

(1) in patients with multiple abscesses; (2) when the abscess is in a location in which surgery could cause damage to vital brain structures; or (3) if the patient is a poor surgical risk. If there are changes in sensorium or evidence of a mass effect, surgery is indicated. Definite clinical improvement should be seen within 1 week if medical therapy alone is used. Lack of improvement or deterioration should dictate neurosurgical intervention. Antibiotic therapy can be discontinued before the CT scan shows resolution of the abscess, which may take from 1 to 11 months (average 3½ months). Antibiotic therapy generally is continued intravenously for a minimum of 6 weeks. When clinical and radiologic improvement is documented, therapy can be discontinued. CT imaging should be done every 2 to 4 weeks until the abscess has resolved, and then every 2 to 4 months for 1 year.

Surgical Therapy

Drainage of a brain abscess can be accomplished by needle aspiration or by total excision. Aspiration is done through strategic burr hole placement. The precise location, shape, and size of the abscess is provided by CT imaging. In selected patients, a single aspirate can provide both accurate microbiologic diagnosis and appropriate therapeutic drainage. In other patients, the abscess needs to be aspirated on multiple occasions. The goal of therapy is to convert the previously purulent-filled cavity to a sterile collagen glial core. Local instillation of antibiotics is not necessary because penetration of the cavity by systemically administered antibiotics is adequate. In addition, local therapy with beta-lactam antibiotics might initiate seizure activity.

Aspiration done in the early stages of disease, before capsules form provides rapid relief of increased intracranial pressure. The risks of aspiration include possible penetration of the ventricle, with the subsequent development of ventriculitis or meningitis, inoculation of additional brain tissue with purulent material, and failure to drain daughter abscesses.

Operative excision provides definitive treatment. It cannot be accomplished if the abscess is very large or involves deep structures such as the thalamus or brain stem. Small abscesses with ill-defined capsules or those with extensive surrounding edema are not removed easily without damaging brain tissue. Many neurosurgeons choose aspiration as the first procedure and follow it with operative excision for those cases that fail to respond to aspiration.

Despite aggressive medical and surgical therapy, the mortality rate continues to approach 30 to 40 percent in some series. As many as 60 percent of patients have neurologic and developmental sequelae, including learning difficulties, visual field defects, seizures, and hemiparesis.

Supportive Care

Brain edema is a frequent concomitant of brain abscess or its operative therapy. Dexamethasone in a dosage of 1 mg per kilogram per day, given in four divided doses, is helpful in reducing cerebral edema. Seizures should be controlled with an appropriate anticonvulsant. Phenobarbital (5 to 7 mg per kilogram per day) or phenytoin (5 mg per kilogram per day) can be given initially. The dosage of these anticonvulsants should be adjusted on the basis of observed clinical effects, and their serum concentrations should be monitored. Anticonvulsant therapy can be tapered gradually when the abscess has resolved. Seizures may recur as a result of cortical scarring.

SUGGESTED READING

Black P, Graybill JR, Charache P. Penetration of brain abscess by systemically administered antibiotics. J Neurosurg 1983; 38:705–709.

Brook I. Bacteriology of intracranial abscess in children. J Neurosurg 1981; 54:484–488.

Everett ED, Strausbaugh LJ. Antimicrobial agents and the central nervous system. Neurosurgery 1980; 6:691–708.

Levy RM, Gutin PH, Baskin DS, Pons VG. Vancomycin penetration of a brain abscess: case report and review of the literature. Neurosurgery 1986; 18:632–636.

Masucci EF, Sauerbrunn BJ. The evolution of a brain abscess. The complimentary roles of radionuclide and computed tomography scans. Clin Nucl Med 1982; 7(4):166–170.

Mathisen GE, Meyer RD, George WL, et al. Brain abscess and cerebritis. Rev Infect Dis 1984; 6:5101–5106.

Nielsen H. Cerebral abscess in children. Neuropediatrics 1983; 14:76–80.

Rennels MB, Woodward CL, Robinson WL, et al. Medical cure of apparent brain abscesses. Pediatrics 1983; 72:220–224.

Spires JR, Smith RJ, Catlin FI. Brain abscesses in the young. Otolaryngol Head Neck Surg 1985; 93:468–473.

Sutton DL, Ouvrier RA. Cerebral abscesses in the under six month of age group. Arch Dis Child 1983; 58:901–905.

SUBDURAL, EPIDURAL, AND SUBGALEAL INFECTIONS

MUTHAYIPALAYAM C. THIRUMOORTHI, M.B., B.S.

Subgaleal, epidural, and subdural infections occur in relation to the coverings and contents of the skull. Epidural space infections can also occur along the spinal cord.

MANIFESTATIONS AND EVALUATION

Subgaleal Abscess

Subgaleal abscess is a purulent infection in the tissue layer between the galea aponeurotica and the pericranium. The most common pathogenesis of subgaleal abscess is direct inoculation of bacterial pathogens into the subgaleal space following trauma to the scalp—whether inflicted accidentally or during a surgical procedure. Subgaleal suppuration usually results in local and regional evidence of inflammation (swelling, warmth, tenderness, fluctuance, and regional adenitis), as well as systemic symptoms and signs. The diagnosis is generally apparent, but at times the clues are subtle. These abscesses contain a polymicrobial flora, usually consisting of aerobic gram-positive cocci and anaerobic cocci.

Cranial Epidural Abscess

A cranial epidural abscess is an accumulation of pus between a cranial bone and the underlying dura mater. These abscesses rarely become large, but have the potential to result in spread of infection to the subdural space or to the brain parenchyma. Cranial epidural abscesses usually form as a consequence of calvarial osteomyelitis, previous craniotomy, parana-sal sinusitis, or middle ear disease. The symptoms and signs of these abscesses are not dissimilar to those of subdural empyemas, although somewhat less pronounced. The microbiology of cranial epidural abscess is similar to that of subdural empyema. Hence, these two entities can be considered together.

Subdural Empyema

A collection of fluid in the potential subdural space is termed subdural effusion or empyema, depending on the nature of the fluid (nonpurulent or purulent). Subdural effusions occur frequently in association with bacterial meningitis in infants. Some of these effusions may become purulent by extention of organisms from the leptomeninges or, rarely, by hematogenous spread of infection to the dura mater. While bacterial meningitis is the most common cause of subdural effusion in infants, in both children and adults, subdural empyema is usually due to extention of infection from an adjacent suppurative focus, such as the paranasal sinuses, the mastoids, or the middle ear space.

Subdural fluid collection should be suspected in a patient with bacterial meningitis when fever or neurologic impairment is prolonged, head circumference increases rapidly, a bulging fontanel persists, focal neurologic signs appear, or secondary fever is noted. Transillumination of the head with a high-intensity light source, when positive, is a simple means of diagnosing a subdural fluid collection. A normal result does not exclude such a collection. In infants with open anterior fontanel, ultrasonagraphy of the head is a relatively inexpensive and readily available diagnostic tool. Computed tomographic (CT) scan with contrast is a definitive means of identifying subdural fluid collections. In young infants subdural taps through the lateral angle of the anterior fontanel provide a sample of the subdural fluid for diagnostic purposes, including chemical and cytologic analysis and culture. Any bacteria found in such fluid is usually the pathogen causing the meningitis.

The presenting features of subdural empyema are different when it occurs in the absence of primary bacterial meningitis. The usual clinical presentation consists of an ill child with fever, severe headache and vomiting, who subsequently develops mental confusion and, sometimes, neck stiffness. Later, features of progressive cerebral dysfunction such as drowsiness, isolated nerve palsies, hemiparesis, seizures (focal or generalized), dysphasia, stupor, and coma may be encountered. The history usually provides evidence of preceding sinusitis (most commonly frontal), chronic otitis, or mastoiditis. Papilledema may be apparent. The constellation of findings is influenced by the size and location of the mass lesion and the degree of involvement of the leptomeninges and the underlying cortex. Systemic findings of an infectious process such as fever and leukocytosis are often present.

A lumbar puncture is of limited value in diagnosing a subdural empyema. The CSF findings are not diagnostic, and the risk of brain stem herniation exists when a lumbar puncture is performed in the presence of increased intracranial pressure. Radiographic examinations are safer and more specific in diagnosing a subdural empyema. A CT scan is the most commonly used diagnostic procedure. However, radioisotopic brain scan and even cerebral angiography are occasionally used for this purpose. Though magnetic resonance imaging (MR) has been used for diagnosing intracranial infections, the availability of and experience with this technique is still rather limited.

Spinal Epidural Abscess

Infections of the spinal epidural space are rare in children. Their importance lies in that they are often difficult to recognize, but prompt diagnosis and therapy are necessary to a good neurologic outcome. The clinical presentation is variable. Back pain, usually near the involved spinal segment, is the most common symptom. Midthoracic and lower lumbar areas are frequently involved, but infection may occur in almost any segment. Fever is usually present. Limping or back stiffness may be apparent. The pain continues to increase, and flexion movements of the spine or cough worsen the pain. Radicular pain, weakness, and finally paralysis follow, but such progression occurs at an unpredictable rate. Significant antecedent events such as a preceding or concomitant site of bacterial infection or blunt trauma to the back are evident in only a few children. The infecting organisms reach the epidural space most commonly by the hematogenous route but, especially beyond childhood, extention of infection from vertebral osteomyelitis and postoperative infections are other likely events.

Staphylococcus aureus is by far the most common pathogen in children, but other organisms such as coagulase-negative staphylococcus and gram-negative bacilli may be responsible in postoperative patients and in intravenous drug users. Fever and localized tenderness over the back are the early signs. Weakness of the lower limbs, abnormalities of bladder or bowel function, and sensory changes indicate progression of the disease. Meningeal signs are rarely present, but signs of systemic sepsis and changes in mental state occasionally suggest meningitis and mask the symptoms and signs referable to the back. The following diagnostic studies are useful. A blood count usually reveals leukocytosis and the erythrocyte sedimentation rate is elevated. A blood culture may provide the etiologic pathogen; it is positive more often when the illness has been acute in evolution. Radiographic examination of the spine is useful in identifying the rare instances of vertebral osteomyelitis and, more often, in excluding other causes of back pain. Lumbar puncture may reveal evidence of a variable degree of spinal block. Frank pus is occasionally encountered during the procedure establishing the diagnosis. Further advancement of the needle into the subarachnoid space should be avoided. The definitive diagnostic procedure for a suspected spinal epidural abscess is myelography. In fact, when the clinical presentation is highly suggestive of epidural abscess, the lumbar puncture could be done as part of a planned myelographic procedure. Myelography establishes the diagnosis and identifies the location of the lesion. CT or MR imaging is often used to define the extent of the disease process, but has not supplanted myelography in the diagnosis of epidural abscess.

THERAPY

In discussing the treatment of subgaleal abscess, I would like to emphasize the preventable nature of this entity. Proper treatment of scalp lacerations is the most important preventive measure. Such wounds should be adequately examined to determine their extent, appropriately debrided, irrigated, and carefully closed. Early recognition of infection of these wounds is also important. The treatment of an established subgaleal abscess consists of incision and drainage of the abscess, with good debridement and cleaning of the subgaleal space and intravenous administration of appropriate antimicrobials. I prefer the combined use of an antistaphylococcal penicillin such as nafcillin, 150 to 200 mg per kilogram daily in six divided doses, and penicillin G, 100,000 to 200,000 U per kilogram daily in six doses. Single-drug therapy with cefazolin, 100 mg per kilogram daily in three doses, cefuroxime, 150 mg per kilogram daily in three doses, or clindamycin, 30 to 40 mg per kilogram daily in four doses, is a reasonable alternative under appropriate conditions. Others have recommended irrigation of the subgaleal space during the first few days of antibiotic therapy. Complications of a subgaleal abscess such as loss of scalp tissue or underlying bone would require appropriate management.

Management of subdural collections associated with bacterial meningitis includes adequate antimicrobial therapy and, when necessary, evacuation of the subdural fluid collection. Although many subdural effusions resolve with antibiotic therapy alone, most large ones and probably all empyemas require evacuation of the fluid. Generally, these fluid collections can be evacuated by needle aspiration of the subdural space. Fluid sometimes tends to reaccumulate, and repeated aspirations are necessary. Surgical interventions such as operative drainage, shunt to drain the subdural collection into the subgaleal space or other sites, or "stripping" of the membranes of the cavity are rarely needed or used these days.

In contrast to the subdural fluid collections associated with meningitis, epidural abscesses and subdural empyemas secondary to adjacent suppurative processes generally require surgical drainage. Drainage through a burr hole is not always adequate. Prompt drainage of a subdural empyema through an adequate craniotomy appears to yield better results. Although some reports have appeared about the successful management of subdural empyema with antimicrobial therapy alone (without surgery), the consensus is that early operative intervention is likely to result in lower mortality and morbidity from subdural empyema. It is important to achieve adequate drainage of the primary focus of infection (sinusitis, mastoiditis) to ensure satisfactory clinical response.

Patients with subdural empyemas associated with meningitis almost always receive antimicrobial therapy directed against the meningeal pathogen. Consideration may be given to the characteristics (such as diffusion into an abscess cavity) of the drug when the infecting organism is susceptible to more than one antimicrobial agent. In the past I have preferred chloramphenicol, 75 to 100 mg per kilogram daily in four doses, given intravenously and later by mouth, with monitoring of serum drug concentrations to maintain them between 15 and 25 μg per milliliter. With the availability of the newer cephalosporins, cefotaxime, 200 mg per kilogram daily in four doses, has become my usual choice under these circumstances. Drugs such as cefuroxime (240 mg per kilogram daily in three doses intravenously) and ceftriaxone (100 mg per kilogram daily in one or two intravenous doses) are other reasonable alternatives. Approximately 2 weeks of therapy is needed, but resolution of clinical signs and symptoms should guide the duration of therapy.

For subdural empyemas associated with sinus or otic infections, chloramphenicol, as mentioned earlier, in combination with nafcillin (150 to 200 mg per kilogram daily in four to six intravenous doses) used to be my choice. At this time I prefer to use cefuroxime, as described earlier. I add metronidazole in a dosage of 30 mg per kilogram daily in four doses (following a loading dose of 15 mg per kilogram), given intravenously, when clinical response is unsatisfactory or when bacteriologic evidence indicates the presence of *Bacteroides fragilis*. Metronidazole may be given by mouth when the child is able to take and retain oral medications. Antibiotic therapy needs to be administered until the inflammatory process has fully resolved, as shown by follow-up CT scans and neurologic evaluations. This may take 4 weeks or longer.

The treatment of spinal epidural abscess also consists of surgical intervention and appropriate antimicrobial therapy. Early decompression of the epidural abscess by adequate drainage is necessary to minimize the effects of pressure and vascular impairment on the spinal cord. This is the most important step in a spinal epidural abscess. There is some disagreement among neurosurgeons about the extent of surgery (fenestration, limited laminectomy, or multisegment laminectomy) that should be performed. The least amount of intervention that is consistent with adequate drainage of the abscess appears to be the choice, so that adverse effects on the growth of the spine are minimized. Nafcillin, in the dosage used for subdural empyema, is my antibiotic of choice. However, when a spinal epidural abscess has occurred following spinal surgery, I initiate therapy with vancomycin, 40 mg per kilogram daily in four divided doses, until bacteriologic data are available. Antimicrobial therapy is administered for 3 to 4 weeks.

The children who have recovered from epidural or subdural infections may have long-term sequelae such as seizures and neurologic deficits. These require appropriate therapeutic and rehabilitative measures.

SUGGESTED READING

Curless RG. Subdural empyema in infant meningitis: diagnosis, therapy and prognosis. Child's Nerv Sys 1985; 1:211–214.

Danner RL, Hartman BJ. Update of spinal epidural abscess: 35 cases and review of the literature. Rev Infect Dis 1987; 9:265–274.

Fischer EG, Greene CS Jr, Winston KR. Spinal epidural abscess in children. Neurosurgery 1981; 9:257–260.

Goodman SJ, Cahan L, Chow AW. Subgaleal abscess—a preventable complication of scalp trauma. West J Med 1977; 127:169–172.

Leys D, Destee A, Petit H, Warot P. Management of subdural intracranial empyemas should not always require surgery. J Neurol Neurosurg Psychiatry 1986; 49:635–639.

Smith HP, Hendrick EB. Subdural empyema and epidural abscess in children. J Neurosurg 1983; 58:392–397.

VIRAL MENINGITIS AND ENCEPHALITIS

MYRON J. LEVIN, M.D.
HARLEY A. ROTBART, M.D.

Virus infections of the central nervous system (CNS) may be asymptomatic or produce only minor systemic symptoms such as fever, malaise, and irritability. Significant meningeal infection (meningitis) produces additional findings such as headache (retro-orbital or frontal), stiff neck and/or other meningeal signs, vomiting, lethargy, and photophobia. Parenchymal brain infection (encephalitis) is associated with a change in affect and/or level of consciousness (confusion, stupor, coma), often with focal neurologic deficits. Seizures, which occur commonly (and are often focal) with encephalitis, are less common with meningitis, and usually generalized. Myelitis is defined by deficits resulting from infection of spinal cord neurons.

Viral CNS infection is typically accompanied by cerebrospinal fluid (CSF) abnormalities, including pleocytosis (10 to 500 cells per cubic millimeter) with a mononuclear leukocyte predominance, a modest elevation of protein (50 to 150 mg per deciliter), and a normal or slightly reduced glucose level. Exceptions are common, however. Early in the illness neutrophils may predominate; hypoglycorrhachia may be present with some infections; and the CSF protein may be very high initially and/or increase progressively with necrotizing infections.

The diagnosis of a viral CNS infection implies that any other treatable disease has been excluded or considered unlikely. Malignancy, collagen–vascular disease, lead poisoning, and Reye's syndrome have been mistaken for virus infections. Important non-viral infectious agents to exclude are rickettsia, leptospira, organisms causing granulomatous infections (fungi, mycobacteria, treponemes, brucella), and listeria. Parameningeal infections (abscess, sinusitis, epidural and subdural collections), partially treated bacterial meningitis, subacute bacterial endocarditis, toxoplasmosis, and nocardiosis must also be considered before concluding that a CNS infection is viral in origin.

Nonspecific therapies are applicable to all severe viral CNS infections (Table 1). Specific treatment is available for herpes simplex and varicella–zoster virus infections (see chapters on *Herpes Simplex Virus Infection* and *Varicella–Zoster Virus Infec-*

TABLE 1 Nonspecific Therapy for Viral CNS Infections

Problem	Management	Comment
Airway obstruction/ respiratory failure	Maintain airway. Tracheal toilet. Assist ventilation.	Artificial airway if necessary
Seizures	Dilantin (15–20 mg/kg IV loading; maintain with bid oral dose); give IV dose slowly over 20–30 min and monitor BP and EKG. Or phenobarbital (5 mg/kg IV); give every 30 min until seizures cease or BP falls.	Dilantin is the drug of choice (does not cloud the sensorium). Seizures may be refractory or persist, especially with herpes simplex and some arboviruses. Status epilepticus may require less commonly used treatments such as paraldehyde. Paralysis is used for uncontrolled seizures (prevents hyperthermia and increased metabolic requirements). Prophylaxis against seizures is not necessary.
Fluid/electrolyte imbalance	Avoid dehydration or dilutional hyponatremia. Monitor electrolytes, and urine and serum osmolality.	Inappropriate secretion of antidiuretic hormone may occur.
Brain swelling	Avoid overhydration. Mannitol (0.5 g/kg of 20% solution IV over 20 min; repeat as needed). Hyperventilation (maintain respiratory rate to reduce P_{CO_2} to 25 mm Hg). Dexamethasone.	Suspect with new deficits, changes in pupil size or extraocular muscle function, falling level of consciousness, CT evidence of swelling. Management of significant swelling is facilitated by the use of an intracranial pressure monitor. Hyperventilation is generally used after other modalities have failed (response may be rapid, but often fails to be effective after 24 hours). The use of glucocorticoids is controversial. In some experimental settings (where infection or ischemia is present) they appear to be harmful.
Bladder atony/ hypotonia	Catheterization.	Common with severe encephalitis and poliomyelitis syndromes.
Skin breakdown	Turn frequently. Use special mattress.	
Malnutrition	Hyperalimentation.	

TABLE 2 Experimental Specific Therapy for Viral CNS Infections

Virus	Agent	Dose	Comment
Cytomegalovirus	Ganciclovir	2.5–7.5 mg/kg IV q8h for 10 days, or longer if symptoms persist.	Available on compassionate plea basis from Syntex Corporation. Should have biopsy diagnosis before therapy. Adjust dose for neutropenia and renal impairment. Not yet used for congenital pediatric infections.
Epstein–Barr	Ganciclovir	As above; duration uncertain.	See above.
Influenza A	Amantadine	5 mg/kg PO to a maximum of 150 mg if <10 years old; 200 mg PO for >10 years old; duration 7–10 days.	Adjust dose for renal impairment.
Human immune deficiency	3′-Azido-3′-deoxythymidine	250 mg PO q4h or 2.5–5.0 mg IV q4h	Available from Burroughs Wellcome Co. under protocol. Important to exclude other concomitant CNS disease.
Arenaviruses (hemorrhagic fevers)	Ribavirin	2 g IV loading; then 1 g q6h for 4 days; then 0.5 g q8h for 6 days. Or 2 g PO loading and 1 g q8h for 10 days may be adequate.	Reported for Lassa fever only. Hemolysis may result.
Measles			
Acute	Ribavirin	2.5 mg/kg PO qid for 7 days.	The dose given has been used for uncomplicated measles. A dose three to five times greater might be considered for encephalitis.
Subacute sclerosing panencephalitis	Ribavirin	10 mg/kg PO tid for 3 days; then 10 mg/kg bid for 6 weeks.	
Enterovirus			
Neonatal (high risk)	Human immunoglobulin for intravenous use.	400 mg/kg IV as a single dose or divided over 2 days.	High risk includes (1) concurrent maternal illness, (2) prematurity, (3) age <6 days at onset.
Immune deficiency disease	Human immunoglobulin for intravenous use.	200–400 mg/kg IV q2–4 weeks, based on response. Intrathecal therapy may be indicated as well.	May want to screen lots for antibody against the infecting virus. Can check patient's serum and CSF for appearance of specific antibody.

tions). There is no established treatment for other CNS viral infections, although experimental therapies are under study for some of them (Table 2).

SUGGESTED READING

Erlendsson K, Swartz T, Dwyer JM. Successful reversal of echovirus encephalitis in x-linked hypogammaglobulinemia by intraventricular administration of immunoglobulin. N Engl J Med 1985; 312:351–353.

Johnson RT. Meningitis, encephalitis, and poliomyelitis. In: Viral infections of the nervous system. New York: Raven Press, 1982; 87–128.

Whitley RJ, Alford CA, Hirsch MS, et al. Vidarabine versus acyclovir therapy in herpes simplex encephalitis. N Engl J Med 1986; 314:144–149.

Yarchoan R, Brouwers P, Spitzer AR, et al. Response of human-immunodeficiency-virus-associated neurological disease to 3′-azido-3′-deoxythymidine. Lancet 1987; 1:132–135.

CEREBROSPINAL FLUID SHUNT INFECTION

MARY ANNE JACKSON, M.D.

Although the management of hydrocephalus has been greatly facilitated by the use of shunts to drain cerebrospinal fluid (CSF) from the ventricles to the peritoneum, shunt infection continues to complicate between 2 and 20 percent of shunt procedures. The majority of infections are caused by strains of coagulase-negative staphylococci, or other skin commensals (including anaerobic *Propionibacterium* [predominantly *P. acnes*], facultative diphtheroids of the genus *Corynebacterium,* facultative *Micrococcus* sp., and coagulase-positive staphylococci), which are introduced at the time of surgery. Gram-negative bacteria such as *Escherichia coli, Klebsiella, Enterobacter, Proteus,* and *Pseudomona aeruginosa* cause infection less commonly, but are associated with more fulminant presentations.

Symptoms in shunt infection are often nonspecific; therefore, a high index of suspicion is necessary when evaluating the shunted patient who has fever, vomiting, lethargy, and irritability. In such cases, examination of the ventricular fluid is indicated; a white blood cell count (WBC) of greater than 10 per cubic millimeter in the ventricular fluid is suggestive of infection. Gram stain of the fluid is generally positive in cases in which infection is caused by *S. aureus* or gram-negative bacilli, but only rarely when infection is caused by the most common pathogen, coagulase-negative staphylococci.

SURGICAL MANAGEMENT

Failure to diagnose and treat CSF shunt infection can lead to serious morbidity, including repeated operations for shunt malfunction, chronic ill health, and impaired intellectual outcome. Case fatality rates of up to 60 percent have been reported, depending on the treatment modality employed. Optimal therapy for CSF shunt infection includes removal of the infected shunt with placement of an extra ventricular drainage (EVD) system and antimicrobial therapy. The high failure rate (70 percent) and increased mortality experienced when shunt infection is treated with antimicrobial therapy alone is consistent with the observations that strains of coagulase-negative staphylococci produce a mucoid glycocalyx, which enhances bacterial adherence to shunts, protects the organisms against normal phagocytic and lysosomal activity, and allows for formation of subsurface colonies on the catheter. Except in selected cases such as meningitis, infected shunts should be removed as part of therapy. Bacterial meningitis caused by *Haemophilus influenzae, Neisseria meningiditis,* or *Streptococcus pneumoniae* probably occurs with normal frequency in shunted patients and symptoms are no more severe. Removal of the shunt in these cases is rarely necessary; organisms can usually be eradicated with the shunt left in situ.

MEDICAL MANAGEMENT

Table 1 outlines antimicrobial therapy based on the common etiologic agents. Because most shunt infections are caused by staphylococci, empiric antimicrobial therapy for CSF shunt infection should be directed against this pathogen. In our institution, where 40 percent of *S. epidermidis* strains are resistant to oxacillin, vancomycin is the drug of choice. (Nafcillin or oxacillin is acceptable therapy when the organism is susceptible.) This provides adequate coverage for the majority of gram-positive pathogens.

Infection caused by gram-negative bacilli is suspected if the onset is more than 2 weeks after surgery and/or when fever and toxicity (suggesting bacteremia and/or peritonitis) are present. In these cases, I recommend one of the third-generation cephalosporins (cefotaxime, ceftazidime, or ceftriaxone), in combination with vancomycin until culture results are known. The excellent penetration into CSF and superior in vitro activity against gram-negative bacilli favor these agents over the aminoglycosides. Dosages for the commonly used antimicrobials are listed in Table 2. Ceftazidime is the only third-generation cephalosporin that demonstrates good antipseudomonal activity.

MONITORING THERAPEUTIC RESPONSE

Placement of an extra ventricular drainage (EVD) system allows not only for continued management of increased intracranial pressure after the shunt has been removed, but also for therapeutic monitoring. A ventricular fluid specimen should be obtained 48 to 72 hours after therapy has been started, to confirm sterility and measure bactericidal activity. If bactericidal activity is less than 1:8, a sec-

TABLE 1 Antimicrobial Therapy for Shunt Infection Based on Etiologic Agent*

	PCN	VANC	OX NAF	Ceftriaxone Cefotaxime	Ceftazidime	Aminoglycosides	Rifampin	T/S
Coagulase-negative staphylococcus	−	+1	−	−	−	+2	+2	+2
S. aureus	−	+	+1	+	+	+2	+2	+2
P. acnes	+1	+	+/−	+	+	−		
Streptococci viridans	+1	+	+	+	+	+2	+2	+2
E. coli	−	−	−	+1	+	+2	−	+
Klebsiella, Enterobacter	−	−	−	+1	+	+2	−	+
P. aeruginosa	−	−	−	−	+1	+2	−	−

* Key to abbreviations:
PCN = penicillin
VANC = vancomycin
OX = oxacillin
NAF = nafcillin
T/S = trimethoprim-sulfamethoxazole
1 = drug of choice
2 = adjunct agent only
− = not useful
+ = usually effective

TABLE 2 Dosages of Commonly Used Antimicrobial for Shunt Infection

Antimicrobial	Dosage (mg/kg/day)	Schedule
Vancomycin	40–60	Divided, q6h
Oxacillin	150	Divided, q6h
Nafcillin	150	Divided, q6h
Cefotaxime	200	Divided, q6h
Ceftazidime	150	Divided, q8h
Ceftriaxone	100	Divided, q12h
Imipenem-cilastatin*	100	Divided, q6h
Rifampin†	20	Divided, q12h
Trimethoprim-sulfamethoxazole†	15–20 (TMP component)	Divided, q6h
Gentamicin	5–7.5	Divided, q8h
Tobramycin	5	Divided, q8h
Amikacin	22	Divided, q8h

* Little information about treatment of shunt infection; not approved for use in children younger than 12 years of age.
† Adjunctive agents only.

ond antimicrobial agent should be added for synergistic effect. Rifampin, trimethoprim–sulfamethoxazole, and an aminoglycoside all have demonstrable in vitro synergy when combined with a beta-lactam antibiotic or vancomycin against staphylococcal strains.

REFRACTORY VENTRICULITIS

When the therapy employed does not appear adequate (persistently positive cultures and/or bactericidal activity less than 1:8), intraventricular antibiotics (vancomycin, 20 μg per milliliter, for gram-positive infections and gentamicin, 12 μg per milliliter, for gram-negative infection) may be used. Only the formulations specifically designated for intrathecal use should be used.

Tolerant strains of staphylococci (those inhibited but not killed by a specific antimicrobial agent) have been reported and are more common with beta-lactam antibiotics than with vancomycin; therefore, for all staphylococcal strains, I recommend that a minimum bactericidal concentration (MBC) be assessed. A MBC greater than 16 times the minimum inhibitory concentration indicates tolerance.

Occasionally the EVD system becomes colonized with bacteria. If cultures remain positive despite apparently adequate therapy, the EVD system should be replaced. Rarely, infected intracranial or intra-abdominal foci occur, and these must be removed to eradicate the infection.

DURATION OF THERAPY AND REPLACING THE SHUNT

Practically speaking, by the time the infecting organism has been isolated in culture, susceptibilities have been reported, and follow-up cultures have been confirmed to be sterile, the patient is 4 to 5 days into the antibiotic course. For infection caused by gram-positive strains, replacement of the shunt may be undertaken at this time, if the clinical course has been satisfactory and antimicrobials continued for a total of 10 days. For infection caused by gram-negative bacilli, antibiotic therapy should be continued longer and shunt replacement deferred until after 10 to 14 days of therapy. When difficulties in achieving sterilization of ventricular fluid are encountered, I favor waiting at least 5 to 7 days after two consecutive cultures are reported to be sterile before replacing the shunt. If the shunt is not removed initially and a satisfactory clinical and bacteriologic response to antimicrobial therapy is demonstrated, I would use a longer course of therapy and be aware that relapse rates are high.

ANTIBIOTIC PROPHYLAXIS

The value of antimicrobial prophylaxis in the perioperative period is unclear. Several prospective, controlled studies suggest that there is no benefit. I do not recommend antibiotic prophylaxis for CNS shunt surgery, but most surgeons use it.

SUGGESTED READING

Congeni BL, Tan J, Salstrom ST, et al. Kinetics of vancomycin after intraventricular and intravenous administration. Pediatr Res 1977; 13:459.

Frame PT, McLauren RL. Treatment of CSF shunt infection with intrashunt plus oral antibiotic therapy. J Neurosurg 1984; 60:354–360.

George R, Leibroch L, Epstein M. Long-term analysis of cerebrospinal fluid shunt infections. J Neurosurg 1979; 51:804–811.

Nelson JD. Cerebrospinal fluid shunt infections. Pediatr Infect Dis 1984; 3:530–532.

Odio C, McCracken GH Jr, Nelson JD. Cerebrospinal fluid shunt infections in pediatrics: a seven year experience. Am J Dis Child 1984; 138:1103–1108.

Schmidt K, Gjerris F, Osgaard O, et al. Antibiotic prophylaxis in cerebrospinal fluid shunting: a prospective randomized trial in 152 hydrocephalic patients. Neurosurgery 1985; 17:1–5.

Schoenbaum SC, Gardner P, Shillito J. Infections of cerebrospinal fluid shunts: epidemiology, clinical manifestations and therapy. J Infect Dis 1975; 131:543–552.

Slight PH, Gundling K, Plotkin SA, et al. A trial of vancomycin for prophylaxis of infections after neurosurgical shunts. N Engl J Med 1985; 312:912.

Walters BL, Hoffman HJ, Hendricks EB, et al. Cerebrospinal fluid shunt infection: influences on initial management and subsequent outcome. J Neurosurg 1984; 60:1014–1021.

Younger JJ, Simmons JCH, Barrett FF. Failure of single dose intraventricular vancomycin for cerebrospinal fluid shunt surgery prophylaxis. Pediatr Infect Dis 1987; 6:212–213.

DISEASES OF THE GENITOURINARY TRACT

INFECTION OF THE FEMALE GENITAL TRACT

THOMAS A. BELL, M.D., M.P.H.

INFECTIONS OF POSTPUBERTAL FEMALES

Neisseria Gonorrhoeae or Chlamydia Trachomatis

Treatment of gonorrhea is complicated by the need for simultaneous treatment for *Chlamydia trachomatis* infection, and treatment should be given even before the results of diagnostic tests are known. Although presumptive treatment for *C. trachomatis* is indicated for persons with *Neisseria gonorrhoeae* infection and for their sexual consorts, the converse is not true if the latter organism has not been found by microscopy and culture of anogenital secretions. The drug of choice for treatment of uncomplicated anogenital *N. gonorrhoeae* infection is ceftriaxone in a single intramuscular dose of 125 mg (regardless of body weight) diluted 1:1 with 1 percent lidocaine. Regimens efficacious against *C. trachomatis* include tetracycline, 500 mg, administered by mouth four times a day for 7 days, doxycycline, 100 mg given by mouth twice a day for 7 days, erythromycin, 500 mg given by mouth four times a day or 666 mg three times a day for 7 days, or sulfamethoxazole, 3,600 mg once a day for 3 days. When given in combination with 720 mg of trimethoprim at each dose (9 single-strength tablets of co-trimoxazole), sulfamethoxazole is quite effective against both *N. gonorrhoeae* and *C. trachomatis*. Test of cure for both infections should occur 1 to 2 weeks after treatment is completed.

Alternative regimens are also required when ceftriaxone is not available and for persons who are allergic to cephalosporins or who refuse injections. For the former group, the treatment of choice would be a single intramuscular dose of 2 g of spectinomycin. For the latter, the aforementioned regimen of co-trimoxazole has the advantage of being the regimen that is effective against both *N. gonorrhoeae* and *C. trachomatis* with which compliance is easiest. This regimen is often accompanied by nausea or lightheadedness for a few hours after the dose is administered and, therefore, may be taken best at night. "Epidemiologic" treatment of consorts is justified by its risk-benefit ratio. Cases should be reported to public health authorities.

Trichomonas Vaginalis

Trichomonas vaginalis infection is usually cured by a single dose of 2 g of metronidazole given by mouth. This should be followed by abstinence from alcohol for 48 hours and may be accompanied by several hours of nausea, lightheadedness, or a metallic taste. Sexual consorts should be treated simultaneously. Metronidazole-resistant strains of *T. vaginalis* may respond to prolonged courses of the drug, such as 500 mg every 12 hours for 7 days. Although the drug is of unproved teratogenicity for human fetuses, most physicians are reluctant to administer it to a woman who is or may be pregnant. This poses difficulties in the treatment of adolescents, who may have irregular menstrual cycles and not use effective contraception. Treatment of them and their consorts with metronidazole should be postponed until a normal menstrual period manifests the absence of pregnancy. Meanwhile, symptomatic relief may be obtained by a daily 100-mg dose of clotrimazole inserted intravaginally. Test of cure is optional if symptoms have resolved.

Bacterial Vaginosis

Bacterial vaginosis is also called nonspecific vaginitis, anaerobic vaginitis or vaginosis, and *Gardnerella* vaginitis. It is characterized by "clue" cells and abnormalities of Gram-stained smears of the vaginal flora, the lack of an inflammatory response in the vagina, an anaerobic and abnormally alkaline vaginal milieu, and the presence of malodorous amines in the vaginal fluid. *Gardnerella vaginalis* is a normal inhabitant of the vagina in half of postpubertal virgins and its presence is not an indication for therapy in the absence of other abnormalities.

Metronidazole is the most effective treatment for bacterial vaginosis, which is usually more of a nuisance than a serious threat to the health of the nonpregnant patient. I offer patients a choice between a single dose of 2-g metronidazole by mouth, which is about 70 percent effective, or a 7-day course of 500 mg every 12 hours, which is still available to those who fail or relapse after the single-dose regimen. Most patients choose the single dose. If metronidazole is not indicated (as in pregnancy), tolerated, or effective, Augmentin is often effective in a dosage of 500-mg amoxicillin/125-mg clavulanate every 8 hours for 7 days. Douching with vinegar or yogurt, although popular, is not of demonstrated efficacy.

Bacterial vaginosis usually occurs in sexually active women, but it does not behave like a sexually transmitted disease in that treatment of sexual consorts seems to have no effect on the incidence of recurrence.

Human Papillomavirus (Condylomata Acuminata)

The human papillomaviruses have been implicated as the etiologic agents of cervical, vulvar, and anal cancer. Their detection is difficult because many cervical warts are visible only with colposcopic magnification and staining of the vagina with acetic acid. Warts may be detected in Papanicolaou-stained smears as koilocytosis. Evaluation of the genitalia with low-power microscopy is warranted for persons of either gender whose sexual consorts have genital warts. Vulvar warts can be treated with liquid nitrogen, but cervical warts should be colposcopically evaluated by a gynecologist because they are not easily distinguished from dysplastic and neoplastic lesions. Cervical warts should be closely monitored and they often require excisional biopsy for accurate diagnosis. They may also be treated by laser cautery. Topical interferon has been promising in clinical trials, but it is not yet commercially available. A woman who has genital warts, or whose consort has them, needs to be carefully observed for several years for early detection of cervical dysplasia and neoplasia.

Candidiasis

Vulvovaginal candidiasis is a common disorder in women of reproductive age, especially those using oral contraceptives. The simplest treatment of acute candidiasis is a single 500-mg vaginal suppository of clotrimazole. A 4- to 7-day course of 200 mg of ketoconazole, given by mouth, is preferred by some patients, especially if the episodes occur during menses.

Recurrent vulvovaginal candidiasis is more difficult to manage. Hygienic measures such as wearing undergarments with a cotton crotch may help, but the principal cause of recurrences seems to be a reversible defect in the host's immune response. One stratagem for preventing recurrences is intermittent use of orally administered ketoconazole. A regimen of proved efficacy is the prophylactic use of a single daily dose of 200 mg every 12 hours for the first 5 days of menses. Smaller doses and shorter courses warrant evaluation in individual patients because intense and protracted use of ketoconazole might be hepatotoxic. Well-informed patients need not seek medical attention for each episode. Most can responsibly treat their recurrences, but they must be warned to seek medical attention if symptoms do not improve within 2 days of starting treatment. Treatment of asymptomatic sexual consorts is not of clear benefit.

Herpes Simplex Genitalis

Primary herpes simplex genitalis is often painful and disabling. Orally administered acyclovir in a dosage of 200 mg, five times daily for 10 days, shortens the patient's misery but does not prevent recurrences. Women suffering their primary episodes may develop temporary bladder dysfunction and require catheterization.

The frequency of recurrences can be reduced by oral administration of 200 mg of acyclovir twice daily. The long-term effects of such use are unknown, but are probably not serious in most patients. Those who have infrequent recurrences may prefer to maintain a supply of acyclovir with which to treat themselves during the prodrome of a recurrence. Such treatment shortens the episode. Alternatively, if recurrences are predictable, such as when they occur with menses, acyclovir can be taken only at those times.

Mucopurulent Cervicitis

Mucopurulent cervicitis is sometimes difficult to detect. It has been defined as the presence of yellow or green endocervical mucopus on a white swab, or of 10 or more leukocytes per 1,000X magnification field in the three fields where the leukocytes are in monolayers in the smear of the endocervical secretions containing fewer than 100 squamous epithelial cells. Mucopurulent cervicitis is a moderately sensitive and fairly specific indicator of the presence of *C. trachomatis* infection, for which presumptive treatment should be given. Mucopurulent cervicitis should not be confused with cervical ectropion or ectopy (sometimes called *cervical erosion*), which is the normal state of the adolescent cervix.

Bartholinitis

Bartholinitis can be caused by *C. trachomatis* or *N. gonorrhoeae,* which should be treated as other lower genital tract infections with these organisms, or, more commonly, by normal vaginal flora. The latter type of infection can be treated with orally administered Augmentin as 500/125 mg every 8 hours. Incision and drainage of the abscess is usually necessary; large abscesses may benefit from surgical "marsupialization."

Pelvic Inflammatory Disease

Treatment of pelvic inflammatory disease (PID) remains controversial and has become a greater therapeutic problem with the proliferation of penicillin- and tetracycline-resistant *N. gonorrhoeae*. Recommendations of the Centers for Disease Control and the World Health Organization differ. Both are based more on expert opinion than on empiric data, which are difficult to generate. The recommendations offered here should be carefully judged for their appropriateness for a given patient and the contemporary patterns of bacterial resistance to antimicrobials.

The clinical diagnosis of PID is notoriously inaccurate. It is most commonly mimicked by ectopic pregnancy, endometriosis, ovarian cysts, and lower genital tract infection with normal fallopian tubes. If the patient fails to respond promptly to broad-spectrum antimicrobial treatment, these other diagnoses should be seriously considered and perhaps confirmed by laparoscopy. Ectopic pregnancy should be excluded by history and by measurement of human chorionic gonadotropin in serum. The diagnosis of PID is supported by demonstration of *N. gonorrhoeae* or *C. trachomatis* in the patient or her sexual consort(s).

One important issue in the treatment of PID is the judgment of the need to hospitalize the patient. Clinical trials that show the superiority of intravenous over oral therapy have not been reported. Hospitalization assures compliance with therapy, but it is difficult to justify if the patient is given only oral therapy. In general, a patient should be hospitalized for treatment of PID if she is pregnant, cannot take medicines by mouth, or has an inflammatory adnexal mass or abscess. Diagnosis of PID in an adolescent requires attention to psychosocial issues because it may compromise the confidentiality of her sexual behavior.

Another unresolved controversy is that of choosing between narrow- and broad-spectrum antimicrobial therapy. All cases should be presumptively treated for both *N. gonorrhoeae* and *C. trachomatis* infection until and unless each can be excluded by appropriate microbiologic tests. Before the proliferation of strains of tetracycline-resistant *N. gonorrhoeae*, this drug was usually sufficient for these organisms. If a single intramuscular dose of ceftriaxone is used to treat a case of PID that may be partly gonococcal in etiology, the dose should be 250 mg instead of 125 mg, again diluted 1:1 with 1 percent lidocaine. This eradicates *N. gonorrhoeae* from the cervix and rectum, but its efficacy against *N. gonorrhoeae* in the upper genital tract is unknown. Against anaerobes or facultative organisms such as *Escherichia coli, Streptococcus agalactiae,* and *Haemophilus influenzae,* similar doses of ceftriaxone on subsequent days of the course of treatment might also be of benefit for managing outpatients (Table 1). Augmentin is an orally administered alternative to ceftriaxone. The dosage is 500 mg/125 mg (amoxicillin/clavulanate) three times a day for 10 days.

For treatment of *C. trachomatis* infection a 10-day course of tetracycline or doxycycline is effective.

TABLE 1 Regimens for Outpatient Treatment of Pelvic Inflammatory Disease

Drug	Dose (mg)	Route	Frequency (h)	Duration (days)
Option 1				
Ceftriaxone	250*	IM	24	1–10
		plus		
Tetracycline (or doxycycline)	500 (100)	PO	6 (12)	10
Option 2		*or*		
Co-trimoxazole (TMP/SMZ)	160/800	PO	12	10
		plus		
Metronidazole	500	PO	6	10
Option 3		*or*		
Augmentin	500/125	PO	8	10
		plus		
Tetracycline (or doxycycline)	500 (100)	PO	6 (12)	10
Option 4		*or*		
Tetracycline (or doxycycline)	500 (100)	PO	6 (12)	10
		plus		
Metronidazole	500	PO	6	10
		plus		
Ceftriaxone	250*	IM	Once	

* Dilute 1:1 with 1 percent lidocaine for intramuscular injection.

These drugs have some activity against anaerobes, coliforms, and *H. influenzae.*

In the absence of tetracycline-resistant *N. gonorrhoeae,* metronidazole is also useful in combination with tetracycline or doxycycline. Co-trimoxazole may also be useful in the treatment of PID in outpatients. The dose is 160 mg of trimethoprim/800 mg of sulfamethoxazole every 12 hours for 10 days. For simultaneous activity against anaerobes, metronidazole, 500 mg every 6 hours, is given.

The emergence of tetracycline-resistant *N. gonorrhoeae* and the need to treat for *C. trachomatis* infection, make combination therapy imperative, even though such therapy is more complicated and more likely to cause unpleasant side effects. Broad-spectrum regimens are probably more likely to prevent tubal damage than are regimens with a narrower spectrum, such as tetracycline or doxycycline.

For treatment of PID in hospital, diverse combinations of parenterally administered drugs offer a useful spectrum of antimicrobial activity (Table 2). Theoretically effective regimens given intravenously include 600 mg of clindamycin every 6 hours plus gentamicin, 2 mg per kilogram every 8 hours (the dosage must be adjusted according to peak and trough serum concentrations of the drug); or doxycycline, 100 mg every 12 hours, plus ceftriaxone, 250 mg daily, or cefoxitin, 2 g every 6 hours. These regimens should be effective against *C. trachomatis,* most anaerobes and facultative bacteria, and almost all strains of *N. gonorrhoeae*. If tetracycline-resistant *N. gonorrhoeae* is not present, doxycycline, 100 mg every 12 hours, plus 500 mg of metronidazole every 6

TABLE 2 Regimens for Inpatients with Pelvic Inflammatory Disease

Drug	Dose (mg)	Route	Frequency (h)	Duration (days)*
Doxycycline	100	IV	12	3–10
plus				
Metronidazole	500	IV	6	3–10
plus				
Ceftriaxone	250	IM†/IV	24	1–10‡
or				
Doxycycline	100	IV	12	3–10
plus				
Cefoxitin (or ceftriaxone)	2000 (250)	IV	6 (24)	3–10
or				
Clindamycin	600	IV	6	3–10
plus				
Gentamicin	2 mg/kg§	IV	8	3–10

* Complete 10-day course with an outpatient regimen.
† Dilute 1:1 with 1 percent lidocaine.
‡ Protracted therapy necessary only for tetracycline-resistant *Neisseria gonorrhoeae.*
§ Adjust according to blood levels.

hours has an adequate spectrum, and it is an easy regimen to continue orally after discharge from the hospital. The necessary duration of parenteral therapy with any of these regimens is uncertain. Most parenteral regimens should be continued until the patient's vital signs and physical findings are nearly normal, but metronidazole can be given by mouth as soon as the patient's gastrointestinal function is normal.

Patients in whom PID develops while an intrauterine contraceptive device is worn (which should be removed) or after a surgical procedure is performed, such as aspiration or curettage of the uterus, should be treated with a regimen active against anaerobes and coliform bacilli as well as *N. gonorrhoeae* and *C. trachomatis.* Doxycycline or co-trimoxazole, plus metronidazole is a suitable regimen.

Counseling, contraception, and consorts are important factors in the management of PID. Patients should be given accurate estimates of the risk of infertility after a single episode of PID which is only about 10 percent. About 25 percent of women have a second episode of PID within 1 year. The second episode triples the risk of infertility, and thus warrants vigorous efforts at prevention. Use of oral contraceptives decreases both the risk and severity of PID and is strongly indicated for contraception after an episode of PID. Such effective contraception may also prevent the patient from becoming pregnant to reassure herself about her fertility. Topical contraceptive spermicides, such as nonoxynol-9, provide some protection against recurrence. Unfortunately, most women who develop PID are not using spermicides when they became ill and are unlikely to use them after they recover.

Sexual consorts of women with gonococcal PID should be sought through the disease-control programs of local health departments. Sexual consorts of women with either gonococcal or chlamydial PID require treatment for these infections regardless of the presence of abnormal signs or symptoms or the results of diagnostic tests in them. The need for treatment of consorts of women with nongonococcal, nonchlamydial PID has not been established.

Patients with perihepatitis (Fitz-Hugh–Curtis syndrome), which usually is a consequence of gonococcal or chlamydial PID, should be treated in the same way as those with PID.

INFECTIONS OF PREPUBERTAL FEMALES

Sexually Transmitted Diseases

Prepubertal females are susceptible to many of the sexually transmitted diseases that afflict adolescents. The disease is usually acquired by sexual abuse. Treatment is similar except that tetracyclines should not be given to children younger than 8 years of age. The appropriate doses of drugs are as follows:

1. For *N. gonorrhoeae,* a single intramuscular dose of ceftriaxone, 5 mg per kilogram (maximum, 125 mg), diluted 1:1 with 1 percent lidocaine.
2. For *Trichomonas vaginalis* or bacterial vaginosis, metronidazole in a single dose of 30 mg per kilogram, given by mouth.
3. For *C. trachomatis,* sulfisoxazole, 150 mg per kilogram in divided doses every 6 hours, or sulfamethoxazole, 50 mg per kilogram divided every 12 hours, for 14 days by mouth, or erythromycin, 12.5 mg per kilogram every 6 hours for 14 days by mouth.

External and introital warts are best treated with liquid nitrogen. The surrounding skin and mucous membranes should be protected with petrolatum jelly. Internal warts require evaluation by a gynecologist.

Infections Other Than Sexually Transmitted Diseases

Vaginitis in a prepubertal female can be caused by a variety of respiratory tract and enteric flora, including *Streptococcus pyogenes, Haemophilus influenzae,* and *Escherichia coli. Shigella* is a cause of bloody vaginal discharge. Treatment should be based on identification of the specific organism. Empiric therapy may be begun with orally administered amoxicillin, 10 mg per kilogram every 8 hours for 7 days. Infection caused by beta-lactamase–producing strains of *H. influenzae* should be treated with the equivalent dose of Augmentin. *S. pyogenes* infection should be treated with oral penicillin V, 10 mg per kilogram every 6 hours for 10 days. Infections caused by *E. coli* and other enteric flora are treated according to their susceptibilities in vitro; Augmentin or co-trimoxazole is good empiric therapy. Many prepubertal patients from whom no specific pathogen is isolated respond to hygienic measures such as careful cleaning after defecation.

Enterobius vermicularis is an occasional cause of vaginitis in prepubertal females. Treatment is with a single oral dose of 100 mg of mebendazole.

Foreign bodies are a common cause of vaginal discharge in prepubertal females, especially if the discharge is bloody. The obvious treatment is removal, for which general anesthesia may be necessary. Antimicrobial therapy is usually not necessary.

SUGGESTED READING

Bell TA, James JF. Computer-assisted analysis of the therapy of acute salpingitis. Am J Obstet Gynecol 1980; 138(Part 2):1048–1054.

Centers for Disease Control. 1985 STD treatment guidelines. MMWR 1985; 34:75S–108S.

Collier AC, Judson FN, Murphy VL, et al. Comparative study of ceftriaxone and spectinomycin in the treatment of uncomplicated gonorrhea in women. Am J Med 1984; 77:68–72.

Eschenbach DA, Critchlow CW, Watkins H, et al. A dose-duration study of metronidazole for the treatment of nonspecific vaginosis. Scand J Urol Nephrol Suppl 1983; 40:73–80.

Johnson RE. Epidemiologic and prophylactic treatment of gonorrhea: a decision analysis review. Sex Transm Dis 1979; 6:159–167.

Sobel JD. Recurrent vulvovaginal candidiasis: a prospective study of the efficacy of maintenance ketoconazole. N Engl J Med 1986; 315:1455–1458.

Stamm WE, Guinan ME, Johnson C, et al. Effect of treatment regimens for *Neisseria gonorrhoeae* on simultaneous infection with *Chlamydia trachomatis*. N Engl J Med 1984; 310:545–549.

Swedberg J, Steiner JF, Deiss F, et al. Comparison of single-dose vs. one-week course of metronidazole for symptomatic bacterial vaginosis. JAMA 1985; 254:1046–1049.

URETHRITIS, MEATITIS, AND BALANITIS

DAVID B. JOSEPH, M.D.

URETHRITIS

Urethritis is uncommon in prepubertal children. It is primarily limited to sexually active males. Urethritis affects the anterior urethra. A thorough history is important, with specific questioning of sexual activity and urethral manipulation with a foreign body. In many cases, children will not admit to sexual activity, especially in the presence of a parent. When the diagnosis of urethritis is confirmed in sexually immature children, consideration must be given to sexual abuse.

In gonococcal or nongonococcal urethritis, symptoms are similar and commonly include dysuria, genital itching, and discharge. Treatment of gonococcal urethritis is discussed in another chapter.

Nongonococcal or nonspecific urethritis (NSU) is more prevalent than gonococcal urethritis. Approximately 60 percent of NSU cases are caused by *Chlamydia trachomatis* or *Ureaplasma urealyticum.* The remainder are caused by *Trichomonas vaginalis, Candida albicans,* or viruses. The urethral discharge in NSU is clear, thin, and watery. In most cases treatment for NSU is based on presumptive diagnosis and a negative gonococcal culture. Both *Chlamydia* and *Ureaplasma* are susceptible to tetracycline and erythromycin. The sulfonamides have also been used effectively to eradicate *Chlamydia* urethritis. *Trichomonas vaginalis* infection is treated with metronidazole, 15 mg per kilogram of body weight per day, every 8 hours. All treatments for NSU are continued for 10 to 14 days. The effectiveness of tetracycline in eradicating most cases of gonococcal and nongonococcal urethritis justifies its use as a first-line drug. Compliance, however, is a significant problem, and treatment must therefore be individualized. Noncompliant patients should be treated with parenterally administered antibiotics.

Herpes simplex virus is the most common cause of vesicular ulcerative lesions of the genitalia, and this virus can cause urethritis. It is most often acquired through sexual intercourse. Newborns are inoculated with the virus during passage through an infected birth canal. Symptoms of herpes usually persist for 7 to 14 days, with subsequent periods of latency and recurrence. Culture and serologic testing are available for diagnosis at some institutions. Symptomatic improvement may be effected with early use of topical acyclovir applied every 3 hours. Severe symptoms are treated with parenteral acyclovir, 30 mg per kilogram per day, in divided doses every 8 hours.

Urethritis has often been diagnosed in prepubertal boys who are now recognized as having *urethrorrhagia.* This is a self-limited condition that lasts 7 to 14 days. It is possibly of viral etiology. Symptoms are mild, and blood-spotted underwear is common. No treatment is necessary. Urethral manipulation should be kept to a minimum of a diagnostic swab for culture in all cases of urethritis and urethrorrhagia. Further urethral intervention in acute states frequently leads to stricture formation.

MEATITIS

Meatitis is associated almost exclusively with circumcision. The inflammatory process is presumed to be secondary to the irritating chemical nature of urine-soaked diapers rubbing on the meatus. Prolonged irritation can lead to meatal stenosis. The meatus appears erythematous, edematous, and weepy. Ulcerations are occasionally present. Dysuria, pencil-thin urinary stream, and postvoiding dribbling are the most common complaints. Local care and improved genital hygiene are the best forms of treatment. Most cases improve with genital cleansing, appropriate diaper changes, and zinc oxide or bacitracin ointment applied to the urethral meatus. If symptoms are severe and meatal stenosis is present, a meatotomy is often required.

BALANITIS

Balanitis (i.e., inflammation of the glans penis) and the associated condition balanoposthitis (i.e., inflammation of the glans penis and foreskin) are usually associated with a redundant foreskin and poor penile hygiene. Normal accumulation of desquamated epithelial cells, glandular secretions, and urine provide a warm, moist culture medium for *Mycobacterium smegmatis.* Frequent penile cleaning eliminates excessive accumulation of smegma. In the infant and young child, cleaning should be confined to the area of the foreskin that is easily retracted. Excessive manipulation of the foreskin can cause disruption of "natural" glanular adhesions, creating localized inflammation and edema of the glans and foreskin and resulting in phimosis. Most cases of balanitis are treated with frequent diaper changes, improved penile hygiene, sitz baths, and use of mildsoap. If this treatment is unsuccessful and there is phimosis, a circumcision is required. Antibiotics are usually unnecessary.

Anaerobic gangrenous balanoposthitis is a serious infection causing necrosis of the glans or shaft of the penis. Fortunately, it is uncommon in children. The disease process begins with an ulcerated and infected glans beneath a tight foreskin. The etiologic organisms are anaerobic Borrelia-like organisms and fusiform spirochetes. The diagnosis is made on stained smears of the penile discharge. Because the organisms are anaerobic, exposure to the air is the most rapid form of treatment. Local cleansing and retraction of the foreskin may suffice. A temporizing dorsal slit is required when the foreskin cannot easily be retracted. The coronal sulcus should be inspected for constricting hairs. Following resolution of the infection, circumcision is advisable. In all cases, penicillin should be administered, either parenterally or orally, depending on the severity of the infection.

SUGGESTED READING

Bowie WR. Nongonococcal urethritis. Urol Clin North Am 1984; 11:55.

Harrison WO. Gonococcal urethritis. Urol Clin North Am 1984; 11:45.

Kramer SA. Genital infections. In: Kelalis PP, King LR, Belman AB, eds. Clinical pediatric urology, Vol. 1. Philadelphia: WB Saunders, 1985; 275–282.

RENAL AND PERIRENAL ABSCESS

DAVID B. JOSEPH, M.D.

Classically, fever, chills, and flank pain are the triad associated with a renal or perirenal abscess. In children, particularly neonates and infants, this is not the case. More commonly fever of unknown origin, failure to thrive, and leukocytosis are the presenting symptoms. The ambiguous nature of these symptoms often causes delay in diagnosis. Gram-negative organisms are responsible for most renal and perirenal abscesses. These are usually related to vesicoureteral reflux and other structural abnormalities in the urinary system. Children with major organ defects, overwhelming sepsis, or immune deficiency syndrome are also more susceptible to abscesses. Gram-positive organisms, particularly *Staphylococcus aureus,* previously accounted for the majority of renal abscesses originating from a hematogenous route. The current use of broad-spectrum antibiotics has significantly decreased the incidence of renal and perirenal abscesses in systemically ill children.

In diagnosing children with a presumed renal or perirenal abscess, the ultrasound examination is used as a screening test. A true abscess can be identified ultrasonographically as a mass with a hypoechoic center and a surrounding rim of increased density. In some cases it may be difficult to plan treatment based solely on a renal ultrasound examination, and a computed tomography (CT) scan should be obtained. The CT scan helps to clarify and determine the extent of the lesion. Intravenous urography and renal arteriography add little to the overall assessment and are seldom obtained. Magnetic resonance imaging (MRI) offers potential in evaluating renal and perirenal masses. However, because of its lack of availability and prolonged examination time, its use in the pediatric population is limited. With current imaging techniques, acute lobar nephronia or acute focal bacterial nephritis (AFBN) can be diagnosed. This condition is an early nonliquified inflammatory process of the kidney that possibly predates an abscess. To complete the child's evaluation, it is necessary to perform a voiding cystourethrogram when the acute illness has subsided.

The most important aspect of successful treatment of an abscess, whether renal or perirenal, is immediate drainage. Depending on the size and nature of the abscess, percutaneous drainage can be performed at the time of a diagnostic tap. Complete aspiration of the abscess may be possible. If not, a small pigtail catheter can be inserted for continuous drainage. For most patients, this is performed with minimal morbidity using sedation and local anesthesia, regardless of age. The use of percutaneous drainage has minimized the need for surgical intervention. However, when children do not respond to the treatment plan described here, surgical debridement and drainage, or possibly nephrectomy, is required. Prompt Gram stain and culture of the aspirate are essential in directing antibiotic treatment. Broad-spectrum antibiotic coverage is used before aspiration. A recommended initial treatment plan combines an aminoglycoside, gentamicin, 6 mg per kilogram per day in divided doses every 8 hours, and a synthetic penicillin, ticarcillin, 200 to 300 mg per kilogram per day in divided doses every 6 hours. The use of a cephalosporin is also acceptable. Within 24 to 48 hours a specific organism can be identified, and antibiotic therapy is adjusted according to susceptibility test results. When an aminoglycoside is used, peak and trough serum concentrations are obtained after the third dose and then every 3 to 4 days, if no changes in dosage are required. Serum creatinine and BUN levels are also routinely monitored. Children who are malnourished secondary to the disease process should have the antibiotic dosage calculated based on body surface area (e.g., gentamicin 60 mg per square meter every 8 hours, ticarcillin 2.5 g per square meter every 6 hours). Antibiotic treatment for AFBN is similar to that of an abscess, but percutaneous intervention is not needed.

Parenteral antibiotics are continued for 10 days. The duration of further antibiotic treatment is dictated by the resolution of the abscess and inflammatory process. Ultrasonography is used for monitoring the resolution of this process. In most cases, an oral broad-spectrum antibiotic (e.g., trimethoprim-sulfamethoxazole) is continued for 2 weeks. Before termination of antibiotic therapy, the precipitating cause for the abscess must be determined. Various urologic abnormalities may require long-term prophylactic or suppressive antibiotic coverage.

SUGGESTED READING

Belman AB. Nonspecific genitourinary infections. In: Kelalis PP, King LR, Belman AB, eds. Clinical pediatric urology, Vol 1. Philadelphia: WB Saunders, 1985; 235–256.

Dairiki Shortliffe LM, Stamey TA. Infections of the urinary tract: introduction and general principles. In: Walsh PC, Gittes RF, Perlmutter AD, Stamey TA, eds. Campbell's urology, Vol 1. Philadelphia: WB Saunders, 1986; 738–796.

Sheinfeld T, Erturk E, Spatar FR, Cockett ATK. Perinephric abscess: current concepts. J Urol 1987; 137:191.

Sty TR, Wells RG, Starshak RT, Schroeder BA. Imaging in acute renal infection in children. AJR 1987; 148:471.

PROSTATITIS

DAVID B. JOSEPH, M.D.

Prostatitis is rare in prepubertal males and has only a slightly increased prevalence in sexually active adolescents. True prostatitis presents with variable symptoms, including fever, perineal pain, generalized malaise, urgency, increased urinary frequency, dysuria, urethral discharge and urinary retention. The diagnosis is often confusing, and the rectal examination is difficult to evaluate in prepubertal males. The presence of a boggy prostate (posterior urethra) may be the only finding. Infrequently, a bulging mass consistent with an abscess is palpable. This mass must be differentiated from a Cowper duct cyst, a müllerian duct cyst, or an enlarged posterior urethra secondary to posterior urethral valves. A normal urinalysis or negative urine culture does not exclude prostatitis. In cases in which the suspicion of prostatitis or a prostatic abscess is high, computed tomography (CT) scanning or aspiration under a general anesthetic may be needed for diagnosis.

Treatment of prostatitis is based on the identification and antibiotic susceptibilities of the offending pathogen which is commonly coliform bacilli. In acute prostatitis, initial treatment with trimethoprim-sulfamethoxazole (TMP/SMZ) (10 to 12 mg TMP, 50 to 60 mg SMZ per kilogram, in two divided doses daily) should provide adequate broad-spectrum antibiotic coverage with good prostatic tissue concentrations of antibiotics. If allergies prohibit use of TMP/SMZ or if severe systemic symptoms are present, a combination of gentamicin, 6 mg per kilogram per day divided doses every 8 hours, and ampicillin, 200 mg per kilogram per day in divided doses every 6 hours, may be substituted. Prostatic abscesses in the infant are usually caused by *Staphylococcus aureus*. Methacillin or nafcillin (150 mg per kilogram per day in divided doses every 6 hours) therapy is recommended. *Ureaplasma urealyticum* and *Chlamydia trachomatis* are the most common pathogens in sexually active males. Erythromycin (40 mg per kilogram per day in divided doses every 6 hours) or tetracycline (50 mg per kilogram per day in divided doses every 6 hours) is effective in treatment; however, erythromycin is believed to offer greater prostatic diffusion and should be used as a first-line drug. Antibiotics are continued for a minimum of 10 days and may be required for 4 to 8 weeks. During the initial period of treatment, bed rest, hydration, antipyretics, and analgesics are essential. Prostatic massage and urethral manipulation should be avoided. If there is no improvement of symptoms related to a prostatic abscess, surgical drainage is required.

Following resolution of acute symptoms, evaluation is recommended to detect a possible congenital urologic anomaly. A voiding cystourethrogram and renal ultrasound evaluation provide adequate screening of the urinary system.

SUGGESTED READING

Kramer SA. Genital infections. In: Kelalis PP, King LR, Belman AB, eds. Clinical pediatric urology, Vol. 1. Philadelphia: WB Saunders, 1985; 275–282

Meares EM. Prostatitis and related disorders. In: Walsh PC, Gittes RF, Perlmutter AD, Stamey TA, eds. Campbells urology, Vol. 1. Philadelphia: WB Saunders, 1986; 868–887.

Pfaw A. Prostatitis: a continuing enigma. Urol Clin North Am 1986; 13:695–716.

EPIDIDYMITIS AND ORCHITIS

GEORGE E. HURT Jr., M.D.

ORCHITIS

Acute infections involving the testes are relatively rare in boys. Orchitis may develop as a result of extension of inflammation of the epididymis, from hematogenous origin, or through lymphatic spread. Orchitis may be pyogenic, viral, or traumatic; it is less often spirochetal, chemical, mycotic, parasitic, or idiopathic in nature. It has been reported in a number of systemic diseases including diphtheria, typhus, influenza, brucellosis, leprosy, dengue fever, syphilis, paratyphoid fever, varicella, variola, mumps, scarlet fever, tuberculosis, amebiasis, schistosomiasis, sporotrichosis, actinomycosis, rickettsial diseases, malaria, filariasis, and mononucleosis.

Mumps orchitis occurs in 18 to 20 percent of boys who develop parotitis, but usually only in those who are postpubertal. Onset occurs 4 to 6 days after parotitis and it may occur without parotid involvement. In 70 percent of cases the orchitis is unilateral, and involvement of the epididymis is common. Currently no drug treatment is available and mumps orchitis usually subsides within 7 to 10 days. The treatment consists of bed rest, scrotal support, hot or cold applications, and use of analgesics. Gamma-globulin given after the onset of parotitis but before orchitis develops has been shown to reduce the incidence of orchitis in postpubertal males by 65 to 70 percent. Occasionally, surgical incision or aspiration of a hydrocele is necessary to reduce the pressure within the tunica vaginalis and alleviate severe disabling pain.

The usual etiologic agents in bacterial orchitis are *Escherichia coli, Klebsiella pneumoniae,* streptococci, staphylococci, and *Pseudomonas aeruginosa.* In this form of orchitis, the testicle is tense and swollen and may have bluish or punctate hemorrhages on the surface. Needle aspiration may be necessary for diagnosis. Scrotal sonography may identify areas of abscess formation and facilitate aspiration of the material for culture and susceptibility studies. Broad-spectrum antibiotics are recommended on the basis of the Gram stain of the aspirate until the culture and sensitivity report becomes available. A lidocaine anesthetic block in the spermatic cord may be used to alleviate severe pain. In the absence of a positive Gram stain, cephalexin can be given as the initial treatment until the results of the culture and antibiotic susceptibility tests are available. Serial scrotal sonograms may be helpful in the evaluation during the treatment period.

Secondary atrophy and resultant sterility from fibrosis and destruction of the tubules of the ductus system may occur in any form of orchitis. Some degree of testicular atrophy occurs in 50 percent of cases of postpubertal mumps orchitis, but sterility is an uncommon sequela of unilateral mumps.

ACUTE EPIDIDYMITIS

Acute epididymitis in prepubertal boys is uncommon, but is important in differential diagnosis of patients with acute scrotal swelling. One must differentiate this condition from torsion of the spermatic cord, torsion of the hydatid of Morgagni, testicular trauma, testicular tumor, orchitis, acute hydrocele, and hernia. Torsion of the spermatic cord demands immediate surgical correction and, unless unequivocal evidence of acute epididymitis can be obtained in acute scrotal swelling, early surgical intervention is mandatory. At Parkland Hospital in Dallas, 50 percent of the testes lost from torsion have been attributed to misdiagnosis on the part of the physician who makes the initial contact with the patient.

After the diagnosis of epididymitis is made in prepubertal boys, urologic investigation is essential. Epididymitis has been shown to be related to vesicoureteal reflux, trauma, urethral valve disorder, urethral diverticulum, urethral stricture, urethral–rectal fistulas, neuropathic bladder managed by intermittent catheterization, ectopic ureteral opening into the seminal vesicle or vas deferens, upper tract anomalies with urinary tract infection, and retrograde flow of urine into the ejaculatory ducts and vas deferens, with or without obstruction of the distal urethra.

When the prepubertal pediatric patient appears with acute scrotal pain and swelling, I feel it is of great importance to watch the patient urinate while catching a clean midstream urine specimen for examination. A poor, interrupted stream, suggesting urethral obstruction or voiding dysfunction, and evidence of infection in the urine suggest the possibility of epididymitis. Infiltration of the cord with 1 percent lidocaine allows a more accurate, painless examination. Occasionally the physical examination can delineate unequivocally the cause of the intrascrotal swelling. An emergency radioisotope scan using technetium-pertechnetate, a Doppler scrotal ultrasonogram, an abdominal sonogram, and/or a scrotal sonogram help in the diagnosis. Nuclear scans are much less accurate in the testicle smaller than 2 cm in diameter.

Acute epididymitis is more common in pubertal males. Treatment should be based on the information obtained from the physical examination, urinalysis, Gram stain, and urine culture. Radionuclide scanning of the scrotum is a very accurate method of diagnosis after puberty.

The most common cause of epididymitis in young men is the organism that causes urethritis in that particular patient. In prepubertal children on intermittent catheterization regimens this would be coliform organisms. In pubertal boys the organisms are more commonly *Chlamydia trachomatis* and *Neisseria* gonorrheae. Occasionally, acute influenza, septicemia, or mumps epididymo-orchitis is the cause. A small group of men have epididymitis caused by systemic diseases such as tuberculosis, cryptococcosis, brucellosis, and other systemic diseases. In most cases of prepubertal epididymitis, no causative organism can be identified. Recently the antiarrhythmic drug amiodarone has been shown to cause acute epididymitis without epididymal infection. Figure 1 illustrates the approaches to treatment of epididymitis, based on the etiology.

The treatment of epididymitis depends entirely on the specific etiologic organism. A urethral specimen smear, Gram stain of the urine, and urine culture should be obtained. After appropriate cultures are obtained, antibiotic therapy should be initiated in the patient with an obvious bacterial etiology. In patients with minimal systemic symptoms associated with the epididymitis, an oral cephalosporin or norfloxacin should be given. (Norfloxacin is not approved for children under 12 years of age.) In patients with evidence of more serious systemic involvement, the antibiotic regimen should be an aminoglycoside such as intravenous gentamicin, 5 to 6 mg per kilogram per day in three divided doses, and a cephalosporin such as cefazolin, 50 mg per kilogram daily, divided into three equal doses.

The treatment of epididymitis in patients with associated urethritis should be based on the findings in the Gram stain of the urine and any urethral discharge that might be present. A Gram stain of the discharge showing gram-negative intracellular diplococci dictates the use of tetracycline, 500 mg four times a day, because the gonococcal urethritis is associated with *C. trachomatis* in approximately 50 percent of the cases. As an alternative treatment, gonococcal epididymitis can be treated with amoxicillin, 500 mg four times a day for 10 days, and, to treat the chlamydial component, erythromycin, 500 mg four times a day for 10 days. Bed rest and cold or warm applications may be used as well as analgesics for pain control.

Scrotal sonography may be used to follow the progression of epididymitis, looking for abscess for-

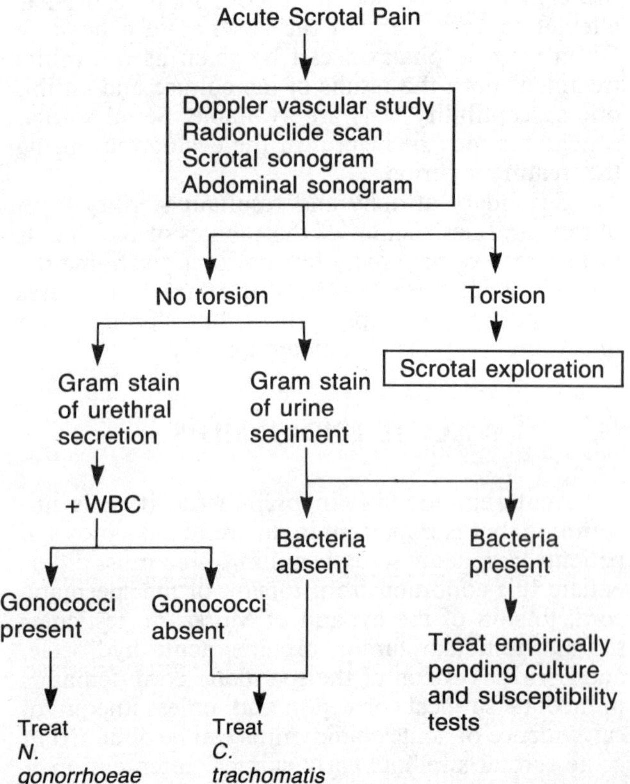

Figure 1 Evaluation of acute scrotal swelling and pain.

mation or extention into the testicle with epididymo-orchitis.

Long-term complications in children with acute epididymo-orchitis are rare unless an underlying genital malformation has contributed to the original infection. In postpubertal epididymitis, mild testicular atrophy or obstruction of the ductus system is not uncommon. Rarely, testicular infarction, infertility, or abscess formation result from epididymitis. Chronic testicular pain may prove to be a vexing problem. The induration of the epididymis itself may persist 4 to 6 weeks before complete resolution occurs. When the pain has completely subsided, the patient may return to limited activity, but heavy lifting or straining should be restricted until the induration is completely resolved. In all cases of epididymitis in children, excretory urography, voiding cystourethrography, and abdominal and scrotal so-nography should be performed when the acute symptoms have resolved.

SUGGESTED READING

Gellis SS, McGuiness AC, Peters M. Study on prevention of mumps orchitis by gamma globulin. Am J Med Sci 1945; 210:661–664.
Kaplan GW, King LR. Acute scrotal swelling in children. J Urol 1970; 104:218–219.
Kaplan GW, King LR. Acute scrotal swelling in children. J Urol 1970; 104:219.
Ransler CW, Allen T. Torsion of the spermatic cord. Urol Clin North Am 1982; 9(2):245–250.
Uremeyama T, Kawamura T, Hasegaua A, Ogawa O. Ectopic ureter presenting with epididymitis in childhood. J Urol 1985; 134:131–133.
Williams CB, Litvak AS, McRoberts WS. Epididymitis in infancy. J Urol 1979; 120:125.

GONORRHEA

PHILIP J. RETTIG, M.D.

Infections with *Neisseria gonorrhoeae* remain the most frequently reported infectious disease in the United States. Incidence rates are larger in teenagers than in any group other than 20- to 24-year-old young adults, and actually may be maximal in 15- to 19-year-olds when the prevalence of sexual activity (50 to 60 percent of this population) is considered. A wide range of clinical infections occur in addition to urethritis in male and cervicitis in female patients. These include salpingitis and endometritis, Bartholin's gland infection, perihepatitis, epididymitis, proctitis, the arthritis-dermatitis syndrome, and ophthalmia neonatorum. Increasingly, genital infection of prepubertal children is being recognized and is now acknowledged to represent an important marker of sexual abuse.

The diagnosis of uncomplicated genital infection in the symptomatic adolescent or young adult may be made by the finding of characteristic gram-negative intracellular diplococci in genital secretions. This finding has a sensitivity of greater than 95 percent in the male (urethral smear) and 50 to 70 percent in the female (cervical smear), with specificities in excess of 98 percent in both instances. Culture confirmation of gonococcal infection is indicated in other settings.

Anal or pharyngeal carriage of meningococci is common in homosexual males, and confirmatory identification of such isolates as *N. gonorrhoeae* by carbohydrate fermentation or immunologic means is necessary. Suspect oxidase-positive isolates from genital or extragenital sites in prepubertal children should likewise be confirmed as gonococci because of the potential medicolegal and social implications of such results.

GENERAL CONSIDERATIONS IN ANTIMICROBIAL THERAPY

The era in which the only consideration in treating gonococcal infection was the amount of penicillin G needed to effect a cure is long since past. A number of different issues now face the clinician in choosing the correct antimicrobial regimen. These include the following:

1. Site of infection.
2. Prevailing local and national in vitro susceptibility patterns and prevalence of beta-lactamase–producing strains.
3. Co-incidence of other sexually transmitted disease (STD) pathogens.
4. Issues of patient compliance.

Uncomplicated extragenital infection (such as pharyngeal or anorectal infection) may not respond to treatment as readily as urethritis or cervicitis. Between the 1950s and the 1970s there was an increase in the relative resistance of gonococci to penicillins and to tetracycline, resistances mediated by gradual chromosomal mutations. In 1976, absolute resistance to penicillin, by virtue of plasmid-mediated carriage of a beta-lactamase, was first reported. By the end of 1986, 1.8 percent of all reported gonorrhea cases in the United States were caused by penicillinase-producing *N. gonorrhoeae* (PPNG). Up to 22 percent of isolates in one area (Dade County, Florida) were PPNG; spread of these strains has become well-established in inner-city minority groups and is no longer linked solely to sexual contacts from Africa or the Far East or contacts with prostitutes. Such strains are also relatively resistant to tetracyclines. Finally, rare isolates with chromosomal resistance to spectinomycin or with chromosomal, high-level resistance to tetracyclines have been confirmed.

Coexistent infectious syphilis continues to be a problem among homosexual males in urban centers. More universal is the concurrence of genital chlamydial infection with gonorrhea in heterosexual patients. *C. trachomatis* genital infection coexists in 15 to 30 percent of men with gonococcal urethritis and in 25 to 50 percent of women with anogenital gonorrhea. These prevalences of chlamydial coinfection, along with the frequent lack of readily available means for diagnosis, have led to current recommendations for combination therapy directed against both pathogens.

Practical issues of medication costs and compliance are the final aspect of choosing an optimal regimen for gonorrhea therapy. Single-dose parenteral or supervised single-dose oral therapy has the advantage of ensured drug administration, but the pain and discomfort of the former may discourage follow-up visits for test-of-cure examination. Multiple-dose tetracycline regimens demand compliance from a patient population in whom this may be problematic; the use of doxycycline twice daily, rather than tetracycline four times a day, considerably increases the cost of medication.

Each of these issues must be considered before an individual regimen is prescribed for a patient with gonorrhea.

UNCOMPLICATED ANOGENITAL INFECTION

Approved regimens for urethral, cervical, and anorectal gonorrhea are listed in Table 1. Because of its activity against incubating syphilis, the procaine penicillin regimen is preferred for homosexual males and others at high risk of concurrent syphilis. I prefer one of the single-dose oral regimens for other patients, because I do not subscribe to the theory that parenteral treatment acts punitively as a deterrent to repeated infection. All heterosexual patients should receive multiple-dose treatment with a tetracycline or, if pregnant or tetracycline-intolerant, with eryth-

TABLE 1 Treatment of Uncomplicated Anogenital Gonorrhea in Adolescents and Adults

A. Single dose of: plus B.*	7 days of:
Amoxicillin 3.0 g PO†	Tetracycline 500 mg PO every 6 hours
or	
Ampicillin 3.5 g PO†	
or	or
Aqueous procaine penicillin G 4.8 million U IM†	Doxycycline 100 mg PO every 12 hours
or	
Cefoxitin 2.0 g IM†‡	
or	or
Ceftriaxone 250 mg IM‡	Erythromycin base 500 mg PO§ every 6 hours
or	
Spectinomycin 2.0 g IM‡	

* An oral antibiotic from column B should be used for all patients at risk of concurrent chlamydial infection.
† Co-administer 1 g of probenicid given orally as a single dose.
‡ Indicated in penicillin-allergic patients *or* patients infected with PPNG.
§ For use in patients unable to take tetracycline or women who are pregnant.

romycin. Symptomatic gonococcal proctitis should be treated with intramuscular administration of procaine penicillin, intramuscular ceftriaxone, or intramuscular spectinomycin. Ampicillin, amoxicillin, and tetracycline are less effective.

All patients should be evaluated for test-of-cure 3 to 5 days after treatment is completed. Follow-up cultures in women should include an anorectal swab, because treatment failures are more often evident at this site than in the cervix.

PHARYNGEAL GONOCOCCAL INFECTION

Pharyngeal infection is usually asymptomatic. It is often a consequence of fellatio and should be sought particularly in patients with disseminated gonococcal infection. Either the procaine penicillin or the tetracycline regimen should be used. Neither spectinomycin nor ampicillin/amoxicillin-probenicid is as effective.

GONOCOCCAL SALPINGITIS

From 20 to 50 percent of pelvic inflammatory disease in American women is associated with gonococcal cervical or tubal infection. Therapy should therefore include antimicrobials active against *N. gonorrhoeae,* including PPNG when indicated (see the chapter on *Infection of the Female Genital Tract*).

DISSEMINATED GONOCOCCAL INFECTION

Migratory polyarthralgias, tenosynovitis (particularly of the wrists and ankles), and papular rashes that evolve to necrotic ulcers on the extremities should suggest disseminated gonococcal infection (DGI). (This entity is also known as the arthritis–dermatitis syndrome.) The diagnosis is usually made on clinical grounds, but can be confirmed by blood culture or by identification of gonococci in the peripheral skin lesions. The latter is best accomplished by immunofluorescent staining (sensitivity 50 to 60 percent) or Gram stain (sensitivity 20 to 40 percent); gonococci can be isolated from these lesions in fewer than 20 percent of cases.

Although PPNG strains rarely cause this syndrome, most isolates from patients with DGI are very susceptible to penicillin G with MICs of less than 0.06 μg per milliliter. Patients should initially receive 10 million U of penicillin G intravenously (divided into doses every 4 hours). Penicillin-allergic patients, or those with the unusual occurrence of DGI caused by PPNG, should be treated with ceftriaxone, 1 g intravenously, given every 24 hours, or cefotaxime, 500 mg intravenously every 6 hours. Parenteral therapy should be given for 3 or 4 days and may be followed by amoxicillin, 500 mg orally every 6 hours, to complete 7 days of treatment. Penicillin-allergic patients should be treated with tetracycline, 500 mg orally every 6 hours, or doxycycline, 100 mg orally every 12 hours, to complete 1 week of antibiotics.

Patients should be carefully evaluated for the rare occurrences of invasive gonococcemia leading to meningitis or endocarditis. These infections should be treated with 20 million U of penicillin G per day, given intravenously in divided doses every 4 hours. Patients who are penicillin-allergic or infected with PPNG strains should receive ceftriaxone, 2 g intravenously every 12 hours. Gonococcal infection may be rapidly destructive of cardiac valves, and patients with endocarditis must be followed closely for the necessity of surgical intervention and possible valvular replacement. (See chapters on *Bacterial Meningitis* and *Infective Endocarditis* for further information.)

INFECTIONS IN PREPUBERTAL CHILDREN

Neonatal Infections

Infants born to mothers with known or suspected untreated cervical infection at parturition should receive 50,000 U of aqueous penicillin G, intravenously or intramuscularly, as soon after birth as possible. (Infants weighing less than 2,000 g should be given 25,000 U of penicillin G.) A single dose of ceftriaxone, 125 mg intramuscularly, should be used if the mother's gonococcal isolate is known or suspected to be a PPNG strain.

Infants born to mothers with gonococcal amnionitis or with documented gonococcemia should be treated with aqueous penicillin G, 50,000 U per kilogram per day, given every 12 hours, for 5 to 7 days. If joint swelling occurs, diagnostic arthrocentesis should be done. Documentation of gonococcal infection of the hip joint mandates open surgical drainage; other joints may be drained by single or repeated needle aspiration.

Gonococcal ophthalmia is treated with intravenous penicillin G, 50,000 U per kilogram per day in divided doses given every 12 hours in the first week of life and every 6 hours thereafter for 5 to 7 days. I do not add topical antimicrobials, but the involved eye(s) should be irrigated with normal saline every 1 to 2 hours until the purulent discharge abates. Persistence of gonococci beyond 24 hours or no decrease in the chemosis and purulent drainage within 36 hours of initiation of therapy should suggest the presence of penicillinase-producing gonococci. Such infection should be treated with intravenous cefotaxime (100 mg per kilogram per day in divided doses given every 12 hours in the first week of life, and 150 mg per kilogram per day in divided doses given every 8 hours thereafter) or ceftriaxone (50 mg per kilogram given once daily) for 5 to 7 days. A single intramuscular injection of ceftriaxone, 125 mg, has been shown to be effective in developing countries. The infant with gonococcal ophthalmia should be isolated with secretion precautions for the first 24 hours of therapy.

Gonorrhea in Prepubertal Children Beyond Infancy

Genital or extragenital infection in prepubertal children may be symptomatic or asymptomatic and usually follows an incident of sexual abuse. Effective therapies are outlined in Table 2. I prefer to use an oral regimen, rather than intramuscularly administered penicillin, whenever possible. These children have been traumatized by the abuser and frightened by the genital examination and specimen collection, and so should be spared the trauma of intramuscular injections. We have found that, similar to adults, 25 to 35 percent of children with gonococcal infection

TABLE 2 Treatment of Gonorrhea in Prepubertal Children*

A. Single dose of:	plus B. 7 days of:
Aqueous procaine penicillin G 100,000 U/kg IM†	Erythromycin base, estolate, or ethyl-succinate 10 mg/kg/dose every 6 hours
or	or
Amoxicillin 50 mg/kg PO†	
or	
Cefuroxime, 25 mg/kg IM‡	
or	
Spectinomycin, 40 mg/kg IM‡	Sulfisoxazole 50 mg/kg/dose, every 12 hours

* Maximum doses should not exceed those listed in Table 1. Ceftriaxone has not been evaluated in prepubertal gonorrhea.

† Coadminister probenicid, 25 mg per kilogram orally as single dose.

‡ Indicated in penicillin-allergic patients *or* patients infected with PPNG.

are coinfected with *C. trachomatis*. These infections may be at genital, anal, or pharyngeal sites and are often asymptomatic. I therefore recommend combination treatment for possible chlamydial infection, unless this can be definitely ruled out. Children older than 8 years of age may receive tetracycline, 10 mg per kilogram per dose, given every 6 hours; erythromycin or sulfisoxazole should be used in younger children.

TOXICITIES OF THERAPY

Single-dose oral therapy is well tolerated without significant side effects. Tetracyclines cause *Candida* vaginitis in some patients; this should be treated locally with clotrimazole suppositories or creams. Tetracyclines occasionally also cause photosensitivity rashes or fixed drug eruptions. A daily dosage of 2 g of oral erythromycin produces nausea, dyspepsia, or bloating in 10 to 15 percent of recipients.

The large volume needed to administer 4.8 million U of procaine penicillin requires two separate injection sites and causes considerable discomfort. Ceftriaxone may be given as a single 0.5-ml injection and, when diluted with 1 percent lidocaine, is well tolerated.

The major toxicity of procaine penicillin is a "procaine reaction," caused by sensitivity to the inadvertent intravenous injection of procaine. Patients may experience extreme agitation, tremors, auditory or visual hallucinations, or, rarely, seizures. Primary treatment is reassurance and restraint of the victim, with anticonvulsants and supportive therapy as needed. True hypersensitivity reactions to penicillin or other beta-lactam antibiotics should be treated with diphenhydramine, epinephrine, and resuscitative measures, as indicated.

PUBLIC HEALTH MANAGEMENT

Gonococcal infections must be reported to local or state health authorities. Contact tracing and referral are the responsibilities of public health personnel, but require reporting and cooperation by the primary physician.

Epidemiologic treatment of sexual contacts of a case of gonorrhea is warranted as a cost-effective control measure. Particularly high priority has been placed on treating contacts of cases of DGI and of gonococcal pelvic inflammatory disease.

Children with gonococcal infection should be assumed to have acquired their infections through sexual routes. All such cases should be reported to child welfare authorities, in addition to STD control workers. Exhaustive social and microbiologic investigations of adult family members and caretakers are indicated. Some authorities have suggested brief hospitalization for all prepubertal children with gonorrhea to facilitate these investigations.

SUGGESTED READING

Judson FN. Treatment of uncomplicated gonorrhea with ceftriaxone: A review. Sex Transm Dis 1986; 13:199–202.

Nelson JD, Mohs E, Dajani AS, et al. Gonorrhea in preschool- and school-aged children. J Am Med Assoc 1976; 236:1359–1364.

1985 STD treatment guidelines. MMWR 1985; 34(45).

Patamasucon P, Rettig PJ, Nelson JD. Cefuroxime therapy of gonorrhea and coinfection with *Chlamydia trachomatis* in children. Pediatrics 1981; 68:534–538.

Rettig PJ, Nelson JD, Kusmiesz H. Spectinomycin therapy for gonorrhea in prepubertal children. Am J Dis Child 1980; 134:359–363.

CHANCROID

THOMAS A. BELL, M.D., M.P.H.

Chancroid is caused by *Haemophilus ducreyi* and typically presents as a painful genital ulcer. Chancroid is rare in the United States, but occasional epidemics have been caused by cases imported from Latin America. Chancroid is the most common genital ulcer in some parts or the world, such as equatorial Africa. Diagnosis of chancroid has been simplified by the use of selective growth media. Optimal culture results are obtained by inoculating material from the ulcer or from fluctuant inguinal nodes onto the two media described by Nsanze et al. Monoclonal antibody stains now under investigation may make diagnosis even easier in the near future.

The treatment of choice for chancroid is a single intramuscular dose of ceftriaxone, 250 mg, diluted 1:1 with 1 percent lidocaine. Other useful drugs include trimethoprim-sulfamethoxazole, trimethoprim-rifampin (not now available in the United States as a fixed-dose combination), erythromycin, spectinomycin, chloramphenicol, and amoxicillin-clavulanic acid. Thus, some patients with chancroid who also require therapy for a concurrent infection can be treated effectively for both with some of the aforementioned drugs. For efficacy against *H. ducreyi* in such mixed infections, the minimal dosages and durations of treatment should be 160 and 800 mg of trimethoprim-sulfamethoxazole, respectively, by mouth every 12 hours for 10 days, or 500 mg of erythromycin, by mouth every 6 hours for 10 days. The World Health Organization recommends only 5 days of treatment with trimethoprim-sulfamethoxazole and 7 days for erythromycin.

Fluctuant lymph nodes should be aspirated with a small-gauge needle through adjacent healthy skin. The clinical response to therapy is the main criterion for cure. Patients with chancroid should be evaluated for other sexually transmitted diseases. Those treated with sulfonamides, which are not effective against *Treponema pallidum,* should be examined for serologic evidence of syphilis for at least 3 months.

Sexual consorts of persons with chancroid should be examined for other sexually transmitted diseases and presumptively treated for chancroid. All cases should be reported to the local health department so that other contacts can be sought and treated. Isolates of *H. ducreyi* from patients who fail therapy should be tested for resistance to antimicrobials.

SUGGESTED READING

Nsanze H, Plummer FA, Maggwa ABN, et al. Comparison of media for the primary isolation of *Haemophilus ducreyi*. Sex Transm Dis 1984; 11:6–9.

Schmid GP. The treatment of chancroid. JAMA 1986; 255:1757–1762.

LYMPHOGRANULOMA VENEREUM

PHILIP J. RETTIG, M.D.

Lymphogranuloma venereum (LGV) is a sexually transmitted disease caused by L-1, L-2, or L-3 serotypes of *Chlamydia trachomatis*. These strains are more invasive than those that commonly cause genital tract or ocular infection, and they cause regional suppurative adenopathy with sequelae of lymphedema and tissue scarring. Infection in prepubertal children has been reported infrequently in the antibiotic era; such a finding should raise the suspicion of sexual exposure.

The primary lesion of LGV occurs at the inoculation site as a papule, vesicle, or small ulcer and often is not clinically noted. A second stage of lymphadenopathy that is tender and often suppurative follows, with the anatomic location depending on the lymphatic drainage from the primary site. Inguinal lymph node infection develops from penile or vulvar sites; deep pelvic and lumbosacral node involvement is a consequence of cervical or anorectal infection. Primary anorectal infection may produce a clinical and endoscopic picture indistinguishable from ulcerative proctitis or Crohn's disease; this has been reported recently in homosexual males. Regional cervical adenopathy has been seen following pharyngeal infection, and mediastinal lymphadenopathy mimicking lymphoma has followed pulmonary inhalation of LGV organisms as a result of laboratory accidents. Scarring of untreated lymph nodes and lymphatics causes late lymphedema of the external genitalia or late rectal structures. A severe form of chronic ulceration and lymphedema of the labia and clitoris is called esthiomene.

Diagnosis should depend on isolation of *C. trachomatis* from a fluctuant lymph node ("bubo") or on demonstration of chlamydial elementary bodies in bubo pus by direct fluorescent antibody staining. Confirmatory serologic tests are (1) a complement fixation titer against chlamydial genus-specific antigen of 1:64 or greater, or (2) a microimmunofluorescence titer against *C. trachomatis* of 1:256 or greater. The traditional intradermal antigen test (Frei test) is no longer generally available in the United States and is less sensitive than contemporary microbiology and serology.

ANTIMICROBIAL THERAPY

LGV strains of *C. trachomatis* are uniformally susceptible in vitro to tetracyclines, erythromycin, and sulfonamides. Antimicrobial therapy is the primary treatment for LGV. Patients older than 8 years of age should receive tetracycline hydrochloride, 10 mg per kilogram per dose (maximum of 500 mg per dose), orally four times daily for at least 14 days. The principal alternative treatment for patients unable to take tetracycline is sulfisoxazole, 50 mg per kilogram per dose (maximum of 1,000 mg per dose), orally twice daily for 2 weeks. Another alternative regimen is erythromycin, 10 mg per kilogram per dose (maximum of 500 mg per dose), orally four times a day for 14 days, although there are few data supporting this drug's efficacy. Clinical experience with other antimicrobials possessing in vitro activity (trimethoprim–sulfamethoxazole, rifampin, chloramphenicol, or ofloxacin) is insufficient to recommend other alternative regimens. A third week of treatment should be given to those patients who are slow to respond in terms of node tenderness, fluctuance, or systemic symptoms.

SURGICAL MANAGEMENT

Aspiration of a fluctuant bubo is indicated for diagnostic purposes; but incision and drainage of involved nodes is contraindicated because this may foster chronic drainage or fistula production.

Women or homosexual men with the sequela of rectal stricture may require rectal dilatation or more extensive surgery. Such procedures should be attempted only by experienced proctologic surgeons and only after adequate antibiotic treatment. Plastic surgery to repair extensive genital scarring or lymphedema and elephantiasis is occasionally necessary.

LGV is a reportable sexually transmitted disease. Recent sexual contacts must be referred for evaluation and treatment. Documentation of LGV in a prepubertal child should initiate an investigation for possible sexual abuse.

SUGGESTED READING

McLelland BA, Anderson PC. Lymphogranuloma venereum. Outbreak in a university community. JAMA 1976; 235:56–57.
Quinn TC, Goodell SE, Mkrtichian E, et al. *Chlamydia trachomatis* proctitis. N Engl J Med 1981; 305:195–200.
Schachter J, Osoba A. Lymphogranuloma venereum. Br Med Bull 1983; 39:151–154.

CYSTITIS AND PYELONEPHRITIS

STANLEY HELLERSTEIN, M.D.

The goals of treatment of pediatric patients with urinary tract infections (UTIs) are (1) the relief of symptoms, (2) the eradication of bacteria from the urinary tract, and (3) the prevention of kidney damage. The pediatric patients with UTIs at greatest risk of kidney damage are those younger than 4 to 5 years of age with severe vesicoureteral reflux and those with obstructive lesions. Because every episode of acute clinical pyelonephritis is probably accompanied by some renal damage, even patients with neither obstruction nor recognized vesicoureteral reflux can incur kidney damage in the course of a UTI. In my experience, the treatment of a patient with a UTI is usually no problem; the challenge is to identify those children with UTIs who are at risk for renal damage and to minimize or prevent the kidney injury.

Most children with vesicoureteral reflux and many with obstructive lesions are identified through an evaluation conducted following a UTI. This is the rationale underlying the recommendation that younger pediatric patients, regardless of sex, have an imaging evaluation of the urinary tract following the first identified UTI. In addition, regardless of age or sex, any pediatric patient who has an episode of acute bacterial pyelonephritis should have an imaging evaluation of the urinary tract if such studies have not already been done.

ACUTE PYELONEPHRITIS

Treatment of an episode of UTI depends on the clinical presentation of the patient and the pathogen cultured from the urine. The neonate with acute pyelonephritis usually has neonatal sepsis with urinary tract involvement as a consequence of bacteremia. With rare exceptions, other infections of the urinary tract are caused by bacteria which are part of the bowel flora. The offending organism is thought to gain access to the urinary bladder and ascend to the renal parenchyma via the ureter, pelvocalyceal system, and collecting ducts. The neonate with sepsis and bacteriuria, the older infant with acute pyelonephritis, and any child with severe systemic symptoms caused by acute pyelonephritis should be hospitalized for treatment. These patients frequently require parenteral fluids for supportive care, along with parenteral antibiotics. For the initial treatment of acute pyelonephritis in pediatric patients, I recommend ampicillin, 50 to 100 mg per kilogram daily in four doses intravenously or intramuscularly, and gentamicin, 5 to 7.5 mg per kilogram daily in three doses intravenously or intramuscularly. For the infant younger than a week of age, the gentamicin dosage should be 5 mg per kilogram daily in two doses. The dosage of gentamicin may also need to be modified in other patients with impaired renal function. Plasma aminoglycoside concentrations should be monitored from the onset of therapy in patients with impaired renal function and in all patients who require aminoglycoside treatment for longer than 4 to 5 days.

A repeat urinary culture—and, if indicated, blood culture—should be obtained after 48 hours of treatment. Assuming that the patient is improving clinically and the repeat urinary culture shows no growth, therapy can usually be modified after a total 4 to 5 days of parenteral antibiotics. If the bacterium isolated from the initial urinary culture was susceptible to ampicillin, a 10-day course of treatment can be completed using oral amoxicillin, 40 mg per kilogram daily in three divided doses. If the blood culture was positive, but the course otherwise uncomplicated, parenteral treatment should be continued for 10 to 14 days.

Younger infants, as well as older pediatric patients with an initial episode of acute pyelonephritis, should have an abdominal ultrasound study within the first few days of treatment to rule out obstructive lesions. Assuming no obstruction is detected, the 10-day course of treatment for acute pyelonephritis should be followed by 3 to 4 weeks of low dosage antibacterial therapy to prevent recurrence of an infection before obtaining a voiding cystourethrogram. The effectiveness of the suppressive antibacterial agent should be monitored with urinary cultures every 2 weeks. Infants younger than 6 to 8 weeks of age can be given amoxicillin, 10 to 20 mg per kilogram daily in two divided doses. Older infants and young children can be given trimethoprim–sulfamethoxazole, 1 to 2 mg TMP/5 to 10 mg SMZ per kilogram daily in two doses, or sulfisoxazole, 20 to 30 mg per kilogram daily in two doses. In case of allergy to or intolerance of sulfonamides, amoxicillin, 10 to 20 mg per kilogram daily in two doses, or nitrofurantoin, 1 to 2 mg per kilogram in two doses, can be used. Because of the potential for pulmonary and hepatic toxicity and the high incidence of gastrointestinal disturbances associated with the use of nitrofurantoin, this agent should be avoided if there are other acceptable alternatives. In the management of patients who are able to void on request, I have found that bladder emptying followed by a single bedtime dose of trimethoprim–sulfamethoxazole, 1 to 2 mg TMP/5 to 10 mg SMZ per kilogram, sulfisoxazole, 20 to 30 mg per kilogram, or nitrofurantoin, 1 to 2 mg per kilogram is usually effective in preventing of reinfection.

CYSTITIS

Although the diagnosis of acute bacterial infection of the kidney is obvious in the patient with fever, flank pain, renal tenderness, and significant bacteriuria, renal bacteriuria is also present in some 20 to 25 percent of girls and women with asymptomatic bacteriuria or clinical cystitis. Pyelonephritic scars are found in 10 to 20 percent and vesicoureteral reflux in 20 to 35 percent of children studied radiologically following a first or second UTI. The incidence of roentgenologic abnormalities of the urinary tract is similar in children who have asymptomatic bacteriuria and in those with symptomatic bacteriuria. These observations make it clear that the child with clinical cystitis—that is, lower urinary tract symptoms, oral temperature not above 38°C, and significant bacteriuria—may have renal bacteriuria and be at risk for kidney damage.

In my opinion, treatment of a pediatric patient with bacterial cystitis depends on the functional and anatomic status of the urinary tract. If the child is being seen for a first diagnosed urinary tract infection and he or, more commonly, she has a normal voiding pattern, treatment can be instituted using one of the antimicrobial agents and dosage intervals shown in Table 1. I often use the morphology of the infecting agent to guide the selection of the agent. If gram-negative bacilli are identified, trimethoprim-sulfamethoxazole or sulfisoxazole is usually chosen. If gram-positive cocci are present, my choice is one of the aminopenicillins, usually amoxicillin.

In most instances symptomatic treatment is not required because of the prompt response to effective antibacterial therapy. Typically both the bacteriuria and the symptoms have cleared before the scheduled 48- to 72-hour follow-up visit. If needed, sitz baths in

TABLE 1 Oral Antimicrobial Agents Useful in the Treatment of Children with Cystitis

Antimicrobial Agent	Daily Dosage and Intervals of Administration
Amoxicillin	20–30 mg/kg/day, in 3 divided doses
Ampicillin	50–100 mg/kg/day, in 4 divided doses
Sulfisoxazole	100–150 mg/kg/day, in 4–6 divided doses
Trimethoprim–sulfamethoxazole	6–12 mg TMP/30–60 mg SMZ/kg in 2 divided doses

warm water for 20 to 30 minutes three or four times a day usually afford prompt relief for urgency, increased frequency of urination and dysuria, and for transient urinary retention. If the bacteriuria has not cleared on the follow-up visit, treatment should be changed based on the antibiotic susceptibility of the bacterium isolated from the initial urinary culture. I usually extend effective antibacterial treatment for 10 days in the patient with clinical cystitis whose urinary tract has not been evaluated previously using imaging studies. These studies should be done after the patient has been free of bacteriuria for 4 to 6 weeks.

The patient with cystitis who has a normal voiding pattern when not infected, normal kidneys by intravenous pyelography or ultrasound examination, and a normal voiding cystourethrogram requires only a few days of treatment with an effective antibacterial agent to clear the symptoms and eliminate the bacteriuria. There appears to be little risk of kidney damage from recurrent cystitis in such patients. If there is no growth in the urinary culture obtained at the 48- to 72-hour follow-up visit, I discontinue treatment and ask the patient to return for a follow-up urinary culture in about 2 weeks. Episodes of cystitis in these children are managed with brief courses of antibiotics, because the goals of therapy—namely, the relief of symptoms and the elimination of bacteriuria—are usually met with this treatment. Patients with dysfunctional voiding, renal anomalies, parenchymal scars, obstructive lesions, or vesicoureteral reflux require different management because they may be at risk for kidney damage during episodes of bacterial cystitis.

SUGGESTED READING

Durbin WA Jr, Peter G. Management of urinary tract infections in infants and children. Pediatr Infect Dis 1984; 3:564.
Hellerstein S. Urinary tract infections in children. Chicago: Year Book, 1982.
McCracken GH Jr. Diagnosis and management of acute urinary tract infections in infants and children. Pediatr Infect Dis 1987; 6:107.
Roberts JA. Pathogenesis of pyelonephritis. J Urol 1983; 129:1102.
Winberg J, Bollgren I, Kallenius G, Mollby R, Svenson SB. Clinical pyelonephritis and focal renal scarring. Pediatr Clin North Am 1982; 29:801.

DISEASES CAUSED BY FUNGI

ASPERGILLOSIS

WALTER T. HUGHES, M.D.

Aspergillosis has a wide range of clinical features and affects both immunocompetent and immunocompromised hosts. Most of the several hundred species in the genus *Aspergillus* are soil and air saprophytes. Certain strains are highly prevalent in the environment of humans. *Aspergillus fumigatus,* and *A. flavus* cause most of the invasive infections, although no clinical manifestation is unique to one species. Less frequently encountered species include *A. niger, A. terreus, A. oryzae, A. glaucus, A. versicolor, A. niderlaus,* and others.

From the standpoint of pathogenesis aspergillosis is classified into three groups: (1) colonization, (2) invasive infection, and (3) allergic responses. Almost all organs of the body have been affected either singly or collectively in invasive aspergillosis; however, the most common sites are the lungs, skin, central nervous system, paranasal sinuses, bone, or a combination of these sites and others in disseminated disease. The allergic type of disease is limited to the respiratory tract as a syndrome of wheezing, transient pulmonary infiltrates, low-grade fever, expectoration of brown plugs of sputum, eosinophilia, and elevated serum immunoglobulin E concentrations. It is especially important to differentiate invasive disease from the allergic form because treatment is strikingly different; for example, corticosteroids are contraindicated in the former and often indicated in the latter type.

The majority of patients with invasive aspergillosis have a severe underlying immunosuppressive disease, or their resistance has been compromised by the use of immunosuppressive drugs. The allergic bronchopulmonary form of aspergillosis is found predominantly in asthmatics and patients with cystic fibrosis.

Aspergilli are not components of the usual microbial flora of humans. Serologic tests for antibody help identify individuals who are or have been infected with this fungus. However, such tests are not diagnostic, and both false-negative caud false-positive tests occur. A definitive diagnosis of invasive aspergillosis requires the histologic demonstration of typical branching septate hyphae in infected tissue and identification of the organism isolated in culture. The typical clinical features plus skin test reactivity and serum antibodies to *Aspergillus* species permit a diagnosis of allergic bronchopulmonary aspergillosis.

TREATMENT

Allergic Bronchopulmonary Aspergillosis

Because of limited studies, no guidelines have been clearly established for the management of bronchopulmonary aspergillosis. Antifungal drugs such as clotrimazole, nystatin, amphotericin B, stilbamidine, and potassium iodide have been tried. Currently, the general opinion is that antifungal therapy is ineffective in this disease, probably because it does not represent an invasive fungal infection. The administration of corticosteroids has been shown to reduce symptoms, pulmonary infiltrates, and the frequency of positive sputum cultures. Complete remission of the disease has been obtained with dosages of 0.5 mg per kilogram of prednisone given on alternate days. A larger dosage of prednisone, e.g., 60 mg daily, has been associated with limited tissue invasion of the fungus. The duration of corticoid therapy has not been established. Irreversible complications of the disease include bronchiectasis and pulmonary fibrosis.

Invasive Aspergillosis

Invasive aspergillosis occurs predominantly in immunocompromised patients with cancer, patients with acquired and congenital immunodeficiency disorders, and organ transplant recipients. Spontaneous resolution of the infection rarely, if ever, occurs. Unfortunately, even with the best of current therapy the prognosis for cure is poor.

Intravenous amphotericin B is the drug of choice. I initiate treatment with a test dose of amphotericin B using 0.25 mg per kilogram administered over a 6-hour period. I use no premedication that might mask reactions to the drug, because the purpose of this test dose is to gauge the magnitude of adverse reactions to expect in a given patient. More than one-half of patients develop fever and chills of varying degrees. Rarely, patients experience hypotensive episodes with the test dose. If the test dose is well-tolerated, the dosage is increased to 0.5 mg per kilogram for the second, 0.75 mg per kilogram for the third, and 1.0 mg per kilogram for the fourth day. With overwhelming life-threatening infections, I attempt to give 1.0 mg per kilogram for the first dose, and this is often possible.

Patients who experience fever and chills with the test dose should be premedicated for subsequent doses. We give an ibuprofen compound or meperidine about 30 minutes before the onset of the infusion. In the treatment of invasive aspergillosis, we aim for a maintenance dosage of 1.0 mg per kilogram per day. Once evidence of resolution is apparent, the dosage of 1.0 mg per kilogram can be given on alternate days. A course of at least 4 to 6 weeks is needed, and some cases require a much longer period of treatment.

Determination of the in vitro minimum inhibitory concentration (MIC) is of no value because methodologies are not standardized and no studies are available to relate the MIC values of isolates to clinical responses of patients to treatment. The optimal blood concentration of amphotericin B is not known.

The most significant life-threatening adverse effects are nephrotoxicity and electrolyte imbalance, especially hypokalemia. Recently it has been observed that in patients receiving rapid infusions of amphotericin B (within an hour) who are anuric, serum potassium concentration may rise rapidly to dangerous levels. In the usual patient undergoing standard treatment, hypokalemia as well as renal toxicity become apparent gradually, over a period of a few days. Serum creatinine, urea nitrogen, sodium, chloride, potassium, calcium, phosphorus, transaminases, and complete blood counts should be done at least every other day. Other adverse effects are mentioned in the package insert with the drug.

We consider carefully the need for surgical resection of localized disease from aspergillosis. In some cases this is easily decided when the primary disease, often cancer, is in a terminal stage. Also, with widely disseminated infection, surgery is not helpful. However, cases with well-localized pulmonary aspergilloma may benefit from surgical excision if the site is not near the hilum or vital vessels. Lobectomy is usually necessary to remove all of the disease. Surgical removal of an infected prosthetic cardiac valve seems to be indicated in most cases if cure of the infection is expected. Less well-established is the benefit from surgical intervention with infections of the

paranasal sinuses, eye, brain, skin, ear, and bone, although at least one or more reports have mentioned patients who responded to surgical management in addition to antifungal therapy. It must be realized that no conclusive studies exist to serve as guidelines for surgical management of aspergillosis.

Some in vitro and animal studies indicate that the combination of certain drugs (such as rifampin, flucytosine, and tetracycline) with amphotericin B may provide additive or synergistic advantages. There are no studies in humans to either support or discount these experimental findings. I usually add rifampin (15.0 mg per kilogram per day, given orally) to the amphotericin B–treated cases with poor prognosis, because the results of treatment with amphotericin B alone are disappointing.

Cancer patients with systemic aspergillosis who are neutropenic (fewer than 500 neutrophils per cubic millimeter) rarely recover from the infection, even with amphotericin B treatment, unless the neutrophil count reaches and maintains a nonneutropenic level. For those in whom neutropenia persists, the use of granulocyte transfusions is considered. Although no studies are available for reference, a single case report describes a favorable response. One must be cautious in administering amphotericin B and granulocyte transfusions concomitantly in neutropenic patients, as episodes of acute respiratory distress and deterioration have been reported. Although no other investigators have been able to confirm these findings, it seems prudent to give these two treatment modalities at least 12 hours apart if they are to be used together.

No other drug has sufficient activity to be considered as an alternative to amphotericin B. Liposomal amphotericin B is under study, but has not reached commercial development. Flucytosine has some in vitro activity, but has not been tested alone in clinical trials. Itraconazole, a triazole derivative of ketoconazole, also has in vitro activity, but clinical studies have not been completed.

SUGGESTED READING

Arroyo J, Medoff G, Kobayashi G. Therapy of murine aspergillosis with amphotericin B in combination with rifampin or 5-fluorocytosine. Antimicrob Agents Chemother 1977; 11:21–25.

Berkow RL, Weisman SJ, Provisor AJ, et al. Invasive aspergillosis of paranasal tissues in children with malignancies. J Pediatr 1983; 103:49–53.

Bow EJ, Schroeder M-L, Louie TJ. Pulmonary complications in patients receiving granulocyte transfusions and amphotericin B. Can Med Assoc J 1984; 130:593.

Rosenberg M, Patterson R, Mintzer R, et al. Clinical and immunologic criteria for the diagnosis of allergic aspergillosis. Ann Intern Med 1977; 86:405–414.

Sugar AM. The polyene macrolide antifungal drugs. In: Peterson PK, Verhoef J, eds. Antimicrobial agents annual 2. New York: Elsevier Science Publishers, 1987; 228–237.

BLASTOMYCOSIS

BRUCE S. KLEIN, M.D.

Blastomycosis, one of the principal endemic systemic mycoses of North America, derives from infection with the thermal dimorphic fungus, *Blastomyces dermatitidis*. The organism is believed to be a soil saprophyte that dwells primarily in the southeastern, south central, and upper midwestern regions of the United States. Primary infection in humans follows inhalation of conidia (asexual spores) into the lungs. At body temperature, the conidia convert to yeast forms that can be distinguished from other yeasts by their size, refractile cell wall, and broad-based buds. The acute primary pulmonary infection can be asymptomatic or produce an influenzal or atypical pneumonia syndrome. Although acute blastomycotic pneumonia may resolve spontaneously, progressive forms of disease involving the lungs, the extrapulmonary organs (usually the skin, bones, joints, or prostate gland), or both develop in some patients. Reactivation of a latent focal infection probably occurs less often than progression of primary infection. Primary cutaneous infection occurs infrequently through direct inoculation from a needle puncture, dog bite, or scalpel wound. Opportunistic infection among immunocompromised patients is uncommon. Although the majority of patients in case series of blastomycosis are 20 to 50 years of age, as many as 10 percent are younger than 20.

The diagnosis of blastomycosis is confirmed by culture of the organism from body fluids such as sputum, pus, or urine, or from biopsied tissue. Cytologic and histopathologic studies with special stains should always be performed on fluid and tissue specimens; the characteristic morphology of the yeast form of *B. dermatitidis* usually allows a presumptive diagnosis well before the results from culture are available.

TREATMENT

Before chemotherapy for blastomycosis was available, patients often had a progressive downhill course and the case-fatality rate approached 80 percent. With the advent of effective antifungal therapy in the 1950s, the case-fatality rate declined to 10 percent and it was accepted that all patients should be treated. This approach came into question after the description of self-limited pulmonary blastomycosis in 1974. To date, at least 76 patients with spontaneously resolving disease have been described. Although some experts now believe selected patients do not require antifungal therapy, others disagree, countering that such patients are at risk of exacerbating and developing miliary disease or endobronchial spread, both associated with high mortality, or developing reactivation of a latent focal infection at a later date. I believe the majority of patients with blastomycosis require specific antifungal therapy.

The decision whether or not to treat and, if so, with what drug should be based on the acuity, severity, and extent of disease (Table 1). Asymptomatic patients, patients who are already improving when the diagnosis is established, and those who present acutely (generally within 3 to 4 weeks of illness onset) with mild symptoms unassociated with respiratory distress or hypoxemia could be observed carefully and antifungal therapy withheld. To date, such patients have been identified mainly during epidemics of blastomycosis. These patients, however, represent the minority of blastomycosis patients, because epidemic disease is far less common than sporadically occurring disease. Observation should include biweekly clinical and roentogenographic evaluation until spontaneous resolution takes place. Progression of pulmonary infection or evidence of extrapulmonary spread should signal the need for treatment.

In the more common subacute or chronically progressive forms of pulmonary blastomycosis and the nonmeningeal extrapulmonary forms, which are mild to moderately severe, ketoconazole therapy is indicated. When pulmonary or extrapulmonary involvement is extensive, particularly if respiratory embarrassment or meningeal spread are documented, amphotericin B is the drug of choice. Serial chest roentogenograms, sputum cultures, or other studies, according to infected sites, should be performed to assess the therapeutic response. Clinical improvement generally occurs by the second week of therapy, but complete healing may not occur until after 2 months or more of therapy.

Accidental lacerations, bite wounds, or needle punctures with *B. dermatitidis* should be treated by careful, vigorous cleansing with tincture of iodine, an iodophor, or chlorhexidine. Systemic antifungal therapy is not indicated for primary cutaneous blastomycosis in the normal host. The lesion should be observed carefully to document resolution.

TABLE 1 Management of Blastomycosis

Disease Form	Severity	Treatment
Acute pulmonary	Asymptomatic, resolving, or mild	Observe
	Mild to moderately severe	Ketoconazole
	Life-threatening	Amphotericin B
Subacute or chronic pulmonary, or extrapulmonary	Mild to moderately severe	Ketoconazole
	Life-threatening	Amphotericin B
Central nervous system (usually meningeal)	——	Amphotericin B

Amphotericin B

Since its introduction in 1956, amphotericin B has remained the most effective antifungal agent available for treatment of blastomycosis. Reported rates of clinical responses to this drug have ranged from 66 to 93 percent, and have been greatest in adults who have received a total of at least 1.5 to 2 g, or 25 to 35 mg per kilogram of body weight.

Amphotericin B may be administered in a variety of schedules. If a 1-mg test dose, infused intravenously over 30 to 60 minutes, is tolerated, an initial therapeutic dose of 0.25 mg per kilogram is administered over a 2- to 4-hour period on the first day. The dosage should be increased in increments of 0.25 mg per kilogram each day to the desired maintenance dosage. In acutely ill patients, 0.3 to 0.6 mg per kilogram (maximum, 50 mg) is administered daily until clinical improvement is noted. For patients less seriously ill, or those who have improved after initial daily therapy (usually by 1 to 2 weeks after treatment is begun), 0.6 to 1.0 mg per kilogram (maximum, 50 mg) can be given three times weekly rather than daily. The latter schedule usually permits treatment to be administered on an outpatient basis. A total dose of at least 25 to 35 mg per kilogram should be achieved. Relapse occurs in 10 to 20 percent of patients within 5 years of completion of treatment (usually within 1 year); in these instances, patients should be treated again with amphotericin B.

Unfortunately, amphotericin B frequently produces side effects and considerable toxicity, including fever, shaking chills, shock, acute respiratory disease syndrome, anemia, and especially azotemia. Most patients treated with amphotericin B in daily doses in excess of 0.3 mg per kilogram, or who have received a total dosage of at least 3 mg per kilogram, show evidence of incomplete renal tubular acidosis with hypokalemia. Amphotericin B side effects can be ameliorated appreciably by pretreatment regimens that include premedication with acetaminophen (10 mg per kilogram orally; maximum, 1,000 mg) and diphenhydramine hydrochloride (1.25 mg per kilogram orally; maximum 100 mg) 30 minutes before the infusion is begun; if rigors persist, an intravenous bolus of meperidine (1.1 mg per kilogram; maximum, 50 mg) is given immediately before the infusion is begun. If severe febrile reactions continue despite these regimens, patients should receive an intravenous bolus of hydrocortisone (0.5 to 0.7 mg per kilogram; maximum, 50 mg) immediately before the infusion is begun. The nephrotoxic effects of amphotericin B are reduced by preventing the insidious dehydration that typically occurs during therapy. This is done by salt and volume loading to maintain urine output (greater than 30 ml per kilogram daily), and by aggressively repleting lost bicarbonate and potassium when the metabolic effects of renal tubular acidosis are apparent in the serum electrolytes ([K^+] less than 4.0 mEq/L; [CO_2] less than 20 mEq/L). The electrolytes and serum creatinine should be monitored closely, especially early in therapy, when the daily dosage is being incremented rapidly, and when other nephrotoxic drugs are being given concomitantly. Temporarily interrupting or decreasing the dosage may be indicated if serum creatinine increases to more than three times normal, or to more than 3.0 mg per deciliter in adolescents.

Ketoconazole

Orally administered, less toxic, and equally effective antifungal agents have long been sought as alternatives to amphotericin B. Ketoconazole, an oral imidazole antifungal drug with broad-spectrum in vitro and in vivo activity against various superficial and deep fungal pathogens, represents a considerable advance in the treatment of blastomycosis. A recent multicenter, prospective, randomized trial of ketoconazole has shown that the drug is a safe, well-tolerated, and effective alternative to amphotericin B for treatment of mild to moderately severe nonmeningeal forms of the disease. In that study, a cure rate of 89 percent was recorded among patients treated for at least 6 months; the rates were 100 percent in those who received a large dosage (800 mg per day) and 79 percent in those who received the smaller dosage (400 mg per day).

Treatment is initiated with a dosage of 400 mg per day (6 mg per kilogram daily in preadolescent children older than 2 years of age). The smaller initial dosage is preferred because of the likelihood that larger dosages will cause more toxic or adverse effects. The drug is administered once daily, preferably each morning with or just after a meal, since absorption from the gastrointestinal tract is enhanced in the presence of gastric acid. In patients who tolerate the initial dose and have no evidence of clinical progression of disease, the 400-mg-per-day dosage should be maintained for a minimum of 6 months. Therapy must be continued until cultures are persistently negative and radiographic resolution, or at least stabilization, is evident. In patients whose disease progresses or who develop a new focus of infection during the initial month of therapy on 400 mg per day, the dosage can be advanced by increments of 200 mg per day (3 mg per kilogram daily in preadolescent children) every 4 to 6 weeks to a maximum of 800 mg per day (12 mg per kilogram daily in preadolescent children). For patients who cannot tolerate ketoconazole or whose disease progresses significantly despite treatment, ketoconazole should be discontinued and amphotericin B begun.

Because *B. dermatitidis* is uniformly susceptible to ketoconazole, routine susceptibility testing of a patient's isolate is not recommended. In patients whose disease progresses, the serum ketoconazole concentration should be determined, and the physician should carefully review concomitant drugs to look for possible causes of decreased absorption of ketoconazole (antacids, anticholinergics, and H_2-blockers), or of an adverse drug–drug interaction (rifampin and isoniazid).

Although ketoconazole is generally well tolerated in the dosage range of 400 mg per day or less, larger dosages may be associated with adverse or toxic effects, especially gastrointestinal and endocrinologic. Anorexia, nausea, and vomiting, the most common adverse effects, may be ameliorated by evening or split-dose administration of the drug. The increased frequency of gynecomastia, impotence, menstrual irregularities, and, rarely, weakness caused by adrenal insufficiency, in adults who have received large doses of ketoconazole derives from the drug's ability to block adrenal and gonadal steroid synthesis. These endocrine-mediated effects are reversible when the drug is withdrawn. Hepatotoxicity, primarily hepatocellular and idiosyncratic but including rare fatalities, has been associated with use of ketoconazole. Hepatic injury is usually reversible upon discontinuation of the drug. Liver function tests should be monitored before treatment is started, and at frequent intervals during treatment. Although transient minor elevations of liver enzymes may occur during therapy, the drug should be stopped if these abnormal elevations persist at greater than three times normal levels, if the abnormalities worsen, or if they are accompanied by symptoms of possible liver injury.

Other Treatment Modalities

2-Hydroxystilbamidine isethionate is a comparably effective alternative to amphotericin B only for treatment of noncavitary pulmonary disease or cutaneous disease. Unacceptably high relapse rates have been noted in the treatment of patients with more extensive disease. The dosage is 3 to 5 mg per kilogram administered by slow intravenous infusion daily to achieve a total dosage of at least 8 g. The availability of ketoconazole, a less toxic but equally effective alternative to amphotericin B, which can be administered orally for treatment of non-life-threatening forms of blastomycosis, would seem to abrogate almost any indication for 2-hydroxystilbamidine.

Surgery plays only a small role in the treatment of blastomycosis, except possibly to drain large abscesses or accumulations of empyema fluid, to repair a bronchopleural fistula, and to debride devitalized bone in some cases of osteomyelitis.

SUGGESTED READING

Chapman SW. Blastomycosis. In: Mandell GL, Douglas RG, Bennett JE, eds. Principles and practice of infectious disease, 2nd ed. New York: John Wiley & Sons, 1985; 1477–1485.

Klein BS, Vergeront JM, Weeks RJ, et al. Isolation of *Blastomyces dermatitidis* in soil associated with a large outbreak of blastomycosis in Wisconsin. N Engl J Med 1986; 314:529–534.

National Institute of Allergy and Infectious Diseases Mycoses Study Group. Treatment of blastomycosis and histoplasmosis with ketoconazole. Results of a prospective randomized clinical trial. Ann Intern Med 1985; 103 (6 pt 1):861–872.

Sarosi GA, Davies SF. Blastomycosis. Am Rev Respir Dis 1979; 120:911–938.

Sarosi GA, Hammerman KJ, Tosh FE, Kronenberg RS. Clinical features of acute pulmonary blastomycosis. N Engl J Med 1974; 290:540–543.

CANDIDIASIS

PHILIP A. PIZZO, M.D.

Candida organisms are ubiquitous and are associated with an array of clinical manifestations and syndromes, ranging from superficial dermatoses and mucositis to invasive and disseminated infections. *Candida albicans* is the predominant pathogen in most centers, but *C. tropicalis, C. glabrata, C. krusei,* and *C. parapsilosis* are also associated with significant infections. The type and severity of the infection(s) that occur are influenced by the host, degree of immunosuppression, route of inoculation, and treatment.

Because *Candida* spp can be readily isolated from mucosal surfaces, particularly in patients who have received antibiotics or immunosuppressive agents, the ability to differentiate simple colonization from infection can be difficult. On the other hand, colonization is an antecedent to local infection or systemic dissemination. The only sure way to establish a diagnosis is to demonstrate evidence of tissue invasion. However, biopsy is not always feasible, because either the site of infection is not readily accessible or the patient is not a good candidate for operation. Treatment of deep-seated infection, however, requires early intervention and, given the diagnostic difficulties that abound, some guidance can be gleaned from defining the hosts that are at highest risk for *Candida* infection and the presenting signs and symptoms that may herald particular infectious syndromes.

Serious infections with *Candida* are most commonly seen in patients receiving immunosuppressive or cytotoxic therapy for the treatment of malignancy or a collagen vascular disease, or as an adjunct to organ transplantation; in children with congenital immunodeficiency or with the acquired immunodeficiency syndrome (AIDS); or in patients with intravascular devices (e.g., Hickman–Broviac catheters) or other central lines.

ANTIFUNGAL DRUGS

The therapeutic options for patients with candidiasis, however, are relatively limited. For patients with invasive or disseminated infections, intravenous amphotericin B remains the gold standard of therapy. Once the decision is made to use amphotericin B, a 1-mg test dose should be given, and if the patient does not experience anaphylaxis (which is exceedingly rare), the remainder of the full daily dose of 0.5 mg per kilogram per day should then be given. I premedicate patients with hydrocortisone (25 to 50 mg) and put another 25 to 50 mg in the infusion. Patients receive the amphotericin infusion over a 2-hour period. When fever, chills, or rigors develop, we do not stop the infusion, but we do administer meperidine, 0.5 to 1 mg per kilogram as an intravenous bolus, to abort the reaction. The complications associated with amphotericin B are notorious, but generally do not limit the ability to deliver a full course of treatment. Unfortunately, in most cases, what defines an "adequate" course of treatment is somewhat arbitrary. The experimental liposome-encapsulated formulation of amphotericin B, it is hoped, will make treatment more tolerable, with fewer side effects. Even though the data are limited, I advocate combining amphotericin B with oral (or if necessary, intravenous) flucytosine (5 FC) in a dosage of 100 to 150 mg per kilogram per day in four divided doses, for high-risk patients who have disseminated *Candida* infection or involvement of particular organs (e.g., liver).

For patients with noninvasive *Candida* infections, either nystatin or imidazole antifungal agents (e.g., clotrimazole, ketoconazole) can be used. Neither nystatin nor clotrimazole are systemically absorbed, but both are available in creams, ointments, troches, suppositories, and liquids. Ketoconazole is systemically absorbed, although this is adversely affected by the coadministration of antacids or H_2-blockers (e.g., cimetidine).

The choices of which antifungal agent to use, when to begin therapy, and how long to continue it are influenced by the site of infection and the degree of patient compromise. The approach that I take to treatment follows.

SUPERFICIAL OR MUCOSAL INFECTIONS

Oral Mucositis (Thrush)

The presence of a patchy white exudate on the buccal mucosa, along the gingiva, tonsillar faucae, or tongue, is relatively characteristic of a superficial oral *Candida* infection. This infection is seen frequently in patients with leukemia or other malignancies who develop chemotherapy-induced stomatitis with a se-

condary *Candida* infection. Thrush may also be the presenting symptom in patients with AIDS or other immunodeficiency states. Symptoms range from mild to severe, and infection can interfere with swallowing and nutrition. Although the patchy exudate is most commonly caused by *Candida,* similar findings can occur with other infections, especially herpes simplex. A scraping and wet mount examination is helpful, but coinfections can occur. In patients with suggestive physical findings, I begin treatment with clotrimazole troches (10 mg, four to five times daily). I have not found nystatin to be helpful in high-risk patients, but it is successful in healthy neonates with thrush. Ketoconazole (200 mg per day or 4 mg per kilogram per day) is our alternative agent, but I do not recommend starting with this imidazole, because it is associated with more complications (e.g., nausea, hepatic enzyme elevations) than clotrimazole. If the patient's infections are progressive, in spite of administration of clotrimazole or ketoconazole, a short course (5 to 7 days) of amphotericin B is generally successful. If patients do not improve with amphotericin B, consideration of other infectious etiologies (e.g., bacteria, herpes) must be renewed.

Chronic mucocutaneous candidiasis is an uncommon disorder in which the hallmarks are severe oral mucosal and cutaneous lesions. Improvement has been noted with clotrimazole and ketoconazole, but therapy must be chronic because relapse occurs when therapy is discontinued. (For further discussion of thrush from the perspective of dentists, see the chapter on *Infections of the Oral Cavity.*)

Esophagitis

Patients with symptoms of retrosternal burning and pain on swallowing, not infrequently with fever, are likely to have esophagitis. This syndrome occurs primarily in neutropenic patients who are receiving antibiotic therapy and in patients with AIDS. *Candida* is the most common etiology. However, bacteria (gram-positive or gram-negative organisms) and herpes simplex also can cause esophagitis. Establishing the diagnosis requires esophagoscopy and biopsy, but I do not advocate this prior to a trial of therapy. Instead, I prefer to determine whether there is evidence of esophagitis by looking for "cobblestoning" on a barium swallow radiographic examination and in symptomatic patients, administering an empiric course of antifungal therapy. I prefer to start with oral clotrimazole troches, and expect a clinical response after 48 hours of therapy. If patients have not improved, a short course of amphotericin B can be given and, again, resolution is expected within 2 days. Although some advocate the use of ketoconazole for patients with esophagitis, I have generally found that patients have difficulty swallowing the pills. If the patient has not improved with antifungal therapy, an etiology other than (or in addition to) *Candida* should be considered. Herpes simplex is the most likely of these and, depending on the patient's clinical status (e.g., degree of thrombocytopenia), either an esophagoscopy should be done to guide subsequent therapy or the patient should be treated empirically with acyclovir (750 mg per square meter per day in three divided doses).

Bladder Thrush

The presence of pseudohyphae in the urine does not necessarily herald systemic infection. More often, it represents superficial infection of the bladder mucosa. These infections are seen most often in patients with indwelling catheters, and they may respond to catheter removal or to the use of intermittent straight catheterization as an alternative to an indwelling catheter. Antifungal agents (including amphotericin B) penetrate the urine poorly. I have not found ketoconazole to be successful in eradicating these infections and prefer to avoid 5 FC to prevent the emergence of resistant organisms. If therapy is necessary, direct instillation of amphotericin B into the bladder (50 to 100 mg per day), using a washout technique, is successful.

Vaginal Infections

The incidence of vaginal *Candida* infection is not increased in high-risk patients. When infection does occur, it is treated successfully with either clotrimazole or miconazole cream or vaginal suppositories. Systemic infection occurs rarely.

Cutaneous Infections

Infections around the perianal area, although common in neonates, are infrequent in immunosuppressed patients. When an erythematous rash with satellite lesions occurs, scrapings of which show yeast or pseudohyphae, topical nystatin, clotrimazole, or miconazole is effective. In the high-risk patient (e.g., with fever and neutropenia), the presence of a pustular rash can herald systemic infection and should always be considered.

INVASIVE OR DISSEMINATED INFECTIONS

Fungemia

As a general rule, any blood culture that is positive for *Candida* in a patient who is neutropenic must be considered a manifestation of systemic infection. If no other site of infection is discerned (i.e., normal chest radiograph, normal abdominal computed tomography [CT] scan and ultrasound), a limited course of amphotericin B (10 mg per kilogram total dose) can be given. If the patient is not neutropenic, but has an intravenous catheter in place when the fungemia is detected, removal of the catheter (whether a Hickman–Broviac or a central line) is an

important part of management, but must be coupled with a limited course of intravenous amphotericin B (10 mg per kilogram total dosage) to avoid endophthalmitis. If cultures remain persistently positive for *Candida* after amphotericin B therapy is begun, a residual intravascular focus (e.g., *Candida* phlebitis or endocarditis) should be sought, because these complications may require surgical intervention in addition to systemic amphotericin B.

Hepatosplenic Candidiasis

Over the past several years, a syndrome named hepatic candidiasis has become increasingly recognized. The disease is characterized by the presence of "bull's eye" lesions in the liver on ultrasound or CT scan. I have found that these lesions are not apparent in patients who are neutropenic, but rather become recognizable at the time of neutrophil recovery. Patients are characterized by the persistence of fever at the time of recovery from an episode of neutropenia, and often have right upper quadrant discomfort, nausea, and an elevated alkaline phosphatase. The lesions are granulomas consisting of an inner core of central necrosis (where the yeast and pseudophyphae can be found) surrounded by a ring of inflammatory cells and then an outer ring of fibrosis. These imaged lesions change over time and with treatment and upon resolution become calcified—an important endpoint of therapy. The diagnosis is based on a high index of suspicion and must be confirmed with liver biopsy. Hepatic candidiasis poses a therapeutic challenge because long courses of amphotericin B are necessary. I have found that the average amount of amphotericin B needed is 5 g. I recommend starting therapy in patients with this syndrome on amphotericin B together with 5 FC, continuing both drugs until the lesions seen with ultrasound have either disappeared or become calcified. Serial biopsy may be necessary to confirm the resolution of infection. It is also worth noting that hepatic lesions may be smaller than the degree of resolution of current imaging techniques; in high-risk patients with negative abdominal ultrasounds, a biopsy may still be necessary to confirm (or rule out) hepatic candidiasis. In the future, liposome amphotericin B might permit a more rapid time to recovery from hepatic candidiasis. Until then, free amphotericin B can be effective in controlling and eradicating this infection if it is administered until the lesions resolve (even if they persist for months after initiation of therapy). I also believe amphotericin B should be combined with 5 FC for this infection.

Gastrointestinal Tract

The gastrointestinal (GI) tract serves as an important portal for infection and occasionally contributes to the primary clinical symptomatology. Ulcerative lesions occur throughout the intestinal tract, and large colonic lesions may contribute to severe bleeding, particularly when patients are also thrombocytopenic. Gastrointestinal bleeding may become so severe that surgical resection is necessary. In such patients, involvement of other organs is not unexpected, and systemic amphotericin B should follow surgical resection. The full therapeutic course is not well defined, but I advocate 30 to 40 mg per kilogram of amphotericin B.

Pulmonary Candidiasis

Primary *Candida* pneumonia may occur, but lung involvement is usually part of generalized infection. The radiographic appearance ranges from a micronodular or interstitial infiltrate to a lobar or consolidative pattern. Diagnosis must be based on histologic examination, this generally requiring an open-lung biopsy. Evidence of *Candida* pneumonia mandates a full course of amphotericin B, generally 30 to 40 mg per kilogram total dosage.

Central Nervous System Infection

Candida meningitis is unusual, and the presence of yeast forms in the spinal fluid should focus on *Cryptococcus*. However, if *Candida* meningitis is diagnosed, systemic amphotericin B should be administered, together with 5 FC. I recommend total dosages of amphotericin B of 30 to 40 mg per kilogram. It is not usually necessary to administer the amphotericin B directly into the cerebrospinal fluid (CSF), but if intrathecal therapy is deemed necessary, I prefer administration by means of an Ommaya reservoir (i.e., into the lateral ventricle).

Disseminated Infection

Candida can involve virtually every organ system. In addition to the sites already noted, subcutaneous tissues, muscle, joints, bone, kidney, and myocardium can all be involved, either as sole sites, or more commonly, as part of a generalized infection. Invasive disease of this magnitude is more likely in patients with phagocytic defects, than in patients with only lymphocyte defects, and this characteristic is helpful in identifying high-risk groups. Patients with disseminated candidiasis require lengthy courses of amphotericin B, usually 30 to 40 mg per kilogram total dosage.

Presumed Infection

Unfortunately, the diagnosis of disseminated infection can be difficult. If treatment is to be successful, therapy must begin early in the course of infection. Diagnosis is exceedingly difficult, and most laboratory measures (including many of the recently developed antigen detection assays) are associated with unacceptably high rates of false-negative results. Accordingly, I believe it is preferable to identify those patients who are at heightened risk for developing disseminated or invasive candidiasis and to treat them empirically—that is, before infection is fully established. I presently advocate beginning amphotericin B empirically in patients who remain persistently febrile and neutropenic following a 7-day course of broad-spectrum antibiotic therapy. Once started, amphotericin B (0.5 mg per kilogram per day) is continued until the patient's neutrophil count recovers.

PREVENTION OF *CANDIDA* INFECTION

Virtually every attempt to prevent candidiasis in high-risk patients has proved fruitless. Antifungal prophylaxis has been the most common approach, and a number of antifungal agents have been studied, including oral nystatin, amphotericin B, clotrimazole (none of which are absorbed), and ketoconazole and miconazole (both of which achieve systemic concentrations). Various studies suggest the ability to decrease colonization with antifungal agents or to decrease the incidence of mucosal infections (e.g., thrush), but none is associated with a reduction in the incidence of invasive candidiasis. For these reasons, I do not currently use antifungal prophylaxis in high-risk patients.

COCCIDIOIDOMYCOSIS

HANS E. EINSTEIN, M.D., F.A.C.P.

In the endemic area of the southwestern United States coccidioidomycosis continues to be a problem commonly encountered by pediatricians and family practitioners. The primary infection, virtually always acquired by the pulmonary route and occasionally accompanied by erythema multiforme or nodosum, is subclinical in about half the cases. The remainder produce the usual cough and fever of a lower respiratory infection, accompanied by chest pain when there is pleuritis (8 percent of primary infections). Supportive care only is required in most primary infections, with chemotherapy limited to those indications listed in the following section.

CHEMOTHERAPY

Most practitioners agree on the following indications for chemotherapy:

1. Any type of coccidioidomycosis in children younger than 2 years.
2. Progressive primary pneumonia (persistent hilar or paratracheal adenopathy accompanied by rising antibody titer).
3. Significant pneumonia in non-Caucasian children, particularly Filipinos, Oriental, American blacks, and Latin-Americans, all of whom have a greater proclivity to dissemination.
4. Complicating congenital or acquired immunosuppression, diabetes, or malignancies.
5. For surgical coverage if disease is extensive, active, or disseminated, or if surgery is being repeated.
6. Mandatory in all forms of metapulmonary infection, combined whenever possible with local amphotericin B.

AMPHOTERICIN B

Amphotericin B, a water-insoluble polyene, remains the drug of first choice after 30 years of use. A 10 percent suspension is given in 5 percent glucose in water (preservative free). The initial dosage is between 1 and 5 mg, (0.25 mg per kilogram) increased daily by 5 mg (0.25 mg per kilogram) until 1 mg per kilogram per day is reached. In severely ill patients one can achieve this in 3 days. The medication is better tolerated by most patients if it is given more rapidly than over the recommended 3 to 6 hours; 1 hour has been found to be optimal. The more rapid infusion also improves the logistics of outpatient therapy. Since the drug has a half-life of 36 hours an every-other-day regimen is acceptable.

Nausea, vomiting, chills, and fever are common adverse effects. Premedication with aspirin, antihistamines, and antiemetics ease these troublesome reactions. Severe shaking chills can be blocked or terminated with meperidine. If severe reactions persist in spite of these measures, corticosteroids can be effective.

Systemic toxicity includes anemia, which is usually self-limited, hypokalemia, and hypomagnesemia responsive to replacement therapy, and renal function changes. The latter is dose-related and best monitored with serial creatinine determinations. Dosage of amphotericin B has to be decreased if creatinine goes above 3 mg per deciliter. Renal function decreases usually return to normal.

The total amount of treatment required for a given lesion is difficult to monitor concurrently. Most workers select a total dosage based on past experience, deliver this dosage, and then monitor the patient carefully for effect. Most syndromes in children can be managed with 30 to 40 mg per kilogram, given during the total course of therapy. If further treatment becomes necessary, emergence of resistance does not usually occur.

Local amphotericin is useful in the treatment of coccidioidal osteomyelitis in which a 10 percent suspension is infused into areas of surgically exposed bone or joint by drip and suction. In meningitis, the most serious form of dissemination, many months of intrathecal therapy is usually required. This therapy is initiated with 0.05 mg in 1 ml of water, which is gradually increased to 0.25 mg or more given every other day at first and then decreased in frequency as the clinical picture improves, as evidenced by decreased spinal fluid pleocytosis and complement-fixing antibody titer in the spinal fluid and serum. Intrathecal injections into the lateral ventricles (Ommaya reservoir), lumbar area, or the cisterna magna have been given; the latter approach is best tolerated, has the fewest complications, and has given the best results. In both meningeal and skeletal disease, 0.5 to 1 g of amphotericin B is given concurrently.

IMIDAZOLES

Miconazole has been available for more than 10 years but has found only limited application in coccidioidomycosis. An orally effective dioxalan derivative, ketoconazole, has been available for 5 years, but experience with it is limited. The drug is moderately effective in some coccidioidal syndromes including primary infection and skin and soft tissue dissemination and synovitis. The incidence of relapses, even after several years of therapy, is high. Toxicity can involve the liver (1 in 10,000 cases) and testosterone suppression, which is usually reversible. Other azoles, itraconazole and fluconazole, are currently undergoing experimental trials.

SURGERY

Children with residual pulmonary cavities after primary infections may need excision if there is persistent bleeding, actual or threatened rupture, or secondary infection. Osteomyelitis is best handled with drainage and removal of sequestra, along with local amphotericin therapy, as outlined previously.

SUGGESTED READING

Catanzaro A, Einstein H, Levine B, et al. Ketoconazole for treatment of disseminated coccidioidomycosis. Ann Intern Med 1982; 96:436–440.
Drutz D, Catanzaro A. State of the art: coccidioidomycosis. Am Rev Resp Dis 1978; 117:727.

CRYPTOCOCCOSIS

JOHN R. GRAYBILL, M.D.

Until recent years, cryptococcosis was a disease rarely seen in children, and then only in scattered patients who had lymphoproliferative disease or were organ transplant recipients. More recently cryptococcosis has appeared in 6 to 9 percent of patients with acquired immunodeficiency syndrome (AIDS). *Cryptococcus neoformans* does not respect age, and as we encounter more and more children with AIDS, pediatric cryptococcosis will probably increase in frequency. Ninety percent of cryptococcosis is meningeal infection, so this is the form we must address therapeutically.

Despite the poor penetration of intravenously administered amphotericin B into cerebrospinal fluid, there is enough antifungal activity that intrathecal amphotericin B is rarely used in treatment of cryptococcal meningitis. The complications of arachnoiditis (dose-dependent, and sometimes progressing to transverse myelitis) and bacterial secondary infection (occurring in as many as half of patients treated with an Ommaya reservoir) are formidable and discourage intrathecal treatment of meningitis. The current "traditional" therapy for cryptococcal meningitis is a 6-week course of intravenously administered amphotericin B (0.3 mg per kilogram per day), coupled with oral flucytosine (100 to 150 mg per kilogram per day in two to four divided doses). The flucytosine concentration in the bloodstream is monitored to approximate 100 μg per milliliter at peak concentration 2 hours after an oral dose. This treatment is given for 6 weeks.

Treatment is rarely uncomplicated. Amphotericin B is not primarily excreted in the kidneys, but is nephrotoxic, producing an early renal tubular acidosis and a late glomerular lesion. Thus, one may have the problems of replacing potassium and bicarbonate to match renal electrolyte losses early in treatment, and later transiently discontinuing amphotericin B briefly for periods with elevated serum creatinine. (Usually 2.5 to 3 mg per deciliter constitute grounds for a pause in treatment.) Much of the nephrotoxicity is reversible, but this is not always so. Complicating this is the primarily renal excretion of flucytosine, such that the dosage must be altered with changing renal function. The most severe toxicities of flucytosine are gastrointestinal distress, hepatitis, and neutropenia. Neutropenia may be severe, has occurred in up to 25 percent of (adult) patients, and is only partly alleviated by adjusting the dosage according to measured serum concentrations. Some have argued that in vivo conversion of flucytosine to 5-fluorouracil occurs, either in the bowel (by bacterial microflora) or in tissue (by mammalian enzymes).

In part because of the toxicities of the 6-week regimen, the Mycoses Study Group conducted a randomized study comparing the results of 6 weeks of treatment with those of 4 weeks of the same regimen; 91 were evaluated at completion of treatment. Of those randomized to 6 weeks' treatment, 15 percent relapsed during a year of follow-up posttreatment. Of those randomized to 4 weeks, 25 percent relapsed (no significant difference). As with prior experience, obtundation and low cerebrospinal fluid (CSF) leukocyte response, and large numbers of cryptococci (positive India ink) were factors favoring poor outcome. Early in the trial, renal transplant recipients were found to have a high relapse rate when randomized to the 4-week regimen. Subsequently this group was removed from randomization, and all were treated for 6 weeks. Therefore, for non-organ-transplant recipients who do not have AIDS, the Mycoses Study Group suggests that 4 weeks of treatment may be adequate.

This study was commenced in 1980 and has not yet been published. However, because of AIDS, it is already out of date for the majority of patients with cryptococcal meningitis. AIDS patients with cryptococcosis may achieve remission with intravenous amphotericin B, but termination of therapy (for no matter how long) is usually followed by relapse. This has led to the recent recommendation to commence treatment with amphotericin B and flucytosine, but to follow initial amphotericin B induction therapy with consolidation treatment of amphotericin B given twice weekly, possibly for the rest of the patient's life. In AIDS patients, flucytosine is extremely myelotoxic, and usually cannot be given for more than a week. We no longer use it at all in these debilitated patients. It is uncertain how many of these patients survive, but the case fatality rate is high no matter what is done.

This experience has led to the attempts to treat cryptococcal meningitis with antifungal azoles. The experience with ketoconazole has been short and not encouraging. On the other hand, itraconazole, despite very little penetration into the CSF, seems to be just as potent as amphotericin B in unpublished foreign series of largely adult patients. The dosage is 6 to 7 mg per kilogram per day, given with meals. Antacids and H_2-blockers may interfere with absorption. Itraconazole is generally much better tolerated than ketoconazole, with neither the depression of steroid synthesis nor the gastrointestinal intolerance that characterize ketoconazole. In animal models the drug does penetrate the brain in measurable amounts, and it is possible that cerebral (rather than CSF) antifungal activity of amphotericin B may be the critical measurement.

Fluconazole has much greater solubility than itraconazole, with virtually 100 percent absorption from the stomach, and 80 percent diffusion into CSF. We have one patient doing well 5 months after induction of remission with amphotericin B and subsequent therapy with fluconazole. In addition, a few other patients have been started with fluconazole therapy, either after amphotericin B initial therapy or instead of amphotericin B. The dosage is presently 1.5 mg per kilogram per day, but it is likely that larger dosages will be in use shortly. At present data are inadequate to indicate the relative efficacy of fluconazole and itraconazole, but it appears that within a short time one or both of these may be used in a major "suppression" therapy for cryptococcosis. We are presently starting our AIDS patients with cryptococcosis on fluconazole therapy. Because the azoles may have a more delayed clinical onset of action, for the more severely ill patients we begin with amphotericin B and after several weeks switch to fluconazole. It is an unhappy comment that treatment of cryptococcosis in AIDS patients has so quickly turned to investigational agents with very limited clinical experience, none yet published.

SUGGESTED READING

Bennett JE, Dismukes WE, Duma RA, et al. A comparison of amphotericin B alone and combined with flucytosine in the treatment of cryptococcal meningitis. N Engl J Med 1979; 301:126–131.
Kovacs JA, Kovacs AA, Polis M, et al. Cryptococcosis in the acquired immunodeficiency syndrome. Ann Intern Med 1985; 103:533–538.
Zuger A, Louie E, Holzman RS, et al. Cryptococcal disease in patients with the acquired immunodeficiency syndrome. Ann Intern Med 1986; 104:234–240.

HISTOPLASMOSIS

H. DAVID WILSON, M.D., F.A.A.P.

The majority of children infected by the spores of *Histoplasma capsulatum* do not come to the physician's attention because of the mild nature of their disease. When a diagnosis of histoplasmosis is made, the doctor must decide whether any treatment is indicated because the otherwise healthy child usually recovers completely without antifungal therapy. The only evidence of past infection usually consists of small fibronodular densities seen on x-ray examination of the lung, spleen, and liver.

DIAGNOSIS

I can make a tentative or definitive diagnosis of histoplasmosis when a child with a history and clinical findings consistent with histoplasmosis is given one or more of the following confirmatory tests:

1. Microscopic evidence of organisms consistent with *H. capsulatum* from biopsy material, blood, phagocytes, or body secretions. Methenamine silver stain is especially useful in identifying the cell wall of intracellular yeast forms in biopsy material. Employing a combination of hematoxylin and eosin stain for tissue morphology plus the methenamine silver stain to demonstrate the cell wall and budding yeast forms usually makes the diagnosis obvious. Microscopic observation of small budding yeasts in wet preparations of respiratory secretions are *not* diagnostic because other yeasts with similar morphology may be present.
2. Positive cultures for *H. capsulatum* from blood, sputum, bone marrow, urine, liver, or other tissues or body fluids provide a definitive diagnosis.

Fresh specimens should be inoculated onto Sabouraud's agar and blood agar plates with and without added selective antibiotics. Sabouraud's agar should never be used alone. When specimens are placed into blood culture bottles containing brain-heart infusion broth or trypticase soy broth, the bottles must be vented to establish an aerobic atmosphere. The Dupont Isolator system is excellent for isolating *H. capsulatum* from blood and does so in a shorter time than do other broth systems. Cultures are generally incubated at room temperature (27°C) and held for 6 weeks before being considered negative.

3. Serum antibodies demonstrated by the following:
   A. *Complement fixation test in a titer greater than 1:8 or showing a fourfold rise over a 2- to 4-week period to the yeast or mycelial form of the organism.* Usually during active infection, antibodies to both antigens are found, but response to the yeast form antigen is generally more sensitive and correlates more closely with the course of clinical disease. The antibodies to the yeast form antigen are less likely to be affected by prior histoplasmin skin testing. These antibodies usually appear within 2 weeks of infection, but may be delayed in some cases of disseminated disease and may remain at low titers in patients with chronic disease. Cross-reacting antibodies to these antigens may occur in patients with blastomycosis and other fungal infections.
   B. *Precipitating antibodies demonstrated by the immunodiffusion to H and M antigens.* Bands to both H and M antigens are present in up to 90 percent of patients with acute infection. Generally the M band occurs earliest and persists for months or years. The H band usually indicates active (recent) infection and disappears in a few months, but is found in only 10 to 20 percent of patients with acute disease.

When an *infant* has either H or M bands or both bands detectable, I feel confident that he or she has active disease. Skin testing for histoplasmosis can be useful in epidemiologic studies, but should not be used as a confirmatory test in making a diagnosis of histoplasmosis. This is especially true in areas where histoplasmosis is endemic. In addition, the use of the skin test may interfere with serologic studies by causing an increase in the complement fixation titer to mycelial antigen and an M band demonstrated by immunodiffusion.

INDICATIONS FOR TREATMENT

Once a diagnosis is made, the question is whether the risks to the patient from the disease are great enough to justify treatment with the potentially toxic drug amphotericin B. Generally, it is the most unusual manifestations of histoplasmosis that benefit from antifungal treatment. I consider the following manifestations as definite or possible indications for treatment.

Disseminated Histoplasmosis in the Infant or in the Immunologically Compromised Patient

The immunologically normal infant with disseminated histoplasmosis can be treated successfully with amphotericin B for a period of about 2 weeks (schedule to be outlined). Improvement is seen in the infant's mood, cessation of fever, recession of hepatosplenomegaly, weight gain, and rising hematocrit values, white blood cell counts, and platelet counts during this period. When clinical and laboratory improvement occurs, I discontinue amphotericin B treatment and follow the baby closely for any signs of relapse. Should signs of disease reappear, a second short course of amphotericin B therapy is undertaken. In patients with lymphoma, leukemia, or other malignant disease in which T-lymphocyte or mononuclear phagocyte function is depressed and in patients recovering from bone marrow or other organ transplantation, a course of 6 to 8 weeks of treatment is needed. Some patients show striking improvement after 4 weeks of treatment, making it possible to halt treatment. Perhaps ketoconazole would be useful in finishing the treatment course in these patients; however, experience is limited in such cases, and I prefer to treat with amphotericin B for the full course of therapy.

Histoplasma Meningitis

This is a rare complication of histoplasma infection in children. The diagnosis may require repeated cultures of large volumes of cerebrospinal fluid (CSF) and the testing of CSF and serum using the serologic tests outlined. Frequently, even when large volumes of CSF are used, the organism is not cultured from spinal fluid. I begin treatment with intravenous amphotericin B (to be described), but if a rapid response in both clinical and CSF measures is not evident in 4 to 7 days and because of its poor penetration into the CSF, I begin to administer amphotericin B directly into the ventricular system by an Ommaya or similar reservoir. For instillation into the ventricle, the amphotericin B is diluted to a concentration of 0.25 mg per milliliter in 5 percent dextrose in water. A test dose of 0.1 ml of this concentration is diluted in CSF and administered. The dose is increased by 0.1-ml (0.025 mg) increments to 0.1 mg, then by that amount until a maximum dose of 0.2 to 0.5 mg is reached. The adult dose is 0.5 mg given three times per week for 6 to 8 weeks. The addition of methylprednisolone, 2 to 3 mg, along with the injection often diminishes fever, headache, and nausea should they occur. In one case of histoplasma meningitis occurring in a child with a ventriculoatrial shunt, I was unable to clear the infection until the shunt was removed.

Lymph Node Compression of the Trachea or Other Organs Caused by Histoplasmosis

I have successfully treated several children with serious compression of the trachea from an enlarged azygous lymph node. *H. capsulatum* has a propensity to involve the lymph nodes in the right paratracheal location. In these children, I have avoided the need for thoracotomy with the following approach. If the symptoms indicate significant and life-threatening airway impairment, I favor treatment with amphotericin B (to be outlined) along with high-dose methylprednisone, 2 mg per kilogram per day in four divided doses given intravenously every 6 hours. Alternatively, one could give prednisone, 2 mg per kilogram per day in two equal divided doses given every 12 hours by mouth. This is done in an attempt to reduce the size of the lymph node rapidly with steroids and to protect against possible dissemination of the histoplasma by treating with amphotericin. The total course of treatment in these immunologically normal children has been 3 to 4 weeks.

Histoplasma Pericarditis

This rare complication of histoplasmosis can result in some degree of cardiac tamponade (approximately 40 percent), but usually resolves without causing constrictive pericarditis. I give a short course (2 weeks) of amphotericin B and steroids, as indicated in the preceding section, because this is believed to be a hypersensitivity response and not actual infection of the pericardium by histoplasma.

Acute Mediastinal Histoplasmosis Resulting in Obstruction of Major Blood Vessels or Pulmonary Airways

I have seen several cases in which fibrosing mediastinitis caused partial or complete obstruction of pulmonary arteries, veins, superior vena cava, or bronchi. For this reason, if a symptomatic patient is found to have acute mediastinal histoplasmosis, I give amphotericin in an attempt to prevent, if possible, this excessive fibrosis with resulting entrapment. This is another condition in which dual treatment with amphotericin and steroids is advisable if treatment is begun early. If the condition is recognized late in its course, amphotericin is not likely to be helpful. Surgical removal of fibrous tissue has, in my experience, been disappointing, but may be the only alternative when the damage has already occurred.

Progressive Primary Histoplasmosis or Heavy-Exposure Acute Pulmonary Histoplasmosis

Children with these forms of histoplasmosis force the physician to individualize treatment. Most, if not all, recover fully if untreated, but I believe that some children benefit from a short course of amphotericin. The child with progressive primary histoplasmosis who continues to have low-grade fever, cough, malaise, hepatosplenomegaly, pulmonary infiltrate with hilar adenopathy, and usually mild anemia and an elevated erythrocyte sedimentation rate after 3 weeks can benefit from 1 to 2 weeks of amphotericin B treatment. The same is true of the child who has had a massive inhalation of spores with high fever, cough, chills, malaise, marked hypoxemia requiring supplemental inspired oxygen, and occasionally, ventilatory support.

GUIDELINES FOR INTRAVENOUS AMPHOTERICIN B ADMINISTRATION

1. Amphotericin B must be suspended in 5 percent dextrose in *water* at a concentration of not more than 0.1 mg per milliliter and the final suspension buffered to pH 5.5. (Amphotericin B is in a colloidal suspension with sodium deoxycholate and precipitates when mixed with electrolyte-containing solutions). It must not be filtered with a 0.22-μm pore membrane filter because it is partially retained. No loss of activity is seen if 0.45-μm pore filters are used.
2. I begin with a test dose of 0.25 mg per kilogram and infuse the solution over a 1- to 2-hour period on the first day of treatment. Close monitoring of heart rate, blood pressure, fever, chills, dyspnea, nausea, and vomiting should be done during this and subsequent infusions until it is demonstrated that the patient tolerates the infusion without hypotensive reactions or cardiac rate irregularities.

3. If serious side effects such as marked hypotension or cardiac arrhythmias do not occur, the dosage is increased by 0.25 mg per kilogram daily until the full dosage of 1 mg per kilogram is reached on the fourth day. Infusion time usually ranges from 1 to 4 hours. Because there are fewer episodes of fever, chills, and nausea with a more rapid infusion, I prefer the 1-hour infusion time provided hypotension or cardiac irregularities do not occur. This dosage is continued on a daily basis unless toxicity occurs.
4. I do not insist that the amphotericin suspension be protected from light as the package insert recommends, since several studies have demonstrated the stability of amphotericin B in light.
5. I premedicate patients with acetaminophen, 10 mg per kilogram per dose given orally (maximum dose 1,000 mg), and diphenhydramine hydrochloride, 1.25 mg per kilogram given orally, 30 minutes before the infusion is begun. The acetaminophen is repeated in 4 hours if a prolonged infusion time is required. If chills are not controlled, methylprednisolone, 0.1 to 0.2 mg per kilogram given intravenously, immediately before the infusion, may be beneficial. For nausea and anxiety, I have found hydroxyzine pamoate, 1 mg per kilogram given orally, 1 hour before infusion, to be effective.
6. I do not routinely use heparin in the amphotericin B infusion, but if thrombophlebitis becomes a problem, I would add heparin sulfate, 1 U per milliliter, to the infusion. However, there are no studies to support its efficacy in reducing the incidence of thrombophlebitis.

The major non-infusion-related toxicities of amphotericin B therapy result in azotemia, hypokalemia, anemia, thrombocytopenia, and neutropenia. Accordingly, I check the BUN, creatinine, urinalysis, serum potassium, and hemogram twice weekly. If the BUN rises to 50 mg per deciliter or the serum creatinine to 3.0 mg or more per deciliter, the dosage of amphotericin B should be reduced to 0.75 mg per kilogram per day and the fluid intake increased, if possible. Further reductions in dosage or temporary discontinuance of therapy may be required. I recommend foods with high potassium content such as bananas and oranges, but if hypokalemia (K^+ less than 3.0 mEq/L) is noted, oral or intravenous potassium supplementation is begun. Anemia resulting from amphotericin B is generally mild, seldom severe enough to require blood transfusion, and is not usually present before 2 weeks of therapy has been completed. If this problem develops, either the dosage of amphotericin B may be reduced or the interval between administrations may be lengthened to alternate days.

In patients with underlying diseases and severe neutropenia requiring white blood cell transfusions, it is prudent to administer amphotericin B at widely different times because of the rarely reported pulmonary leukocyte aggregation that seems to occur when the infusions are not adequately spaced.

There is obviously a need for a less toxic drug than amphotericin B to treat histoplasmosis. Accordingly, there has been considerable interest in the use of ketoconazole for treatment of this disease. Experience has been limited, primarily in adults, in treating chronic pulmonary and mild chronic disseminated histoplasmosis with this drug. Use of the drug has often proved successful only over the short term. However, failures with reactivation have been reported, and the long-term effectiveness of ketoconazole in these forms of histoplasmosis is not yet known. Use of ketoconazole in unusually severe or prolonged acute pulmonary histoplasmosis has not yet been extensively studied. Furthermore, no comparative studies have been reported. Ketoconazole is not without its own toxicity (primarily nausea, vomiting, elevation of serum transaminases, and, rarely, fatal hepatotoxicity and decreased androgen

synthesis) and must be used for a prolonged period of time when employed as a sole agent in treating systemic mycoses. Although its use might be indicated in mildly ill patients without underlying immunosuppression, I favor the use of amphotericin B in patients who are not in these categories.

In addition to ketoconazole, recent studies using liposome-encapsulated amphotericin B look promising. This form of the drug appears to be more effective with fewer infusion-related adverse reactions and less nephrotoxicity. Both of these two agents may prove less toxic for the children who may benefit from treatment for histoplasmosis.

SUGGESTED READING

Fosson AR, Wheeler WE. Short-term amphotericin B treatment of severe childhood histoplasmosis. J Pediatr 1975; 86:32–36.
Goodwin RA, Loyd JE, Des Prez RM. Histoplasmosis in normal hosts. Medicine 1981; 60:231–266.
Wilson R, Feldman S. Toxicity of amphotericin B in children with cancer. Am J Dis Child 1979; 133:731–734.

ZYGOMYCOSIS AND PHAEOHYPHOMYCOSIS

JOHN R. GRAYBILL, M.D.

Zygomycosis is most often caused by members of the genera *Mucor, Absidia,* and *Rhizopus,* with *Cunnighamella* and others occurring less frequently. These fungi are molds that grow very rapidly in an acid milieu, especially in the presence of high glucose concentrations. Zygomycetes are readily killed by polymorphonuclear leukocytes. They are uncommon pathogens of adults, and even less common in children. The population at risk includes diabetics, especially those with ketoacidosis, burn patients, and severely neutropenic patients. Once established, most commonly in the paranasal sinuses or the lungs, the organism spreads rapidly without respect for tissue planes, causing necrosis of tissues and thrombosis of blood vessels. Sinusitis, proptosis, and blindness are hallmarks of rhinocerebral disease. Mortality may be upwards of 50 percent, and depends largely on how promptly the disease is diagnosed and how aggressively the patient is managed. Mortality is higher in pulmonary disease, which occurs more commonly in neutropenic patients.

When the disease is suspected, the diagnosis is made by *deep* biopsy of the affected tissues; when confirmed by frozen section, the surgeon must debride the involved sinus promptly and aggressively,

and often the orbit as well. Repeated debridement may be necessary. Debridement is coupled with amphotericin B therapy. In the case of pulmonary disease, segmental or lobar resection of the involved lung should be undertaken, if possible.

Regarding medical therapy, immediately after a 1-mg test dose is given, if there is no hypotension, the dosage should be increased to 0.7 to 1 mg per kilogram of amphotericin B intravenously; this dosage should be continued daily. I rarely use doses larger than 50 mg per day in adults. The outcome is usually determined early in the course of treatment. A total course of 15 to 25 mg per kilogram of amphotericin B should be administered. If the patient is neutropenic, I recommend continuing amphotericin B throughout the period of leukopenia. In the case of rhinocerebral disease, the wound can be packed with gauze impregnated with amphotericin B (50 mg per liter of water). Zygomycetes are resistant to the azoles, and there is no place for ketoconazole or its cogeners in therapy of zygomycosis.

Management of the underlying diabetic ketoacidosis or of the cause of neutropenia is also important for successful outcome.

Phaeohyphomycosis is caused by dematiacious (darkly pigmented) fungi of the genera *Bipolaris* and *Exserohilum.* This is less common than zygomycosis and it is a more slowly invasive process. Phaeohyphomycosis is more often subject to relapses than zygomycosis, especially in immunosuppressed patients. Disease presents as sinusitis, corneal ulcers, pneumonia, skin nodules and abscesses, and encephalitis.

Debridement is a major part of therapy. In the case of sinusitis this can be accomplished by a Caldwell–Luc procedure, often without systemic antifungals. Corneal ulcers may resolve with topical amphotericin B therapy. Flucytosine has been used, usually in conjunction with amphotericin B, but its role is uncertain. Although the organisms are susceptible to azoles, there is little experience with their use. Amphotericin B is given at a total dosage of 10 to 20 mg per kilogram. Phaeohyphomycosis is one of the more recently appreciated causes of peritonitis in patients undergoing continuous ambulatory peritoneal dialysis. It is treated with intravenously administered amphotericin B and removal of the dialysis catheter. Amphotericin B has been given through dialysis catheters, but I do not recommend this practice because it causes intense peritoneal irritation. Prolonged treatment may be warranted in the immunosuppressed patient, especially if relapse has occurred.

SUGGESTED READING

Adam RD, Paquin ML, Petersen EA, et al. Phaeohyphomycosis caused by the fungal genera *Bipolaris* and *Exserohilum*. Medicine 1986; 65:203–217.

Lehrer RI, Howard DH, Shepherd PS, et al. Mucormycosis. Ann Intern Med 1980; 93:93–108.

SPOROTRICHOSIS

WILLIAM S. FOSHEE, M.D.

Sporotrichosis is a relatively rare cause of infection in children. The etiologic agent *Sporothrix schenckii* has a worldwide distribution. The most common clinical presentation is with cutaneous lesions on the extremities or face. These skin lesions are described as either fixed or lymphocutaneous. The initial lesion at the inoculation site often ulcerates and less frequently remains confined to a single site, which is referred to as *fixed cutaneous sporotrichosis.* Classically, and more commonly, new lesions appear along the path of the lymphatics; this is referred to as *lymphocutaneous sporotrichosis.* Extracutaneous sporotrichosis (pulmonary, joint, bone, central nervous system, etc.) is extraordinarily uncommon in children and is usually associated with immunosuppression or immunodeficiency.

SPECIFIC THERAPY

Potassium Iodide

The treatment of choice for cutaneous sporotrichosis is saturated solution of potassium iodide (KI), 1.0 g per milliliter. The usual starting dose is 1 or 2 drops per year of age three times daily. This dosage can be increased gradually 1 to 2 drops per dose to a maximum of 10 drops three times daily for a small child or 20 to 40 drops three times daily for a teenager. The maximum dosage for a 50- to 70-kg person is 30 to 40 drops three times daily. The KI is often given with fruit juice or milk to disguise the bitter taste. A response to therapy is usually apparent within 7 to 10 days, with healing of the lesions occurring in 2 to 4 weeks. Therapy is continued for 4 to 6 weeks after clinical healing has taken place. The response to KI is usually good, with rare recurrences. Relapse may respond to a second course of KI.

Adverse reactions to KI include acneiform rash, increased lacrimation, excessive salivation, salivary gland swelling, nausea, vomiting, epigastric pain, headache, or facial edema. These toxic effects can be reduced by discontinuing therapy for a few days and restarting at a lower dosage. The use of KI during pregnancy is cautioned because hypothyroidism and thyromegaly of the fetus can develop with airway obstruction of the infant at birth.

KI is absorbed well from the gastrointestinal tract with 98 percent of the oral dose excreted in the urine. Recently it has been ascertained that the therapeutic effect of potassium iodide is mediated through the direct antifungal action of molecular iodine. As little as 20 μg per milliliter of iodine kills the yeast form of *S. schenckii,* whereas 10 percent potassium iodide failed to inhibit the organism.

Amphotericin B

Amphotericin B is recommended as the drug of choice for patients who are intolerant to KI, have serious iodide sensitivity, fail therapy with KI, or have extracutaneous sporotrichosis. The amphotericin B dosage is 0.5 mg per kilogram per day for 6 to 12 weeks. In refractory cases flucytosine, 150 mg per kilogram per day given in four divided doses, has been combined with amphotericin B with reported efficacy. When meningitis is present amphotericin B must be given intrathecally or by way of an Omaya reservoir.

Ketoconazole

Oral ketoconazole has been used in managing sporotrichosis with limited success. Adult patients treated for cutaneous infection have required 400 mg per day to achieve a therapeutic response. For extracutaneous infections, the response has not been successful even with larger dosing schedules of 800 mg daily. The dosage in children is 5 to 10 mg per kilogram of body weight daily, usually given as a single dose. The rare case of fatal hepatitis and the endocrine side effects limit consideration of ketoconazole use as initial therapy for sporotrichosis in children. Its use in refractory or extracutaneous disease has been disappointing.

Itraconazole

Oral itraconazole, an investigational triazole, has demonstrated good in vitro activity (minimum inhibitory concentration [MIC] 0.1 to 1.0 μg per milliliter) and experimental efficacy against *S. schenckii*. Preliminary data indicate excellent clinical efficacy for cutaneous sporotrichosis, but there is no published information on treatment of extracutaneous sporotrichosis. Itraconazole is poorly absorbed after oral administration, but absorption is better when it is given with a meal. The serum concentrations are low but because of the long half-life (15 hours) accumulation occurs with continuing therapy. An 18-month-old child we treated with itraconazole, 150 mg per day, achieved a peak serum concentration of 2.2 μg per milliliter. Itraconazole has a particular affinity for tissue, especially skin and liver. This drug does not penetrate the cerebrospinal fluid in sufficient concentrations to treat fungal meningitis.

Itraconazole does not have an effect on androgen or cortisol metabolism as occurs with ketoconazole. Adverse reactions to this drug are few (2.8 percent) and are primarily gastrointestinal. It is only slowly metabolized in the body. With the clinical experience thus far there has been no case of hepatitis associated with itraconazole therapy. Because this is not an approved drug, its use has to be under an investigational protocol. Itraconazole is manufactured by Janssen Pharmaceutica.

ADJUNCTIVE THERAPY

In extracutaneous sporotrichosis, adjunctive surgery in addition to antifungal chemotherapy is usually required to effect a cure. Synovectomy, pulmonary lobectomy, pneumonectomy, or bone debridement is frequently required with infection of the respective sites.

MONITORING RESPONSE TO THERAPY

Looking for clinical changes in the skin lesions is the primary means of monitoring the response to therapy, since superficial fungal cultures are frequently negative. Although biopsy or needle aspiration may have been necessary to make the initial diagnosis, repeat biopsy is usually unnecessary. Careful follow-up for at least a year is recommended to detect the rare case of relapse.

In extracutaneous sporotrichosis the erythrocyte sedimentation rate is frequently elevated and is a useful marker of disease activity in the face of antifungal therapy. Serum antibody titers are highly specific indicators of disease activity, but unfortunately they are unreliable in monitoring the response to therapy. The latex agglutination and immunodiffusion assays are more sensitive than the complement fixation test. Although the antibody titers are higher in extracutaneous disease than for cutaneous disease, a negative or falling titer does not ensure resolution of the infection.

Culture of tissue, body fluids, or secretions is the most sensitive means of monitoring response to extracutaneous sporotrichosis. The organism grows on most fungal media in 3 to 5 days after inoculation. Direct immunofluorescence of tissue specimens is highly specific but less sensitive than culture. Other tissue-staining techniques are much less sensitive because of the small number of organisms present.

Long-term follow-up is required for patients with extracutaneous sporotrichosis because chronicity and relapse is more common.

PREVENTION

Horticulturists should wear protective gloves and clothing because they are at significant risk for inoculation of this organism into their skin. Transmission of feline sporotrichosis to humans has recently been reported. All of the involved cats had ulcerating or draining skin lesions. Avoidance of direct contact with cats that have such lesions is important, because these lesions contain a large number of organisms. Human-to-human transmission from cutaneous lesions has occurred, but is an unimportant mode probably because the lesions contain a small number of organisms. Large outbreaks of sporotrichosis have occurred from contact with highly contaminated sphagnum moss, bales of hay, and mine timbers. It is important to identify the source in outbreaks, because avoidance, decontamination with formaldehyde solution, or destruction of the involved material can abort the epidemic.

SUGGESTED READING

Dunstan RW, Langham RF, Reimann KA, Wakenell PS. Feline sporotrichosis: a report of five cases with transmission to humans. J Am Acad Dermatol 1986; 15:37–45.

Hay RJ, Dupont B, Graybill JR. First international symposium on itraconazole. Rev Infect Dis 1987; 9(Suppl 1):S1-S152.

Orr RE, Riley Jr HD. Sporotrichosis in childhood. J Pediatr 1971; 78:951–957.

Pluss JL, Opal SM. Pulmonary sporotrichosis: review of treatment and outcome. Medicine 1986; 65:143–153.

Powell KE, Taylor A, Phillips BJ, et al. Cutaneous sporotrichosis in forestry workers: epidemic due to contaminated sphagnum moss. JAMA 1978; 240:232–235.

DERMATOPHYTOSIS

DAVID A. WHITING, M.D., M. MED. (DERM.), F.A.C.P., F.R.C.P.

The key to successful treatment of dermatophytosis is an accurate diagnosis. This is especially true in prepubertal children, in whom the site of fungal infection often differs from that of the adult. The futility of prolonged ringworm therapy in children with atopic eczema of the feet or groins is only too evident. Conversely, prolonged treatment with immunosuppressive agents such as strong, topical corticosteroids for eczema or psoriasis can encourage secondary fungal invasion, and a diminished therapeutic response should suggest that possibility. Confirmation of active, fungal invasion by direct, microscopic examination of skin, hair, or nails treated with 10 to 20 percent potassium hydroxide (KOH) is essential, and species identification by culture should follow. Wood's light examination may be helpful in some cases. Positive KOH and culture results depend on sampling tissue that is actively involved by the fungus, and experience is needed to ensure that skin scrapings are taken from the scaly borders of lesions or that actively damaged hair or nail fragments are obtained.

TINEA CAPITIS

The most common cause of tinea capitis today in urban areas in Western countries is *Trichophyton tonsurans,* which causes a large-spore endothrix infection. It invades and weakens the hair shaft and causes it to break off at the skin surface, leading to scattered or diffuse patches of alopecia, containing small black dots that are sometimes hard to find. These dark fragments of proximal hair shaft must be extracted with hair tweezers or a pointed (No. 11) scalpel blade for KOH examination or culture. *T. tonsurans* is an anthropophilic fungus and tends to produce lesions that are noninflammatory and therefore easy to overlook. It is important to identify and treat this infection because it is contagious to other humans and can even infect adults, unlike most other forms of tinea capitis. Black dot ringworm can also be caused by *T. violaceum,* but is usually more inflammatory in nature. The other major causes of tinea capitis are the small-spore ectothrix infections *Microsporum canis* and *M. audouinii.* Here the hairs are less brittle, so that the areas of alopecia contain a stubble of gray, lusterless hairs that break off a few millimeters away from the scalp surface. The patches of alopecia are often well-circumscribed and easy to find, and may show varying degrees of scaling and inflammation.

M. canis is zoophilic and therefore not contagious from human to human to any extent. Small-spore ectothrix infections fluoresce bright green under Wood's light, but so does other material, and it is important to be sure that the fluorescence emanates from the hair shaft itself. Other rarer causes of tinea capitis include large-spore ectothrix infections such as *T. verrucosum* and *T. mentagrophytes,* which tend to be inflammatory but are nonfluorescent, and the rare favic type of invasion caused by *T. schoenleinii,* which fluoresces pale green under Wood's light and can also affect adults.

The zoophilic fungi *T. verrucosum* and *T. mentagrophytes,* and occasionally a geophilic or even an anthropophilic species, can lead to intense hypersensitivity with the formation of the boggy, pustular mass that characterizes a kerion. Kerion should be suspected in any child with persistent pustules, folliculitis, or abscesses of the scalp that does not respond to antibiotic therapy.

Systemic therapy is required to eradicate tinea capitis because topical preparations do not penetrate the hair shaft. Griseofulvin is the drug of choice. Microsize griseofulvin is adequate, and the usual dosage for children is approximately 5 mg per pound (or 10 to 15 mg per kilogram) per day, given in one or two doses, preferably with a fatty meal such as whole milk. On this basis, the usual daily dosage for children weighing 30 to 50 pounds is 125 to 250 mg, and for children over 50 pounds it is 250 to 500 mg. It may be given as tablets (Fulvicin U/F, Schering, 500 mg; Grisactin, Ayerst, 500 mg), as capsules that may be pulled apart and the powder dispersed in milk or ice cream (Grisactin, Ayerst, 125 mg or 250 mg) or as a suspension (Grifulvin V, Ortho, 125 mg per 5 ml). Ultramicrosize griseofulvin can be used instead, and is given in a dosage of approximately 3.3 mg per pound per day, although the dosage has not been established for children younger than 2 years of age. It is available as tablets (Fulvicin P/G, Schering, 125, 250, 165, and 330 mg; Grisactin Ultra, Ayerst, 125, 250, and 330 mg; Gris-PEG, Herbert, 125 and 250 mg), but these confer no particular advantage over the ordinary microsize griseofulvin. Griseofulvin should be given until new hair has grown out in all patches of alopecia and Wood's light, KOH examinations, and cultures are negative. This usually takes 2 to 3 months, but longer treatment may be necessary. Griseofulvin is a remarkably safe drug and serious side effects are rare. Headaches, nausea, vomiting, diarrhea, urticaria, photosensitivity, and other minor side effects may be seen.

Griseofulvin is contraindicated in hepatocellular failure, porphyria, chronic renal failure, and cases of hypersensitivity to griseofulvin. In nonresponders you should ensure that the drug is properly ingested regularly after meals, and if necessary increase or even double the dosage. If griseofulvin resistance is suspected, or the drug is contraindicated, oral ketoconazole is the alternative. It has not been studied in children younger than 2 years of age, but if strongly indicated may be given in older patients in a single daily dose of approximately 1.5 to 3.0 mg per pound

(3.3 to 6.6 mg per kilogram). It is available in tablet form (Nizoral, Janssen, 200 mg scored tablets), which can be divided and crushed in milk or ice cream. It should also be given until clinical and mycologic cure is obtained, which may take 3 months. Because idiosyncratic hepatitis has been reported in 1 in 15,000 patients taking the drug, liver function tests should be monitored during therapy. Ketoconazole is contraindicated in patients who have shown hypersensitivity to the drug.

Kerion is treated as described earlier with griseofulvin or, if necessary, with ketoconazole. If the inflammatory stage is unusually severe or prolonged, oral prednisone in a dosage of 1 to 2 mg per kilogram per day for 3 to 4 weeks hastens resolution. If small lesions less than 3 cm in diameter are present, intralesional injections of triamcinolone acetonide, 10 mg per milliliter may suffice. In my experience concomitant antibiotics such as erythromycin are rarely necessary or useful.

The hair should be shampooed each morning to help remove infected scales and hairs. The hairs bordering on active lesions can be cut shorter and a topical antifungal agent (see later) applied to reduce contagion. Keratolytic agents are sometimes useful for softening thick scales. The patient's towels, combs, or other toilet articles should not be used by others. Patients with zoophilic infections such as *M. canis* need not be isolated, but their pets should be checked by a veterinarian. Those with anthropophilic infections may return to school once oral griseofulvin therapy has been started.

TINEA CORPORIS

Tinea corporis ranges from typical ringworm lesions with spreading, scaly borders and clear centers, through erythematous, scaly macules, to irregular lesions showing scattered pustules or folliculitis. The lesions are invariably asymmetric. The most common cause of tinea corporis in children is *M. canis,* followed by *T. mentagrophytes. T. rubrum* and *Epidermophyton floccosum* infections also occur; these are usually acquired from parents.

Tinea corporis usually responds to local therapy when only a few early lesions are present. Topical therapy is generally necessary for 3 to 4 weeks. I prefer imidazole preparations and usually prescribe miconazole nitrate (Monistat-Derm, Ortho, 2 percent cream) twice daily, although clotrimazole (Lotrimin, Schering, Mycelex, Miles) or econazole (Spectazole, Ortho) is equally useful. Ketoconazole cream (Nizoral, Janssen, cream) has the advantage that it can be administered once daily. A different compound, ciclopirox olamine (Loprox, Hoechst-Roussel, cream), can be applied twice daily with equally good results. In my opinion these products are superior to haloprogin and tolnaftate. Low cost and a vanishing-cream base have prompted a return to popularity of a salicylic and benzoic acid combina-

tion (Antinea, American Dermal), related to the old standard, Whitfield's Ointment. All of these preparations should be applied well beyond the visible margins of the lesions, to control the outward spread of fungus that cannot be seen clinically but is demonstrable microscopically. If lesions of tinea corporis are chronic, widespread, or unresponsive to 1 month of topical therapy, then systemic treatment with griseofulvin is indicated, as outlined previously. Treatment should be continued until complete clearing occurs, usually in 2 to 4 weeks, but sometimes several months in cases of *T. rubrum* infection. In chronic, resistant cases, ketoconazole may be indicated, as described earlier.

Tinea faciei is a special form of *T. corporis* that is often difficult to diagnose and must be confirmed by KOH examination or culture. Topical treatment may be inadequate, especially if the lesions have a follicular component, and oral griseofulvin may be necessary.

TINEA PEDIS

Tinea pedis is rare in prepubertal children and should be diagnosed only after positive KOH examinations or cultures are obtained. It is much more common after puberty, when it can occur as an interdigital intertrigo, usually starting in the lateral toewebs; as a blistered variety, caused by *T. mentagrophytes,* occurring on the foot sole under the long arch; or as a widespread, scaly, moccasin variety affecting both feet, caused by *T. rubrum.* The first two forms of tinea pedis are often unilateral or asymmetric.

Eczematous or secondarily infected forms of tinea pedis should be treated with twice-daily soaks of Burow's solution or of potassium permanganate diluted to a light pink color. Antibiotics may be necessary for secondary infection. Topical antifungal agents should be applied, as outlined earlier, as creams or lotions, and regular treatment is often necessary for 1 to 2 months. A powder applied between the toes or in the socks in the morning is often useful during the day against sweating, and my preference is undecylenic acid powder (e.g., Desenex, Pharmacraft). Castellani's Paint (Carbol-Fuchsin Solution USNF), or colorless Castellani's Paint are also useful for daytime drying. Resistant toeweb infections, vesicular lesions of the soles, and the dry, moccasin type of tinea require prolonged griseofulvin therapy, sometimes for 2 to 3 months. Ketoconazole may be useful in resistant cases.

TINEA CRURIS

Tinea cruris is also rare in prepubertal children, but may affect adolescents. Definitive diagnosis depends on positive KOH examination or culture. Topical treatments, as outlined previously, should suffice for mild cases, but resistant or severe infections require administration of oral griseofulvin for 3 to 4 weeks for cure.

TINEA UNGUIUM

Tinea unguium occurs infrequently in prepubertal children and is usually acquired from adults in the household. The most common causative organism is *T. rubrum.* Tinea unguium occurs more frequently after puberty, when the incidence of tinea pedis rises sharply. Oral therapy with griseofulvin is required for 3 to 6 months, or with ketoconazole in resistant cases. Topical therapy under and around the nail plate should also be given, and continued for as long as necessary after oral treatment is stopped. The affected nail plate should always be trimmed back as far as possible to allow maximum penetration of the topical medication. This is especially relevant in treating toenails, in which the slow nail growth makes maintenance of oral treatment for too long a period undesirable.

OTHER FORMS OF TINEA

Deeper or more extensive and persistent forms of ringworm such as tinea barbae, tinea profunda (Majocchi's granuloma), and the infections seen in immunocompromised patients usually require oral therapy with griseofulvin or ketoconazole as primary treatment.

SUGGESTED READING

Hay RJ, Clayton YM, Griffiths WA, et al. A comparative double blind study of ketoconazole and griseofulvin in dermatophytosis. Br J Dermatol 1985; 112:691–696.

Hurwitz S. Clinical pediatric dermatology. Philadelphia: WB Saunders, 1981; 277–287.

Logan RA, Hay RJ, Whitefield M. Antifungal efficacy of a combination of benzoic and salicylic acids in a novel aqueous vanishing cream formulation. J Am Acad Dermatol 1987; 16:136–138.

Roberts SOB, Mackenzie DWR. Mycology. In: Rook A, Wilkinson DS, Ebling FJG, et al, eds. Textbook of dermatology, 4th ed. Vol 2. Oxford: Blackwell Scientific, 1986; 885–936.

SYSTEMIC DISEASES

ACTINOMYCOSIS

GREGORY A. FILICE, M.D.

Actinomycosis is an indolent infectious disease caused by *Actinomyces israelii* or one of several other anaerobic or microaerophilic actinomycetes that normally inhabit the human oral cavity. The disease is characterized by intense fibrosis and discharge of pus containing characteristic granules.

Actinomycosis takes one of several distinct clinical syndromes. The most common is cervicofacial disease, which is the result of direct spread from an oral lesion, usually a dental or gingival infection. Thoracic actinomycosis results from aspiration of infected material from the oral cavity or, less commonly, from direct spread through the mediastinum. Usually, there is clinical evidence of tooth decay or other oral pathology in cases of thoracic actinomycosis. Since good oral hygiene is difficult to maintain in mentally subnormal children, they suffer from cervicofacial and thoracic actinomycosis more commonly than other children. Actinomycetes are passed transiently through the gastrointestinal tract, and abdominal disease follows escape of the organisms into surrounding tissues or spaces, frequently from the appendix. Perianal disease follows escape of organisms from the rectum. *A. israelii* frequently colonizes intrauterine devices or other foreign bodies in the female genital tract. Rarely, such colonization gives rise to genitourinary actinomycosis. Bloodborne, disseminated actinomycosis occurs rarely.

A. israelii is the most common organism associated with actinomycosis, but *Actinomyces naeslundii*, *Actinomyces viscosus*, *Actinomyces meyeri*, and *Arachnia propionica* have all been implicated in typical cases of human actinomycosis. Lesions of actinomycosis often contain other bacteria, referred to as "concomitant bacteria," which are usually from the same mucosal niche as the actinomycetes. These concomitant bacteria may contribute to the pathogenesis of actinomycosis.

Certain features are common to all forms of actinomycosis. The disease begins insidiously and pursues a chronic, indolent course. The typical lesion is an abscess surrounded by intense fibrosis and eventual scarring. Actinomycosis tends to spread across tissue planes, and draining sinuses are common. The disease typically presents with swelling and induration. Lesions contain characteristic granules up to 4 mm in size, which consist of masses of filaments. Granules are often found in the drainage from lesions and are important clues to the etiology. They can often be detected in gauze dressings placed over draining lesions. Granules are also observed in drainage from cases of mycetoma, including cases associated with *Nocardia* and *Streptomyces* that might be confused morphologically with *Actinomyces* species. Granules are occasionally found in infected tissues of patients with other forms of nocardiosis, but they are rare in pus from such patients.

The diagnosis of actinomycosis depends on recognition of the typical clinical signs and symptoms along with microbiological evidence of disease with *Actinomyces* species or *A. propionica.* The presence of typical granules is a strong clue to the diagnosis, but they are often not found. Since the organisms associated with actinomycosis are part of the normal flora, their isolation from mucosal surfaces or lesions that might be contaminated with such flora does not establish the diagnosis. Instead, organisms must be isolated from otherwise sterile body sites or they must be seen within tissue sections. Surgical biopsy for histopathology and culture is often necessary to make the diagnosis.

Organisms associated with actinomycosis are sometimes found in association with cases of other syndromes (e.g., periapical tooth abscess, tonsillitis, anaerobic empyema). Unless the symptoms or signs are suggestive of actinomycosis, these cases should be considered anaerobic or mixed infections and treated like infections associated with other anaerobic oral flora.

SPECIFIC THERAPY

Penicillin is the drug of choice and should be given in large dosages and for a prolonged period (Table 1). For extensive, well-established infections, 250,000 U of aqueous penicillin G per kilogram should be given intravenously in four to six divided doses until the infection is substantially improved, usually a period of 2 to 4 weeks. In less extensive infections, intravenous therapy can be given for a shorter time or 50 mg penicillin V per kilogram can be given orally in four divided doses. I administer 40 mg probenecid per kilogram per day in two divided doses (up to 1 g twice daily) in conjunction with oral

TABLE 1 Antimicrobial Therapy for Actinomycosis

Antimicrobial	Parenteral Therapy		Oral Therapy	
	Daily Dosage	Interval (hr)	Daily Dosage	Interval (hr)
Drug of choice				
Penicillin	250,000 U/kg	4–6	50 mg/kg	6
Preferred alternatives*				
Tetracycline†	30 mg/kg	6	50 mg/kg	6
Clindamycin	40 mg/kg	6–8	25 mg/kg	6
Other alternatives‡				
Erythromycin	50 mg/kg	6	40 mg/kg	6
Chloramphenicol	50 mg/kg	6	50 mg/kg	6
Rifampin	Unavailable		10 mg/kg	12–24
Sulfadiazine	75–100 mg/kg	4–6	150 mg/kg	6–8

* Substantial clinical experience indicates that these antimicrobials are likely to be effective.
† Tetracycline should not be given to children under 8 years of age.
‡ Limited clinical experience and/or in vitro susceptibility testing indicate that these drugs are likely to be effective.

penicillin to slow excretion of the drug. Some authors recommend that antibiotic concentrations in blood be measured to ensure that absorption is adequate. Intravenous therapy should be used initially in cases of central nervous system infection or disseminated infection. Side effects of penicillin are most commonly allergic and include rash, hives, anaphylaxis, gastric upset, seizures, and other central nervous system (CNS) dysfunctions. Among other beta-lactams, ampicillin and cephalothin are active in vitro. Cephalexin and semisynthetic penicillins are considerably less active.

Other drugs that may be useful are listed in Table 1. Tetracycline has been used with good results, but it should not be given to children younger than 8 years of age because it interferes with normal bone development. Side effects of tetracycline include gastrointestinal irritation, hepatitis, fatty liver, azotemia, and hypersensitivity. Other tetracycline derivatives appear active in vitro, but there is less clinical experience with them. Clindamycin is effective, but it is sometimes associated with diarrhea, including *Clostridium difficile* colitis, and it is expensive. Clindamycin also can cause skin rashes and other forms of hypersensitivity.

There is less experience with other drugs, but sulfadiazine, erythromycin, and chloramphenicol have been associated with success in a few cases. Optimal dosages of these other drugs are not well established. Metronidazole is not effective. Crystalluria can occur with sulfonamide therapy and adequate hydration should be maintained. Other side effects of sulfonamides include hypersensitivity, hemolytic anemia, myelotoxicity, and hepatitis. Side effects of erythromycin therapy include gastrointestinal irritation, hypersensitivity, cholestatic jaundice, and reversible hearing loss with large dosages. Side effects of chloramphenicol therapy include hypersensitivity, reversible erythroid suppression, idiosyncratic aplastic anemia, and the gray syndrome.

In vitro tests of susceptibility of *A. israelii* and related organisms to antimicrobials are used in research, but methods are not standardized, and the tests have not been shown to be reliable guides to therapy in individual cases. The choice of antimicrobials in individual cases should be based on clinical experience.

Patients should be followed carefully and appropriate therapy should give rise to steady improvement. Since actinomycosis results in tissue destruction and fibrosis, the response to therapy is usually slow. Failure of the disease to respond usually indicates that a lesion has not been adequately drained (see following) or that adequate medication is not being taken. Occasionally, concomitant bacteria are present that do not respond to the primary therapy. If drainage has been established and the disease does not respond to appropriate antimicrobials, antimicrobials active against any concomitant bacteria that have been isolated from the patient should be added.

Therapy should be continued for 6 to 12 months because actinomycosis has a marked tendency to relapse. The exact duration should depend on the location and extent of the disease and the rapidity of the response to therapy. Central nervous system, abdominal, bone, or disseminated disease should be treated for 12 months or longer.

Uterine colonization with *Actinomyces* in women with intrauterine devices is common, but the risk of actinomycosis is very small. Whether the device should be removed in asymptomatic colonized women is unknown. The decision should take into account the appropriateness of other birth control strategies for each patient. The device should be removed when symptoms are attributable to *Actinomyces* infection of the uterus. In addition, mild endometritis associated with *Actinomyces* should be managed by short-term antibiotic therapy. More extensive infection should be managed like other cases of actinomycosis.

SURGICAL MANAGEMENT

Surgical biopsy may be necessary to establish the diagnosis. Beyond that, surgical therapy should be used as it is for other infectious diseases. Abscesses in most locations should be drained, but lung abscesses usually respond to medical therapy. Sinus tracts resistant to antimicrobial therapy rarely require radical excision.

SUGGESTED REFERENCES

Golden N, Cohen H, Weissbrot J, Silverman S. Thoracic actinomycosis in childhood. Clin Pediatr 1985; 24:646–650.
Lerner PI. Susceptibility of pathogenic actinomycetes to antimicrobial compounds. Antimicrob Agents Chemother 1974; 5:302–309.
Nelson JD, Hermann DW. Oral penicillin therapy for thoracic actinomycosis. Pediatr Infect Dis 1986; 5:594–595.
Weese WC, Smith IM. A study of 57 cases of actinomycosis over a 36-year period. Arch Intern Med 1975; 135:1562–1568.

ANTHRAX

LAURENCE B. GIVNER, M.D.

Anthrax is rare in the United States, occurring primarily among textile workers. The disease occurs in three forms: cutaneous, inhalation, and gastrointestinal. Cutaneous disease accounts for 95 percent of all cases; gastrointestinal disease has not been reported in this country. Cutaneous anthrax is associated with little morbidity and no mortality if it is recognized and treated appropriately. Inhalation anthrax is almost always fatal. Any form of anthrax can be complicated by sepsis or meningitis, which are fatal in most cases.

ANTIMICROBIAL THERAPY

Penicillin is the drug of choice for infections caused by *Bacillus anthracis*. Penicillin resistance is extremely rare. Alternative drugs for penicillin-sensitive patients include erythromycin and, for patients at least 8 years of age, tetracycline. Chloramphenicol also may be used.

Mild cases of cutaneous anthrax can be treated orally with potassium penicillin V, 7.5 mg per kilogram of body weight given every 6 hours for 1 week. If extensive local lesions or moderate systemic symptoms are present, initial therapy should be administered by the intramuscular route, 35,000 U of procaine penicillin G per kilogram per day in two divided doses. As the edema subsides (usually after a few days), therapy can be administered orally. While local edema and systemic symptoms respond to antimicrobial therapy, the evolution of the anthrax pustule is not altered by such therapy. Also, regional adenopathy may persist for weeks and is not an indication for continued antibiotic therapy.

Inhalation anthrax requires penicillin G administered by continuous intravenous drip, 80,000 U per kilogram of body weight over the first hour and then 320,000 U per kilogram per 24 hours. In light of a synergistic effect in experimental disease, streptomycin, 15 to 30 mg per kilogram per day, should be administered in conjunction with penicillin. Antimicrobial therapy for inhalation anthrax should be continued for at least 14 days.

Gastrointestinal disease, sepsis, or meningitis should be treated with penicillin, as outlined for inhalation anthrax.

SUPPORTIVE CARE

Topical antibiotics have no effect on the lesions of cutaneous anthrax, which should be covered with a dry, sterile dressing. If the patient is hospitalized, secretion precautions should be observed and contaminated dressings should be sterilized to destroy spores. Within 6 to 24 hours of initiation of appropriate antimicrobial therapy, the lesions are sterile. Surgical excision during the acute phase should be avoided because this can intensify symptoms. Reconstructive surgery can be considered after convalescence. Systemic steroid therapy may be of benefit to patients with extensive edema of the head, neck, or upper thorax. Because such edema can compromise the airway, patency of the airway should be monitored closely.

Patients with inhalation anthrax may require respiratory support because of impingement on the airway of mediastinal lymph nodes or because of primary lung involvement. Inhalation anthrax requires strict isolation.

Systemic steroid therapy is sometimes of benefit to patients with anthrax meningitis. Close monitoring of fluids is vital in patients with meningitis and in patients demonstrating signs of shock, which can complicate any form of anthrax. Fluid losses may be extensive in gastrointestinal anthrax.

PREVENTION

High-risk employees in the textile industry and veterinarians should receive anthrax vaccine. The value of antibiotics administered prophylactically after exposure is uncertain. Human-to-human transmission of anthrax has not been documented.

SUGGESTED READING

Brachman PS. Anthrax. In: Hoeprich PD, ed. Infectious Diseases, 3rd ed. Philadelphia: Harper & Row, 1983; 939–944.

Christie AB. Anthrax. In: Infectious Diseases: Epidemiology and Clinical Practice. 3rd ed. New York: Churchill Livingstone, 1980; 703–721.

Knudson GB. Treatment of anthrax in man: history and current concepts. Milit Med 1986; 151:71–77.

BARTONELLOSIS

BARBARA W. STECHENBERG, M.D.

Bartonella bacilliformis, besides producing subclinical asymptomatic infection, can cause Oroya fever, a disease characterized by a severe febrile hemolytic anemia or, later, verruga peruana, an eruption of hemangiomalike lesions. The disease is restricted in its distribution to parts of Peru, Ecuador, and Colombia, which are areas inhabited by the sand fly vector.

Patients are either totally asymptomatic or have nonspecific findings such as headache, malaise, and occasional fever; in these patients the diagnosis is made on the basis of blood cultures. In patients who develop severe hemolytic anemia, peripheral blood smears usually demonstrate organisms parasitizing the erythrocytes. The presence of typical verruga in patients from the endemic area is pathognomonic of the disease.

The *B. bacilliformis* is susceptible to many antibiotics including penicillin, tetracycline, streptomycin, and chloramphenicol. However, the choice of antibiotics must be guided by considerations other than simple eradication of the *B. bacilliformis,* particularly the risk of intercurrent infection. Because concurrent salmonellosis has been associated with a high mortality rate in this disease, chloramphenicol is the drug of choice, since it is usually effective against both organisms. Chloramphenicol should be used in a dosage of 50 to 75 mg per kilogram per day given in four divided doses, either orally or intravenously, depending on the severity of the illness. The fever usually abates within 24 hours, but patients should be treated for 7 to 10 days. Blood transfusions may be helpful during the period of severe anemia; it is preferable to obtain blood from patients who have recently recovered from bartonellosis as their erythrocytes appear to be more resistant to parasitism.

Specific treatment for verruga peruana usually is not necessary, although oral tetracycline, 30 mg per kilogram per day in four divided doses for 10 to 14 days, may aid the healing of the cutaneous lesion. Lesions that are particularly large or interfere with function may need to be surgically excised.

Prevention of infection requires control of the sand fly. For the community, this usually means spraying the interiors and exteriors of dwellings with insecticides. For the person, protection may be obtained by the use of insect repellent and bed netting and by removing oneself from endemic areas at night.

SUGGESTED READING

Stechenberg BW. Bartonellosis. In: Feigin RD, Cherry JD, eds. Textbook of pediatric infectious diseases. Philadelphia: WB Saunders, 1987; 1096–1098.

BOTULISM

SARAH S. LONG, M.D.

INFANT BOTULISM

Botulism occurs in infants under 1 year of age when seemingly natural events can allow both the acquisition of spores and the temporary susceptibility of the intestine to colonization by *C. botulinum,* elaboration of toxin in vivo, and absorption. Rapidly progressive symptoms occasionally result in sudden infant death, but the more common form of illness is paralysis, which descends progressively and symmetrically from muscles innervated by cranial nerves to muscles of the trunk and limbs. Atony of the bowel and bladder is also present. Organisms are confined to the lumen of the gut, and toxin is usually not present in measurable amounts in serum. The majority of cases are caused by *C. botulinum,* producing neurotoxin types A and B. Recently, disease resulting from types E and F as well as disease caused by botulinal neurotoxins produced by other *Clostridium* species have been reported. Diagnosis is confirmed when a sterile filtrate of the patient's stool is positive in the mouse lethality-neutralization assay (available almost exclusively at State Laboratories and at the Centers for Disease Control, Atlanta, Georgia).

Although infant botulism is a toxicoinfection, no specific anti-infective or antitoxic agents are routinely given for treatment. Most patients have paralysis of the muscles of respiration and require mechanical ventilation for 2 to 3 weeks. Nutritional and respiratory support are sufficient to effect complete recovery, which occurs with ultrasprouting of new nerve endings. Peculiarly, clinical recovery proceeds despite continued proliferation of botulinal organisms and toxin in the intestine. The success of supportive therapy has made it difficult to use specifically anticlostridial therapies, which incur risk of adverse effects.

Antitoxin is not generally given because (1) by tests performed on serum, there is usually no toxin "available" for neutralization, (2) no benefit has been noted in the few instances when it has been used, and (3) the only product available is an equine preparation, which can cause anaphylaxis or serum sickness. Recent reports from Italy and the Centers for Disease Control in Atlanta suggest that more patients than was previously appreciated have toxin in serum (as many as 15 percent) and could theoretically benefit from administration of botulinal antitoxin. Adults whose guts have presumably been made susceptible by disease and antibiotics are being recognized as having the infant form of botulism. Their prognosis does not appear to be as favorable as that of infants. We eagerly await the availability of human botulinal immune globulin currently under development.

Antibiotics are not generally given. Penicillin and its derivatives, clostridicidal in vitro, have been administered to infants with botulism; their use has neither hastened clinical recovery nor halted proliferation of clostridia or toxin in the intestine. Orally administered vancomycin (which is not absorbed systemically) would be expected to be rapidly clostridicidal. Some speculate, however, that a massive release of toxin consequent to cell death could suddenly lead to adverse clinical effects. I think this is unlikely, considering other models of clostridial disease and vancomycin usage. Aminoglycosidic agents are contraindicated as they also cause neuromuscular blockade, and their administration to infants with botulism has been temporally associated with respiratory failure. Otitis media, aspiration pneumonia, and urinary tract infection (catheter-related or not) are the major infective complications of botulism and require antimicrobial therapy.

The patient need not be isolated, and contacts need not be treated in any special way. Although the offending botulinal spores can usually be found in the patient's home environment, honey is the only practically avoidable source of spores. Reinfection or second cases in family members or close contacts have not been recognized.

FOODBORNE BOTULISM

Foodborne botulism, a neurologic disorder that results from the pure intoxication of eating tainted food, rarely occurs in childhood because children usually do not enjoy foodstuffs that are subject to contamination. Clinical diagnosis is confirmed when toxin is identified in the patient's serum or stool and in the contaminated food. Trivalent antitoxin (types A, B, and E) of equine origin should be obtained through the Centers for Disease Control (404/329-3753 from 8 AM to 4:30 PM; 404/329-2888 on nights, weekends, and federal holidays) and administered immediately. One vial of antitoxin (approximately 10 ml) is administered intravenously, and one vial is given intramuscularly. The stomach should be emptied if ingestion of contaminated food has occurred within a few hours in a symptomatic individual, or regardless of time elapsed in an asymptomatic individual. Purgatives and high enemas are recommended unless paralytic ileus is present. Guanidine hydrochloride has been used in adults in an attempt to antagonize neuromuscular blockade. Recently studied in a double-blind crossover fashion, it had no beneficial effect. Supportive care is the mainstay of therapy. Despite this, the mortality in foodborne botulism is significant.

WOUND BOTULISM

Wound botulism occurs when spores contaminating a wound germinate and produce toxin. Neurologic abnormalities are much more impressive than the appearance of the wound. Diagnosis is confirmed when *C. botulinum* is recovered from the wound or toxin from the serum. Thorough debridement, irrigation, and drainage of the wound and supportive care during paralysis are the most important aspects of therapy. Trivalent antitoxin is given prior to debridement. Dosage and administration are the same as for foodborne botulism. Anticlostridial agents such as penicillin or vancomycin are usually given parenterally, although they may not penetrate into these wounds, which are characteristically avascular. Their therapeutic usage is not clearly beneficial. At the time of injury, the prophylactic usage of antibiotics does not prevent the development of wound botulism. Neither antitoxin nor toxoid is routinely given prophylactically. Cleansing and vigorous irrigation of wounds are the most effective forms of prophylaxis and may have greater efficacy than the limited spectrum of bug–drug interactions.

SUGGESTED READING

Arnon SS. Infant botulism: anticipating the second decade. J Infect Dis 1986; 154:201–206.

Long SS. Botulism in infancy. Pediatr Infect Dis 1984; 3:266–271.

BRUCELLOSIS

JAY P. SANFORD, M.D.

Brucellosis is a zoonosis, a disease of animals transmissible to humans, but not transmissible from human to human in nature. It is a systemic disease with acute or insidious onset, characterized by fever and nonlocalizing symptoms, headache, insomnia, anorexia, myalgia, and arthralgia. In contrast with the frequency of symptoms, objective physical signs are usually absent. Leukocyte counts are usually normal. Brucellosis is one of the infections typically categorized as being associated with normal erythrocyte sedimentation rates.

Of the six species of *Brucella*, *B. melitensis*, *B. abortus*, *B. suis*, and *B. canis* are pathogenic for humans while *B. ovis* and *B. neotomae* are not. *B. melitensis* is the most invasive and produces the most severe disease. *B. suis* often causes localized suppurative disease. In the United States, infection is most often associated with consumption of unpasteurized milk or milk products such as cheese from cows, goats, or sheep. Abbatoir workers are exposed occupationally. Children may also be exposed to *B. canis* through contact with stray dogs.

In the United States as a result of adoption of dairy product pasteurization and the bovine brucellosis eradication program, brucellosis has become uncommon; only 84 cases were reported to the Centers for Disease Control in 1986. The proportion of cases in children and adolescents is 2 to 10 percent. In children as in adults, there is a male predominance (6:1). Because of its overall low rate of occurrence and even lower frequency in children, diagnosis depends on a high index of suspicion and a detailed history of contacts with animals and food habits. Specific laboratory diagnosis is based on isolation of the organism from blood, other body fluids, or tissues. Primary isolation of *B. abortus* requires a 10 percent carbon dioxide atmosphere, and growth may require up to 4 weeks incubation. An agglutination titer of greater than 1:160, especially with IgG antibodies, provides for a strong presumptive diagnosis. A "routine" brucella agglutination test does not detect antibodies to *B. canis.*

SPECIFIC TREATMENT

Recovery from brucellosis without treatment is usual, but morbidity is often pronounced. Fatality is 2 percent or less.

Brucellae are amongst the classic intracellular parasites, where they may be protected from the lethal effects of some of the antibiotics that are effective in vitro. Early institution of specific antimicrobial therapy significantly reduces morbidity and complications. It is unclear as to whether antimicrobial therapy alters the course of chronic brucellosis. The regimens recommended are based on historic controls; no randomized double-blind studies have been reported.

Tetracyclines have been the agents of choice. Initial clinical response—that is, defervescence and resolution of symptoms within 3 to 10 days—is reported in 72 to 100 percent of adults. Relapse occurs in 10 to 20 percent of patients. In children over 7 years of age, the dosage of tetracycline is 40 mg per kilogram per day, given orally or intravenously in divided doses every 6 hours. The intravenous dosage should not exceed 2.0 g per day regardless of weight because of the potential for serious hepatotoxicity. Doxycycline (100 mg twice daily) has been effective in adults; however, data in children are lacking. Treatment with tetracycline should be continued for 21 days. With severe disease or infections with *B. suis,* combined therapy with tetracycline plus streptomycin, 20 to 30 mg per kilogram per day intramuscularly in divided doses every 12 hours for the first 10 days of the 3-week regimen, reduces the rate of relapse and development of localized complications. Aside from the hazard of dental staining in young children, tetracycline treatment has been less successful than in adults. Trimethoprim–sulfamethoxazole (TMP 10 mg per kilogram/SMZ 50 mg per kilogram per day) orally in divided doses every 12 hours for at least 4 weeks has resulted in excellent clinical response (90 percent) with low relapse rates (5 percent). Side effects included mild anemia in one-quarter of patients. Administration of folinic acid prevents the hematotoxicity. In experimental infections rifampin has been superior to tetracycline. In Europe, rifampin has been used as sole agent therapy in *B. melitensis* infection. However, because of the potential for emergence of rifampin-resistant organisms, use in combination with tetracycline or trimethoprim-sulfamethoxazole has been recommended. Although data are limited, a regimen of rifampin, 15 to 20 mg per kilogram per day given orally in divided doses every 12 hours, plus tetracycline for 3 weeks or rifampin plus trimethoprim-sulfamethoxazole for 4 weeks should be considered if the patient relapses after tetracycline-streptomycin or trimethoprim-sulfamethoxazole. Rifampin should also be used in the rare patient with brucella meningitis.

In adults, antimicrobial therapy may be associated with a worsening of symptoms, an increase in fever, and hypotension analagous to the Jarish-Herxheimer reaction in the treatment of spirochetal disease. Such reactions have been minimized with corticosteroid therapy, prednisone 1 mg per kilogram per day given orally in divided doses every 8 hours. In my experience, corticosteroids are seldom indicated.

In localized brucellosis, surgical drainage of abscesses should be performed. An antibiotic regimen of tetracycline–streptomycin or trimethoprim–sulfamethoxazole should be administered in conjunction with surgical drainage.

SUGGESTED READING

Buchanan TM, Faber LC, Feldman RA. Brucellosis in the United States. 1960–1972. Medicine 1974; 53:403–413.
Daikos GK, Papapolyzos N, Manketos N, et al. Trimethoprim-sulfamethoxazole in brucellosis. J Infect Dis 1973; 128:5731–5733.
Havas L. Problems and new development in the treatment of acute and chronic brucellosis in man. Acta Tropica 1980; 37:281–286.

CAT SCRATCH DISEASE

ANDREW M. MARGILETH, M.D.

Cat scratch disease (CSD) characteristically presents as a chronic (3 weeks or longer) lymphadenopathy caused by a gram-negative bacillus and is usually a benign, self-limited illness. Management consists of reassurance, supportive care, and use of analgesics for symptoms such as headache, malaise, and fever. Specific treatment is difficult because no chemotherapeutic agent has been effective to date. In the majority of patients no active therapy is needed.

Once the diagnosis is made, the parent and/or patient should be reassured that the cause of the lymphadenopathy is not a malignancy and that the disease will regress spontaneously over a 2- to 4-month period. Lymph node tenderness usually decreases and disappears within 1 to 2 weeks. If suppuration occurs, needle aspiration relieves painful adenopathy and provides material for culture and for skin test antigen. After one or two aspirates the patient usually becomes symptom-free within 24 to 48 hours. If fluid reaccumulates, reaspiration may be needed. Suppuration occurs in about 12 to 15 percent of patients. I do not recommend incision and drainage because chronic sinus tract discharge may persist for several months. The technique for needle aspiration follows: after washing with Betadine cleanser, an 18- or 19-gauge needle is inserted through 1 to 2 cm of normal unanesthetized skin at the base of the mass to avoid a chronic sinus tract in the event that a tuberculous lesion is present. Surgical excision of the nodes is usually not indicated unless one suspects a noninfectious etiology such as a neoplasm.

No antimicrobial drugs can be recommended because patients with CSD consistently do not respond to antibiotics. One possible documented exception to this was an adult with severe cat scratch disease who was treated with intravenous trimethoprim-sulfamethoxazole and appeared to respond. Initially if the patient presents with moderate to severe acute lymphadenitis, an antibiotic against beta-hemolytic *Streptococcus* and *Staphylococcus aureus* may be prescribed for 7 to 10 days. The use of steroids to reduce lymphadenopathy is not recommended. Excisional biopsy of the node may be necessary in selected patients, particularly adults, for diagnostic purposes or to relieve persistent pain. We advise the patient to avoid direct trauma to the area of lymphadenitis because in our experience spontaneous drainage has occurred in about 5 percent of our patients after trauma.

In patients with oculoglandular disease of Parinaud, treatment should be symptomatic. Secondary infection of the eye is rare. Surgical removal of the conjunctival granuloma or polyp appears to shorten the course of the illness.

In the patient who develops encephalopathy, supportive care is the primary treatment since spontaneous recovery over a 5- to 10-day period is expected. Complete recovery from this rare complication has occurred in about 98 percent of reported patients; therefore, invasive procedures should be avoided. Initially an electroencephalogram is usually abnormal. Recently, computed tomographic scans have shown transient nonspecific abnormalities suggestive of cerebritis.

If families are concerned about the advisability of keeping the cat or kitten that may have been the vector of the cat scratch bacillus, I recommend keeping the cat. About 5 to 8 percent of family members develop the disease and the healthy animal seems to carry the organism for only a few weeks. Generally the prognosis for patients with CSD is excellent. Recurrences have been documented in two or three cases, but are extremely rare. No fatalities from CSD have been reported.

The opinions and assertions contained herein are the private views of the author and are not to be construed as official or as reflecting the views of the Uniformed Services University of the Health Sciences or of the Department of Defense.

SUGGESTED READING

Black JR, Harrington DA, Hatfield TL, et al. Life threatening cat scratch disease in an immunocompromised host. Arch Intern Med 1986; 146:394.
Lewis DW, Tucker SH. Central nervous system involvement in cat scratch disease. Pediatrics 1986; 77:714–721.
Margileth AM, Wear DJ, English CK. Systemic cat scratch disease: report of 23 patients with prolonged or severe recurrent bacterial infection. J Infect Dis 1987; 155:390–402.

CLOSTRIDIAL SEPSIS

JAY P. SANFORD, M.D.

Clostridial bacteremia poses a clinical paradox. Based on knowledge of the organisms and the toxins that they elaborate, one would anticipate that patients with clostridial bacteremia would be profoundly toxic. However, such is not necessarily the case. Several reports have noted a poor correlation between bacteremia and the clinical features of sepsis. Many patients with positive blood cultures recover without ever having the source detected. Management must be based on the clinical status of the patient. If the patient is not immunocompromised and does not appear clinically toxic, observation without initiation of specific treatment is appropriate.

SPECIFIC THERAPY

In the patient who is clinically septic or in the immunocompromised patient, especially the patient undergoing antineoplastic chemotherapy, prompt empiric therapy should be initiated.

Antibiotic Therapy

The antimicrobial regimen should be that employed in patients with gas gangrene. (See the chapter on *Gas Gangrene.*)

Hyperbaric Oxygen Therapy

As with gas gangrene, proof of the clinical efficacy of hyperbaric oxygen therapy is lacking. However, based on logic and analogy with gas gangrene, such therapy would appear to be reasonable. (See the chapter on *Gas Gangrene.*)

SUGGESTED READING

Nelson RM, Wilson RF, Osmer RL. Clostridium perfringens bacteremia, opportunist or killer? Am Surg 1985; 51:301–303.

Tikko SK, Distenfield A, Davidson M. Clostridium septicum septicemia with identical metastatic myonecroses in a granulocytopenic patient. Am J Med 1985; 79:256–258.

CYTOMEGALOVIRUS INFECTIONS

GAIL J. DEMMLER, M.D.

Cytomegalovirus (CMV) can cause severe illness in congenitally infected newborns, producing jaundice, hepatosplenomegaly, thrombocytopenia and petechiae, pneumonia, and severe central nervous system damage with microcephaly, intracerebral calcifications, chorioretinitis, and sensorineural deafness. In immunocompromised hosts, especially bone marrow and organ transplant recipients and patients with acquired immunodeficiency syndrome, CMV causes interstitial pneumonia, fever, leukopenia, colitis, hepatitis, and retinitis, and it may also enhance the host's susceptibility to superinfection.

TREATMENT OF ESTABLISHED CYTOMEGALOVIRUS INFECTIONS

Congenital Infection

Treatment of asymptomatic, congenitally infected infants is not currently indicated because the risk of experimental antiviral chemotherapy is not justifiable, even though 10 to 17 percent of these infants may later develop deafness and learning problems. Antiviral agents have been tried, however, in severely symptomatic infants congenitally infected with CMV because up to 90 percent of these infants may develop severe neurologic sequelae and deafness. It is hoped that by reducing or eliminating viral replication and, therefore, the length of illness and viral shedding in these infants, sequelae may be prevented. Idoxuridine, cytosine arabinoside, vidarabine, acyclovir, human leukocyte interferon-alpha, interferon inducers, and transfer factor all have been used on an experimental basis to try to treat a small number of symptomatic congenitally infected infants. None of these antivirals has demonstrated clinical efficacy, and only inconsistent and transient effects on viral excretion have been observed. The possible clinical benefits of a new, as yet unlicensed, antiviral agent, 9-(1,3-dihydroxy-2-propoxymethyl)-guanine (DHPG), an acyclic nucleoside analog of guanine with significant anticytomegalovirus activity, are unknown, but its pharmacokinetics, antiviral effects, and toxicities may soon be studied experimentally in small numbers of infants.

Organ and Bone Marrow Transplant Recipients

Cytomegalovirus commonly infects patients who have undergone marrow transplantation. It may cause myalgias, arthralgias, arthritis, fever, leukopenia, gastritis, colitis, hepatitis, and most important, interstitial pneumonia, which has a mortality rate up to 90 percent. Unfortunately, treatment of established CMV infections in bone marrow transplant recipients has not been encouraging. Vidarabine, human leukocyte interferon-alpha, acyclovir, vidarabine in combination with interferon, acyclovir in combination with interferon, CMV-specific hyperimmune globulin, and trisodium phosphonoformate have not shown any consistent antiviral or therapeutic effects. Even treatment with DHPG, alone or in combination with high-dose corticosteroids, has not decreased mortality or increased the duration of survival in these patients. However, some patients treated with DHPG show very impressive reduction in viral titer (more than 99 percent) in quantitative culture of lung tissue obtained before and after therapy. This significant antiviral effect suggests a potential role for this new antiviral agent, especially if the diagnosis of severe CMV disease is made early and therapy is instituted promptly.

A DHPG dosage regimen of 2.5 mg per kilogram given every 8 hours (7.5 mg per kilogram per day) has been shown to give mean peak and trough plasma concentrations of 30 and 6 micromol per liter, respectively, exceeding the in vitro mean inhibitory dose of DHPG for most strains of CMV. Higher-dosage regimens of 5 mg per kilogram every 12 hours (10 mg per kilogram per day) or even 15 mg per kilogram per day may be associated with marrow toxicities, especially neutropenia and thrombocytopenia. For children under 2 years of age, dosages of 100 mg per square meter every 8 hours and higher regimens up to 200 mg per square meter every 12 hours may be employed, though the pharmacokinetics of DHPG in young children have not yet been extensively studied. The drug should be infused over at least 1 hour in a solution containing a maximum concentration of 50 mg per milliliter. An initial 14-day course of therapy is recommended with a maximum recommended therapy of 30 days.

Antiviral response to DHPG should be monitored with twice-weekly urine, saliva, and bood cultures for CMV. Because the drug is excreted by the kidneys, a lower starting dosage regimen should be used in patients with renal insufficiency and adjusted according to creatinine clearance. The drug DHPG is also myelotoxic and should be used with extreme caution in patients with a past or present exposure to myelotoxic drugs. Daily complete blood counts and platelet counts should be performed and, if they fall to 30 to 50 percent of the baseline count (or an absolute neutrophil count of 500 or a platelet count less than 25,000), the dosage of DHPG should be decreased or treatment suspended. Because overwhelming viral infections may also cause neutropenia and thrombocytopenia, the distinction between drug toxicity and the effects of infection may be difficult. Though DHPG has been shown to produce testicular atrophy in laboratory animals, no accumulation of

the drug in the testes has yet been shown in humans. This potential toxicity is, however, an important consideration when treatment of children is considered. In addition to specific antiviral chemotherapy, general supportive measures, as well as a decrease in or withdrawal of immunosuppressive therapy when feasible, also may be helpful.

Renal and cardiac transplant recipients also may suffer from severe CMV disease, including fever, arthralgias, arthritis, malaise, leukopenia, hepatitis, retinitis, and pneumonia. Secondary bacterial and fungal infections, as well as graft rejection, may also occur in association with CMV infections in organ transplant recipients. Because the degree of immunosuppression is less in these patients than in bone marrow transplant patients, there is more hope therapeutic intervention may be successful.

Organ transplant recipients treated with vidarabine (10 mg per kilogram per day for 7 days) show a decrease in viral shedding but no clinical improvement. It is therefore doubtful that vidarabine will ever have a role in the treatment of CMV infections in transplant recipients. Intravenous acyclovir (ACV) (500 mg per square meter administered three times daily for at least 7 days) has been shown in a small randomized, placebo-controlled, double-blind trial to improve survival, accelerate resolution of fever and other clinical symptomatology, and clear viremia in renal transplant recipients with symptomatic CMV infections. Although CMV does not code for thymidine kinase and is therefore substantially less susceptible to ACV than the other herpesviruses, inhibition of some strains of CMV by ACV has been demonstrated in vitro. Therefore, in certain transplant recipients with severe or life-threatening CMV disease, high-dose ACV may prove of some benefit. Acyclovir causes renal toxicity, an important consideration in treating these patients. Renal function should be monitored closely and the ACV dosage adjusted according to creatinine clearance. Acyclovir should be administered by slow intravenous infusion (at least 1 hour) to avoid local phlebitis and precipitation of crystals in the renal tubules. The investigational drug DHPG also may be helpful in organ transplant recipients with severe life-threatening CMV infections. Early diagnosis and prompt institution of therapy are important, as well as supportive care and decrease or elimination of immunosuppressive therapy when feasible.

Acquired Immunodeficiency Syndrome Patients

Cytomegalovirus causes life-threatening pneumonia and colitis and sight-threatening retinitis in adult and pediatric patients with the acquired immunodeficiency syndrome (AIDS). The antiviral agent DHPG has been studied on a "compassionate use" basis in adult patients, as well as in a few children with AIDS, and treatment results in clinical and virologic improvement or cure in certain subgroups of patients. Sixty-nine to 100 percent of patients with CMV retinitis treated with DHPG respond favorably, with increased visual acuity and decreased retinal inflammation when treated with dosages varying from 7.5 to 15 mg per kilogram per day in divided doses every 8 to 12 hours for 14 days. Similarly up to 63 percent of patients with AIDS and CMV infections of the gastrointestinal (GI) tract may respond favorably, with decreased diarrhea and pain and virologic cure. However, only about 40 percent of patients with CMV pneumonitis and AIDS have shown a clinical or virologic response. Relapse of infection occurs in 80 to 100 percent of patients with AIDS and CMV retinitis, colitis, or pneumonia, so a repeat full course of therapy may be required, followed by a maintenance regimen. The success of maintenance regimens has been variable, with two to three doses per week of 2.5 mg per kilogram being associated with a high rate of relapse and regimens of 2.5 mg per kilogram given five times weekly being associated with neutropenia. The experience of using DHPG in children with AIDS and other immunodeficiencies, both congenital and acquired, is limited, but dosages of 100 mg per square meter every 8 hours to 200 mg per square meter every 12 hours may be tried. Dosages must be adjusted according to creatinine clearance (similar to ACV) and hematologic parameters should be monitored closely. Neutropenia or thrombocytopenia are indications for cessation of therapy, either temporarily or permanently.

PREVENTION OF CYTOMEGALOVIRUS INFECTIONS

Because treatment with antivirals for established CMV infections remains experimental, measures to prevent CMV infection should be employed whenever possible. Transplant recipients who are CMV seronegative and receive kidney, heart, or bone marrow transplants from CMV seropositive donors are at significant risk for acquiring symptomatic, primary CMV infections. Therefore, whenever possible, CMV seronegative recipients should receive transplants from CMV seronegative donors. Similarly, blood product transfusions, especially granulocyte transfusions but also red blood cell and platelet transfusions, from CMV seropositive donors may transmit CMV, and these products also should be from CMV seronegative donors. However, the large quantities of blood product transfusions required by transplant recipients, especially bone marrow transplant patients, makes this approach not always practical.

Passive immunization in bone marrow transplant recipients with cytomegalovirus immune plasma or globulin remains controversial mainly because studies have used different dosages (100 to 200 mg per kilogram) administered at different intervals (1 week before transplant and every 1 to 3 weeks following transplant) for varying lengths of time (60 to 120 days). Although the administration of cytomegalovirus immune globulin probably does not decrease the overall incidence of CMV infections, it does appear to decrease the incidence of symptomatic CMV infections, including CMV pneumonia, in seronegative bone marrow transplant recipients who do not receive granulocyte transfusions or marrow from seropositive donors.

Active immunization with a live CMV vaccine using Towne strain appears to lower the incidence of severe CMV disease in renal transplant recipients, even in CMV seronegative patients who receive renal allografts from seropositive donors. In experimental trials, the vaccine induces both humoral and cellular immunity, is well-tolerated, and does not appear to reactivate during immunosuppression for renal transplantation. Clinical trials are in progress to answer questions of efficacy and of the long-term effects of the vaccine, such as oncogenicity, during prolonged immunosuppression.

The prophylactic use of antiviral agents, such as vidarabine, ACV, and interferon, has also been investigated. Although ACV administered before bone marrow transplantation and for 3 months after transplantation prevents recurrent herpes simplex infection in HSV-seropositive patients, it does not appear to affect the incidence of CMV infections in these patients. However, prophylactic administration of human leukocyte interferon-alpha has been shown in at least one trial to reduce the incidence of severe CMV disease in renal transplants.

Methods to prevent congenital CMV infections have not yet been developed. However, CMV-seronegative women who are pregnant probably should avoid intimate contact and wash their hands carefully after casual contact with persons known to be shedding CMV or who are very likely to be shedding the virus, such as young children who attend group day care. Infection with CMV can also be prevented in seriously ill CMV-seronegative neonates by using blood products from CMV-seronegative donors or products such as frozen-thawed-deglycerolized red blood cells.

SUGGESTED READING

Balfour HH Jr, Bean B, Mitchell CD, et al. Acyclovir in immunocompromised patients with cytomegalovirus disease: a controlled trial at one institution. Am J Med 1982; 73(1A):241–248.

Bowden RA, Sayers M, Flournoy N, et al. Cytomegalovirus immune globulin and seronegative blood products to prevent primary cytomegalovirus infection after marrow transplantation. N Engl J Med 1986; 314:1006–1010.

Collaborative DHPG Treatment Study Group. Treatment of serious cytomegalovirus infections with 9-(1,3-dihydroxy-2-propoxymethyl)guanine in patients with AIDS and other immunodeficiencies. N Engl J Med 1986; 314:801–805.

Plotkin SA, Friedman HM, Fleisher GR, et al. Towne-vaccine-induced prevention of cytomegalovirus disease after renal transplantation. Lancet 1984; 1:528–530.

Shepp DH, Dandliker PS, deMiranda P, et al. Activity of 9-[2-hydroxy-1-(hydroxymethyl)ethoxymethyl]guanine in the treatment of cytomegalovirus pneumonia. Ann Intern Med 1985; 103:368–373.

EPSTEIN-BARR VIRUS INFECTION (INFECTIOUS MONONUCLEOSIS)

CIRO V. SUMAYA, M.D., M.P.H.T.M.

Epstein-Barr virus (EBV) infections manifesting as infectious mononucleosis occur in all age groups of children. In the very young, the diagnosis is more likely to require Epstein-Barr virus–specific serologic testing because the characteristic heterophil antibody response may not be detected. Primary Epstein-Barr virus infections that present as isolated manifestations, i.e., tonsillopharyngitis, thrombocytopenia purpura, acute neurologic disorders, or an incomplete infectious mononucleosis picture, may not be recognized as being caused by EBV unless specific serologic testing is used. The comments in this section are directed to EBV infectious mononucleosis, but could pertain to other EBV-induced disorders as well.

ROUTINE INFECTIOUS MONONUCLEOSIS

Children, like adults, with routine or uncomplicated infectious mononucleosis are managed principally by measures to control or minimize symptomatology. Aspirin or acetominophen can be used to control fever as well as to alleviate discomfort from headache and throat inflammation. Gargling with warm saline water also provides some relief from pharyngeal discomfort. Reduction of activity and bed rest usually are dictated by the tolerance of the patient. It is generally agreed that contact sports or activities with a potential for trauma or stress to the abdomen (vigorous exercise, heavy lifting) should be avoided during the period that the spleen is palpable, and thus presumably enlarged.

Earlier findings of an increased frequency of group A streptococci in the throat of patients with acute infectious mononucleosis has not been supported by recent reports. It remains unclear, therefore, if those patients with a positive throat culture should be treated with an antibacterial drug. This author believes it is prudent to treat these patients with a 10-day course of oral penicillin V, 125 to 250 mg given four times a day, or alternately, erythromycin at equivalent doses, because it is not possible to distinguish an acute streptococcal pharyngitis from the colonized state or from the EBV precipitated inflammation of the pharynx. Parenteral benzathine penicillin, 600,000 U given intramuscularly for children weighing less than 60 lb and 1.2 million U for larger children, may be necessary if the patient refuses to swallow. Ampicillin is not recommended because it may elicit a hypersensitivity-related maculopapular rash. The latter hypersensitivity phenomenon has not been as noticeable in the young childhood patient, possibly because of the high rate (approaching 25 percent) of "spontaneous" rashes that develop in acute EBV infectious mononucleosis episodes in this age group.

Corticosteroids have been administered to alleviate some of the symptomatology experienced during routine infectious mononucleosis. Recommendations for their use are unclear, at best, because of insufficient data showing definite substantial efficacy. The apparent advantage of an earlier resolution of pharyngitis reported in steroid-treated patients may be minimized by the similar degree of clinical symptomatology noted in the steroid- and placebo-treated groups within 3 days of treatment. Corticosteroid therapy showed a tendency to decrease the stay of hospitalized patients compared with placebo-treated patients, but the difference was not statistically significant. On the other hand, the mean number of febrile days is probably significantly decreased in moderately ill patients receiving steroids instead of placebo therapy. Even in these cases, however, the patients may become febrile after the steroids are discontinued. Moreover, careful consideration must be given to the potential adverse effects of corticosteroid administration, such as bacterial superinfection, before using them in patients with routine infectious mononucleosis.

The administration of oral acyclovir may reduce the duration of excretion of infectious virus in saliva from patients with acute infectious mononucleosis, but it does not significantly alter the course of the clinical illness from that with placebo therapy.

Many other treatments have been advocated or used, but without proved success, including gamma globulin, convalescent serum, and methisazone. Recent reports of the efficacy of metronidazole and tindazole require more critical evaluation before their general use is considered.

COMPLICATED INFECTIOUS MONONUCLEOSIS

Approximately one of every five children with infectious mononucleosis develops one or more significant complications, usually involving the respiratory tract, neurologic, or hematologic systems (Table 1).

Severe airway obstruction necessitating intensive care monitoring has been treated with a short course (2 to 5 days) of corticosteroids, with reportedly excellent results. The corticosteroids are given orally or parenterally at dosages equivalent to about 2 mg per kilogram per day of prednisone. Unfortunately, critically controlled studies evaluating the true efficacy of corticosteroids in this situation have not been adequate. This author recommends their use with progressively worsening respiratory distress. Supplemental oxygen and blood gas determinations may be necessary adjunctive measures. If the airway embar-

TABLE 1 Complications Present in Childhood Epstein-Barr Virus Infectious Monoculeosis

Complications	No. of Children (% in Parentheses)
Respiratory tract	
Pneumonia	6 (5.3)
Severe airway obstruction*	4 (3.5)
Neurologic	
Seizures	4 (3.5)
Meningitis/encephalitis	2 (1.8)
Peripheral facial nerve paralysis	1 (0.9)
Guillain-Barré syndrome	1 (0.9)
Hematologic	
Thrombocytopenia with hemorrhages	4 (3.5)
Hemolytic anemia	1 (0.9)
Infectious	
Bacteremia	1 (0.9)
Recurrent tonsillopharyngitis	3 (2.7)
Liver: jaundice	2 (1.8)
Renal: glomerulonephritis	1 (0.9)
Genital: orchitis	1 (0.9)
Total	31†

* Criteria consisted of nasal alar flaring, suprasternal retractions, or stridor.
† Because four children had more than one of these complications, this total is composed of 24 different children, or 21.2 percent of the study group [from Sumaya & Ench, 1985. Reprinted by permission of the American Academy of Pediatrics.]

rassment progresses in spite of this treatment, an artificial airway (endotracheal tube) may need to be inserted. A tracheostomy is an alternative measure to relieve the airway obstruction; an emergency tonsillectomy is now an obsolete consideration.

Some degree of thrombocytopenia is a common manifestation of infectious mononucleosis. This complication, including cases with platelet counts less than 20,000 per cubic millimeter or associated with hemorrhagic manifestations, normally resolve spontaneously within 2 to 4 weeks. Uncommonly, and only in quite severe or persistent forms of thrombocytopenia, is oral corticosteroid therapy indicated. Splenectomy is a last resort in recalcitrant cases. A similar therapeutic approach should be used with the rare and usually transient episodes of significant hemolytic anemia. Blood transfusions may be necessary in selected patients with these hematologic complications.

The efficacy of corticosteroids in the management of systemic neurologic complications is even less clear. Again, adequate controlled studies evaluating their potential usefulness are lacking. Moreover, these complications also are usually transient and resolve spontaneously within several weeks after onset. If brain edema is associated with the neurologic problem, then costicosteroids should probably be administered.

Splenic rupture is an uncommon complication that is more likely to occur in the early convalescent state. Abdominal pain of any sort, but particularly pain that radiates to the left shoulder or pain in the left upper quadrant, should alert the physician to this possibility. Obtaining a hematocrit is not of much assistance in early stages, and may even give false assurance because the red cell volume decreases slowly following hemorrhaging.

Equivocal results have been obtained from the intravenous administration of acyclovir to a small group of patients with severe, often disseminated, forms of EBV infections. However, since no other viral-specific drug is available, it still should be used in these rare cases.

Despite the frequent occurrence of neutropenia in children with infectious mononucleosis, significant bacterial superinfections are quite uncommon. The neutropenia, not uncommonly below 500 cells per cubic millimeter, normally resolves spontaneously within 2 to 4 weeks. Nonetheless, patients with granulocyte counts that drop extremely low should be under close surveillance for bacterial superinfections, particularly if corticosteroids are being administered. Peritonsillar abscesses have gained increased attention recently as bacterial complications during the infectious mononucleosis episode. Drainage and antimicrobial therapy, based on the Gram stain and later culture results of the removed pus, are needed to treat this effectively.

Several reports now present specific laboratory data suggesting that chronic or continually reactivated EBV infections may produce a significant clinical syndrome in both adults and children. The more common clinical manifestations include fatigue, neuropsychological abnormalities, recurrent fever, and weight loss. Less common manifestations include arthritis, rashes, and at times, hepatosplenomegaly. A low level of serum gamma globulins found in some of these patients has been used as a rationale for evaluating the therapeutic efficacy of intravenous gamma globulin. Unfortunately, neither this form of therapy, the administration of oral and intravenous acyclovir, nor any other therapeutic modality tried thus far has been shown to have any significant efficacy in patients with suspected chronic EBV infections. The physician needs to be aware that other possibly treatable disorders, i.e., autoimmune or collagen–vascular diseases or tumors, may produce similar manifestations and should not be overlooked.

CONTROL OF TRANSMISSION

Isolation procedures generally are not indicated because (1) virus is secreted in saliva for many months following infectious mononucleosis, (2) a small amount of virus is secreted in saliva in 5 to 15 percent of healthy children and adults with prior, old EBV infections, and (3) low infection rates are seen in susceptible contacts. Moreover, the majority of adults and older children have already been exposed to the virus as young children.

The transmission of EBV through blood product transfusions, with the subsequent development of an infectious mononucleosislike illness, has been well documented. However, the frequency of this phenomenon is much less than that seen with cytomegalovirus. Blood banks routinely do not accept blood donations from individuals who have had infectious mononucleosis within 6 months.

There is limited interest in developing a vaccine against EBV. Recently, a glycoprotein of EBV, free of viral DNA, was found to be immunogenic and without significant side effects when inoculated into experimental animals. Clinical trials in human subjects may be forthcoming but not in the immediate future.

SUGGESTED READING

Klein E, Cochran JF, Buck RL. The effects of short-term corticosteroid therapy on the symptoms of infectious pharyngotonsillitis: a double blind study. J Am Coll Health Assoc 1969; 17:446–452.

Sumaya CV, Ench Y. Epstein-Barr virus infectious mononucleosis in children. I. Clinical and general laboratory findings. Pediatrics 1985; 75:1003–1010.

Sumaya CV, Ench Y. Epstein-Barr virus infectious mononucleosis in children. II. Heterophil antibody and viral-specific responses. Pediatrics 1985; 75:1011–1019.

Wolfe JA, Rowe LD. Upper airway obstruction in infectious mononucleosis. Ann Otol Rhinol Laryngol 1980; 89:430–433.

HERPES SIMPLEX VIRUS INFECTION

STEVE KOHL, M.D.

The diagnosis of herpes simplex virus (HSV) infection in typical situations, such as oral or genital disease, is usually not difficult on a clinical basis. It may be easily confirmed by Tzanck smear, cytology (both about 50 percent positive), new antigen detection tests (which are specific, but often not very sensitive, e.g., ELISA), or culture (taking 2 to 5 days). It is in the immunocompromised patient with atypical or chronic skin or mucosal lesions (ulcerative, hemorrhagic, vesicular, pustular), in the neonate, and in the patient with febrile encephalitis with focality (by clinical or electroencephologram criteria) that a high index of suspicion for HSV infection must be maintained. In the patient with encephalitis, a brain biopsy is strongly recommended to exclude other clinically similar conditions (over 50 percent of cases), which are often amenable to specific therapy.

In treating HSV infection, it is critical that the type of infection, defined both by anatomic setting (mucocutaneous, visceral, central nervous system) and by previous patient experience (i.e., primary illness versus recurrent illness), be known. Also important is the category of the host as normal or immunocompromised.

THERAPEUTIC ALTERNATIVES

Two agents are currently licensed for therapy of systemic or mucocutaneous HSV infections. These are acyclovir (Zovirax) and vidarabine (Vira-A). Several drugs are also licensed for therapy of ocular HSV infection (Table 1).

Because well-controlled clinical studies show acyclovir to be equal to, or superior to vidarabine,

TABLE 1 Therapy for HSV Infection in Children

Genital disease	Primary: acyclovir—oral, 200 mg 5 times a day for 10 days (1 capsule = 200 mg), intravenous—15 mg/kg/day in 3 divided doses for 5–7 days Recurrent: acyclovir—oral, 200 mg, 5 times a day for 5 days Suppressive: acyclovir—oral, 200 mg, 3 to 5 times a day for 6 months
Oral disease (primary)	As in primary genital infection, the oral dosage for children should not exceed 50 mg/kg/day*
Encephalitis	Acyclovir—intravenously, 30 mg/kg/day in 3 divided doses, for 10–14 days†
Neonatal	Acyclovir—intravenously, 30 mg/kg/day in 3 divided doses, for 10–14 days† (20 mg/kg divided q12h for premature infants) Vidarabine—intravenously, 30 mg/kg/day in 1 dose over 12-hour infusion for 10–14 days
Immuno-compromised patients	Acyclovir—intravenously, 15 mg/kg/day in 3 divided doses, duration as warranted clinically; orally, 200 mg, 3 to 5 times a day, not to exceed 50 mg/kg/day, duration as warranted clinically* Vidarabine—intravenously, 10 mg/kg/day in 1 dose over 12 hours
Ocular infection	Trifluorothymidine (Viroptic) 1% ophthalmic solution—1 drop every 2 hours, maximum 9 drops, then 1 drop every 4 hours (5 drops per day), not to exceed 21 days Vidarabine (Vira-A) 3% ophthalmic ointment—5 times a day, change to different agent if no healing in 7–9 days Idoxuridine (Stoxil) 0.1% ophthalmic solution or 0.5% ophthalmic ointment solution, 1 drop every hour during the day and every 2 hours during the night; ointment, 5 times a day every 4 hours and before bedtime, change to different agent if no healing occurs in 7–9 days

* This is an unlicensed use, and controlled trials in children have not been performed.

† Note the large dosage, which is the dosage found to be effective and nontoxic in these particular clinical conditions and patients.

and because it is relatively easy to administer, acyclovir has become the drug of choice for treating non-ocular HSV infection. The main dilemma for the practitioner is what manifestations of HSV warrant therapy and with which form of acyclovir (topical, oral, or intravenous). I outline the different types of HSV infections in normal hosts, immunocompromised hosts, and neonates, and specify my preferred therapy (see Table 1).

NORMAL HOST

Genital Disease—Primary Infection

This is often a moderately severe illness that lasts 2 to 3 weeks. In this clinical setting, all three forms of acyclovir have been shown to be of benefit. The topical form is the least useful (messy), and I can advise it only for individuals who want therapy but refuse oral medication ("must keep the body pure"). Oral acyclovir is the drug of choice for all forms of genital HSV. In patients ill enough to necessitate hospital admission, therapy often begins with intravenous acyclovir. These treatments reduce the duration of signs and symptoms by approximately 50 percent, and may prevent or modify complications. Local treatment should be aimed at keeping lesions dry and clean. Urinating while sitting in a bathtub may decrease urethral pain. Therapy of primary disease does not reduce the incidence of subsequent recurrent HSV infection and may make the first recurrence more severe (see the subsection on Immune Response under Acyclovir).

Genital Disease—Recurrent Infection

Although recurrent disease is a milder illness than the primary infection, use of oral acyclovir shortens the duration of signs and symptoms by approximately 50 percent and also decreases viral shedding. Its use should be individualized and is generally reserved for patients with severe or very frequent recurrences. Topical acyclovir has no efficacy in this setting.

Genital Disease—Suppressive Therapy

In patients with very severe or frequent recurrences or whose life-styles are altered by their illness, chronic suppressive therapy can markedly reduce the incidence of recurrence (75 to 90 percent reduction) in almost all patients. Use for this purpose must be carefully discussed with the patients and individualized. One must also remember that, although patients may not experience a clinical recurrence, they may still shed virus intermittently. To date there is no good explanation for the etiology of occasional breakthrough recurrences while patients are taking acyclovir. It does not appear to be associated with poor patient compliance or with acyclovir-resistant HSV

isolates. The drug is currently licensed only for 6-month periods of use, but studies over 12 months have shown continued efficacy without increased side effects. The main problem with the use of suppressive acyclovir is the patient's reluctance to stop its use. This is not irrational because, in most patients, cessation of therapy is associated with the onset of recurrences in 1 to 2 months or less. Often the first recurrence is more severe than the remembered severity of earlier episodes.

Oral Infections

There are no data as yet documenting the efficacy of acyclovir in primary oral infections (either gingivostomatitis or pharyngitis). Nevertheless, in patients ill enough to be hospitalized, especially when they are unable to swallow, we have used intravenous (15 mg per kilogram per day in three divided doses), and then oral (200 mg, three to five times a day, but not to exceed 50 mg per kilogram per day) acyclovir. There are no dosage recommendations or studies of oral acyclovir in pediatric patients. The recommended dosage given here is based on a 15 to 20 percent bioavailability of oral acyclovir and extrapolation to intravenous levels, as well as extrapolation from preliminary studies with an oral pediatric suspension. The oral preparation can also be used as the initial therapy of HSV in the outpatient setting, as described earlier. It must be emphasized that, to date, no studies have proved efficacy, and FDA licensure does not exist for this use. The physician may want to obtain informed consent before giving acyclovir for this use.

Miscellaneous Infections of Skin and Extremities (Whitlow)

Miscellaneous infections of the skin and extremities have been treated as oral infections with intravenous or oral acyclovir if the severity warrants treatment. Use of acyclovir in these settings demands careful individualization and explanation to the parents and patient regarding the lack of proven efficacy and licensure.

Central Nervous System Infection

HSV encephalitis is a highly lethal disease with a 75 to 80 percent mortality rate when untreated. Two large, well-controlled studies have shown acyclovir to be superior to vidarabine in therapy of HSV encephalitis. It reduces the overall early mortality rate to 20 percent. A critical factor determining morbidity and mortality of HSV encephalitis is the degree of alteration of mental status at onset of therapy. The lethargic patient does much better than the comatose patient. Thus, we begin acyclovir before the diagnosis is proved in any patient with a febrile encephalitis, with a lymphocytic spinal fluid pleocytosis, and with signs of neurologic focality or a focally abnormal electroencepholegram or brain scan (computed tomography or magnetic resonance imaging). A biopsy is performed within 24 hours of onset of therapy. This amount of antiviral therapy usually does not sterilize the brain or prevent antigen detection by fluorescent antibody or other immunohistologic techniques. The dosage of acyclovir is twice that usually utilized for other forms of HSV infection in the normal host, namely, 30 mg per kilogram per day divided every 8 hours. Duration of therapy is 10 to 14 days.

Vidaradine is less effective than acyclovir, but in patients doing poorly while receiving acyclovir, we and others have been tempted to use a combination of both drugs based on in vitro and animal data suggesting additive or synergistic effects. To date, no human studies support combined therapy or alert us to unusual toxicities caused by combined therapy with these DNA inhibitors.

We and others have seen smoldering cases of encephalitis and cases with clinical recrudescence after cessation of therapy. Although several groups have suggested long-term oral therapy to reduce the late damage, there are no controlled studies to support this approach.

Ancillary intensive care measures to monitor and lower intracranial pressure, treat seizures, and avoid respiratory complications are critical in these very ill patients. Survivors generally need extensive rehabilitation.

Ocular Infection

Three topical preparations are effective for the therapy of ocular HSV. In the order of clinical efficacy, these are trifluorothymidine, vidarabine, and idoxuridine. In addition, corticosteroids are occasionally used by ophthalmologists with concommitant use of an antiviral. It is my belief that ocular HSV infection should be treated by an ophthalmologist experienced in its clinical vagaries, and not by a pediatrician or primary care physician. The latter two groups should avoid the use of steroid-containing eye drops, which may exacerbate unsuspected HSV ocular infections.

NEONATE

Studies have documented the efficacy of vidarabine versus placebo in the therapy of neonates with HSV infection, especially before the virus disseminates. The dosage of vidarabine was usually 15 mg per kilogram given as a 12- to 24-hour IV infusion, but I prefer 30 mg per kilogram per day because, in a comparative study, fewer patients getting the larger dosage experienced progression of lesions. A recent study has shown that the efficacy of acyclovir for the acute episode is similar to that of vidarabine. Again, because of the ease of administration, I begin therapy of any form of neonatal HSV infection with acyclovir. This includes treatment of the most trivial form of HSV infection (as a single skin vesicle) because of the propensity of this mild illness to progress rapidly to central nervous system involvement and visceral dissemination.

As with HSV encephalitis, there is a temptation to use combined therapy (acyclovir plus vidarabine) in the neonate who fails to respond to single-agent therapy. No clinical studies support combined therapy. Similarly controversial is the use of human immunoglobulin. Although the currently available intravenous preparations contain large concentrations of anti-HSV antibody, and this has been shown to be effective when used early in several animal models, there are no clinical studies to support its use. Indeed, results of the studies to determine whether or not maternal antibody has an effect on the neonate's illness are contradictory.

Perhaps the most controversial issue regarding the neonate is what to do with the healthy neonate who has been born vaginally to a mother with active lesions or with a positive vaginal culture for HSV obtained at delivery. The attack rate appears to be linked to whether the mother has symptomatic primary disese (50 percent attack rate) or recurrent disease (2 to 5 percent attack rate). There are no data on the attack rate in asymptomatic viral shedding.

I have chosen to culture (1 to 2 days postpartum, from the eyes or mouth) and carefully observe the infant born to a mother with recurrent illness. If either the baby's culture is positive or the baby has any signs suggestive of HSV, he or she will receive a full course of treatment. In the infant born to a woman with primary genital disease, I have elected to treat the infant for a full course, after culturing, and to administer human immunoglobulin by the intravenous route (300 mg per kilogram, once). No controlled studies support these recommendations. In view of the lack of predictive value of weekly predelivery maternal cultures, we no longer perform them, but rely on careful examination of the birth canal and on cultures obtained at delivery to determine the need for cesarean section or for subsequent infant cultures and therapy.

The majority (90 percent) of infants who survive HSV neonatal infection suffer recurrent episodes of cutaneous vesicular eruptions. In general, these are mild. The rare infant with other concomitant signs or symptoms as well should be treated for a second course. There are no data in this patient population with frequent cutaneous recurrences to support the use of oral suppressive acyclovir therapy, although one would expect this therapy to prove efficacious. The continuous use of a DNA inhibitor in a developing infant or young child may lead to currently unrecognized and serious side effects not encountered in adults and older children receiving chronic suppressive therapy.

Intensive care support to treat the respiratory, neurologic, and hematologic problems that often arise, especially in the infant with central nervous system or disseminated disease, is crucial to optimize outcome.

IMMUNOCOMPROMISED HOST

Any manifestation of HSV infection must be treated in the immunocompromised host because of the inability of these individuals to eradicate the virus and often to even keep the infection localized. Immunocompromised hosts tend to have chronic erosive spreading skin or mucocutaneous lesions and, less commonly, involvement of the esophagus, lungs, central nervous system, and other visceral organs. In the most trivial illness in mildly compromised patients the topical ointment has some benefit. In general, the choice is between the oral and intravenous form of acyclovir. This is a clinical judgment based on the degree of immunocompromise and the extent of infection. If there is doubt, I tend to use the intravenous form and, as the infection improves, move to the oral form while observing the patient either in the hospital or with daily clinic or office visits. Intravenous vidarabine is also effective, but less convenient to administer than acyclovir. It may have a role in the immunocompromised patient who has received multiple courses of acyclovir and who seems not to respond. This may be the result of an acyclovir-resistant strain of HSV. In this setting, it is important to isolate the organism and to obtain acyclovir susceptibility testing. (The manufacturers of acyclovir, Burroughs-Wellcome, have been helpful in these matters.)

Acyclovir has been used to prevent HSV in the HSV seropositive patient or in the patient with a history of HSV infection who is about to undergo major immunosuppression (as for bone marrow transplantation or renal transplantation in the first month). Both the oral and the intravenous forms are efficacious, the form used being based on patient convenience and tolerance. In several groups of very immunocompromised patients (e.g., those with AIDS), chronic suppressive oral acyclovir administration prevents frequent recurrences of moderately severe HSV infection. This requires patient individualization gained from close supervision and communication.

DRUGS

Acyclovir

Mechanism of Action

Acyclovir is a fairly specific antiviral that must be converted in vivo by a viral enzyme, thymidine kinase, to the monophosphate, which is then further phosphorylated by cellular enzymes to the active antiviral (acycloguanosine triphosphate). The triphosphate inhibits the viral DNA polymerase and also acts as a DNA chain terminator. The concentration of acyclovir producing 50 percent inhibition of HSV type 1 is 0.2 μg per milliliter and of HSV-2 is 0.5 μg per milliliter among susceptible strains in one type of assay.

Pharmacokinetics

Intravenous acyclovir (5 mg per kilogram per dose) achieves peak serum concentrations of 9.8 (5 to 13) μg per milliliter. An oral dosage of 200 mg to an adult achieves a mean steady state peak serum concentration of 0.6 (0.4 to 0.7) μg per milliliter. Oral acyclovir is 15 to 20 percent bioavailable. Excretion is primarily by renal routes. For intravenous use, dosage adjustment is suggested in patients with renal insufficiency (Table 2). For oral use in adults with a creatinine clearance of less than 10 ml per minute per 1.73 M^2, one capsule each 12 hours is recommended (two-fifths the normal dose). This may be helpful to extrapolate to an oral dose in the child with renal insufficiency.

Side Effects

The major side effects of intravenous acyclovir are phlebitis (15 percent), elevation in serum creatinine (5 percent), and rash (5 percent). Less frequent complications include headache, gastrointestinal upset, hypotension, and, especially in patients with renal insufficiency, neurologic symptoms including lethargy, confusion, tremor, seizures, and coma. These can usually be reversed by stopping use of the drug. Elevations in serum creatinine and nephrotoxicity can usually be avoided by maintaining a state of good hydration.

The major side effects of oral acyclovir include nausea and vomiting (3 percent) and headache (1 percent). In long-term suppressive therapy, side effects include headache (13 percent), diarrhea (9 percent), nausea and vomiting (8 percent), and, uncommonly, vertigo and arthritis.

Viral Resistance

There are several mechanisms of resistance to acyclovir, the most common being viruses that lack thymidine kinase. These are occasionally found in patients receiving chronic acyclovir and have been rarely associated with failure to respond to acyclovir, especially in immunocompromised hosts. The vast majority of clinical isolates are susceptible to acyclo-

TABLE 2 Dosage of Intravenous Acyclovir for Patients with Renal Insufficiency

Creatinine Clearance (ml/min/1.73 M²)	Dosage (mg)	Dosing Interval (hr)
>50	5	8
25–50	5	12
10–25	5	24
0–10	2.5	24

vir, even after long-term administration. The role of viral susceptibility testing remains to be ascertained.

Immune Response

Several studies have shown that acyclovir-treated individuals with primary HSV infection fail to mount as exuberant an antibody response as placebo-treated patients. The acyclovir-treated patients may also experience a significantly more severe first recurrence, after which their subsequent antibody response and recurrences are similar to those in untreated patients. In marrow transplantation patients, acyclovir therapy of HSV recurrence was associated with a low lymphocyte response to HSV and more frequent and earlier subsequent recurrences of HSV. It is not clear what implications these data have for the therapy of pediatric patients. For instance, will therapy of primary oral disease increase the risk or severity of recurrent fever blisters? Will therapy of neonates with acyclovir (versus vidarabine) intensify the cutaneous outbreaks or even predispose the neonate to more severe HSV disease when the agent is stopped (as has been seen anecdotally in several cases)? Careful investigation and follow-up studies are necessary to answer these questions.

Vidarabine

Mechanism of Action

Vidarabine is a nucleoside derivative. It is phosphorylated to the triphosphate and inhibits herpes virus DNA polymerase, thereby acting as a chain terminator of viral DNA. It inhibits HSV at a concentrate of 3 μg per milliliter.

Pharmacokinetics

It is difficult to evaluate vidarabine pharmacokinetics because its metabolites, such as arabinosyl hypoxanthine (ara-Hx), are also antiviral. Peak ara-Hx and vidarabine levels range from 3 to 6 μg per milliliter and from 0.2 to 0.4 μg per milliliter, respectively, after a 10-mg-per-kilogram infusion. The agent is primarily excreted by the kidneys, but there are no good guidelines for its use in renal insufficiency. It is a relatively insoluble agent (1 mg requires 2.2 ml of infusion fluid), and the fluid load necessary for infusion often makes it inconvenient.

Side Effects

Side effects include anorexia, nausea, vomiting, diarrhea, elevated liver function tests, suppression of the hematopoietic system, and neurologic symptoms (tremor, dizziness, hallucination, ataxia, seizures). Neurologic problems have been encountered especially in leukemics who have previously received intrathecal antineoplastic therapy. Vidarabine should be avoided in these patients. The large fluid volume necessary for delivery has resulted in overhydration, a special problem in patients with encephalitis.

Ocular Preparations

All three ocular preparations (trifluorothymidine, vidarabine, and idoxuridine) have similar side effects, including punctate epithelial keratopathy, contact dermatitis, drug sensitization, lacrimation, and edema. Of the three, trifluorothymidine is the best tolerated. Their basic antiviral mechanism is the same as for acyclovir. In young children the ointment preparations may be a bit easier to use because of the longer periods between administration. These drugs should generally be used with the assistance of an experienced ophthalmologist.

SELECTED READING

Kohl S. Postnatal herpes simplex virus infection. In: Feigin RD, Cherry JD, eds. Textbook of pediatric infectious diseases, 2nd ed. Philadelphia: WB Saunders, 1987; 1577–1601.
Kohl S, James AR. Herpes simplex virus encephalitis during childhood. The importance of brain biopsy diagnosis. J Pediatr 1985; 107:212–215.
Whitley RJ, Hutto SC. Therapy of viral infections in children. In: Aronoff SC, Hughes WT, Kohl S, et al, eds. Advances in pediatric infectious diseases, vol 2. Chicago: Year Book Medical Publishers, 1987; 35–53.

KAWASAKI SYNDROME

WILBERT H. MASON, M.D.
MASATO TAKAHASHI, M.D.

Since it was first described in Japan in 1967, Kawasaki syndrome (KS) has been recognized in increasing numbers throughout the world. Certain epidemiologic characteristics of the illness, such as a seasonal occurence and an appearance in temporally and geographically related clusters, suggest an infectious etiology. Several microbial pathogens are infrequently associated with the illness, but as yet no organism has been definitively proved to be the cause. Antimicrobial agents are ineffective in altering the course of the illness, and until recently treatment has been largely symptomatic. Recent reports, however, show treatment with immunoglobulin to be effective therapy for this disorder.

The diagnosis of KS is made by fulfilling the diagnostic criteria (Table 1). In the United States, the

TABLE 1 Kawasaki Syndrome Diagnostic Criteria*

1. Fever persisting for 5 days or more
2. Changes of peripheral extremities:
   Acute phase: reddening of palms and soles, indurative edema
   Subacute phase: membranous desquamation from fingertips
3. Polymorphous exanthema
4. Bilateral conjunctival congestion
5. Changes of lips and oral cavity: reddening and fissuring of lips, strawberry tongue, diffuse injection of oral and pharyngeal mucosa
6. Acute nonpurulent cervical lymphadenopathy

* At least five of items 1 through 6 should be satisfied for a diagnosis of Kawasaki disease. However, patients with four of the principal symptoms can be diagnosed as having Kawasaki disease when coronary aneurysm is recognized by two-dimensional echocardiography or coronary angiography.
Source: Japan Kawasaki Disease Research Committee. Diagnostic guideline of Kawasaki disease, 4th ed. Japan, 1984.

Centers for Disease Control suggest that cases of KS should have fever for longer than 5 days, four of the five remaining criteria, and no more reasonable explanations of the illness. In addition to the diagnostic criteria, numerous other associated symptoms, signs, and laboratory findings have frequently been observed during the illness (Table 2). KS affects nearly every body organ, with the possible exception of the kidneys. The organ system that suffers the most significant damage is the cardiovascular system (Table 3).

Clinically, KS presents as an acute febrile illness with dramatic mucocutaneous features, lymphadenopathy usually in the cervical area, and widespread visceral involvement. The clinical course usually occurs in three phases: acute, subacute, and convalescent. The acute phase encompasses the period of

TABLE 2 Associated Noncardiac Symptoms or Findings in Kawasaki Syndrome

Gastrointestinal	Diarrhea (50%),* hydrops of gallbladder (16%), hepatitis
Genitourinary	Urethritis (~50%), orchitis
Central nervous system	Aseptic meningitis (~25%), coma (rare), stroke (rare)
Ocular	Uveitis (66%)
Pulmonary	Pulmonary infiltrates (9%)
Musculoskeletal	Arthralgia (55%), arthritis (38%)
Changes in laboratory tests	Leukocytosis (95%)
	Mild to moderate anemia (>50%)
	Thrombocytosis (in subacute phase) (90–100%)
	Elevated acute-phase reactants (sedimentation rate, C-reactive protein, alpha-1-antitrypsin) (95%)
	Elevated aspartate aminotransferase or alanine aminotransferase (43%)
	Elevated serum bilirubin, alkaline phosphatase
	Decreased serum albumin (88%)
	Hyponatremia (19%)

* Percentages are from the literature or from Children's Hospital of Los Angeles experience.

TABLE 3 Cardiac Features of Kawasaki Syndrome

Feature	Percent*
Myocarditis and/or pericarditis	15–50*
Mitral regurgitation	8–11
Aortic regurgitation	<5
Conduction abnormalities or arrythmias	
Coronary artery aneurysms	15–20
Aneurysms of other arteries	~10

* Percentages are from the literature or from Children's Hospital of Los Angeles experience.

fever, rash, and mucocutaneous manifestations, usually lasting 1 to 2 weeks. Myocarditis is most commonly seen in the acute phase. The subacute phase lasts from the time of defervescence until all laboratory tests, including acute-phase reactants and platelet count, have normalized. It may be as long as 6 to 8 weeks in some cases. The characteristic membranous desquamation of the palms and soles occurs in this phase. Convalescence extends for up to 6 months, and during this phase the patients regain their full strength and vitality.

GENERAL MANAGEMENT

Since there are other illnesses that can closely mimic clinical presentation of KS, we usually attempt to rule out some of the more common diseases in the differential diagnosis. Infections such as those caused by *Streptococcus pyogenes* and Epstein-Barr virus are assessed for by means of culture or serologic assay. In some areas of the country, leptospirosis also might be confused with KS, and a history of contact with animals should be sought. Finally, in unimmunized children, measles should be considered. The presence of severe cough and Koplik's spots usually allow for the accurate diagnosis of this infection.

Initial evaluation of the patient should include assessment for dehydration, which is common because of poor oral intake and fluid losses from diarrhea and from increased insensible loss. Fluid replacement is essential, but it should be done cautiously because of the common presence of myocardial dysfunction. Chest roentgenography, electrocardiography, and two-dimensional echocardiography should be performed to evaluate myocardial performance and to obtain baseline information regarding the status of the coronary arteries. In addition, laboratory data should be obtained to assess the hematologic and hepatic systems and the electrolyte status. Finally, careful palpation of the axillary and femoral arteries should be performed to evaluate for aneurysms.

MEDICAL MANAGEMENT

Kawasaki syndrome has been treated with a variety of antimicrobial agents without noticeable effect on the course of the illness. Because the pathogenesis of the disorder seems to involve a diffuse vasculitis, possibly mediated by perturbation of the immune system, the approach to medical management has focused on measures to ameliorate the inflammatory response. Steroids have been used, but appear to increase the risk of coronary artery aneurysm formation. Nonsteroidal anti-inflammatory agents have been tried, but offer no significant relief in most cases. The two modalities that offer the greatest benefit to patients with KS have been salicylates and, more recently, intravenous immunoglobulin.

Aspirin therapy given in large dosages (80 to 100 mg per kilogram per day in divided doses every 6 hours) appears to decrease the fever and arthralgia in some cases and may shorten the symptomatic course. Although it has been suggested by some that aspirin therapy may reduce the occurrence of coronary artery abnormalities, this has not been our experience. The mechanism of action of aspirin in KS is not known, although it is presumably through the anti-inflammatory properties.

Preliminary studies in Japan suggested that infusions of immunoglobulin reduce the occurrence of coronary artery aneurysms in Kawasaki patients. We participated in a multicenter randomized trial in the United States that compared aspirin alone with aspirin and four daily infusions of gamma globulin in patients treated within 10 days of onset. There was a fivefold decrease in prevalence of coronary artery abnormalities in patients who received gamma globulin. Moreover, these gamma globulin–treated patients experienced a more rapid fall in temperature, most becoming afebrile after the first infusion, and a more rapid normalization of the total white blood cell and absolute granulocyte counts.

The mechanism of action of gamma globulin is speculative, but can involve correction of one or more alterations of the immune response, which may be of pathophysiologic importance in the illness (Table 4). An increase in the $T_4{:}T_8$ cell ratio has been reported during the acute and subacute phases of the illness. In addition, circulating immune complexes are frequently found in sera of patients with Kawasaki syndrome. Thus, immunoglobulin may modulate the abnormal immune response by altering, in some way, immunoregulatory cells or their chemical mediators (e.g., gamma interferon or interleukin-1). Alternatively, it may act by blocking the inflammatory effect on vessel walls by immune complexes.

At the time of this writing, the gamma globulin preparation used in the multicenter trial is not approved for use in the United States, and none of the presently available preparations has been approved by the Food and Drug Administration for treatment of Kawasaki syndrome. This creates a dilemma for the practitioner who desires to treat a particular patient with gamma globulin in this situation. The physician might consider consultation with one of the centers that participated in the clinical trial. Alternatively, administration of one of the second-generation intravenous immunoglobulin preparations could be considered after the family is fully informed of the therapeutic options and risks.

PREFERRED APPROACH

The diagnosis of KS should be established as early as possible, preferably within 10 days of onset. Aneurysms usually are not evident until 10 days after the onset of illness. To be effective, treatment should be instituted early to reduce inflammation within the arterial wall before dilatational changes occur. Patients who present beyond 10 days from onset may be treated if they continue to demonstrate significant symptoms of acute inflammation.

At the time of diagnosis, we obtain the appropriate laboratory data and cardiologic consultation. We then initiate aspirin therapy (80 to 100 mg per kilogram per day given in divided doses every 6 hours). We also initiate infusion of gamma globulin in a dosage of 400 mg per kilogram per dose, infused over 2 hours. During the infusion, the patients are monitored closely for evidence of cardiac decompensation and for reactions to the gamma globulin preparation (Table 5). This dosage is repeated daily for 4 days.

We continue large-dosage aspirin therapy until the fever and systemic symptoms subside, usually for about 2 weeks. Serum concentrations of salicylate are monitored to prevent salicylism. The aspirin dosage is then abruptly decreased to 3 to 5 mg per kilogram per day as a single dose. This is the period of the illness during which the numbers of circulating platelets increase, aneurysms begin to develop, and the risk of coronary artery thrombosis emerges. Small-dosage aspirin therapy provides anticoagulation because it inhibits platelet aggregation by inhibiting platelet thromboxane synthesis while not inhibiting prostacycline synthesis by the endothelial cells. Prostacycline inhibits platelet aggregation and is a potent vasodilator. Small-dosage aspirin therapy is continued for the next 4 to 6 weeks.

Repeat echocardiograms are obtained at the end of immunoglobulin therapy and again at about 3 and 8 weeks after initial evaluation. If no coronary artery abnormalities are appreciated, and if the sedimentation rate and platelet count have returned to normal, aspirin therapy is discontinued. If aneurysms are present, small-dosage aspirin therapy is continued until echocardiographic or angiographic evidence of arterial abnormalities has resolved.

TABLE 4 Immunologic Abnormalities in Kawasaki Syndrome

Elevated IgE, IgM levels
Increased numbers of activated T_4 helper cells
Decreased numbers of T_8 suppressor cells
Circulating immune complexes
Increased C3 levels

TABLE 5   Adverse Effects of Immunoglobulin Infusions*

Adverse Effect	Cause	Frequency (%)	Treatment
Fever Flushing Chest tightening Vomiting Pain in back and hips Hypotension	Vasomotor effects possibly resulting from aggregates of immunoglobulin in solution	~1	Slow infusion or interrupt and restart more slowly
Anaphylaxis	Allergic reaction in individuals lacking IgA, but with anti-IgA antibodies. Most commercially available immunoglobulin has small amounts of IgA.	Rare ≪1	Stop infusion, epinephrine, fluid support
Phlebitis	Irritation?	Uncommon	Slow infusion
Congestive heart failure	Fluid overload caused by weakened myocardium	4†	Slow infusion, treat heart failure (diuretics, inotropic support)
Transmission of infectious agents (i.e., hepatitis B virus, HIV)	Not reported with any preparation of immunoglobulin used in the United States for any indication	0	

* Reactions listed (except for heart failure) are those reported in patients treated for conditions other than Kawasaki syndrome.
† Of 84 immunoglobulin-treated patients with KS, 4 percent developed mild heart failure after the first dose in a multicenter trial. A similar number (4.5 percent) of aspirin-treated patients had heart failure.

MANAGEMENT OF COMPLICATIONS

Gastrointestinal

Diarrhea is a common finding in KS and contributes to dehydration and electrolyte abnormalities. Supportive care with parenteral rehydration is effective in correcting these problems. Mild to moderate elevations of serum transaminases are frequently noted at the time of admission, thus suggesting the presence of hepatitis. Serum enzyme concentrations usually decrease following the institution of aspirin therapy. However, if enzyme values rise during large-dosage salicylate treatment or if aspirin toxicity develops, hepatitis resulting from salicylism is probably the cause and aspirin should be discontinued or radically decreased in dosage.

Hydrops of the gallbladder is the most significant gastrointestinal complication of KS. It is associated with severe abdominal pain, distention, and a palpable mass in the right upper abdominal quadrant. Elevation in serum total and direct bilirubin and alkaline phosphatase values are also indicative of this complication. Although hydrops may cause considerable discomfort and last as long as 3 to 4 weeks, rupture has never been reported and surgical intervention is not necessary.

Musculoskeletal

Arthritis of the hands and feet is a prominent sign in KS, but arthritis of other joints, most notably the knees, hips, wrists, and elbows, occurs in up to 40 percent of patients. Arthritis is often noted as a late complication, appearing after the first week of illness. When aspirin therapy fails to ameliorate the arthritic symptoms or when they persist beyond the usual period of large-dosage aspirin treatment, nonsteroidal anti-inflammatory agents such as tolmetin (15 to 30 mg per kilogram per day in three divided doses) may be of some benefit.

Myocarditis

Most children with KS show some evidence of myocarditis in the first week to 10 days of illness. Signs of myocarditis may be manifested only as persistent tachycardia, gallop rhythms, muffled heart sounds, or electrocardiographic evidence of myocardial inflammation such as reduced QRS voltages, prolonged PR intervals, flattened T-waves, or ST-segment abnormalities. In a small number, but possibly in as many as 5 to 10 percent of patients, more severe involvement of the myocardium occurs, thus resulting in cardiac decompensation with congestive heart failure and hypotension. Intensive care is required for adequate management of these patients. Diuretic therapy and the cautious use of inotropic agents such as dopamine or dobutamine have been successful in maintaining cardiac output until the myocardial inflammation has subsided.

Central Nervous System

Aseptic meningitis has been noted in up to 25 percent of children who have undergone lumbar puncture during KS. Cerebrospinal fluid findings usually include a mononuclear pleocytosis, a normal sugar concentration, and a normal to slightly elevated protein content. Gram stain and culture are uniformly negative. Encephalopathy with seizures, obtundation, and strokelike syndromes have been described. Rarely, permanent neurologic sequelae have resulted. No specific therapy is known for these complications.

Coronary Artery Aneurysms

During the late acute and subacute phases of KS, inflammatory changes occur within medium and large arteries, beginning in endothelial and perivascular areas and progressing to panvasculitis in some cases. Inflammation weakens vessel walls and aneurysms form as a result.

Dilatation or frank aneurysm formation in coronary arteries occurs in 15 to 20 percent of patients with KS. Aneurysms usually become detectable by echocardiography after 10 to 14 days of illness, but may not appear until 4 to 6 weeks after onset. Aneurysm formation is usually noted in the proximal portions of the major coronary arteries. More distal aneurysms occur, but are virtually always associated with abnormalities in the proximal segments. There is no satisfactory treatment for aneurysms once they have formed, therefore prevention is of utmost importance. After aneurysms are established, medical management is directed at preventing thrombosis within the aneurysm, and small-dosage aspirin therapy is the recommended treatment. If a patient is felt to be at high risk for coronary thrombosis because of multiple or very large aneurysms, 3 to 6 mg per kilogram per day of dipyridamole, in two to three divided doses, may be given. If so-called giant aneurysms (measuring greater than 8 mm in diameter) are present, the addition of heparin may be necessary to maintain patency of the vessel.

If a patient taking small doses of aspirin develops varicella or influenza, we recommend substituting dipyridamole for aspirin until the infection resolves in order to minimize the very small risk of the complication of Reye's syndrome.

If we detect coronary artery changes by echocardiography, we generally recommend angiography to better characterize the lesion, to evaluate for more peripherally located aneurysms, and to assess for the presence of stenotic lesions. This is particularly important in cases in which large or multiple aneurysms are suspected. In some centers, progression and regression of coronary artery changes are followed with echocardiography alone.

Fortunately, aneurysms tend to regress, and 50 to 75 percent of patients with coronary artery changes show partial or complete resolution over a 1- to 2-year period, based on angiographic evaluation.

Peripheral Vascular Complications

Occasionally, other arteries undergo aneurysmal change. Approximately 5 percent of our patients have had palpable aneurysms of the axillary, brachial, or femoral arteries. When children with axillary aneurysms are lifted under the arms, care should be taken not to apply excessive pressure on the involved vessels.

Aneurysms of other visceral arteries including the aorta, mesenteric, hepatic, renal, and iliac arteries have been reported. Rarely occlusive phenomena occur during the acute phase of the illness and involve arteries in the extremities. This can result in cyanosis or even gangrene of the involved limb. We have observed this only once in a patient with a transient decrease in flow in a femoral artery, but the event resolved spontaneously. Others have treated severe episodes of this type with steroids with or without anticoagulants.

Myocardial Infarction

Death occurs in 0.5 to 1 percent of children with KS. Rarely, death occurs in the acute or subacute phases because of arrhythmia or severe myocarditis. Equally uncommon is death resulting from rupture of a coronary artery aneurysm.

Most fatalities from myocardial infarction result from thrombosis within a coronary artery aneurysm. Approximately three-quarters of infarcts occur within 1 year from onset of illness. When thrombosis occurs, death may be prevented through the prompt use of thrombolytic therapy with streptokinase or urokinase. We have successfully lysed a coronary artery thrombosis in one patient using streptokinase infusion. Management of myocardial infarction obviously requires intensive care and the expertise of a cardiologist.

Mitral and Aortic Regurgitation

A small number of children have been reported to have mitral and/or aortic insufficiency following KS. In a few instances, surgery was necessary. Pathologic specimens revealed degeneration and microvascular proliferation in valve tissues.

LONG-TERM MANAGEMENT

Patients who develop aneurysms require long-term cardiologic follow-up and indefinite anticoagulant therapy to prevent thrombosis. Bypass surgery using saphenous veins or internal mammary arteries has been performed on a very small number of patients with varying, but generally discouraging, results. Internal mammary artery grafts have been reported to have better patency rates and greater growth potential than saphenous vein grafts.

The long-term consequences of KS in patients with coronary artery lesions or healed aneurysms remain unknown. Recent studies suggest prolonged abnormal diastolic function of the left ventricle unrelated to coronary artery disease in some patients. Autopsy data from patients with "healed" aneurysms show intimal hyperplasia and other changes that predispose to atherosclerotic disease in later life. There is also some question whether these arteries are able to vasodilate in response to exercise or stress. We recommend periodic cardiac evaluation of patients following KS because of these unanswered questions. As children mature and reach an age at which participation in competitive sports is desired, treadmill testing or other stress-related evaluation of cardiac performance may be indicated in those individuals who demonstrated coronary artery abnormalities.

Parental anxiety is very high following the diagnosis of KS. Reassurance is important to those parents whose children demonstrate no cardiac sequelae of the disease, and we encourage them not to restrict the children's activities in any way. For parents of children with cardiovascular complications, adequate explanation and psychologic support is vital so that the children can understand the need for long-term treatment and follow-up. In addition, we recommend that the parents learn the techniques of cardiopulmonary resuscitation. Children with coronary artery aneurysms can tolerate normal physical activity, but we discourage participation in contact sports while the child is on anticoagulant therapy.

Finally, we reassure parents that, although KS is an infectious disease, it is not contagious and siblings and schoolmates cannot acquire the illness from their child.

SUGGESTED READING

Hicks RV, Melish ME. Kawasaki syndrome. Pediatr Clin North Am 1986; 33:1151–1175.
Leung DYM, Collins T, Lapierre LA, et al. Immunoglobulin M antibodies present in the acute phase of Kawasaki syndrome lyse cultured vascular endothelial cells stimulated by gamma interferon. J Clin Invest 1986; 77:1428–1435.
Mason WH, Jordan SC, Sakai R, et al. Circulating immune complexes in Kawasaki syndrome. Pediatr Infect Dis 1985; 4:48–51.
Newburger JW, Takahashi M, Burns JC, et al. Treatment of Kawasaki syndrome with intravenous gamma globulin. N Engl J Med 1986; 315:341–347.
Takahashi M, Mason WH, Lewis AB. Regression of coronary aneurysms in patients with Kawasaki syndrome. Circulation 1987; 75:387–394.

LEPROSY

F. KEVIN MURPHY, M.D., F.A.C.P.
TRUDY V. MURPHY, M.D.

Leprosy occurs among Asian and Hispanic immigrants throughout the United States and in an endemic zone along the western Gulf coast in Texas and Louisiana.

The clinical finding suggesting early or "indeterminate" leprosy is a hypopigmented or erythematous macule accompanied by paresthesia or pruritus. At this stage, pain and temperature sensation may be impaired at the site of lesion, but light touch sensation is preserved initially. After several months or years, there is either spontaneous resolution or progression to one of the forms of "determined" leprosy (Table 1): lepromatous, tuberculoid, or borderline.

Lepromatous leprosy is a predominantly cutaneous disease characterized by infiltrated patches and nodules, usually accompanied by impairment of sensation, hair loss, and a decrease in sweating. Enlarged, pressure-sensitive nerves develop later in lepromatous leprosy. As the disease progresses, skin folds and earlobes thicken, and perforating ulceration of the nasal, palatal, or laryngeal mucosa may develop. Face, ears, and pressure points are particularly affected.

Tuberculoid leprosy, in contrast, predominantly affects nerve function, thus producing more anesthesia and less infiltration of nerves or skin. The classic skin lesion is a large, anesthetic, hypopigmented macule; tuberculoid skin lesions are often lichenoid, scaly, and anhidrotic.

Diagnosis is confirmed by biopsy of the affected tissue or by skin scraping of the earlobe, knee, or elbow and demonstration of *Mycobacterium leprae* in histologic section or smear. Nasal swabs for organisms are infrequently positive and difficult to obtain

TABLE 1   Classification of Leprosy

Clinical Type	Clinical Features	Cutaneous Histologic Features	Lepromin Skin Test
Tuberculoid	Neuropathy Hypopigmented anesthetic macule Exposure keratitis Nerve abscesses	Epithelioid cell predominance Dense lymphocytic infiltrate Few or rare bacilli Necrosis of nerves	Positive at 4 weeks
Lepromatous	Maculonodular skin lesions Nasal and palatal mucosal ulcers Thickening of skin folds Palpable nerve trunks	Histiocyte predominance Scant lymphocytes Many bacilli Preservation of nerves but invaded by AFB	Negative
Borderline	Moderate neuropathy Annular punched-out ("upside down saucer") hypesthetic plaques Hypertrophic nerves	Scattered bacillis in dermis	Variable

in children. Early diagnosis and treatment eliminate infectivity, prevent deformity, and are associated with a good prognosis for complete recovery.

The discussion that follows is intended to familiarize pediatricians with the major approaches to therapy of leprosy. Because of the complexities of management, therapy should be guided by consultants with experience. The National Hansen's Disease Center (NHDC) at Carville, Louisiana, provides initial and follow-up screening of patients and household contacts. The Center also provides drugs for therapy. Questions can be directed to the Chief of the Clinical Branch, NHDC, at 1-800-642-2477.

In index cases, the initial choice of treatment regimen is based on disease classification. Classification of disease is based on the form and extent of skin and peripheral nerve involvement (see Table 1). Classification is further aided by the patient's late reactivity to the lepromin skin test (Mitsuda reaction). Patients with tuberculoid leprosy have strongly positive reactions to this test. Those with borderline, indeterminate, or lepromatous disease have weak or negative responses.

Before therapy is initiated, patients should be screened for preexisting causes of anemia, including G6PD deficiency. Anemia amenable to therapy should be corrected. Baseline liver function tests and complete blood count, including platelet count, are helpful in assessing changes resulting from therapy. Nerve conduction studies should be obtained in patients with neuropathy.

SPECIFIC THERAPY

For the first 6 months to 2 years of therapy, at least two drugs are used, depending on the classification of disease (Tables 2 and 3). For midborderline to lepromatous cases, three drugs are used. Although dapsone is usually given daily, a three-times-per-week regimen can be substituted. In the past, some physicians initiated dapsone therapy in small graduated doses. Reduced dosage is not recommended, as it appears to be associated with development of dapsone-resistant *M. leprae* and does not reduce the rate of reactions. Acedapsone is a repository derivative of dapsone reserved for noncompliant patients or those remote from health care centers. It may have a role in chemoprophylaxis of household contacts.

Rifampin, which is rapidly bactericidal, is recommended as the second drug in initial therapy; the rapid reduction in total body burden of viable bacilli that occurs with the combination of dapsone and rifampin is thought to reduce the risk that dapsone resistance will develop. World Health Organization recommendations differ from American recommendations in advocating monthly, rather than daily, doses of rifampin for reasons of cost. The disadvantages of intermittent rifampin therapy are a reduced bactericidal effect and hypersensitivity reactions. These include a flulike syndrome and interstitial nephritis with renal failure.

Clofazimine has the special advantage of suppressing leprous reactions, in addition to its antimicrobial activity. It is therefore used preferentially in treatment of reactions to therapy, in substitution for dapsone, and for management of dapsone-resistant cases. However, the darkening and discoloration of skin it produces precludes its use in primary treatment. Thiacetazone is a weakly bacteriostatic drug, inexpensive, and sometimes used in patients intolerant of clofazimine. However, without assured compliance, it is unlikely to be effective.

Ethionamide is bactericidal in large dosage, but dosage in children is not well established, and it is generally reserved for dapsone-resistant leprosy. Since both ethionamide and rifampin are hepatotoxic, the combination of these drugs for prolonged periods is generally avoided.

TABLE 2   Oral Antibiotic Therapy for Leprosy

Drug	Dosage		Major Side Effects
Dapsone	Child:	0.9–1.4 mg/kg/day	Hemolytic anemia, especially in patients with G6PD Allergic dermatitis
	Adult:	100 mg/day*	Agranulocytosis Gastrointestinal complaints Hepatotoxicity
Rifampin	Child:	10–15 mg/kg/day	Nausea, vomiting Hepatotoxicity
	Adult:	600 mg/day	Thrombocytopenia Allergic reactions precipitated by intermittent use
Clofazimine	Child:	1 mg/kg/day	Reversible skin pigmentation Gastrointestinal complaints (enteritis, small bowel obstruction)
	Adult:	50–100 mg/day†	Reduced sweating, tearing
Ethionamide	Child:	(Not established)	Gastrointestinal complaints Hepatotoxicity
	Adult:	250–500 mg/day	Peripheral neuritis and CNS toxicity (seizures)

* Alternative schedule: 200 mg three times per week.
† Up to 300 mg per day for severe reactive episodes.

TABLE 3   Treatment Regimens for Leprosy

Disease Classification	Dapsone-Susceptible M. leprae	Dapsone-Resistant M. leprae
Indeterminate and tuberculoid	Dapsone: 3 years beyond negativity; and rifampin: at least 6 months	Clofazimine: 3 years beyond negativity; and rifampin: about 6 months
Borderline-tuberculoid	Dapsone: 5 years beyond negativity; and rifampin: at least 6 months	Clofazimine: 5 years beyond negativity; and rifampin: about 6 months
Midborderline	Dapsone: 10 years beyond negativity; and rifampin: at least 2 years; and clofazimine or ethionamide: at least 2 years	Clofazimine: 10 years beyond negativity; and rifampin: at least 2 years; and ethionamide: at least 2 years
Borderline-lepromatous and lepromatous	Dapsone: for life; and other drugs: as for midborderline leprosy	Clofazimine: for life; and other drugs: as for midborderline; or rifampin plus ethionamide: for life

Adapted from National Hansen's Disease Center Regimen, 1985.

Patients are considered noncontagious within a week after therapy is initiated.

Therapy of leprous reactions requires a clear understanding of the reaction type (Table 4). Downgrading or worsening of untreated borderline tuberculoid leprosy is an indication for cautious initiation of standard therapy. Reversal reactions (type 1), in contrast to downgrading reactions, result from delayed hypersensitivity during therapy. Reversal reactions are treated with large dosages of corticosteroids tapered rapidly. Clofazimine may be helpful in reducing or eliminating the need for steroids if the reaction becomes chronic.

TABLE 4   Therapy of Lepromatous Reactions

Reaction	Therapy
Reversal (type 1)	Acute: Analgesics Prednisone: 2 mg/kg/day (maximum 60–80 mg) PO. Taper over several weeks and discontinue. Chronic reactions: use alternate-day steroids at the lowest possible dosage and consider clofazimine. Chronic: Clofazimine: 300 mg (adult dose)* PO daily until controlled off steroids (4–6 weeks); then reduce to 100 mg/day (adult dose) and adjust as needed.
Erythema nodosum leprosum (type 2)	Acute: Analgesics Prednisone: As above. Chronic or recurrent: Thalidomide†: 25–100 mg/dose (adult dose)* 4 times daily. Tapered over 2–3 weeks after the reaction is controlled. Regulate with the lowest alternate-day to twice-daily dosage. Clofazimine: As above if thalidomide is contraindicated or if the reaction is not controlled by thalidomide and steroids alone.

* No established dosage for children.
† Contraindicated in pregnancy.

Erythema nodosum leprosum (ENL or type 2) reaction is a complication of both lepromatous and borderline lepromatous leprosy. It is a result of immune complex injury and can be severe, resulting in fever, hepatosplenomegaly, arthritis, iritis, and necrotic skin ulceration. Milder reactions in patients with borderline and borderline tuberculoid leprosy may consist of hypesthesia or worsening of preexisting lesions. Arthritis is subtle and painless in insensitive joints, which should be examined carefully for synovial thickening. Large dosages of steroids, clofazimine, thalidomide (in nonpregnant patients), and analgesics are useful in modifying this reaction. Patients must be monitored closely for evidence of iridocyclitis, which can have a sudden onset and a rapid progression to blindness. Inflammation and swelling of peripheral nerves are sometimes severe enough to cause vascular compromise and require surgical release of fibro-osseous tunnels to prevent permanent nerve injury. Painful swollen limbs should be splinted in positions of function. Care should be given to necrotic ulcerated skin to prevent progressive destruction. A severe form of ENL, characterized by widespread necrotic ulcers, is seen in treatment of diffuse lepromatous leprosy (Lucio phenomenon) and is said to be uncommon in children.

MONITORING THE RESPONSE TO THERAPY

To quantify response to therapy, skin scrapings are taken in a standardized manner from designated sites before therapy and at intervals throughout treatment. From these scrapings, the number of positive samples, a bacteriologic index, and a morphologic index are determined. The bacteriologic index (BI) is an estimate of the number of acid-fast bacilli on a logarithmic scale by which 1.0 corresponds to a count of 1 to 10 per 100 oil-immersion fields and 6.0 corresponds to a count of 1,000 per microscopic field. The morphologic index (MI) is the percentage of bacilli that are viable or solid-staining. Within a few months of initiation of therapy, the MI, which may begin as high as 20 percent, should fall below 1 percent. Because of poor phagocytic clearance, however, the BI generally falls slowly, especially in lepromatous patients in whom leprous bacilli may persist indefinitely despite clinical remission.

Clinical improvement, as judged by physical examination and nerve conduction studies, should occur within 2 to 3 months of therapy. Patients who fail to respond may have dapsone-resistant *M. leprae,* which can be demonstrated by inoculation of biopsy tissue into the footpads of dapsone-treated mice. Clinical relapses are caused by either sensitive or resistant strains and are usually confined to cases of lepromatous leprosy in which therapy has been discontinued. Dapsone-susceptible cases of relapse respond as rapidly to renewed dapsone as do new cases. Dapsone resistance arises in patients treated irregularly or with small doses and can be managed with a combination of rifampin and either clofazimine or ethionamide, depending on disease classification (see Table 3). Lepromatous leprosy is generally treated for life. Patients treated for 20 years with dapsone alone at the Sungei Buloh Leprosarium in Malaysia exhibited a relapse rate of 1 percent per year during 8 to 9 years of follow-up after discontinuation of treatment. There is hope that lifetime maintenance therapy may not be necessary if currently advocated multidrug therapy is used.

Close monitoring of patients for leprous reactions and side effects of drug therapy is essential during the first months of treatment, although children generally tolerate therapy well. Gastrointestinal complaints associated with therapy are common, and the ability of the patient to comply with the treatment regimen must be assessed. Patients should be warned that intermittent rifampin therapy can precipitate allergic reactions. They must be counseled to seek medical attention at the first sign of oral ulceration or rash, which may herald the onset of Stevens-Johnson syndrome. Clinical and laboratory monitoring for blood dyscrasias and hepatotoxicity should be carried out weekly for the first month, monthly for 6 months, and at least biannually therafter. Except for mild, early elevation of liver enzymes, evidence of any one of these complications is indication for discontinuation of the suspect drug.

Patients with mild G6PD deficiency, but not the Mediterranean variety, may be treated with dapsone if the anemia resulting from hemolysis is not symptomatic. Dapsone should be given initially under close supervision if anemia becomes profound. Patients taking ethionamide may develop neurotoxicity, and this must be differentiated from the neuropathy of leprosy. Clofazimine-induced discoloration of skin is reversible and does not require discontinuation, except for cosmetic reasons.

Education of the patient in protection of the anesthetic limb and splinting of weak limbs in positions of function is of major importance in preventing the complications of leprosy. Plantar ulcers, analogous in every way to those associated with diabetic or luetic neuropathy, can be prevented by a threefold program of (1) preventing and trimming callus, (2) fitting the patient with orthopaedic shoes with rigid soles and resilient form-fitted insoles, and (3) frequently inspecting for preulcerative signs of pressure.

Orthopaedic surgery to restore mechanical function or neurosurgery to preserve peripheral nerve function is sometimes required in late or advanced leprosy. Elective surgery should generally be avoided in borderline and lepromatous leprosy until the bacteriologic index is below 0.5 to avoid precipitating leprous reactions. There are three indications for neurosurgical intervention: nerve abscess, acute mononeuritis with severe pain unresponsive to anti-inflammatory agents, and nerve pain in an irreversibly functionless nerve. In addition, some authorities believe that nerve decompression by incision of constrictive fibro-osseous tunnels is effective for selected cases of chronic neuritis. Decompression of the posterior tibial nerve and artery has been advocated for treatment of plantar ulcers, but is of unproven value.

Tendon transfers and grafts can be used to restore finger-thumb apposition and, in conjunction with stabilization of the wrist, can restore grasp in median nerve lesions. Footdrop, deformities of limbs and face, and contractures are also indications for surgery, but to be effective, intervention must include an intensive program of rehabilitation.

FOLLOW-UP

At present, patients with lepromatous leprosy are treated for life. In other types of leprosy, therapy is discontinued 3 to 10 years after negativity (see Table 3), but reexamination for evidence of relapse should be continued for 10 years. Relapse may indicate dapsone-resistant *M. leprae,* which can be detected by mouse footpad inoculation.

MANAGEMENT OF CONTACTS

A contact of a patient with leprosy is defined as anyone living in the same household during the 3-year period preceding diagnosis of the patient's disease. Contacts should have annual examinations for 5 years following adequate treatment of the patient. Examination should include survey of the skin for lesions or areas of numbness, palpation of peripheral nerves for tenderness or enlargement, and sensory testing of the distal extremities. Prophylactic therapy usually is not indicated after negative physical examination, although some authorities recommend that contacts exposed to patients with multibacillary (lepromatous or borderline) disease receive prophylaxis with dapsone for 3 years.

SUGGESTED READING

Jacobson RR. Antibiotic therapy for leprosy. In: Peterson PK, Verhoef J, eds. The antimicrobial agents annual II. New York: Elsevier, 1987.

Levis WR. Treatment of leprosy in the United States. Bull NY Acad Med 1984; 60:696–711.

Murphy FK, Mackowiak P, Luby J. Management of infections affecting the nervous system. In: Rosenberg RN, ed. The treatment of neurological diseases. New York: SP Medical & Scientific Books, 1979.

Noussitou FM, Sansarricq H, Walter J. Leprosy in children. Geneva: World Health Organization, 1976.

WHO Study Group. Chemotherapy of leprosy for control programs. WHO Technical Report Series, No 675 Geneva: World Health Organization, 1982.

LEPTOSPIROSIS

DOUGLAS H. JONES, M.D.
DONALD C. ANDERSON, M.D.

Pathogenic leptospires are parasites of an array of wild and domestic mammals, the most important of which are rodents, livestock, and domestic dogs. Asymptomatic infected animals, including cattle, previously immunized domestic dogs, and wild carnivores, may excrete leptospires in urine for several months, and these organisms can remain viable in fresh water and moist soil for up to several weeks. The majority of human disease arises from direct or indirect contact with animal carcasses or, more commonly, urine of infected animals (Figure 1). Leptospires demonstrate the capacity to invade through cutaneous lesions or intact mucous membranes, including conjunctivae, to cause systemic disease in humans. In recent years exposure to domestic dogs in the home and recreational exposure to contaminated water has replaced occupational exposure (veterinarians, slaughterhouse workers, farmers) as the predominant means of acquisition of disease. A suburban outbreak has clearly shown that the adequately immunized and asymptomatic pet dog may shed leptospiral organisms, thus serving as both a reservoir and a vector for the transmission of disease to humans.

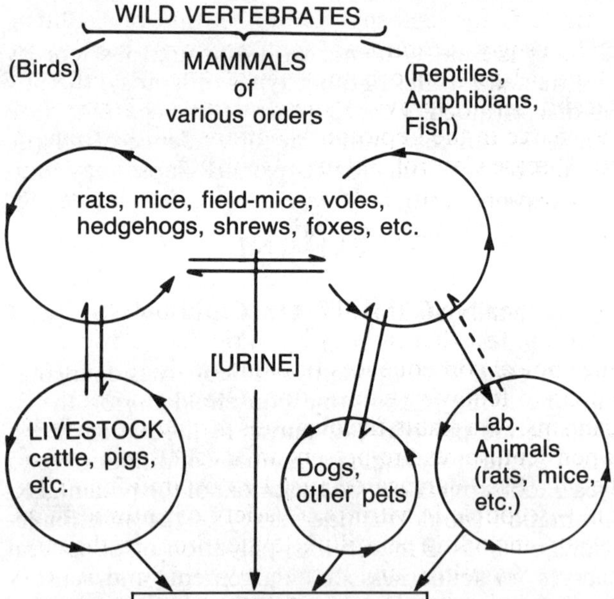

Leptospirosis is an acute systemic infection characterized by an extensive vasculitis. In the United States, *Leptospira icterohaemorrhagiae, L. pomona, and L. canicola* are some of the most prevalent of many pathogenic strains in humans. Many infections are asymptomatic, and serologic surveys of slaughterhouse workers suggest that the majority of infections do not come to medical attention. Among symptomatic cases, the diverse spectrum of nonspecific presenting clinical features often suggests other common diagnostic considerations, such as viral syndrome. The incubation period of leptospirosis averages 7 to 12 days, with a range of 2 to 26 days. The disease occurs in two forms: the more common and benign anicteric presentation and the rare, but severe, icteric form, termed Weil's syndrome. Both anicteric and icteric cases generally demonstrate a biphasic course (Figure 2). The initial or septicemic phase is characterized by 3 to 7 days of high-grade remittent fever, myalgia, headache, abdominal pain, and/or vomiting. Conjunctival suffusion (injection without exudate) may provide a specific diagnostic clue. During this stage, cultures of blood, cerebrospinal fluid (CSF), and other tissues may yield leptospires even in the absence of an inflammatory response. A 1-to 3-day afebrile and relatively asymptomatic period precedes the second, or immune, stage, which is ushered in by a brisk humoral immune response and is characterized by the onset of fever, headache, vomiting, and CSF pleocytosis. Weil's syndrome is distinguished from anicteric forms of disease by the presence of severe renal and hepatic dysfunction, hemorrhagic complications, vascular collapse, severe alterations in cerebral function, and a 5 to 10 percent mortality rate. Vascular collapse and death is usually attributed to complications of diffuse vasculitis, but is

Figure 1 Interrelations of the principal reservoir hosts of leptospires and man. (From Turner LH. Leptospirosis. Br Med J 1973; 1:537.)

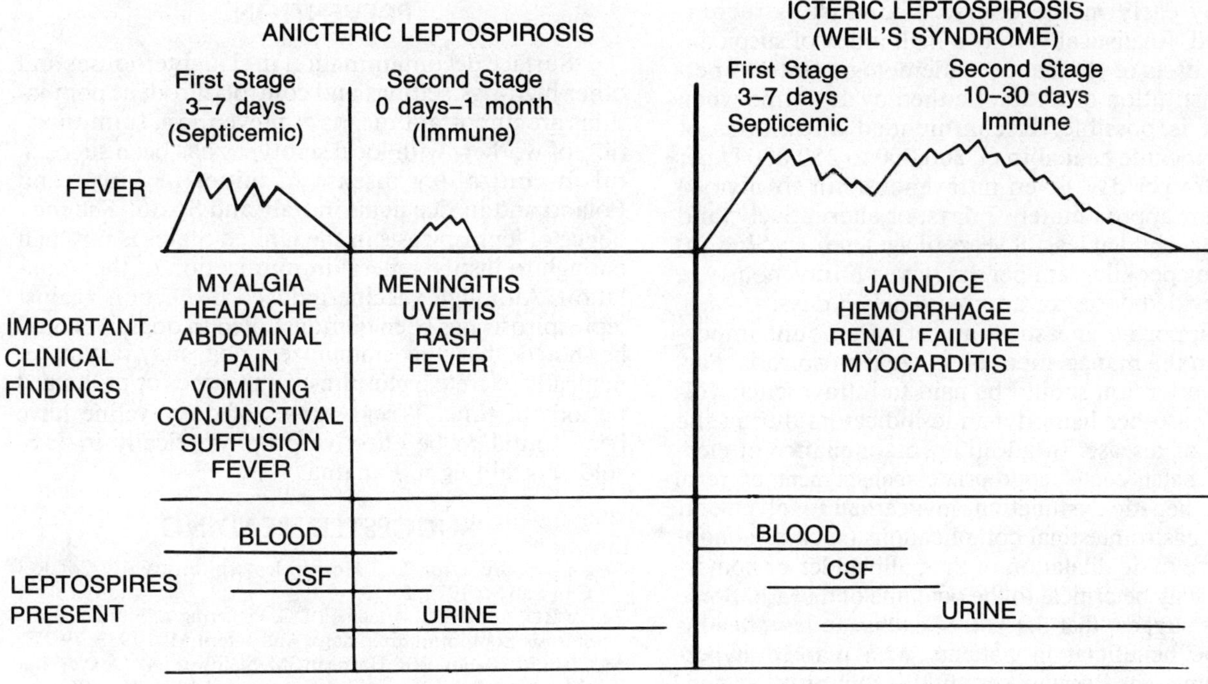

Figure 2 The stages of anicteric and icteric leptospiroses. Correlation between clinical findings and presence of leptospires in body fluids. (From Feigin RD, Anderson DC. Human leptospirosis. CRC Crit Rev Clin Lab Sci 1975; 5:413.)

rarely caused by myocarditis or massive gastrointestinal or other hemorrhagic events. Generally, during the immune phase of disease, leptospires are recoverable only from the urine or aqueous humor. With respect to most target organs, clinical and histopathologic features of leptospirosis are most apparent following the elimination of leptospires from these tissues.

A confirmed case of leptospirosis is established by one of the following criteria: (1) a clinical specimen that is culture positive for leptospires, or (2) the occurrence of clinical symptoms compatible with leptospirosis, such as the combination of fever, headache, myalgia, jaundice, oliguria, and conjunctivitis, *and* either a seroconversion *or* a fourfold or greater rise or decrease in the microscopic agglutination (MA) titer between acute and convalescent serum specimens obtained 2 or more weeks apart and studied at the same laboratory. A presumptive case of leptospirosis is defined as a patient whose clinical symptoms are compatible with a diagnosis of leptospirosis and who has either an MA titer of 1:100 or greater, a positive macroscopic agglutination slide test (SA) reaction on a single serum specimen obtained after the onset of symptoms, *or* a stable MA of 1:100 or greater in two or more serum specimens obtained after the onset of symptoms. The isolation of leptospires by direct culture from blood obtained from patients during the septicemic stage of illness or from urine during the immune phase is, if properly

executed, the most reliable of all laboratory procedures available for the diagnosis of leptospirosis. Whenever possible, the clinician should attempt to use laboratory facilities in which cultural and serologic tests for leptospirosis are routine procedures. We strongly recommend that specimens be sent to standard reference laboratories. The U.S. Public Health Service provides these laboratory services at no charge in the Leptospirosis Branch of the Centers for Disease Control, Atlanta, Georgia.

TREATMENT

Difficulty in treatment of leptospirosis arises from the fact that in both anicteric and icteric cases the clinical consequences of tissue invasion are most apparent following elimination of the pathogenic organisms. As a result, the diagnosis is rarely considered when leptospires are present in most tissues and/or before tissue damage occurs. Leptospiral organisms are susceptible in vitro to a variety of antimicrobial agents, including penicillin, tetracycline, erythromycin, cephalothin, and streptomycin. Several controlled studies have found no differences between antibiotic treatment and placebo with respect to the duration or severity of disease. However, two studies suggest that antimicrobial therapy, when provided within the first 4 days of disease, can favorably alter the course of disease. For this reason antimicrobial therapy early in the course of disease is recommended. Realistically, only a high index of suspicion on the basis of clinical or epidemologic features permits institution of antibiotic therapy at a time when benefit is possible. Recommended antibiotics of choice include penicillin G, 200,000 to 250,000 U per kilogram per day, given intravenously in six divided doses for approximately 7 days, or alternatively (and only in a child at least 8 years of age), tetracycline, 10 to 20 mg per kilogram per day, given intravenously in four divided doses for approximately 7 days.

Supportive measures are of paramount importance in the management of severe leptospirosis. Particular attention should be paid to intravascular volume and other hemodynamic indicators during the course of disease. In addition, maintenance of electrolyte balance and appropriate management of renal failure, hepatic dysfunction, myocardial involvement, and/or gastrointestinal complications (such as nonobstructive toxic dilatation of the gallbladder or hemorrhage) may be critical to the outcome of disease. Some reports suggest that the use of exchange transfusions may be beneficial in patients with marked hyperbilirubinemia. Because serum bilirubin or other nondialyzable serum factors may be present in excess and may aggravate renal failure, these investigators have suggested that exchange transfusion might provide a useful adjunct to hemodialysis in patients with renal failure associated with hyperbilirubinemia.

PREVENTION

Surface decontamination in slaughterhouses and other high-risk settings and control of rodent populations are important means of prevention. Immunization of workers with local serotypes has been successful in controlling disease in mines in Japan and Poland and in rice fields in Italy and Spain. The incidence of leptospirosis in the United States is not high enough to justify general immunization of the population. Although vaccine-induced protection against leptospirosis has been demonstrated in dogs, it should be noted that the immunized dog may asymptomatically excrete leptospires in the urine for prolonged periods of time. Weekly doses of doxycycline have been found to be effective prophylactically in U.S. soldiers training in Panama.

SUGGESTED READING

Feigin RD, Anderson DC. Human leptospirosis. CRC Crit Rev Clin Lab Sci 1975; 5:413.
Feigin RD, Lobes LA, Anderson DC, Pickering L. Human leptospirosis from immunized dogs. Ann Intern Med 1973; 79:777.
McClain BL, Ballou WR, Harrison SM, Steinweg DL. Doxycycline therapy for leptospirosis. Ann Intern Med 1984; 100:696.
Sulzer CF, Jones WL. Leptospirosis: methods in laboratory diagnosis. Centers for Disease Control, US Department of Health, Education and Welfare, Publication No. (CDC) 74-8275.
Turner LH. Leptospirosis. Br Med J 1973; 1:537.
Wong ML, Kaplan S, Dunkle LM, et al. Leptospirosis: a childhood disease. J Pediatr 1977; 90:532.

LISTERIOSIS

KEITHA FARMER, M.B., Ch.B., F.R.C.P.(U.K.), F.R.A.C.P., Ph.D.

Listeria monocytogenes is a gram-positive bacillus that can cause abortion, stillbirth and neonatal death in animals and humans. There is no correlation between the incidence of disease in humans and animals except isolated veterinary contacts. There are racial and geographic differences in infection rates. Practically speaking, in my experience listeriosis is a perinatal problem, although disease is seen in the elderly and the immunocompromised.

The typical history is that of a woman who has an influenzalike illness, abdominal pain, or urinary symptoms within a few weeks of delivery, which is premature in many cases. Bacteremia may be documented antepartum. There are frequently signs of amnionitis and the amnionitis is the apparent cause of onset of labor. The diagnosis can be made antepartum by finding gram-positive bacilli on amniocentesis in women with unexplained fever.

The infected infant usually has a clinical picture of respiratory distress and a chest roentgenogram suggestive of meconium aspiration. In addition to septicemia, multiple organs are frequently involved with microabscesses manifested by hepatosplenomegaly, a petechial, red macular rash, or, more rarely, white microabscesses in the skin. Laboratory features are a blood polymorphonuclear leukocytosis or neutropenia with immature granulocytes. The disease may present as meningitis in the late-onset form.

Routine laboratory culture media such as sheep's blood agar are satisfactory for culture of *Listeria* from sites not expected to be contaminated by other organisms, but selective media or the cold enrichment technique is used to improve isolation from heavily contaminated sites.

SPECIFIC THERAPY

In the event that maternal septicemia is diagnosed, ampicillin, 1 g given intravenously every 6 hours, is indicated and should be continued for a minimum of 5 days after the time of defervescence. Delivery of normal infants after treatment of maternal septicemia has been recorded. As with all pathogens causing amnionitis, viable infants must be delivered urgently in view of the difficulty of treating the fetus.

Ampicillin is the drug of choice for the infant. The dosage for an infant under the age of 7 days is 50 mg per kilogram twice daily and 50 mg per kilogram every 8 hours thereafter as a bolus injection by the intravenous route. I use amikacin, 7.5 mg per kilogram, twice daily as a 20-minute intravenous infusion initially while awaiting confirmation of culture because of a synergistic effect of aminoglycosides in vitro. In infants whose birth weight is less than 1,200 g the interval between doses of amikacin is 18 to 24 hours. Ampicillin is continued for a minimum of 10 days for septicemia and 2 weeks for meningitis. Amikacin is continued only if meningitis is present. Another aminoglycoside used routinely in a unit to treat neonatal sepsis of unknown origin would be suitable.

Penicillin, 50,000 U per kilogram every 12 hours, is the second choice. It has been less effective than ampicillin according to some reports. Late-onset meningitis is treated by the foregoing regimen for a minimum of 2 weeks.

Listeria monocytogenes is usually susceptible in vitro to erythromycin and tetracycline. The former is bacteriostatic and less effective; the latter is contraindicated in the newborn. Trimethoprim-sulfamethoxazole is effective in vitro, but has not been tried extensively in vivo and should be reserved for the improbable event of lack of response to ampicillin and aminoglycoside and in the absence of significant jaundice. Rifampin is also effective in vitro, but has not been adequately studied. Cephalosporins are ineffective, and when *Listeria* is a possibility, they should not be used alone. Chloramphenicol is bacteriostatic, is frequently ineffective, may interfere with ampicillin, and should not be used in the newborn.

If I were treating listeriosis in a child other than a neonate, I would use ampicillin 200 to 400 mg per kilogram per day, given intravenously in divided doses every 6 hours for at least 2 weeks, with an aminoglycoside because such a child would probably be immunocompromised.

SUPPORTIVE THERAPY

Supportive therapy includes maintenance of fluid and electrolyte balance, blood products for shock and sepsis, oxygen for the severe congenital pneumonia, and mechanical ventilation.

MONITORING RESPONSE TO THERAPY

In the presence of cerebrospinal fluid (CSF) pleocytosis, lumbar puncture should be performed daily until the CSF is sterile (usually within 24 hours) and repeated when therapy is completed. The trough concentration of amikacin in serum should be checked at least after the first 24 hours, at 5 days, and weekly thereafter. Trough concentrations should be between 3 and 5 μg per milliliter and dosage adjusted to achieve this.

FOLLOW-UP

The prognosis of early-onset disease depends on the control of shock, septicemia, and congenital pneumonia. If there is control of sepsis and respiratory support is not necessary in the first 24 hours, survival can be expected and the outlook is good if oxygenation is possible with ventilatory assistance. If 100 percent oxygen and full ventilatory support are necessary for more than a day or two (when appropriate antibiotics are given), the prognosis is guarded.

The late-onset meningitis has a prognosis similar to that of meningitis caused by other gram-positive organisms, and in my experience, it is good. However, sequelae have been described in the literature, as might be expected with late treatment, and careful neurologic assessment is indicated on recovery and at least every 6 months in the first 2 years of life. As with all newborns who have received an aminoglycoside or who have had meningitis, a hearing test should be performed before discharge and at age 9 months. The long-term prognosis appears good. I have not observed sequelae, although they have been described. There is a limited follow-up in our area in view of the migratory habits of our Polynesian population, the group most frequently affected with the disease.

PREVENTION AND MANAGEMENT OF CONTACTS

Although possible cross-infection has been observed only in adult immunocompromised hosts, the usual isolation techniques, with special attention to fecal and oral secretions, are carried out in newborn nurseries. No studies have been done of the value of treatment of rectal or vaginal disease in carrier mothers. I am unaware of studies of transmission between sexual partners. However, as with group B streptococcus, it is improbable that treatment would be of value. If a carrier mother has lost a fetus from *Listeria,* it has been suggested that she should receive erythromycin, 250 mg every 6 hours for 10 days; this is reasonable, although not proved to be effective in preventing further fetal loss.

Symptomatic pregnant women should be investigated by means of genital, rectal, and blood cultures, and if there is evidence of *Listeria,* they should be treated in view of the case reports suggesting that treatment can prevent infection of the fetus. Signs of amnionitis call for diagnostic amniocentesis and delivery if the diagnosis is confirmed. Cultures should be obtained from infants of asymptomatic colonized mothers, but treatment is not justified unless the infant is symptomatic, in which case ampicillin is indicated pending results of cultures. I did not find asymptomatic colonized infants in the prospective study of more than 1,000 infants admitted to the special care unit during an "epidemic period."

SUGGESTED READING

Evans JR, Allen AC, Stinson DA, et al. Perinatal listeriosis: report of an outbreak. Pediatr Infect Dis 1985; 4:237–241.
Ceeliger HPR. Listeriosis. New York: Hafner, 1961.
Teberg AJ, Yonekura ML, Salminen C, et al. Clinical manifestations of epidemic neonatal listeriosis. Pediatr Infect Dis J 1987; 6:817–820.
Tim MW, Jackson MA, Shannon K, et al. Non-neonatal infection due to *Listeria monocytogens*. Pediatr Infect Dis 1984; 3:213–217.

LYME DISEASE

BARBARA W. STECHENBERG, M.D.

Lyme disease, recognized initially in 1975 in Connecticut as a new kind of arthritis, is an infectious disease syndrome that can involve skin, nervous system, joints, and heart. It has been diagnosed subsequently in many states and countries, although it is seen mainly on the Eastern seaboard, in the upper Midwest, and in the West. A distinct pattern of signs and symptoms has emerged; most characteristic is the early rash, erythema chronicum migrans (ECM). The causative agent is a spirochete, *Borrelia burgdorferi.* It usually is transmitted by the bite of the *Ixodes dammini* or related ticks.

The clinical findings of Lyme disease are divided into three stages on the basis of chronologic relationship to the original bite. The most common manifestation is the rash, which usually begins 4 to 20 days after the tick bite. An erythematous macule or papule forms and gradually enlarges to form a large plaque-like, erythematous annular lesion. Multiple secondary annular lesions are often seen. These lesions may be associated with a wide variety of systemic symptoms such as malaise, fatigue, headache, and arthralgias. Fever and lymphadenopathy are common.

Neurologic abnormalities occur roughly within 4 weeks after the tick bite occurs. The spectrum of involvement is wide and includes aseptic meningitis, cranial neuritis, radiculopathies, and myelitis. Cardiac abnormalities occur in a small percentage of patients, commonly young adult males, within several weeks after the bite. The duration is usually brief, but may include myopericarditis and atrioventricular block.

The second most common manifestation of Lyme disease is arthritis, which typically begins about 5 to 6 weeks after the bite. Some patients with arthritis do not recall any skin lesions. The arthritis is usually of sudden onset, monoarticular, or oligoarticular and involves the large joints. Recurrent attacks are common.

The diagnosis of Lyme disease is best made on clinical and epidemiologic grounds, particularly early in the course of the illness, from the gross appearance of the skin lesions. Routine laboratory testing is usually nonspecific and not helpful. Specific serologic diagnosis can be used for patients who present with late complications and/or without a history of erythema chronicum migrans. Indirect fluorescent antibody (IFA) testing and enzyme-linked immunosorbent assay (ELISA) have both been used to make the diagnosis, particularly in patients with neurologic problems or arthritis. An elevated IgG response, which may persist for many months or years, is usually demonstrated in these patients.

TREATMENT

Early Lyme Disease

Even before the spirochete was identified as the causative agent, antibiotic treatment with penicillin or tetracycline was associated with more rapid resolution of the rash and its associated symptoms. Both antibiotics have been shown to prevent late complications of the disease. However, nearly half of all treated patients do have minor late symptoms such as headache, musculoskeletal pain, and lethargy.

Early treatment on the basis of characteristic clinical findings is imperative to prevent complications. Treatment regimens are listed in Table 1. The treatment of choice is tetracycline, but this should not be used in children younger than 8 years of age because of its adverse effect on teeth and bones. The duration of treatment is usually 10 days. If symptoms of disease persist or if immediate relapse occurs after treatment is stopped, the antibiotic should be continued for 20 days.

Late Lyme Disease

Adult patients with neurologic complications treated with large dosages of intravenous penicillin G (20 million U per day for 10 days) have been reported to show improvement. Therapy was begun a mean of 6 weeks after the neurologic symptoms developed.

TABLE 1   Therapy of Lyme Disease

Drug	Dosage	Comments
Early Lyme disease		
Tetracycline	25–50 mg/kg/day in 4 divided doses orally for 10 days	For children > 8 years of age; maximum dose 1 g/day
Penicillin V	50 mg/kg/day in 4 divided doses orally for 10 days	For children < 8 years of age; maximum dose 2 g/day
Erythromycin	30–50 mg/kg/day in 4 divided doses orally	For penicillin-allergic children; efficacy not certain
Late Lyme disease		
Neurologic disease		
Penicillin G aqueous	300,000 U/kg/day IV in 6 divided doses for 10 days	Not for patients with isolated facial palsy not previously treated for ECM (use early regimens above)
Tetracycline	50 mg/kg/day po in 4 divided doses for 30 days	Use only in penicillin-allergic patients
Ceftriaxone	100 mg/kg/day IV in 2 divided doses for 10 days	For cases refractory to penicillin; information limited; use with caution in penicillin-allergic patients
Cardiac disease		Effectiveness of treatment uncertain
Established arthritis		
Penicillin G aqueous	300,000 U/kg/day IV in 6 divided doses for at least 10 days	
Benzathine penicillin	50,000 U/kg weekly for 3 weeks	Maximum: 2.4 million U/dose; use only if IV therapy is impossible
Ceftriaxone	50–75 mg/kg/day in 2 divided doses for at least 10 days	For use in cases refractory to penicillin; limited information

Duration of meningitic symptoms was shortened, but time to resolution of motor deficit was not affected. No large studies of pediatric patients with neurologic complications has been reported, but parenteral penicillin has been efficacious in selected patients.

Patients with established Lyme arthritis also have been treated successfully with penicillin. In one trial, half the patients given intramuscular benzathine penicillin (2.4 million U weekly for 3 weeks) had complete resolution of arthritis without recurrence.

By both in vitro and in vivo susceptibility studies, *B. burgdorferi* has been shown to be exquisitely susceptible to ceftriaxone. Its use in cases of refractory neurologic and arthritic complications recently has confirmed these observations. Further studies are in progress to determine its comparative efficacy to penicillin, but in the meantime it is a reasonable alternative in those patients who do not respond to penicillin.

The importance of antibiotic treatment in patients with carditis is unclear. The involvement is usually self-limited, although those with heart block may need temporary pacing.

The efficacy of steroids and nonsteroidal anti-inflammatory agents in patients with established arthritis is not clear. Initial episodes of arthritis may be treated symptomatically with analgesics such as acetaminophen along with antibiotic therapy.

The prompt recognition of this disease, with its diverse manifestations, should lead to early treatment and resolution. Prevention occurs only with avoidance of contact with the tick vector. Knowledge of areas where the ticks are found, avoidance of such areas, and, if bitten, prompt removal of the tick are the primary preventive measures.

SUGGESTED READING

Andiman WA. Lyme disease: epidemiology, etiology, clinical spectrum, diagnosis and treatment. In: Aranoff SC, ed. Advances in pediatric infectious diseases. Chicago: Year Book, 1986; 1:163–187.

Stechenberg BW. Borrelia: Lyme disease. In: Feigin RD, Cherry JD, eds. Textbook of pediatric infectious diseases. Philadelphia: WB Saunders, 1987; 1102–1107.

Steere AC, Green J, Schoen RT, et al. Successful parenteral penicillin therapy of established Lyme arthritis. N Engl J Med 1985; 312:869–874.

Steere AC, Hutchinson GJ, Rahn DW, et al. Treatment of the early manifestations of Lyme disease. Ann Intern Med 1983; 99:22–26.

MELIOIDOSIS

JAY P. SANFORD, M.D.

Melioidosis is an infection with a protean clinical spectrum caused by the aerobic gram-negative bacillus, *Pseudomonas pseudomallei*. Melioidosis is endemic in Southeast Asia and northern Australia (North Queensland). It is being recognized more frequently in Africa and is probably endemic there as well. Human melioidosis has been described only rarely in the Western Hemisphere: Panama, Ecuador, Mexico, a neonatal case in Hawaii, a case in Georgia, and a possible case in Oklahoma. With these exceptions, confirmed melioidosis has occurred in U.S. or European residents only when they have traveled in endemic areas.

Clinical presentations are varied. Acute pulmonary infection varying from mild bronchitis to overwhelming necrotizing pneumonia is most common. Acute septicemic infection with rapid development of respiratory, hepatic, and renal failure, disorientation, shock, and death is not uncommon. Chronic suppurative infection with abscesses that can involve virtually any organ is yet another presentation. Melioidosis is unusual in that activation of inapparent or quiescent infection can occur following triggering by events such as influenzal pneumonia, diabetic ketoacidosis, surgery, or trauma many years after probable time of exposure (infection).

Melioidosis has been uncommon in children, even in endemic areas, hence it is seldom considered in a clinical differential diagnosis and often represents a surprise provided by the laboratory.

Pseudomonas pseudomallei is usually susceptible in vitro to the tetracyclines, chloramphenicol, novobiocin, kanamycin, trimethoprim-sulfamethoxazole, imipenem, and some of the cephalosporins such as ceftazidime, ceftriaxone, and cefsulodin. In most instances, strains are resistant to penicillins, most cephalosporins, aminoglycosides, rifampin, colistin, and the fluoroquinolones.

SPECIFIC TREATMENT

The treatment regimen should vary according to the form of the disease. Individuals with low-titer positive serologic tests, but with no evidence of disease, do not require treatment.

In patients with acute or subacute pulmonary melioidosis, effective therapy has included tetracycline, 40 mg per kilogram per day given orally in divided doses every 6 hours, chloramphenicol, 40 mg per kilogram per day given orally, or trimethoprim-sulfamethoxazole (8 mg TMP per kilogram and 40 mg SMZ per kilogram) given orally in divided doses every 12 hours. Treatment should be continued for at least 2 months. The mean interval until sputum cultures become negative has been 6 weeks. Because of the need for long-term treatment with the potential hematotoxicity of chloramphenicol and dental staining in children younger than 7 years with tetracycline, my recommendation has been the trimethoprim-sulfamethoxazole regimen. If sputum cultures remain positive for 6 months, surgical lobectomy should be considered.

With chronic extrapulmonary suppurative disease, the same regimen or regimens are recommended; however, treatment should be continued for 6 months to 1 year. The usual principles of surgical drainage should be followed.

With severe pneumonitis or the acute septicemic form, the case fatality rate is 50 to 95 percent. Under these circumstances, multiple parenteral antibiotics are usually administered. Various regimens have been used. One regimen is chloramphenicol, 50 to 75 mg per kilogram per day, given intravenously or orally in divided doses every 6 hours, *plus* trisulfapyrimidines or sulfisoxazole, 120 to 150 mg per kilogram, given orally in divided doses every 6 hours, *plus* an aminoglycoside for 10 to 14 days, although the value of triple therapy has not been established. While experience with it is limited, a regimen of trimethoprim-sulfamethoxazole (9 mg TMP per kilogram–45 mg SMZ per kilogram) intravenously divided into a 12-hourly dosage, *plus* ceftazidime (150 mg per kilogram per day), given intravenously in divided doses every 8 hours, is currently being used in the endemic areas of Thailand. This regimen has the advantage of both agents being bactericidal and relatively nontoxic. An alternative agent to ceftazidime is ceftriaxone, which can be used in a dosage of 100 mg per kilogram per day, given intravenously in divided doses every 12 hours. Currently I recommend the TMP/SMZ plus ceftazidime or ceftriaxone regimen.

Isolation of the patient is not necessary because human-to-human transmission has been reported in only one instance of sexual transmission. In the patient with a draining abscess, wound and secretion precautions are logical.

SUGGESTED READING

Barnes PR, Appleman MD, Cosgrove MM. A case of melioidosis originating in North America. Am Rev Resp Dis 1986; 134:170–171.

Patamasucon P, Schaad UB, Nelson JD. Melioidosis. J Pediatr 1982; 100:175–182.

Sanford JP. Melioidosis and glanders in Harrison's principles of internal medicine, 11th ed. Braunwald E, Isselbacher KJ, Petersdorf RG, et al, eds. New York: McGraw-Hill, 1987; 589–592.

NOCARDIOSIS

EDGAR O. LEDBETTER, M.D.

Nocardiae are gram-positive, variably acid-fast, filamentous aerobic actinomycetes commonly present in the soil worldwide. They are generally acquired by inhalation or by traumatic transcutaneous tissue inoculation. *Nocardia asteroides, Nocardia brasiliensis,* and *Nocardia caviae* are the major pathogenic species isolated from diseased individuals.

CUTANEOUS, LYMPHOCUTANEOUS, AND LOCALIZED INFECTIONS

Cutaneous or lymphocutaneous *Nocardia* infections are the most common form of disease in otherwise normal children, most often introduced accidentally in the course of active play. *N. brasiliensis* has been isolated from a majority of the cutaneous and lymphocutaneous lesions, and causes disease in immunologically normal individuals. This organism's capacity for local invasion is thought to relate to its increased pathogenicity over that of other *Nocardia.* Dissemination from a cutaneous pustule or secondary to the lymphangitic form of this disease is rare in nonimmunocompromised individuals. The nocardial lymphocutaneous syndrome most closely mimics cutaneous sporotrichosis, but could be confused with suppurative lymphadenitis caused by *Staphylococcus aureus* or group A streptocococci, actinomycosis, cat scratch disease, plague, tularemia, or cutaneous diphtheria. Cutaneous lesions are often cervicofacial in distribution, being commonly located just below the nares, but may occur anywhere. *Nocardia* pericarditis and shunt-associated ventriculitis have been reported to occur secondary to surgical intervention with suspected surgical contamination in most of these cases.

Post traumatic keratitis can be caused by *Nocardia* species. In addition to receiving systemic therapy, patients with *Nocardia* keratitis should receive benefit from topical 30 percent sodium sulfacetamide every 2 hours. Ophthalmology consultation is encouraged. The source for nontraumatic localized disease such as osteomyelitis or panophthalmitis is usually pulmonary, although the site of origin may be obscure.

Nocardia madurae, other *Nocardia* and other actinomycetes, and some fungi can cause mycetomas, which I shall not discuss because of their rarity.

SYSTEMIC INFECTION

Pulmonary nocardiosis, is the most common systemic manifestation of this disease, and is usually acquired by inhalation. *N. asteroides* is the most frequent offender and may spread to involve any organ, most often the brain or meninges, kidneys, bone, muscle, and the eye. Although outbreaks of infection caused by *Nocardia* species have occurred in renal and heart transplant units, there is no direct evidence for man-to-man transmission, and respiratory isolation is generally not recommended. Normal individuals seldom, but occasionally, harbor these organisms, and it is important to attempt to verify or exclude pulmonary and other forms of systemic disease whenever *Nocardia* species are isolated from sputum specimens. Children with lymphocutaneous nocardiosis, who appear otherwise healthy with no past history of chronic or recurrent infection and who exhibit a prompt response to treatment, do not require an extensive immunologic evaluation. Nocardiosis is sometimes the initial manifestation of chronic granulomatous disease and may occur in association with other pathogens such as *Aspergillus* species or atypical mycobacteria. Should an otherwise healthy-appearing child develop pulmonary or systemic nocardiosis, a nitroblue-tetrazolium dye test and/or other tests to determine the bactericidal capability of the patient's neutrophiles should be performed.

ANTIMICROBIAL THERAPY

Sulfonamides have long been considered the mainstay of therapy and have been my initial choice in the management of children with a cutaneous or lymphocutaneous syndrome. A loading dose of 75 mg per kilogram of sulfamethoxazole followed by 150 mg per kilogram per day in four to six divided doses usually suffices to achieve peak serum concentrations of 15 to 20 mg per deciliter. Pulmonary and other deep *Nocardia* infections may also be responsive to a sulfonamide preparation.

Several investigators have demonstrated synergistic activity with trimethoprim–sulfamethoxazole (TMP/SMZ) against *Nocardia* species, noting reduction in the total concentration of each drug required to inhibit growth. Although there is no proven superiority of TMP/SMZ over sulfonamide therapy alone, collective experience for TMP/SMZ-treated systemic *Nocardia* infections, even in the immunocompromised patient, has been quite favorable. Therapeutic trimethoprim concentrations are achieved in sputum, pleural fluid, lung, bone, aqueous humor, and most other body sites. Therapeutic concentrations of both drugs are regularly achieved in the cerebrospinal fluid (CSF), even in the absence of inflammation. Sulfonamides are also well distributed throughout the body, with 60 to 80 percent of the serum concentration present in the CSF and other major body fluids. Therapeutic concentrations of both agents are achieved within infected brain tissue by oral dosage when administered in the standard fixed 1:5 ratio of the TMP/SMZ combination (40 mg of TMP–200 mg of SMZ or 80 mg of TMP–400 mg of SMZ). Most treated patients have received 6 to 12 mg of TMP–30 to 60 mg of SMZ per kilogram per day, in two to four divided doses. Intravenous TMP/SMZ may be advantageous for the patient with serious infection in whom an oral preparation is poorly tolerated or unreliably absorbed. A loading dose of 250 mg of TMP and 1,250 mg of SMZ per square meter, followed by maintenance doses of 150 mg of TMP and 750 mg of SMZ per square meter every 8 hours for children aged 10 years or younger and every 12 hours for adults with normal renal function, has been recommended. Dosage reduction or less-frequent administration is required for patients in renal failure. The patient's renal and electrolyte status must be accurately assessed and monitored. Adequate fluid intake and alkalinization of the urine minimizes the potential for crystalluria and secondary urinary obstruction, which is most often seen with sulfadiazine therapy.

In addition to the well-known potential side effects of the sulfonamides, which include Stevens-Johnson syndrome, TMP/SMZ may cause hepatotoxicity (rarely fulminant hepatic necrosis), megaloblastic anemia, thrombocytopenia, aplastic anemia, agranulocytosis, and toxic epidermal necrolysis. The antifolate activity of TMP/SMZ may be prevented by the administration of folinic acid, 0.2 mg per kilogram per day, in an attempt to obviate marrow suppression. Toxicity should be treated with larger amounts of folinic acid, 0.8 mg per kilogram per day in four divided doses. Hemolysis may occur in patients with glucose-6-phosphate dehydrogenase deficiency. Striking rashes have been related to TMP/SMZ administration in patients with the acquired immunodeficiency syndrome (AIDS).

The sulfonamides and/or trimethoprim should be discontinued at the first appearance of skin rash or any sign of adverse reaction. These drugs are contraindicated late in pregnancy and during the first 2 months of life. The intravenous preparation of TMP/SMZ has not been approved for use in infants or children under 2 years of age.

The clinical outcome depends on the site and extent of disease, the host response, the susceptibility of the offending organism, and associated disease(s). Early recognition and treatment may allow for a more rapid clinical response, prevent dissemination, alleviate the need for surgery, and allow for a shorter course of treatment. Surgical drainage or excision of abscess cavities can be an important adjunct to medical treatment. Discontinuation of immunosuppressive agents may be of value, but is not always feasible.

Seriously ill patients may also deserve an additional antimicrobial agent until susceptibility test results are available and/or a clinical response has been achieved. Occasional failure of response to sulfonamides or TMP/SMZ therapy has provoked a continued search for more effective agents. Drugs utilized with varying success include ampicillin, minocycline, erythromycin, chloramphenicol, cycloserine, and amikacin sulfate.

Experience with other aminoglycosides, third-generation cephalosporins, imipenem, and fusidic acid is limited. Selection is governed primarily by the site of infection, the potential diffusion of the various agents available and their sensitivity patterns, and the known side effects of these antimicrobials. The need for long-term treatment limits the value of the aminoglycosides because of potential renal and otic damage. Amikacin dosage is 15 to 30 mg per kilogram per day, in two or three divided doses given intravenously or intramuscularly, with a maximum recommended dosage of 600 mg per square meter per day. Monitoring of serum concentrations is mandatory for patients with any degree of renal insufficiency. Dental staining and/or pseudotumor cerebri may result from tetracycline therapy, and in addition minocycline may cause vestibular toxicity. The hematopoietic toxicity of chloramphenicol is well known. Experience with cycloserine in children is limited, and it cannot be recommended. *Nocardia* are consistently resistant to nafcillin and oxacillin.

It is important to note that *Nocardia* infection may coexist with other diseases such as tuberculosis or alveolar proteinosis.

DURATION OF THERAPY

No clear treatment guidelines are available regarding the required duration of therapy. Cutaneous lesions are generally treated for 6 to 12 weeks, depending on how rapid the response is. Some prefer to continue therapy for 6 weeks or longer following resolution of cutaneous lesions and/or lymphadenitis. Patients with systemic disease such as pneumonia or brain abscess deserve treatment for 6 to 12 months or longer, depending on the clinical course and associated conditions and complications.

Treatment failures are most commonly observed with *Nocardia* meningitis and/or brain abscess. Patients managed with chemotherapy alone must be carefully monitored with serial computed tomography scans in addition to sequential CSF examinations. Patients with systemic nocardiosis may show evidence of recurrence months or years after their initial *Nocardia* infection, and are best evaluated periodically over a prolonged period of time. Unfortunately, the common predisposing conditions are usually nonremedial.

PROGNOSIS

Most nonimmunocompromised patients with *Nocardia* infection should benefit from therapy. Treatment failures among children with cutaneous or lymphocutaneous disease have not been reported. The mortality in patients with central nervous system disease approximates 50 percent. Patients with systemic disease without central nervous system involvement have a relatively good prognosis with early recognition and appropriate treatment, and depending on the severity of their predisposing and associated conditions.

SUGGESTED READING

Curry WA. Human nocardiosis: a clinical review with selected case reports. Arch Intern Med 1980; 140:818.

Lampe RM, Baker CJ, Septimus EJ, Wallace RJ Jr. Cervicofacial nocardiosis in children. J Pediatr 1981; 99:593.

Law BJ, Marks MI. Pediatric nocardiosis. Pediatrics 1982; 70:560.

Overturf GD. Use of trimethoprim-sulfamethoxazole in pediatric infections: relative merits of intravenous administration. Rev Infect Dis 1987; 9:S168.

Wallace RJ Jr, Septimus EJ, Williams TW Jr, et al. Use of trimethoprim-sulfamethoxazole for treatment of infections due to noncardia. Rev Infect Dis 1982; 4:315.

NONTUBERCULOUS (ATYPICAL) MYCOBACTERIAL DISEASE

KEITH KRASINSKI, M.D.

Since the recognition of nontuberculous mycobacteria as pathogens in the 1950s, experience and understanding of nontuberculous (atypical) mycobacterial disease has undergone an evolution. Most recently, treatment of infections has changed because of recognition of the limitations of familiar drugs, the potential application of new drugs and biologicals, and the prevalence of these infections among persons infected with human immunodeficiency virus.

An important obstacle in formulating therapeutic recommendations for nontuberculous mycobacterial disease is the lack of controlled experience with drug combinations and durations of therapy. Another obstacle is the absence of long-term posttreatment observations to assess efficacy. In this and like situations, the experience and judgment of the treating physician, who considers the particular aspects of the individual patient, assumes paramount importance.

General considerations in the treatment of nontuberculous mycobacterial disease include the use of surgery to remove well-localized foci of infection, and the use of potentially synergistic drug combinations for treatment of widespread or disseminated disease, as well as the use of drug combinations to prevent the emergence of resistant organisms. Antimycobacterial chemotherapy is predicated on empiric therapy for likely agents with drugs to which they are usually susceptible (Table 1). Mycobacterial culture and susceptibility testing are always indicated, and when susceptibilities become available, therapy must be tailored to include drugs to which the organisms are susceptible.

LYMPHADENITIS

The most common syndrome in children attributable to nontuberculous mycobacteria is lymphade-

nitis, usually caused by *M. scrofulaceum* or *M. avium-intracellulare,* although *M. kansasii* and *M. chelonei* can also cause lymphadenitis. These organisms tend to be resistant to the usual antimycobacterial drugs; only *M. kansasii* is regularly susceptible to rifampin, and it is also susceptible to erythromycin. Although these agents do not ordinarily cause disseminated disease in immunocompetent children, they are associated with unsightly illness that persists for many months, and foci that drain spontaneously.

In view of the lack of efficacy or uncertainty of drug therapy, I favor total surgical excision of involved lymph nodes, and involved skin and sinus tracts if present. Surgical therapy, however, does not necessarily imply extensive removal of uninvolved contiguous nodes. The availability of a skilled and experienced surgeon is critical to this approach. For

TABLE 1 Predicted Antimycobacterial Drug Susceptibilities*

Organism	Usually Susceptible to:	Sometimes Susceptible to:
M. kansasii	Rifampin Erythromycin Streptomycin Ethionamide	Amikacin Cycloserine Ethambutol
M. marinum	Rifampin Amikacin Kanamycin	Minocycline
M. scrofulaceum	Amikacin Kanamycin Streptomycin Erythromycin	Rifampin
M. avium-intracellulare	Amikacin Ansamycin Ciprofloxacin† Ofloxacin†	Clofazimine
M. ulcerans	Rifampin Streptomycin	Clofazimine
M. fortuitum	Imipenem† Ciprofloxacin†	Cefoxitin Amikacin Sulfamethoxazole
M. chelonei		Amikacin Kanamycin Erythromycin

* Based on achievable serum levels.

† No clinical experience with these drugs exists in the treatment of nontuberculous mycobacterial disease.

resection of the submandibular nodes, identification preservation of the mandibular branch of the facial nerve is essential. Identification of the nerve can be facilitated with the use of electrical stimulation. The cure rate with surgery alone should approach 95 percent. In children with widespread involvement, in whom total excision would be disfiguring, the larger nodes should be removed. Incision and drainage and needle aspiration have been attempted, but can result in sinus tract formation, and this approach is not recommended. I recommend rifampin (10 to 20 mg per kilogram per day) for patients with extensive nodal involvement in whom total excision is not practical and for patients declining surgery.

An alternative approach is no therapy. The natural history of such infection is that resolution occurs following a period of disease lasting from 9 to 15 months, and often only after sinus drainage lasting for as long as 4 months. Because of the duration of disease and the temporary or permanent disfigurement that may result, I do not recommend this approach.

CUTANEOUS INFECTION

Skin and soft tissue infections usually follow traumatic inoculation with *M. marinum,* and are known as "swimming pool granulomas." The rapid growers *M. fortuitum* and *M. chelonei,* as well as the photochromogen *M. kansasii,* also produce this syndrome. *M. ulcerans* is a nonchromogen that is responsible for chronic ulcerative disease, known in Africa as Buruli ulcer and in Australia as Bairnsdale ulcer.

Infections caused by *M. marinum* and the rapid growers are frequently self-limited. If they persist for more than several months or are progressive, local excision is effective therapy. Infection with *M. marinum* can also be treated with rifampin, 10 to 20 mg per kilogram per day, and ethambutol, 15 mg per kilogram per day. Some strains are susceptible to sulfamethoxazole and tetracyclines. If either ethambutol or tetracyclines are used, the usual cautions and proscriptions apply to their use in children. The rapid growers are frequently resistant to antimycobacterial chemotherapy. *M. ulcerans* infections are also best treated with excision and grafting. The application of local heat may improve the outcome because these organisms grow only at between 30 and 35°C.

SKELETAL DISEASE

Nontuberculous mycobacteria are rare causes of bone and joint disease in children. *M. avium-intracellulare* and scotochromogens, presumably *M. scrofulaceum,* have been recovered. Surgical excision of localized disease should be curative.

TABLE 2 Use of Antimycobacterial Drugs in Children

Drug	Dosage (mg/kg)	Interval (hr)	Cautions
Isoniazid	10–20†·‡	12–24	Rash, nephrotoxicity, peripheral neuritis, hepatitis
Streptomycin	20–30‡	12	Auditory and/or vestibular damage, nephrotoxicity, fever, rash
Amikacin	15–30‡	8	
Capreomycin	20‡	24	
Rifampin	10–20†	12–24	Orange discoloration of body fluids, hepatotoxicity, leukopenia, thrombocytopenia, drug interactions
Ansamycin	5†*	12–24	
Ethambutol	15†	24	Rash, optic neuritis, age use limited to those in whom visual screening is possible
Ethionamide	10–20†*	12	Gastrointestinal irritation, neurologic disorders, hepatotoxicity, interference with control of diabetes
Cycloserine	7–10†*	12	Peripheral and central nervous system dysfunction, contraindicated in patients with seizure disorder
Erythromycin	40†	6	Gastrointestinal intolerance
Minocycline	4†	12	Not indicated for children less than 7 years of age
Cefoxitin	80–160‡	4–6	Limit to known susceptible organisms
Imipenem	60–100‡	6	Neurologic disorders
Sulfamethoxazole	60†	12	Hypersensitivity, bone marrow suppression in HIV-infected patients, can substitute trimethoprim–sulfamethoxazole
Clofazimine	2–5†*	24	Gastrointestinal intolerance, skin pigmentation, suspend in sesame oil and dispense dropwise
Ciprofloxacin	30–35†*	12	Hepatotoxicity, not indicated for children because of effects on formation of cartilage
	5–10‡*	12	

* No established dosage for children.
† Oral.
‡ Parenteral.

PULMONARY AND DISSEMINATED DISEASE

Pulmonary disease and disseminated infection are very rare in immunologically normal children. In children with immunodeficiency, whether congenital or acquired as a result of neoplastic disease, cytotoxic chemotherapy, or transmissible agents, widespread infections with nontuberculous mycobacteria, are associated with fatal illness. Disease in immunodeficient children is also complicated by the presence of other opportunistic pathogens. Diagnosis usually requires an invasive test such as bronchoalveolar lavage or lung biopsy in patients with pulmonary syndromes. Blood cultures using the Dupont Isolator have been useful adjuncts for the diagnosis of disseminated infection. Multiple regimens have been used with little success in immunodeficient patients. The usual etiologic agents, *M. avium-intracellulare* and *M. scrofulaceum,* tend to be multiply drug resistant. Traditionally a regimen of three or four drugs has been used in these patients. Such a regimen should include rifampin and ethionamide. Isoniazid is usually not active against these agents in vitro, and need not be included in the treatment regimen. Table 2 shows antimycobacterial drugs and dosages.

Experience with human immunodeficiency virus–infected patients with opportunistic infections caused by *M. avium-intracellulare* has shown that traditional regimens fail. Newer drugs (pyrazinamide, ansamycin, and clofazimine) with improved activity against nontuberculous mycobacteria have also been used, and have been associated with decreasing bacterial burdens, as determined by blood culture. Despite this activity, the organisms have not been eradicated and the clinical outcome of such patients has been disappointingly poor. This lack of efficacy is an indicator of the role of cell-mediated immunity in recovery from mycobacterial disease, and indicates that disseminated disease is a marker for immunologic attrition and not the principal cause of disease. Lack of efficacy can also be attributed to the failure to kill at achievable serum concentrations with these drugs. The in vitro activity of the 4-quinolones against *M. intracellulare* suggest these may be useful agents; however, because of their adverse effects on cartilage, their use in children is currently limited (see Chapter on *Acquired Immunodeficiency Syndrome*).

Nontuberculous mycobacteria are not transmitted from person to person, and no special measures of prevention are recommended.

SUGGESTED READING

Hawkins CC, Gold JWM, Whimbey E, et al. *Mycobacterium avium* complex infections in patients with the acquired immunodeficiency syndrome. Ann Intern Med 1986; 105:184–188.

Lincoln EM, Gilbert LA. Disease in children due to mycobacteria other than *Mycobacterium tuberculosis.* Am Rev Resp Dis 1972; 105:683–714.

Schaad UB, Votteler TP, McCracken GH, Nelson JD. Management of atypical mycobacterial lymphadenitis in childhood: a review based on 380 cases. J Pediatr 1979; 95:356–360.

Wolinsky E. State of the art: nontuberculous mycobacteria and associated diseases. Am Rev Resp Dis 1979; 119:107–159.

PLAGUE

ALICE H. CUSHING, M.D.

The most difficult part of treating plague is suspecting it. Even in an endemic area, 65 percent of patients with a discharge diagnosis of plague were not suspected of having that disease when they entered the hospital. Antibiotic therapy directed nonspecifically against lymphadenitis or fever of unknown origin is unlikely to be effective against *Yersinia pestis.* Failure to diagnose plague and to treat it appropriately contribute to the disease's high morbidity and mortality.

Once the diagnosis is made, specific treatment is limited to a very small number of drugs which have been shown to be clinically efficacious. The selection of drug, dosage, and route of administration depends on the age of the patient, the clinical presentation, and the severity of the illness (Table 1).

Plague may be treated as an outpatient disorder in third world countries, but it is our policy to hospitalize any patient in whom we suspect the diagnosis even if he or she is no more than moderately ill. We place these patients in strict isolation until they have been treated for 72 hours or another diagnosis has been established. Therapy should be started on the basis of clinical suspicion, because valuable time may be lost waiting for verification of the diagnosis.

The mildest form of plague is the bubonic type. The bubo itself is a regional lymph node, most often inguinal, which is enlarged, inflamed, exquisitely tender, and overlaid by erythematous, edematous soft tissue and skin. It is, in itself, evidence of vigorous host defense. If the host response is adequate, the patient may not be very ill. In patients treated as suggested in the table, the bubo can be expected to become less tender within 24 to 48 hours, but objective signs of improvement may not be evident for several days. Not only may the bubo persist for days in appropriately treated patients, but it may point and drain spontaneously, or it may persist until the managing physician resorts to excising it surgically.

TABLE 1 Plague Treatment

Clinical Presentation	Drug	Dose (mg/kg/day)	No. of Doses per Day	Route	Duration (days)
Bubonic	Streptomycin and	20–40 (2 g max)	2–3	IM	10
<8y	chloramphenicol	50*	3	PO	7–10
≥8y	Streptomycin and	20–40 (2 g max)	2–3	IM	10
	tetracycline	20–40 (2 g max)	4	PO	10
Bubonic-septicemic Primary septicemic Pneumonic					
	Streptomycin or	20–40 (2 g max)	2–3	IM	10
<8y	gentamicin and	3–7.5*	3	IM, IV	10
	chloramphenicol	50–75*	4	IV, PO	7–10
	Streptomycin or	20–40 (2 g max)	2–3	IM	10
≥8y	gentamicin and	3–7.5*	3	IM, IV	10
	tetracycline	10–20	2–4	IV†	10
Meningitis or	Chloramphenicol	50–100* (4 g max)	4	IV	7–10
endophthalmitis,	and				
all ages	streptomycin or	20–40 (2 g max)	2–3	IM	10
	gentamicin	3–7.5	3	IM, IV	

* Monitor serum concentrations.
† May change to oral administration at 20 to 40 mg per kilogram per day, pending clinical improvement.

Although the material drained from the bubo may be positive by fluorescent antibody staining, we have been unable to recover viable organisms after 48 hours of treatment.

Patients who have buboes may be more seriously ill. This presentation is called bubonic-septicemic. It is usually accompanied by positive blood cultures and, in some cases, further complications such as pneumonia. Treatment is as suggested in Table 1. I would expect these patients to improve within 48 to 72 hours, but patients with this presentation may progress in severity over the first 12 to 24 hours of treatment, and they may require additional support modalities.

If pneumonia is present, as it commonly is in patients with prolonged bacteremia, respiratory secretions should be handled with extreme care because they may contain plague bacilli (not in the astronomical numbers seen in patients with primary plague pneumonia resulting from inhalation of organisms). We culture the secretions daily and isolate the patient until cultures have been negative for 48 hours. We treat these patients with an aminoglycoside and chloramphenicol. Radiologic resolution may require a long period, up to a month. One of our patients exhibited cavitation of pulmonary lesions. This slow radiologic resolution does not mandate prolongation of antibiotic treatment.

Many patients with plague have changes of mental status out of proportion to the other manifestations of illness. In such a patient—as well as in any patient with lethargy, any patient with a positive blood culture, or any patient with prolonged illness before diagnosis and institution of appropriate antibiotic therapy—it is mandatory to examine the spinal fluid. If meningitis is proved, or if the diagnosis cannot be ruled out, I would treat with "meningeal" dosages of chloramphenicol. I give such a patient an aminoglycoside as well, for its extraneural bactericidal activity. I give this patient chloramphenicol, monitoring the serum concentrations, until the cerebrospinal fluid (CSF) pleocytosis has clearly improved and sugar and protein values are near normal or normal. This has usually required 7 to 10 days of therapy. In our experience patients improve markedly within 24 to 48 hours after they receive chloramphenicol. Temperature resolution has lagged behind improvement of mental status and diminution of headache. CSF has been sterile in 48 hours in our patients.

Many patients with plague are severely ill. They may have physiologic derangements characteristic of endotoxic shock, disseminated intravascular coagulation, adult respiratory distress syndrome, and renal failure. The usual methods of management of those derangements have been employed to manage plague patients with varying degrees of success. The use of large dosages of steroids in this condition is no less controversial than it is in other life-threatening conditions, but I know of no specific contraindication to their use. Mortality is high in spite of all support modalities employed.

Alternative drugs include the other aminoglycosides, of which kanamycin has been directly compared with streptomycin and found to be equally effective. We use gentamicin because we have had more experience with it than with streptomycin, serum drug concentration testing is readily available, and we have found it to be efficacious. We have not compared it directly with streptomycin.

Sulfonamides fell out of use in plague therapy after sulfa-resistant *Yersinia pestis* strains were identified. Streptomycin-resistant isolates have been identified elsewhere in the world, but have not been a problem in the United States.

Trimethoprim-sulfamethoxazole has been compared with streptomycin in treatment of pneumonic plague. Although patients treated with trimethoprim-sulfa were cured, they had a longer median duration of fever and more complications than did those treated with streptomycin. It may therefore be considered an acceptable alternative drug only if there are compelling reasons not to use the first-line drugs: streptomycin or other aminoglycosides and tetracycline or chloramphenicol.

"Overlapping" therapy is often mentioned in textbooks. This involves treating 7 to 10 days with the aminoglycoside and giving a second drug for the last 3 days of aminoglycoside treatment. The second drug is then given for an additional 7 days. This provides a total duration of therapy of 10 to 14 days. I know of no advantage to this dosing regimen and, accordingly, do not recommend it.

SUGGESTED READING

Ai NV, Hanh ND, Dien PV, Le NV. Co-trimoxazole in bubonic plague. Br Med J 1973; 4:108–109.
Cantey JR. Plague in Vietnam. Arch Intern Med 1974; 133:280–283.
Mann JM, Shandler L, Cushing AH. Pediatric plague. Pediatrics 1982; 69:762–767.

RAT-BITE FEVER

PENELOPE G. SHACKELFORD, M.D.

Rat-bite fever (RBF) is the common name shared by two clinically similar diseases of separate etiologies. Streptobacillary rat-bite fever is caused by *Streptobacillus moniliformis,* a gram-negative pleomorphic rod of the Bacteroidaceae. This organism grows best in a microaerophilic environment, requires enriched media, and does not appear in culture until 2 to 6 days of incubation. Spirillary rat-bite fever is caused by a spirochete, *Spirillum minus,* which can be seen by darkfield examination or on Wright-stained smears of blood, but has never been recovered on artificial media. Considering the difficulty in confirming the specific microbiologic etiology of RBF, it is fortunate that both of these organisms are susceptible to penicillin G.

Spirillum minus is very susceptible to penicillin. In contrast to the 3- to 8-week course of relapsing fever, myalgia, and rash in untreated patients, penicillin treatment results in marked improvement within 24 to 72 hours.

In untreated patients with streptobacillary RBF, rash, fever, and joint involvement are characteristically present for 10 to 20 days, and some patients develop severe persistent arthritis. In addition, streptobacillary RBF may be complicated by pneumonia, brain abscesses, and endocarditis. These complications are frequently found in the 10 percent of patients who die with untreated disease. As with spirillary RBF, penicillin therapy produces dramatic recovery from streptobacillary RBF.

Streptobacillus moniliformis is less susceptible to penicillin than *S. minus,* and thus all pediatric patients with the uncomplicated syndrome of RBF should receive 20,000 to 50,000 U per kilogram every 24 hours (adult dosage is 1.2 million U) of procaine penicillin, given intramuscularly, or 1 to 2 g of oral penicillin V given in divided doses for 7 to 10 days. Shorter courses of therapy have been associated with relapse. Patients allergic to penicillin may be treated with streptomycin (20 mg per kilogram per day in two divided doses) or tetracycline (30 to 50 mg per kilogram per day). A few patients have also responded to therapy with clindamycin or chloramphenicol, but experience with these drugs for the treatment of RBF is very limited.

Patients with endocarditis should receive intravenous penicillin G (160,000 to 240,000 U per kilogram every 24 hours) for at least 4 weeks. The adult dosage is 20 million U daily. Some physicians also recommend a combination of streptomycin and penicillin for patients with endocarditis, particularly during the initial phase of therapy. As usual in the treatment of bacterial endocarditis, the in vitro susceptibility of the infecting organism should be determined, and adequate serum bactericidal activity should be documented (see the Chapter on *Infective Endocarditis*).

SUGGESTED READING

Anderson LC, Leary SL, Manning PJ. Rat-bite fever in animal research laboratory personnel. Lab Anim Sci 1983; 33:292–294.
Raffin BJ, Freemark M. Streptobacillary rat-bite fever: a pediatric problem. Pediatrics 1979; 64:214–217.
Rat-bite fever in a college student—California. MMWR 1984; 33:318–320.
Shackelford PG. Rat bite fever. In: Feigin RD, Cherry JD, eds. Textbook of pediatric infectious diseases, Vol 1. Philadelphia: WB Saunders, 1987; 1257–1260.

RELAPSING FEVER

PENELOPE G. SHACKELFORD, M.D.

Relapsing fever occurs in two distinct but clinically similar forms, louse-borne (epidemic) and tick-borne (endemic). Both illnesses are caused by spirochetes of the genus *Borrelia,* and are characterized by repeated (up to 10) episodes of high fever alternating with afebrile, asymptomatic periods.

The louse-borne disease, caused by *Borrelia recurrentis,* requires a human reservoir and is spread by *Pediculus humanis.* There have been no cases of louse-borne relapsing fever in the United States for many years, but the disease remains common in the North African countries of Ethiopia and Sudan.

In North America, the disease occurs in the western United States where wild rodents are the reservoir for three *Borrelia* species (*B. hermsii, B. parkeri,* and *B. turicatae*). These organisms are transmitted from rodents to human by ticks of the genus *Ornithodoros.* The most commonly occurring tick species, *O. hermsi,* is found in the coniferous forests of over 5,000 feet elevation. Patients are most frequently exposed while staying in cabins inhabited by rodents, especially chipmunks and pine squirrels. Other persons have been exposed while working with wood piles or animal hides. Infection with *Borrelia* can also be acquired transplacentally. Because *O. hermsi* ticks feed at night, taking blood meals within 15 to 30 minutes and inflicting only a small painless bite, few patients recall having been bitten.

The clinical manifestations of relapsing fever are nonspecific and closely resemble those of a viral infection. Following an incubation period of about 7 days (range, 4 to 18 days), the patient experiences the sudden onset of fever accompanied by headache, myalgia, arthalgia, photophobia, and vague abdominal distress. Although organ involvement, manifested by jaundice, hepatosplenomegaly, and neurologic symptoms, is frequently mentioned in the literature, these have been uncommon features of pediatric cases of tick-borne disease reported in the United States. The symptoms last about 3 days and then resolve by crisis. The patient feels better and is afebrile for about a week. The most characteristic feature of relapsing fever is the cyclic return of fever. Relapses with similar, but usually milder symptoms may be repeated up to 10 times. The cyclic nature of the illness appears to be caused by antigenic variation in the surface proteins of the *Borreliae,* followed by the production of antibodies against the new variant.

The mortality of relapsing fever ranges from 2 to 70 percent, with the highest figures being reported in malnourished infants with louse-borne disease. With treatment, the mortality of tick-borne relapsing fever in the United States is very low. No fatalities have occurred in 462 cases reported in California since 1931.

The most important clue to the diagnosis of relapsing fever is a history of exposure. When a patient presents with fever of unknown origin within 3 weeks of travel to an endemic area, efforts to diagnose relapsing fever should be made. The organisms are fastidious and have only recently been recovered on artificial media. However, the high grade of spirochetemia (10^5 to 10^8 organisms per milliliter), has permitted the diagnosis by visualization of organisms on Wright or Giemsa-stained blood smears in 70 percent of cases. The diagnosis frequently has been made by alert technicians observing spirochetes on the routine peripheral blood smear. Increased sensitivity may be obtained using a "thick," dehemoglobinized blood smear stained with acridine orange. Blood, urine, or cerebrospinal fluid (CSF) also can be sent to the state laboratory for culture by animal inoculation.

SPECIFIC THERAPY

Because it is difficult to cultivate *Borrelia,* in vitro, data on antibiotic susceptibility are not available. Present recommendations for clinical therapy are based on animal studies and clinical trials performed in patients with epidemic (louse-borne) disease. In North Africa, considerations such as epidemic spread, efficacy against other louse-borne diseases (e.g., typhus), and limited medical resources favor cheap, single-dose regimens. Under these circumstances, oral single-dose therapy using 500 mg of tetracycline or erythromycin (or 100 mg of doxycycline) is considered optimal therapy for *B. recurrentis* infection. In severe cases, intravenous tetracycline (250 mg) has been used. To avoid staining of teeth by tetracycline, erythromycin has been the drug of choice in pregnant women and children 7 years of age or younger. In children, a single dose of 10 mg of erythromycin per kilogram of body weight is used.

Based on its safety and proven efficacy, I consider erythromycin the drug of choice for treatment of relapsing fever in children in the United States. Because occasional cases of relapse have been reported in patients treated for both louse-borne and tick-borne disease, I would recommend a 7- to 10-day course of therapy. In a febrile patient, administration of an initial dose of oral phenoxymethyl penicillin (7.5 mg per kilogram) should be considered. This is done to lessen the risk of a Jarisch-Herxheimer reaction by more gradually clearing spirochetes from the circulation than would be done with erythromycin. Following the initial dose of penicillin, treatment should be continued with erythromycin, as in the case of afebrile patients. The dosage of oral erythromycin estolate is 40 mg per kilogram per day in divided doses given every 6 hours.

SUPPORTIVE THERAPY

In addition to selection of the proper antibiotic, a major consideration in the therapy of relapsing fever is the almost universal occurrence of the Jarisch-Herxheimer reaction. In epidemic (louse-borne) relapsing fever, the Jarisch-Herxheimer reaction occurs in nearly 100 percent of patients, with a mortality rate as high as 12 percent. In tick-borne disease, the reaction is less severe and occurs in only one-third of patients. The reaction usually begins within 1 hour of starting intravenous therapy and within 2 to 3 hours of beginning oral therapy. The initial phase of the reaction is characterized by a rise in temperature, often to 41°C, an increase in blood pressure, and hyperventilation. This phase, which lasts from 10 to 30 minutes, ends abruptly with a sharp fall in temperature and blood pressure, often to shock levels. The second phase (defervescence) coincides with clearance of spirochetes from the blood. It may last up to 12 hours, and is the period when mortality occurs. The cause of mortality most often appears to be myocardial failure. The most important supportive measure during defervescence appears to be administration of large volumes of normal saline. In adults, 2 to 3 liters are usually infused over 12 hours.

Attempts to control the Jarisch-Herxheimer reaction have included supportive measures such as volume expansion and use of antipyretics. In addition, several studies of alternative antibiotics that eliminate circulating organisms more gradually (e.g., penicillin) have been performed. These regimens have produced less severe but more prolonged reactions. In general, it was felt the total physiologic stresses were equivalent, and thus the more effective antibiotics that produce rapid clearance of spirochetes are generally preferred. Finally, pharmacologic blockade of the reaction has been attempted unsuccessfully, using steroids and opioid antagonists (e.g., naloxone). Recently, the opioid antagonist and partial agonist (meptazinol) has been shown effectively to block the reaction. This drug, which is available in the United Kingdom, is not licensed in the United States.

In the United States, I would recommend that physicians initiate therapy for tick-borne relapsing fever in an office, emergency room, or hospital. During the first 8 hours of therapy, close nursing supervision should be provided with an intravenous infusion in place. In most patients, therapy can be initiated with oral erythromycin estolate. In an extremely ill, febrile child, oral penicillin should be considered as initial therapy. Positioning, volume expansion, and acetaminophen should be used as necessary to control blood pressure, pulse, and temperature.

MONITORING RESPONSE TO THERAPY

After the first 8 hours, additional monitoring is not necessary. After 24 hours, an uneventful recovery should be expected. Clearing of spirochetes from blood smears should occur within the first 8 hours. Patients should be reevaluated if fever recurs within 2 months of therapy.

PREVENTION

Prevention of louse-borne disease most fundamentally depends on prevention of conditions of poverty, crowding, and malnutrition. Epidemic control involves control of louse infection in individual patients and their environment.

Although tick-borne disease is not epidemic, many cases can often be traced to a particular rodent-infested cabin. In this situation, it is necessary to remove nesting materials and spray the walls, floors, ceilings, and crawl spaces with insecticide. Resources for information regarding these problems are the Vector-borne Diseases Division of the CDC (Fort Collins, Colorado, 303-221-6420) and the Rocky Mountain Laboratories of the National Institutes of Health (Hamilton, Montana, 406-363-3211). Reporting cases of tick-borne disease is important, particularly in public recreational settings such as state or national parks, where many individuals may be exposed.

SUGGESTED READING

Boyer KM. Borrelia: relapsing fever. In: Feigin RD, Cherry JD, eds. Textbook of pediatric infectious diseases, Vol 1. Philadelphia: WB Saunders, 1987; 1099–1102.

Butler T. Relapsing fever: new lessons about antibiotic action. Ann Intern Med 1985; 102:397–399.

Butler T, Jones PK, Wallace CK. *Borrelia recurrentis* infection: single-dose antibiotic regimens and management of the Jarisch-Herxheimer reaction. J Infect Dis 1978; 137:573–577.

Horton JM, Blaser MJ. The spectrum of relapsing fever in the Rocky Mountains. Arch Intern Med 1985; 145:871–875.

Le CT. Tick-borne relapsing fever in children. Pediatrics 1980; 66:963–966.

RHEUMATIC FEVER

ELIA M. AYOUB, M.D.

Treatment of a patient with acute rheumatic fever comprises a general and a specific aspect. The general aspect involves the administration of a course of antibiotics to all patients with acute rheumatic fever to eradicate group A streptococci. The specific aspect addresses the acute manifestations the patient presents with. All patients are initiated on a prophylaxis program to prevent future streptococcal infections and recurrences of rheumatic fever. Patients with cardiac involvement should be instructed about the need for prophylaxis against bacterial endocarditis. The importance and significance of these prophylactic measures should be stressed initially and at future follow-up visits.

ANTIBIOTIC THERAPY FOR ERADICATION OF STREPTOCOCCI AND PROPHYLAXIS AGAINST GROUP A STREPTOCOCCAL INFECTION

Streptococcal Eradicating Course

The regimens outlined for the use of antibiotics in the treatment of streptococcal pharyngitis can be used (see chapter on *Acute Tonsillopharyngitis and Scarlet Fever*). For patients not allergic to penicillin, my preference is to give the patient benzathine penicillin (Bicillin-LA), 1.2 million U intramuscularly, particularly if the patient has carditis. This form of therapy, in addition to providing treatment for the eradication of the streptococcal infection that precipitated the acute attack of rheumatic fever, initiates the patient into the most effective form of prophylaxis. Erythromycin should be given to patients allergic to penicillin. One should again emphasize that sulfonamide derivatives should not be used for the eradication of streptococci from host tissues.

Group A Streptococcal Infection Prophylaxis

Antibiotic prophylaxis to prevent streptococcal infections and recurrences of rheumatic fever should follow the treatment course for eradication of streptococci. For patients who are not allergic to penicillin, the most effective regimen consists of intramuscular administration of benzathine penicillin, 1.2 million U monthly (600,000 U for children weighing less than 30 kg). This regimen should be used for at least 5 years following the acute illness, particularly in patients with cardiac involvement, who are at highest risk for recurrences during this period of time. The patient can be maintained on this regimen or

changed to oral prophylaxis after this interval if compliance can be assessed.

Oral regimens that can be used include penicillin, 125 mg, erythromycin, 250 mg, and sulfadiazine, 500 mg, taken twice daily. Either sulfadiazine or erythromycin can be given to patients allergic to penicillin. Sulfadiazine is more effective than penicillin as an oral prophylactic agent and is less expensive than erythromycin. Although other antibiotics could be equally effective in eradicating streptococci from the tissue of the patient, their efficacy as prophylactic agents remains to be determined. Because oral prophylaxis carries with it the hazard of noncompliance, it should be monitored closely.

TREATMENT OF ACUTE MANIFESTATIONS

Of the five major manifestations of acute rheumatic fever, the three that require "specific" therapy are arthritis, carditis, and chorea. Anti-inflammatory agents, salicylates or steroids, are used for the treatment of arthritis and carditis. Sedatives are usually helpful in the treatment of choreiform symptoms.

Arthritis

The arthritis of rheumatic fever is characteristically quite responsive to salicylates. Patients presenting with arthritis as the only symptom should be treated with aspirin, 75 to 80 mg per kilogram body weight per day. Most patients respond promptly to this dosage or to even smaller dosages of aspirin, with rapid resolution of their joint symptoms. The lack of response after 24 to 72 hours should suggest the possibility of another disease as the cause of the arthritis. Blood salicylate concentrations are usually determined after 4 to 5 days of therapy. The dosage should be adjusted if the concentration is lower than 20 mg per deciliter and the patient has not responded. The blood salicylate concentration should not exceed 30 mg per deciliter. For patients whose only manifestation is arthritis, treatment with the full dose of salicylates is continued for about 2 weeks, followed by gradual withdrawal over the following 4 weeks.

Carditis

The choice of therapy for carditis is based on the severity of this manifestation. Mild or even moderate carditis is treated initially with salicylates, 80 to 100 mg per kilogram body weight per day, for 2 to 4 weeks. With a good clinical response and a return of acute-phase reactants to normal, salicylate therapy is withdrawn gradually over the following 4 to 6 weeks. In patients with severe carditis, and in particular patients with pancarditis manifested by the presence of myocarditis, pericarditis, and cardiac failure, initial therapy with corticosteroids is preferable to salicylate therapy. Steroids offer the advantage of a more prompt therapeutic effect and avoidance of a large salt load. Prednisone is given in a dosage of 1 to 2 mg per kilogram body weight per day for 2 to 4 weeks, followed by gradual withdrawal over 2 to 4 weeks. One week before prednisone withdrawal starts, salicylate therapy should be started, using the preceding regimen, to minimize clinical and laboratory rebounds.

Digitalis is administered to patients with severe carditis and congestive heart failure. The total initial digitalizing dosage is 0.02 to 0.03 mg per kilogram body weight of digoxin, with a maximum total dosage of 1.5 mg. This is followed by a maintenance dosage equal to one-fourth the digitalizing dose, given in two equal doses daily. Because patients with rheumatic myocarditis are often overly reactive to the effects of digitalis, some physicians prefer to start with the smaller digitalizing dosage; others omit the digitalizing dosage and start the patient on the maintenance dosage.

The need for confinement to bed for patients with acute rheumatic fever is limited to those with carditis and is dictated by the severity of the cardiac disease. Bed rest is advisable for patients with active carditis or heart failure. The average patient is restricted to bed for 2 to 3 weeks after the onset of the acute illness. Gradual ambulation should be started shortly after the cardiac disease is stabilized and signs of failure have resolved. Extreme measures, such as restoring the patient to full activity too quickly or restricting the patient to bed for months after the cardiac status has stabilized, should be avoided.

Sydenham's Chorea

The efficacy of therapeutic intervention in patients with this manifestation is questionable. Chorea is self-limiting, and patients with mild symptoms respond to rest and avoidance of stress. Patients with more severe choreiform activity should be confined to a padded bed in a quiet room and receive sedation in the form of either phenobarbital or haloperidol. Phenobarbital is given in doses of 15 to 30 mg every 6 to 8 hours. Haloperidol is started at 0.5 mg, given every 8 hours, and is gradually increased to 2.0 mg every 8 hours if the patient fails to respond to the smaller dosage. The choice of either of these agents is empirical. The patient may respond to one or the other, or to neither of the two agents. Patients who do not respond to phenobarbital after 2 weeks of therapy should be tried for the same length of time on haloperidol. If there is no response to either agent, reassurance of the patient or parents about the self-limiting nature of this manifestation is very important. Steroids and other anti-inflammatory agents have no therapeutic role in patients with chorea as the only manifestation of rheumatic fever.

FOLLOW-UP CARE

Prior to discharge of the patient who has recovered from an acute episode of rheumatic fever, the physician should make sure that the patient is made aware of the importance of future compliance to prophylaxis. The rationale for daily prophylaxis to prevent streptococcal pharyngitis and recurrences of rheumatic fever should be explained to all patients, regardless of which organ is involved in the rheumatic disease. In addition, patients with cardiac involvement should be informed about the necessity for prophylaxis against bacterial endocarditis before certain dental or surgical procedures (see recommendations in chapter on *Infective Endocarditis*). Our patients are given the American Heart Association recommendations for prophylaxis against endocarditis, in the form of a pocket card, to be presented to the physician before dental or surgical procedures are done. Patients with residual cardiac damage should also be informed about the types of physical activities they can engage in. It is important to educate the patient about the prognosis of his or her disease and the factors that influence its eventual course. Arrangements for regular follow-up care should be undertaken prior to discharge of the patient, to ensure proper compliance to prophylaxis. The latter is perhaps the most important facet in the care of patients with this disease.

SUGGESTED READING

Ayoub EM, Schiebler GL. Acute rheumatic fever. In: Kelley VC, ed. Practice of pediatrics. Philadelphia: Harper & Row, 1985.

Combined Rheumatic Fever Study Group. A comparison of short-term intensive prednisone and acetylsalicylic acid therapy in the treatment of acute rheumatic fever. N Engl J Med 1965; 272:63–70.

Shulman ST, Amren DP, Bisno AL, et al. Prevention of rheumatic fever. A statement for health professionals prepared by the Committee on Rheumatic Fever and Infective Endocarditis of the Council of Cardiovascular Disease in the Young. Circulation 1984; 70:1118A–1122A.

RICKETTSIAL DISEASES

JACOB A. LOHR, M.D.

THE SPOTTED FEVERS

Rocky Mountain Spotted Fever

Rocky Mountain spotted fever (RMSF) is usually diagnosed on the basis of a history of tick exposure, suggestive symptoms and signs, and supportive laboratory findings. Specific confirmatory serologic tests are uncommonly positive at the time of presentation. Therefore, treatment is usually initiated on the basis of a presumptive rather than an established diagnosis.

RMSF is caused by *Rickettsia rickettsii* (Table 1). The prolonged bite of an infected tick precedes invasion of the bloodstream by the causative organism and development of a diffuse endovasculitis. Up to 40 percent of patients have no known recent exposure to ticks. In those that do, the time from the tick bite to onset of illness is usually 3 to 12 (average 7) days. Typical clinical presentation includes fever, rash, malaise, headache, abdominal symptoms, myalgias, neurologic deficits, edema, and conjunctivitis. The rash usually begins 2 to 3 days after the onset of fever. Characteristically, it initially appears as a macular or maculopapular eruption on the wrists and ankles and soon thereafter is apparent on the palms and soles. It progresses, especially in the untreated patient, to involve the proximal parts of the extremities and the trunk and becomes petechial or hemorrhagic.

Several laboratory studies, though nonspecific, support the diagnosis of RMSF. Serum sodium equal to or less than 130 mg per deciliter is seen in about half the patients. Abnormally low platelet counts are found in about 75 percent of cases.

The time-honored Weil–Felix agglutination titers and the RMSF complement fixation antibody test have been supplanted by tests that are more sensitive, more specific, and positive earlier in the course. Such tests include the microimmunofluorescent test and the latex agglutination test. However, none of the serologic tests is reliably positive before the second week of the illness. Confirmation may be provided as early as the fourth day of illness with a direct immunofluorescent stain of punch biopsy specimens of active skin lesions; but this test is not available in most hospitals.

Treatment of RMSF must be definitive even though initiated on the basis of a presumptive diagnosis. The more seriously ill patients should be hospitalized to provide effective antibiotic therapy and detect and treat complications. When the diagnosis is suspected in a mildly ill patient, outpatient care can

TABLE 1 Etiology, Laboratory Diagnosis, and Prevention of Rickettsial Diseases

Disease	Organism	Insect Vector	Laboratory Diagnosis	Preventive Therapy

Spotted fever group
  Rocky Mountain spotted fever
	R. rickettsii	Tick	Immunofluorescence (IF)
			Latex agglutination
			Complement fixation (CF)
			Weil–Felix OX-19
			        OX-2
				Avoidance of ticks
				Vaccine

Tick typhus fevers	*R. conorii* *R. australis* *R. sibericus*	Tick	IF CF Weil–Felix OX-19 OX-2	Avoidance of ticks
Rickettsialpox	*R. akari*	Mite	IF CF	Rodent control
Typhus group Epidemic typhus	*R. prowazekii*	Body louse	IF CF Weil–Felix OX-19	Louse control Vaccine
Brill–Zinsser disease	*R. prowazekii*	None	IF CF	None
Murine typhus	*R. typhi* (formerly, *R. mooseri*)	Flea	IF CF	Rodent control
Scrub typhus	*R. tsutsugamushi*	Mite	IF Weil–Felix OX-K	Mite control Chemoprophylaxis for high-risk persons
Other Q fever	*Coxiella burnetii*	Tick	IF CF	Vaccine

sometimes be justified, but antibiotic treatment should not await the development of additional signs. The disease can progress at an unpredictable pace, and the case fatality rate in untreated patients approaches 25 percent.

Antibiotic treatment is effective when initiated early. The case fatality rate of 4 percent in treated patients can be attributed to delayed therapy in patients whose diagnosis was unrecognized. Chloramphenicol and the tetracyclines are the agents of choice. In ill patients, the drugs should initially be given parenterally, because intestinal absorption may be altered by vomiting, diarrhea, or vasculitis involving the gastrointestinal tract. Intramuscular therapy would be ill-advised in the presence of thrombocytopenia. Oral therapy can be used in most patients after they are stable. The total duration of therapy should be a minimum of 7 days, and at least 3 days after the patient becomes afebrile. Clinical improvement may be evident as early as 24 hours after initiation of therapy, and fever usually subsides within 3 days. Resolution of the rash is variable.

Chloramphenicol has the advantage of treating RMSF as well as meningococcal disease, the headliner of the differential diagnoses. Therapy should be administered at a dosage of 50 to 100 mg per kilogram per day, in divided doses every 6 hours (Table 2). The drug may be given intravenously or orally. In patients younger than 2 years of age and in patients with liver or renal dysfunction, the drug should be used cautiously, preferably while monitoring serum chloramphenicol concentrations. The maximum daily dosage is 3 g.

The tetracyclines are equivalent to chloramphenicol in therapeutic efficacy. Their advantage is they avoid the rare bone marrow depression or aplasia seen with exposure to chloramphenicol. Their disadvantage is they produce discoloration and hypoplasia of tooth enamel in children younger than 8 years old. Exposure to only a few short courses of

tetracycline probably presents no measurable risk of such toxicity in this age group. Doxycycline is potentially less destructive to tooth enamel than tetracycline, because it is less bound to calcium. If a patient younger than 8 years of age has a completely negative history for tetracycline or doxycycline exposure, either drug (preferably doxycycline) is acceptable for treatment of RMSF in that patient. In patients of any age treated with tetracycline or doxycycline, penicillin should be added until meningococcal disease is ruled out.

Tetracycline therapy is given intravenously, intramuscularly, or orally. The intravenous dosage is 20 to 30 mg per kilogram per day, given in divided doses every 12 hours in a 2-hour infusion (see Table 2). The intramuscular dosage is 15 to 25 mg per kilogram per day, given in divided doses every 12 hours. This route is a secondary choice because of associated pain and variable absorption. The oral dosage is 25 to 50 mg per kilogram per day, given in divided doses every 6 hours. Oral doses of tetracycline are optimally absorbed if given 1 hour before meals or milk intake. In addition, absorption is impaired by antacids containing chelating or pH-elevating agents such as aluminum hydroxide, magnesium hydroxide, bicarbonate, or calcium salts, which may be given to patients with gastric bleeding secondary to gastrointestinal endovasculitis or thrombocytopenia. Tetracycline should not be used in patients with hepatic or renal insufficiency.

Doxycycline therapy should be initiated with two loading doses of 2.2 mg per kilogram, given at 12-hour intervals orally or intravenously (see Table 2). Maintenance therapy is given at a dosage of 2.2 mg per kilogram per day, in divided doses every 12 hours orally or intravenously. Intravenous infusions are given slowly over 2 to 4 hours, with careful avoidance of extravasation. The maximum daily dose is 300 mg. The drug is contraindicated in patients with decreased renal or hepatic function.

Other antibiotics are either ineffective or untested in the treatment of RMSF. The sulfonamides can adversely affect outcome.

Corticosteroid therapy may shorten the febrile period. Corticosteroids have also been used to treat central nervous system involvement, but benefits are not documented. I do not recommend their use.

The seriously ill patient with RMSF requires careful supportive care. The fever responds poorly to antipyretics, and the headache is relieved minimally by analgesics. Aspirin should be avoided because it can induce platelet dysfunction, and many patients are already thrombocytopenic. The presence of hyponatremia dictates that intravenous fluid and sodium be restricted. It is usually not possible to correct the hyponatremia until disease activity subsides, and cardiac decompensation and pulmonary or cerebral edema can result from overly aggressive intravenous therapy. Disseminated intravascular coagulopathy is a severe complication that remits only as the endo-

TABLE 2 Therapy of the Rickettsial Diseases

Chloramphenicol	
Maintenance dose	50-100 mg/kg/day IV or PO, divided q6h
Maximum dose	3 g daily
Doxycycline	
Loading dose	4.4 mg/kg/day IV or PO, divided q12h for 1 day
Maintenance dose	2.2 mg/kg/day IV or PO divided q12h
Maximum dose	300 mg daily
Tetracycline	
Maintenance dose	20–30 mg/kg/day IV, divided q12h or
	15–25 mg/kg/day IM, divided q12h or
	25-50 mg/kg/day PO, divided q6h
Maximum dose	2 g daily

vasculitis subsides. The value of heparin in this setting is unproved, and its use is not recommended. Gangrene of the earlobes, scrotum, and extremities provides fertile sites for secondary infection, but additional antibiotics are not indicated until infection develops. Other potential complications necessitating monitoring and supportive care are numerous, including renal failure, which requires fluid and nutrient restriction and alteration of antibiotic choice or dosage.

Available preventive measures include avoidance of ticks, early removal of ticks, and use of a killed vaccine. Wearing proper clothing while in tick-infested areas and exercising caution in handling tick-carrying dogs are reasonable means of preventing tick attachment. Tick repellents are either ineffective or potentially toxic and are not recommended. During tick season, children should have their skin, including hair-covered areas, searched carefully daily. Embedded ticks are best removed by grasping them as close to the head as possible with tweezers or protected fingers and forcefully extracting them. The wound should be cleansed with alcohol to prevent bacterial infection.

Although the vaccine may prevent death, it does not always protect from the disease. The need for annual boosters further limits the vaccine's usefulness. It is not recommended for routine use in children.

Tick Typhus Fevers

Fièvre boutonneuse, Siberian tick typhus, and Queensland tick typhus are other tick-borne spotted fevers that are antigenically distinct but serologically related to RMSF. *Rickettsia conorii, R. sibericus,* and *R. australis* are the etiologic agents, respectively (see Table 1). These three tick typhuses are similar to RMSF, but the clinical disease is much milder, with a reported case fatality rate of less than 1 percent in untreated cases.

One distinctive feature of this group of diseases is the small indurated lesion, the *tache noire,* at the site of the tick bite, which becomes necrotic, causing prominent regional lymphadenopathy.

Therapy is the same as that for RMSF (see previous section).

Rickettsialpox

Rickettsialpox is a mild, nonfatal rickettsial infection caused by *R. akari,* which is antigenically related to the other tick typhus rickettsias (see Table 1).

Clinically, the patient has a history of a red papule at the site of the mite bite, which precedes the systemic illness by approximately 1 week. Regional lymphadenopathy is generally present. The fever pattern, which lasts for 1 week, is irregular and varies between 37.8 and 39.5°C. Headache and myalgia are prominent clinical findings. The rash is the most characteristic finding. It develops within several days of the onset of fever as scattered macules, which progress to maculopapules surmounted by vesicles. The lesions may involve the oral cavity, but rarely the palms and soles. The major differential diagnosis is chickenpox.

Laboratory confirmation can be made with complement fixation or immunofluorescent tests. Weil-Felix tests are of no use because no *Proteus* agglutinins are produced.

Therapy is the same as that for RMSF, but the duration of therapy differs in that only 3 to 5 days is required for cure.

THE TYPHUS GROUP

Primary Louse-Borne Typhus Fever

Typhus fever is an acute infection caused by *R. prowazekii* and transmitted to humans by the body louse (see Table 1). In untreated patients, death is uncommon in children, but case fatality rates are 10 percent in young adults and as high as 60 to 70 percent in patients older than 50 years of age.

The clinical disease is similar to that of RMSF, with fever, headache, and rash being the prominent presenting findings. The rash usually presents on the trunk, and spreads to the extremities, sparing the face, palms, and soles. Severe untreated cases progress to a petechial and hemorrhagic rash, coma, and terminal myocardial and renal failure.

Laboratory diagnosis is confirmed with a positive Weil–Felix *Proteus* OX-19 and specific *R. prowazekii* complement fixation and immunofluorescent tests.

Therapy is identical to that described for RMSF (see previous section), early initiation of therapy being the only means of preventing the systemic sequelae.

Preventive therapy is limited to use of a vaccine and louse control. The vaccine is a killed vaccine produced from yolk sacs in chick embryos; it is not effective in preventing infection, but it does decrease the mortality. Insect control is an important and effective preventive measure, particularly in epidemic disease.

Brill–Zinsser Disease

Brill–Zinsser disease is relapsing louse-borne typhus fever (see Table 1). Because of partial immunity, the disease is the same, but the recrudescent disease is a much milder, shorter, and less debilitating form of the primary typhus infection.

Therapy is the same as that for the primary infection—i.e., tetracycline or chloramphenicol. Therapy should be continued for a minimum of 1 week.

Murine Typhus

Murine typhus is caused by *R. typhi* (formerly *R. mooseri*), and infection in humans results from infected rat flea bites (see Table 1). The disease is similar to louse-borne typhus but milder and of shorter duration. The fever rarely rises above 39°C, is remittent, and terminates by 2 weeks. The headache is less severe, and the maculopapular rash is less extensive than that in louse-borne typhus. Complications are uncommon, and mortality in untreated cases is less than 1 percent.

The diagnosis is made serologically with complement fixation and immunofluorescent tests specific for the *R. typhi* antigen.

Therapy is the same as that described for RMSF (see previous section). Prevention is directed at control of the rat population.

Scrub Typhus

Scrub typhus, or tsutsugamushi disease, is spread by mites and caused by the organism *R. tsutsugamushi* (see Table 1).

An initial lesion, which progresses to a necrotic eschar at the site of the mite bite, develops at the same time as the fever. Generalized lymphadenopathy is common in the axilla, neck, and inguinal regions. A macular rash generally presents between the fifth and eighth days of illness. Hepatosplenomegaly and conjunctival infection are common. Tinnitus and deafness are diagnostically helpful when they occur. Myocarditis and disseminated intravascular coagulation are unusual manifestations.

Laboratory diagnosis is aided with a positive Weil–Felix OX-K; and although definitive immunofluorescent studies are available, the multiple antigenic strains make this a difficult study to perform; therefore, the tests are not routinely available.

Treatment with tetracycline or chloramphenicol, as described for RMSF, is highly effective. However, because antibody production does not develop until the second week of illness, patients who have been treated early in their disease may abort their own immune response and require repeated sporadic

short courses of chloramphenicol or tetracycline during convalescence, to avoid relapse.

Because the case fatality rate from this disease varies from 1 to 60 percent as a result of antigenic differences among strains, early initiation of therapy is mandatory.

Preventive efforts are twofold: (1) vector control by means of brush clearing, insecticides, and clothing is required, and (2) chemoprophylaxis in adults in high-risk areas for short periods has been shown to be effective. The adult dosage is 1 g chloramphenicol or tetracycline every other day while the patient is at risk, and for 1 month after he or she leaves the high-risk area.

No vaccine is available.

Q FEVER

Q Fever is an acute rickettsial disease caused by *Coxiella burnetii* and is unique among the rickettsial diseases because it is caused by inhalation of the agent rather than by an arthropod bite (see Table 1).

The clinical features of this disease are fever, headache, hepatosplenomegaly, and, in more than 50 percent of patients, interstitial pneumonitis. The disease is usually mild and self-limited. The severe complications of myocarditis, pericarditis, and endocarditis are unusual.

Laboratory diagnosis is made with complement fixation or immunofluorescent tests. This organism fails to stimulate cross-reacting *Proteus* agglutinins.

Therapy is the same as that described for RMSF (see previous section).

Preventive therapy consists of vaccinating animals and nonimmune persons at high risk.

SUGGESTED READING

Bradford WD, Hawkins HK. Rocky Mountain spotted fever in childhood. Am J Dis Child 1977; 131:1228–1232.
Feigin RD, O'Neil JH Jr. Rickettsial diseases. In: Feigin RD, Cherry JD, eds. Textbook of infectious diseases. 2nd ed. Philadelphia: WB Saunders, 1987;1878–1895.
Linneman CC, Janson PJ. The clinical presentations of Rocky Mountain spotted fever. Clin Pediatr 1978; 17:673–680.
Riley HD. Rocky Mountain spotted fever. Hosp Pract 1977; (April):51–57.

SYPHILIS

LAURENE MASCOLA, M.D., M.P.H.

Syphilis is a very ancient and complex disease and is still very much a part of our present-day society. Although acceptable treatment has been used for

the last four decades, changes in the therapeutic regimens for syphilis continue to be made. In fact, in 1982, when the Centers for Disease Control (CDC) Sexually Transmitted Diseases (STDs) Treatment Guidelines were being updated, more questions were raised about the treatment of syphilis than about any of the other 26 sexually transmitted diseases.

One cannot discuss the treatment of syphilis without a firm understanding of the various clinical stages. The incubation period for syphilis is an average of 21 days (range, 3 to 90 days). Primary syphilis, which usually occurs after this incubation period, is manifested by a painless chancre and some local lymphadenopathy. After 6 to 8 weeks, the secondary stage of syphilis occurs. This stage is characterized by fever, lymphadenopathy, malaise, sore throat, and cutaneous or mucosal rashes.

Without treatment, these secondary symptoms either regress spontaneously or last up to 8 weeks. The next stage, latency, is defined as the period when a person has historical or serologic evidence of syphilis but no clinical manifestations. Early latency is considered as occurring up to 1 year from onset of infectious syphilis. During this stage, mucocutaneous lesions might still recur and infection may still be transmitted. After 1 year, the term *late latent* is applied. Tertiary syphilis is the destructive stage of the disease and usually includes cardiovascular syphilis, benign gummatous syphilis, and neurosyphilis. Finally, congenital syphilis has been traditionally and arbitrarily divided into two stages: early and late. Clinical manifestations appearing within the first 2 years of life are designated early, and those occurring after this time are considered late.

The causative organism, *Treponema pallidum*, cannot be readily cultured. Although it is easily seen by darkfield microscopy, this technology is not available to all clinicians. Therefore, the diagnosis of syphilis is usually made through a combination of clinical and serologic evaluations. These surrogates usually work quite well, except in the diagnosis of congenital syphilis in which the process is significantly more complicated.

THERAPY

Except in special circumstances, penicillin is still the drug of choice for all stages of syphilis. Penicillin in dosages causing a serum concentration of 0.03 μg per milliliter is treponemicidal. Because of the long generation time of the spirochete (around 30 hours), 1 to 2 weeks of effective serum concentrations of antibiotic must be maintained for treatment to be successful. Therefore, benzathine penicillin is used to treat syphilis in all stages except for central nervous system syphilis. Benzathine penicillin does not provide adequate treponemicidal levels of penicillin in sequestered anatomic sites, such as the central cerebrospinal fluid.

No direct evidence exists that *T. pallidum* has become resistant to penicillin, although newly recognized plasmids in *T. pallidum* might increase the potential for the subsequent development of penicillin resistance. Other drugs, such as ampicillin, appear to be as effective as penicillin G against treponemes in vitro. First-generation cephalosporins have also been tried, and more recently third-generation cephalosporins, such as ceftriaxone, have been used in treating central nervous system syphilis because of their better penetration into inflamed meninges. Although no published clinical trials to date have reported solid evidence, one penicillin-allergic patient with asymptomatic neurosyphilis was treated successfully with ceftriaxone.

Early Syphilis

The recommended treatment for early syphilis (incubating, primary, secondary, latent syphilis of less than 1 year's duration) should include the following: benzathine penicillin G 2.4 million U total, given intramuscularly at a single session; two intramuscular injections of 1.2 million U each can be given.

Recently, reports of treatment failures with this regimen for early syphilis have been documented in the literature. Earlier studies showed the failure rate of therapy for early syphilis to be 0 to 7 percent. For this reason, some authors recommend treating primary and secondary syphilis with 2.4 million U of benzathine penicillin weekly for 2 weeks. However, this regimen has not been evaluated in large, clinical settings.

Syphilis of More Than 1 Year's Duration

Treatment of syphilis of more than 1 year's duration (latent syphilis of indeterminate or more than 1 year's duration, cardiovascular or late benign syphilis), excluding neurosyphilis, should consist of the following: benzathine penicillin G (2.4 million U), given intramuscularly once a week for 3 successful weeks (7.2 million U total). Syphilis of longer duration requires more prolonged therapy, and optimal treatment schedules are less well established.

Syphilis in Pregnancy

Prevention and treatment of congenital syphilis begins with the identification of the pregnant woman with syphilis. Ideally, a decreased rate of syphilis in pregnant women could be achieved by decreasing the rates of primary and secondary syphilis in the community. However, prenatal screening early in the first trimester and early treatment of infected women also cures the fetus in utero and prevents the late sequelae of congenital syphilis. In areas of high prevalence of syphilis, a second screening, nontreponemal test should be performed during the third trimester of pregnancy.

For patients at all stages of pregnancy who are not allergic to penicillin, this drug should be used in dosage schedules appropriate for the stage of syphilis as recommended for the treatment of nonpregnant patients. However, I agree with others, that a course of oral amoxicillin, 500 mg three times a day for 7 days, should also be administered to ensure adequate concentration of antibiotics in the fetal circulation.

Treatment failures have been reported in pregnant women, especially those treated in the third trimester of pregnancy, even with appropriate penicillin regimens. Therefore, pregnant women should be followed more closely after treatment with monthly, quantitative nontreponemal tests for the remainder of their pregnancy.

Treated women who do not show a fourfold decrease in titer in a 3-month period should be retreated. Also, all infants born to women treated in the third trimester of pregnancy should be closely monitored at birth.

Congenital Syphilis

Congenital syphilis is still very much a disease of the present. The number of reported cases of congenital syphilis in infants younger than 1 year of age rose, from 108 to 268 during the period of 1978 to 1985. This recent increase probably represents underutilization and inadequacy of prenatal care.

The diagnosis of congenital syphilis is still difficult to make. Many infants are asymptomatic at birth and may even be seronegative if maternal infection occurred late in gestation. An adequately treated infant may have a positive nontreponemal test at birth (up to 3 to 4 months), because of passive transfer of maternal antibodies. Ideally, the diagnosis is made in the child with congenital syphilis by identifying treponemes by darkfield examination. However, one usually needs to evaluate the maternal clinical and epidemiologic information such as past history of stillbirths or abortions, history of signs and symptoms consistent with syphilis, maternal serology, and maternal treatment history along with the examination of the placenta and an evaluation of the infant, both clinically and serologically.

Any infant in whom follow-up cannot be guaranteed, in whom maternal treatment was inadequate or unknown or did not include penicillin, or in whom treatment was provided during the last 4 weeks of pregnancy should be considered congenitally infected and treated as such.

Recently, the therapeutic regimen for congenital syphilis recommended by the Centers for Disease Control was changed. Various case reports revealed that treatment with benzathine penicillin in prior recommended dosages did not prevent the progression of disease. These latest CDC recommendations differ in some aspects from those of the American Academy of Pediatrics. Both groups agree that all infants with congenital syphilis should have a cerebrospinal fluid (CSF) examination before being treated, to provide a baseline for future follow-up. The CDC advocates that, regardless of CSF results, all children should be treated with a regimen effective for neurosyphilis. This regimen for symptomatic or asymptomatic infants includes aqueous crystalline penicillin G, 50,000 U per kilogram, given intramuscularly or intravenously daily in two divided doses for a minimum of 10 days, or aqueous procaine penicillin G, 50,000 U per kilogram, given intramuscularly daily for a minimum of 10 days. Other experts, including the American Academy of Pediatric's Red Book Committee on Infectious Diseases, feel that asymptomatic infants, in whom central nervous system involvement is ruled out, may be treated with benzathine penicillin G, 50,000 U per kilogram, given intramuscularly in a single dose.

However, data on the efficacy of this regimen in congenital neurosyphilis is lacking. After the neonatal period, penicillin for congenital syphilis should be used in the same dosages as for neonatal congenital syphilis. For older children, the total dosage of penicillin should not exceed that used in adult syphilis of more than 1 year's duration.

Neurosyphilis

All patients with clinical signs and symptoms consistent with neurosyphilis or patients with syphilis of greater than 1 year's duration should have a cerebrospinal fluid examination to exclude asymptomatic neurosyphilis. Treatment of neurosyphilis still remains a problem. Without meningeal inflammation, only 1 to 2 percent of serum penicillin concentrations reach the cerebrospinal fluid system. With neurosyphilis, meningeal inflammation is low. However, in over 90 percent of patients with neurosyphilis, a total dosage of 6 to 9 million U of penicillin G over a 3- to 4-week period results in a satisfactory clinical response. Some authors also recommend using probenecid because it helps achieve higher serum concentrations by interfering with renal excretion and blocking active transport of penicillin out of the cerebrospinal fluid space. *T. pallidum* persists in cerebrospinal fluid after treatment with benzathine penicillin in standard dosages, procaine penicillin in dosages of less than 2.4 million U daily, and tetracycline and erythromycin.

Therefore, potentially effective regimens proposed for neurosyphilis, none of which have been adequately studied, include the following:

Aqueous crystalline penicillin G, 12 to 24 million U per day, given intravenously (2 to 4 million U every 4 hours) for 10 days, followed by benzathine penicillin G, 2.4 million U weekly, given intramuscularly, for three doses.

Aqueous procaine penicillin G, 2.4 million U daily, given intramuscularly, plus probenecid, 500 mg given by mouth four times daily, both for 10 days, followed by benzathine penicillin G, 2.4 million U weekly, given intramuscularly, for three doses.

Benzathine penicillin G, 2.4 million U weekly, given intramuscularly, for three doses.

Alternatively, other authors suggest using ceftriaxone, a third-generation cephalosporin, in cases of neurosyphilis. The drug has proved active against *T.*

pallidum in animal studies, and has a long serum half-life and good penetration into the CSF.

ALTERNATIVE THERAPY

For early syphilis (incubating, primary, secondary, latent syphilis of less than 1 year's duration), patients allergic to penicillin can be treated with tetracycline hydrochloride (HCL), 500 mg given by mouth four times a day for 15 days. If a patient cannot tolerate tetracycline, another option is to treat the patient with erythromycin, 500 mg given orally four times a day for 15 days. This regimen is only recommended, however, if compliance and serologic follow-up can be ensured.

The effective use of erythromycin and tetracycline for all stages except primary syphilis has been poorly documented. Problems also occur as a result of adverse side effects and the multiple-dose regimens required for a 2- to 4-week period. In addition, tetracycline should not be used in children younger than 8 years of age or in pregnant women.

For treatment of syphilis of more than 1 year's duration, except neurosyphilis, in patients allergic to penicillin, therapy should consist of tetracycline HCL, 500 mg given by mouth four times daily for 30 days. For pencillin-allergic patients who cannot tolerate tetracycline, their drug allergy should first be confirmed. Otherwise, if compliance and serologic follow-up can be ensured, erythromycin, 500 mg given by mouth four times daily for 30 days, can be employed. For patients with neurosyphilis who claim to be allergic to penicillin, their penicillin allergy should first be confirmed because alternative therapy, except perhaps for the third-generation cephalosporins, is not considered to be as effective. Other specialists consider ceftriaxone to be the drug of choice for persons allergic to penicillin. The duration of therapy should be the same as with penicillin regimens.

For pregnant women with a documented penicillin allergy, desensitization should be performed with penicillin, given either orally or parenterally. Such desensitization procedures should be accomplished in an intensive care setting with adequate monitoring equipment. Other antibiotic alternatives for pregnant women, such as erythromycin, do not effectively treat the fetus because they do not readily cross the placenta.

For neonatal congenital syphilis, only penicillin regimens are recommended. For late congenital syphilis, in children older than 8 years of age, tetracycline can be administered.

CONTACT TREATMENT (EPIDEMIOLOGIC TREATMENT)

Clinical and serologic evidence of syphilis can take from 10 to 90 days to become apparent. Ten to 90 percent of contacts to early syphilis cases may become infected with the disease. If one treats contacts before they develop lesions, further transmission of the disease is prevented. Therefore, epidemiologic treatment refers to the treatment of contacts to early syphilis even if they do not have symptoms of the disease. Treatment is the same as for incubating syphilis.

JARISCH-HERXHEIMER REACTION

The Jarisch-Herxheimer reaction is a febrile reaction seen following treatment in fewer than 10 percent of patients treated for primary or secondary syphilis. Occasionally, it occurs in the treatment of congenital syphilis. The reaction starts within 4 hours after initiation of treatment, peaks at 8 hours, and dissipates within 24 hours. The reaction consists of fever, arthralgia, myalgia, worsening of secondary lesions of syphilis, and increased swelling of the lymph nodes. In addition, some people may experience vasoconstriction with an increase of blood pressure, nausea, and vomiting, followed by vasodilatation and a decrease in blood pressure. In pregnant women, Jarisch-Herxheimer is often associated with fetal heart rate decelerations, decrease in fetal motion and, occasionally, spontaneous abortion. The reaction does not decrease if the initial penicillin dosage is reduced. Whether or not a short course of corticosteroids concurrent with therapy prevents this reaction is unproved.

RESPONSE TO THERAPY AND FOLLOW-UP

All patients with early syphilis and congenital syphilis should return for repeat, quantitative nontreponemal tests at least 3, 6, and 12 months after treatment.

Seroconversion after treatment is more rapid if the duration of infection is shorter. For people with early syphilis after treatment, the VDRL (or RPR) titer has declined fourfold by 3 months and eightfold by 6 months. Ninety-seven percent of effectively treated patients with primary syphilis are seronegative 2 years after therapy. Most infants with neonatal congenital syphilis are also seronegative 1 year following treatment. Fluorescent treponemal antibody-absorption (FTA/ABS) antibodies persist indefinitely.

Serologic response with latent syphilis or in patients who have had a previous syphilitic infection is less predictable. Patients with syphilis of longer than 1 year's duration should also have a repeat serologic test 24 months after treatment. Careful follow-up of serologic testing is particularly important in patients treated with antibiotics other than penicillin. Examination of the CSF should be planned as part of the last follow-up visit in patients treated with alternative antibiotics.

All patients with neurosyphilis should be followed carefully with repeat CSF examinations within 3 months after treatment, at 6-month intervals until the CSF is normal, and then annually for at least 3 years.

The possibility of reinfection should always be considered when retreating patients with early syphilis. A CSF examination should be performed before retreatment unless reinfection and a diagnosis of early syphilis can be established.

Retreatment should be considered in the following situations:

1. Clinical signs or symptoms of syphilis persist or recur.
2. There is a fourfold increase in the titer of a nontreponemal test.
3. An initially high-titer nontreponemal test fails to decrease fourfold within a year. Patients should be retreated with the schedules recommended for syphilis of more than 1 year's duration.

In general, only one retreatment course is indicated because patients may maintain stable, low titers in nontreponemal tests or may have irreversible anatomic damage.

SUGGESTED READING

American Academy of Pediatrics. Report of the committee on infectious diseases, 20th ed. Elk Grove Village, IL: AAP, 1986; 346–352.
Centers for Disease Control. 1985 STD treatment guidelines. MMWR 1985; 34(Suppl 4S):75–108S.
Hook EW, Baker-Zander SA, Moskovitz BL, et al. Ceftriaxone therapy for asymptomatic neurosyphilis. Sex Transm Dis 1986; 3:185–188.
Ingall D, Norins L. Syphilis. In: Remington JS, Kean JO, eds. Infectious diseases of the fetus and newborn infant. Philadelphia: WB Saunders, 1976; 414–463.
Rathbun KC. Congenital syphilis: a proposal for improved surveillance, diagnosis, and treatment. Sex Transm Dis 1983; 10:102–107.

TETANUS

DUANE L. DOWELL, M.D.

Despite adequate preventive measures, tetanus remains an important cause of morbidity and mortality worldwide. It is uncommon in the United States, but there are about 300,000 cases per year worldwide, with a mortality approaching 45 percent. An infectious disease caused by the organism *Clostridium tetani*, tetanus behaves more like an environmental hazard than a contagious disease. A soluble exotoxin, tetanospasmin, is responsible for the clinical manifestations of the disease. When the patient initially presents, the severity of the disease can be judged by the presence or absence of convulsions, the length of the incubation period, the rapidity with which the symptoms progress, and the presence or absence of apneic episodes.

SUPPORTIVE MANAGEMENT OF THE PATIENT

The key to successful management and survival of the patient is constant and attentive nursing care. A principal cause of death in this disease is asphyxia during laryngospasm in the midst of frequent and prolonged muscle spasms. Whether in a sophisticated intensive care unit or in a more simply appointed hospital ward in a developing country, the continuous monitoring of the patient with ready access to suctioning and an AMBU bag has a direct relationship to morbidity and mortality.

Sedative-relaxant therapy is directed at the control of seizures and muscle spasm. In severe tetanus, the line between control of these symptoms and respiratory depression becomes very thin. The use of a single agent enables the physician to exert maximal control over seizure activity while avoiding excessive sedation and respiratory depression. During the past 20 years, diazepam (Valium) has become the most useful drug in the control of the neuromuscular manifestations of tetanus. It can be given orally, intramuscularly, or intravenously, can be titrated to individual patient needs, and is useful in all age groups. The broad dosage range is 2 to 20 mg every 1 to 8 hours. Initially 0.1 mg per kilogram may be used, but the key is individual titration of dosage. Tetanus spasms are painful, and morphine can be a very useful adjunct for sedation and pain control in a dosage of 0.1 to 0.15 mg per kilogram every 3 to 6 hours.

Airway management is equally important and closely related to the control of spasms. In mild to moderate cases, gentle suctioning and easy access to oxygen and an AMBU bag suffices to maintain the airway. In the severe case, because the frequency and severity of seizures and spasms increase, the decision for tracheostomy should be made early. It is possible and desirable to manage a tracheostomy and feeding gastrostomy, if necessary, in a rural hospital without an intensive care unit and without sophisticated artificial ventilation equipment. When facilities and trained personnel are available, the severe case of tetanus requires neuromuscular blockade and mechanical ventilation. *D*-tubocurarine, 0.2 to 0.3 mg per kilogram given intravenously every 1 to 3 hours, has been the mainstay of the neuromuscular blocking agents in the treatment of tetanus. In neonatal tetanus, however, it is best to avoid tracheostomy unless a modern, well-equipped neonatal intensive care unit is available with personnel skilled in the use of respirators.

CARE OF THE WOUND

A portal of entry is not discovered in 20 to 30 percent of cases. When a wound is identified, it should be thoroughly cleansed and debrided. Radical, disfiguring excision is not helpful and should be avoided. There has been no evidence that local infiltration of immune globulin or antitoxin around the wound offers any benefit, and it should not be done. Remember that by the time the patient presents with symptoms, the toxin has traversed the neuronal pathways and is fixed either centrally or at the nerve endings. Nevertheless, it does make sense to cleanse dirty wounds and excise necrotic tissue, which may still harbor organisms.

ANTISERUM THERAPY

Cost and availability continue to prevent the universal use of human tetanus immune globulin (TIG). TIG is preferrable to equine and bovine tetanus antitoxin (TAT) because of the more serious side effects of antitoxin such as anaphylaxis and serum sickness. The dosage of TIG is 500 U for tetanus neonatorum and 500 to 5,000 U, given intramuscularly, in older children and adults. When TAT must be used, 10,000 U intramuscularly is sufficient for all cases. Some authors are enthusiastic about intrathecal therapy. I have no experience with it and clinical trials have been inconclusive, therefore, I cannot personally recommend its use.

ANTIBIOTIC THERAPY

Penicillin G is the drug of choice. It is effective against both vegetative and spore forms of the organism. The dosage is 100,000 U per kilogram per day, given intravenously at 6 hourly intervals, or procaine penicillin G, given intramuscularly once daily. Treatment should be continued for 7 to 10 days. Alternatively, tetracycline, erythromycin, and chloramphenicol are effective, although the tetracyclines are limited to use in children over 8 years of age.

PREVENTION

Inexpensive, effective prevention in the form of a toxoid has been available for 60 years, yet tetanus remains an important cause of mortality, especially neonatal mortality, in the world today. Active immunization is readily achieved by the use of alum-precipitated toxoid, using three injections, given 4 weeks apart. A booster dose given 6 months or more after the initial series completes the primary immunization. A second booster is given on entry into school at the age of 4 to 6 years. In children under age 7, this should be accomplished with diphtheria–tetanus–pertussis (DTP) vaccine. In older children and adults, two or three doses of adult-type tetanus diphtheria vaccine (Td), given 1 to 2 months apart, followed by a booster in 6 to 12 months accomplishes the primary series. Further boosters at 10-year intervals ensures lifelong protection.

Prevention at the time of injury includes wound management and attention to immunization status. The wound should be thoroughly cleansed and debrided where necessary, to eliminate necrotic tissue. With a clean, minor wound and a complete primary immunization series, no further prophylaxis is necessary other than the routine booster at 10-year intervals. All other wounds require a booster if more than 5 years have elapsed since the previous injection. If the initial series is incomplete (fewer than three doses), 500 U of TIG should also be given at the time of injury.

Prevention of neonatal tetanus can be accomplished by administering two doses of tetanus toxoid, 1 month apart, to women of child-bearing age before or during pregnancy. Infants of unimmunized mothers delivered without skilled attendance, should receive TIG and TAT as soon after birth as possible.

SUGGESTED READING

Alfrey D, Rauscher LA. Tetanus: a review. Crit Care Med 1979; 7:176–181.

Garnier Muller J. Tetanus in children three years of age and up. Am J Surg 1975; 129:459–463.

Marshall F. In: Gellis, Kagan, eds. Tetanus, in current pediatric therapy. Philadelphia: WB Saunders, 1976; 567–571.

Weinstein L. In: Feigen R, Cherry J, eds. Textbook of pediatric infectious disease. Philadelphia: WB Saunders, 1980; 843–850.

TOXIC SHOCK SYNDROME

RONALD M. PERKIN, M.D.

Toxic shock syndrome (TSS) is an acute febrile illness with mucocutaneous manifestations and multisystem involvement that is often associated with focal staphylococcal infection. Although many TSS cases are associated with menstruation, a substantial number of cases in men, children, and nonmenstruating women have been reported. These reports clearly show that TSS can be associated with various types of staphylococcal infections including empyema, bacteremia, deep and superficial wound infections, infected burns, adenitis, osteomyelitis, tracheobronchitis, septic abortion, and staphylococcal colonization of mucous membranes. The site of staphylococcal infection is often subtle in appearance. Surgical TSS cases are notable because signs of inflammation are absent; many of the surgical wounds have been described as benign in appearance.

Although focal infection or colonization with *Staphylococcus aureus* appears to be a necessary precondition for the development of TSS, the exact mechanism by which it mediates TSS is not known. The fact that most patients do not have disseminated infections suggests that TSS is mediated by one or more staphylococcal toxins. The toxin that appears to be very important is called toxic shock syndrome toxin-1 (TSST-1). Recent studies suggest that another group of toxins, enterotoxins, may be implicated in a smaller portion of cases, especially those associated with the nonmenstrual form of the disease. An intriguing component in the pathophysiology is the demonstration that sera from most patients with the acute syndrome show no detectable antibody to TSST-1. The implication of these observations is that patients who acquire TSS are either antigenically naive or have an ill-defined immunodeficiency that inhibits either the production or maintenance of TSST-1 antibodies.

No rapid diagnostic test is available to aid in making a definitive diagnosis. The diagnosis of TSS is based on a strict case definition, which is outlined in Table 1. A strict definition has been necessary because TSS has features in common with several other diseases such as leptospirosis, streptococcal scarlet fever, Rocky Mountain spotted fever, atypical measles, Kawasaki disease, and the Stevens–Johnson syndrome. TSS can, however, be distinguished as a clinical entity distinct from all of these illnesses. Although they are variable in intensity, the order in which clinical manifestations develop in TSS is relatively constant and does not differ in the menstrual and nonmenstrual forms.

TABLE 1 Case Definition of Toxic Shock Syndrome

Mayor Symptoms and Signs	
Fever	Temperature ≥ 38.9°C (102°F).
Rash	Diffuse macular erythroderma. Desquamation occurs 1–2 weeks after onset of illness, most prominently on the palms and soles.
Hypotension	Systolic blood presure ≤ 90 mm Hg for adults of below the fifth percentile by age, for children less than 16 years of age.
Multisystem Involvement—3 or More of the Following	
Gastrointestinal	Vomiting or diarrhea at onset of illness.
Muscular	Severe myalgia or creatine phosphokinase level greater than or equal to twice the upper limit of normal.
Renal	Blood urea nitrogen or creatinine level greater than or equal to twice the upper limit of normal, or pyuria in the absence of a urinary tract infection.
Hepatic	Total bilirubin, serum aspartate aminotransferase, and serum alanine aminotransferase values twice the upper limit of normal.
Mucous membrane	Vaginal, oropharyngeal, or conjunctival hyperemia.
Hematologic	Platelets ≤ 100,000/mm³.
Central nervous system	Disorientation or alteration of consciousness without focal neurologic signs when fever and hypotension are absent.
Reasonable Evidence for Absence of Other Etiologies	

Negative blood, throat, or cerebrospinal fluid cultures for organisms other than *Staphylococcus aureus*.

No rise in antibody titers to Rocky Mountain spotted fever, leptospirosis, or measles.

THERAPY

TSS is a devastating illness because it occurs primarily in young, healthy individuals and has a mortality rate of 3.5 and 9 percent in menstrual and nonmenstrual cases, respectively. The mainstays of therapy are identification and control of the infection and supportive care aimed at preservation of cardiopulmonary function (see also the chapter on *Septic Shock*).

Eradication of Infection

A successful outcome of TSS may be most dependent on early recognition of the syndrome and elimination of the source of presumed staphylococcal infection and toxin production. This might involve removal of a tampon or other foreign body from the vagina, drainage of an abscess, or debridement and irrigation of a wound. Antistaphylococcal antibiotics such as nafcillin (150 mg per kilogram per day, given intravenously in four divided doses) should be started based on clinical factors and not withheld pending the results of cultures.

In patients with severe TSS, vasodilation and increased capillary permeability with extravasation of fluid and serum proteins results in hypotension, oliguria, low central venous pressures, pulmonary and peripheral edema, low serum albumin with hypocalcemia, and metabolic acidosis. The severity of hypovolemia and hypotension may be augmented by large gastrointestinal volume losses, which some patients display. Enormous quantities of fluid are required to restore intravascular volume, alleviate metabolic acidosis, improve urine output, and restore peripheral perfusion. These large volumes of fluid should be given with careful monitoring of central venous pressure, arterial pressure, physical examination, and urine output. Isotonic crystalloid solution (normal saline or Ringer's lactate) may be used in the initial period of stabilization, but as fluid resuscitation continues, blood, fresh frozen plasma, or albumin may be required. Despite appropriate therapy, some patients continue to lose substantial volumes of fluid into the extravascular space, so that peripheral and pulmonary edema develop, often with impressive weight gain. Intravascular volume must be maintained during this period.

The initial hemodynamic presentation of TSS is hyperdynamic, with elevated cardiac index and decreased systemic vascular resistance. Provision of an adequate intravascular volume usually maintains the hyperdynamic state, and the patient improves rapidly after the focus of infection is identified and removed. Some patients, unfortunately, do not follow this relatively benign course, and progressive myocardial failure develops 12 to 48 hours into the treatment of TSS, despite appropriate fluid management. These patients become tachycardic, often with a gallop rhythm, as central venous pressure rises, urine output falls, and peripheral perfusion and blood pressure decrease. Echocardiographic evidence of depressed shortening fraction and ejection fraction is usually evident. This observed myocardial dysfunction is usually reversible and may represent a toxic cardiomyopathy. Inotropic support must be provided, to improve cardiovascular performance. Dobutamine alone or in combination with small-dosage dopamine is a reasonable initial inotropic selection. Electrolyte abnormalities, hypoxemia, metabolic acidosis, hypocalcemia, hypophosphatemia, and hypoglycemia may be seen in TSS and should be treated. Correction of these biochemical aberrations helps optimize myocardial function. Hypocalcemia may be related to hypoalbuminemia; therefore, ionized calcium serum concentrations should be measured. Patients who remain hypotensive may require vasoconstrictor dosages of dopamine, epinephrine, or norepinephrine to maintain perfusion pressure.

Other Supportive Measures

Complications of this syndrome include renal failure, respiratory failure, tachydysrhythmias, coagulopathies, and cerebral edema. Children appear more prone to require respiratory support than adults. Development of pulmonary edema, pleural effusions, hypoventilation secondary to respiratory muscle fatigue, and adult respiratory distress syndrome are the common causes of respiratory problems. Supplemental oxygen, intubation, and mechanical ventilation may all be required supportive procedures.

Impaired renal function is usually prerenal in origin and responds to volume replacement, inotropic support, and judicious use of diuretics. In rare cases, persistent oliguric renal failure necessitates dialysis.

Recent evidence suggests that corticosteroids may reduce the severity of illness and duration of fever in patients with TSS if they are given early in the course of illness. Methylprednisolone is given in a dosage of 10 mg per kilogram of body weight every 8 to 12 hours. The dosage is tapered after the patient is afebrile and no longer needs cardiovascular support. Prospective studies supporting the use of corticosteroids in TSS have not been conducted. Other suggested adjuncts to therapy, including immunoglobulin infusion, plasmapheresis, renal ultrafiltration, and naloxone, remain of unproved value and cannot be recommended.

SUGGESTED READING

Buchdahl R, Levin M, Wilkins B, et al. Toxic shock syndrome. Arch Dis Child 1985; 60:563–567.

Chesney PJ, Davis JP, Purdy WK, et al. Clinical manifestations of toxic shock syndrome. JAMA 1981; 246:741–748.

Crass BA, Bergdoll MS. Toxin involvement in toxic shock syndrome. J Infect Dis 1986; 153:918–926.

Fisher CJ, Horowitz BZ, Albertson TE. Cardiorespiratory failure in toxic shock syndrome: effect of dobutamine. Crit Care Med 1985; 13:160–165.

Wiesenthal AM, Todd JK. Toxic shock syndrome in children aged 10 years or less. Pediatrics 1984; 74:112–117.

TUBERCULOSIS

RICHARD F. JACOBS, M.D., F.A.A.P.

The basic principles for the treatment of tuberculosis in children are essentially the same as those for adults. The ongoing investigations of short-course chemotherapy for pulmonary and extrapulmonary tuberculosis in adults and children have demonstrated that treatment regimens of 12 to 18 months are no longer necessary for a successful outcome. Nine-month regimens containing at least isoniazid and rifampin have been demonstrated to have a high rate of success in children.

Before initiating therapy with antituberculous agents, the clinician must address the issue of whether the treatment of tuberculous disease or skin test conversion without disease is required. Children are usually infected by a family member, caretaker, or frequent visitor to the home. Most cases of tuberculosis in children in the United States are asymptomatic and are diagnosed as a result of screening contacts of known active tuberculosis cases. Infection with *Mycobacterium tuberculosis* should be suspected in any child with a positive tuberculin skin reaction. The standard intermediate-strength Mantoux intracutaneous test using 0.1 ml containing 5 tuberculin units of purified protein derivative (PPD) is the standard diagnostic approach in suspected cases. Measurement of the induration of the reaction in millimeters is taken at 48 to 72 hours. A reaction of 10 mm or more is positive in any child, and a 6 to 9-mm reaction probably represents a significant skin test.

The next consideration is to determine whether the child has tuberculous disease or is only a tuberculin reactor. In children, this requires a high-quality posterior-anterior (PA) and lateral chest roentgenogram. Evidence of hilar adenopathy, often detectable only in the lateral view, is the hallmark of primary tuberculosis in children and should be present for this diagnosis. A thorough physical examination, and evaluation of bony detail on the chest roentgenogram may allow the clinician to detect extrapulmonary tuberculosis. The child with a normal physical examination and a normal chest roentgenogram is a tuberculin reactor and therefore infected but without symptomatic disease. This child requires isoniazid prophylaxis for preventive therapy.

Tuberculous disease is assumed in the presence of a positive PPD skin test, an abnormal chest roentgenogram, or physical findings suggestive of extrapulmonary tuberculosis. Bacteriologic confirmation is generally not necessary in children. In uncomplicated primary cases, one can use culture and drug susceptibility test results, which are available from the active index case in the child's environment. For this same reason, bacteriologic examinations are less useful in evaluating the response to treatment; thus, clinical and radiographic examinations are of relatively greater significance in children. It has recently been shown that drug susceptibility testing on the isolate from the adult contact is usually identical to susceptibility data on the child's isolate.

If no isolate is obtained from the patient contact, and the child is seriously ill or is from an endemic population strongly suspected of harboring drug-resistant mycobacteria, an attempt should be made to obtain cultures. Gastric aspirates collected from a fasting child early in the morning on 3 successive days yield positive cultures in more than 60 percent of cases with primary disease. In new cases of miliary tuberculosis, organisms can be identified in bone marrow, urine, or liver biopsy. Older children and adolescents suspected of having pulmonary tuberculosis, especially of the adult type, should submit five sputum specimens for smear and culture. Drug susceptibility studies should be done on all organisms. Acid-fast bacilli obtained from extrapulmonary cases of tuberculosis manifesting as cervical lymphadenitis should always be tested for susceptibility to antituberculous drugs.

A child who is profoundly ill with progressive primary tuberculosis or disseminated disease may not react to PPD skin testing. In any child with pneumonia and hilar adenopathy that is unresponsive to empiric antibiotic therapy, especially when a cavity is present or when a child is the contact of a known active case, antituberculous therapy should be instituted at that time. Presence of miliary lesions on chest roentgenogram or meningitis with compatible cerebrospinal fluid findings should also suggest tuberculosis. In these situations, cultures should be obtained from all possible sources and empiric antituberculous therapy instituted. A PPD skin test should be repeated in 2 to 6 weeks in these cases because many of these patients will convert their PPD reaction after clinical improvement has occurred.

TREATMENT OF TUBERCULOSIS

In the years since the advent of antituberculous chemotherapy, controlled clinical trials have yielded two basic principles on which recommendations for treatment are based: (1) regimens for treatment of disease should contain multiple bactericidal drugs to which the organisms are susceptible, and (2) drug ingestion must continue for a sufficient period of time. The aim for antituberculous therapy is to provide the most effective therapy in the shortest period of time. This allows for the maximum utilization of resources available. The currently accepted regimen for short-course chemotherapy in children with tuberculosis uses a 9-month regimen of isoniazid (INH) and rifampin (RIF). The 9-month regimen with INH and RIF has been recently shortened to 6 months for some cases of pulmonary tuberculosis in children.

Extrapulmonary tuberculosis can most likely be treated with the same 6-month regimen. Regimens using INH and RIF have been successful because these two bactericidal drugs have been shown to kill rapidly multipling extracellular organisms within 6 to 9 months and eliminate persisting organisms that are slow growing and/or dormant. A recent investigation showed that bactericidal drugs administered once daily for 1 to 2 months are equally effective in consolidation therapy (months 2 to 9) when they are given twice weekly. There are many advantages to the shorter, largely intermittent modern treatment. The advantages of intermittent chemotherapy are better patient compliance, fewer side effects, lower cost of drugs, less supervisory time, and the added advantage of direct administration of medication by health care personnel in cases of proved or suspected noncompliance.

Bactericidal drugs that kill the tubercle bacillus during replication are INH, RIF, streptomycin, capreomycin, and pyrazinamide (Table 1). Ethambutol has been shown to be bacteriostatic at a dosage of 15 mg per kilogram but to have bactericidal activity at the dosage of 25 mg per kilogram. All of these bactericidal drugs are best administered as a single morning dose. Drugs that make up the second-line antituberculous chemotherapeutic regimens are primarily bacteriostatic drugs that inhibit replication of the organism but have to be administered in divided daily doses for more than 18 to 24 months to produce an effective cure. These drugs include ethionamide, cycloserine, para-aminosalicylic acid, and ethambutol at the 15-mg-per-kilogram dosage. These drugs are second-line agents because of their bacteriostatic nature and increased toxicity over the bactericidal drugs. They should be used only in cases of drug-resistant organisms and only after consultation with a tuberculosis expert.

SPECIFIC TREATMENT

Several important generalizations can be made regarding combinations of antituberculous treatment regimens from more than 25 years of clinical studies. Observations include the following ideas:

1. INH possesses the best combination of effectiveness, fewer side effects, and lower cost of any of the antituberculous agents and should be used for the duration of whatever regimen is used.
2. Despite some scattered reports of good results with regimens of less than 6 months, in general relapse rates are unacceptably high.
3. With regimens of less than 9 months, INH and RIF are central components of at least the initial 4 to 8 weeks; the outcome of regimens of less than 8 months is probably better if INH and RIF are used throughout.
4. Pyrazinamide (PZA), given in the initial phase, improves the efficacy of regimens of less than 9 months duration. Continuing PZA beyond the initial 2 months does not seem to improve the outcome in regimens containing both INH and RIF.
5. At least in the dosages usually given, substituting ethambutol or streptomycin for PZA in the initial phase decreases the effectiveness of a regimen.
6. It also appears that continuation of streptomycin

TABLE 1 Recommended Drugs for the Initial Treatment of Tuberculosis in Children

Drug	Dosage Forms	Daily Dose	Maximal Daily Dose in Children and Adults	Twice-Weekly Dose	Major Adverse Reactions
Isoniazid	Tablets: 100 mg, 300 mg; Syrup: 50 mg/5 ml; Vials: 1 g	10–20 mg/kg PO or IM	300 mg	20–40 mg/kg, max. 900 mg	Hepatic enzyme elevation, peripheral neuropathy, hepatitis, hypersensitivity
Rifampin	Capsules: 150 mg, 300 mg; Syrup: formulated from capsules, 10 mg/ml	10–20 mg/kg PO	600 mg	10–20 mg/kg, max. 600 mg	Orange discoloration of secretions and urine; nausea, vomiting, hepatitis, febrile reaction, purpura (rare)
Pyrazinamide	Tablets: 500 mg	15–30 mg/kg PO	2 g	50–70 mg/kg	Hepatotoxicity, hyperuricemia, arthralgias, skin rash, gastrointestinal upset
Streptomycin	Vials: 1 g, 4 g	20–40 mg/kg IM	1 g	25–30 mg/kg	Ototoxicity, nephrotoxicity
Ethambutol	Tablets: 100 mg, 400 mg	15–25 mg/kg PO	2.5 g	50 mg/kg	Optic neuritis (decreased red/green color discrimination, decreased visual acuity), skin rash

beyond the initial 2 months does not improve the outcome.

In summary, this information indicates that the current minimal acceptable duration of treatment is 6 months. The initial phase of the 6-month regimen must consist of at least a 2-month period of daily INH and RIF. The consideration for the addition of pyrazinamide to 6-month regimens should be entertained. The second phase of treatment should consist of INH and RIF given daily or twice weekly for 4 months. Nine-month regimens using INH and RIF are equally effective. These generalizations apply only when the organisms are susceptible to the agents used. The prevalence of initial drug resistance is generally low in the United States and Canada, but in some areas the rate is considerably higher than the national average. Patients in these areas tend to have come from parts of the world where the prevalence of tuberculosis and drug resistance are high. In such areas, drug susceptibility testing on an individual isolate or a contacts isolate should be done as part of the routine treatment.

I currently recommend either a 9-month course of INH and RIF or a 6-month course of INH and RIF with or without PZA for the treatment of tuberculosis in children and adolescents. The use of a 6-month regimen of INH and RIF alone for children with a positive PPD and hilar adenopathy on chest roentgenogram as the only manifestation of disease has been successful. The addition of pyrazinamide to this 6-month regimen would be considered for cases with symptomatic disease or extrapulmonary tuberculosis. There is also excellent support for the use of INH and RIF alone for the treatment of extrapulmonary tuberculosis in Arkansas. Since extrapulmonary tuberculosis represents infection with a much smaller organism population than is found in cavitary pulmonary tuberculosis, there is no logical reason for a more prolonged treatment in these disease forms. If there are collections of infectious fluid anywhere, such as in an empyema, paravertebral abscess, psoas abscess, or brain abscess, the lesions may need to be drained.

The antituberculous drugs used for the treatment of disease in children are depicted in Table 1. The dosage of INH is 10 to 20 mg per kilogram daily, to a maximum dose of 300 mg; the RIF dosage is also 10 to 20 mg per kilogram daily, to a maximum dose of 600 mg. These drugs can be given daily for the full 6 to 9 months of treatment, but it is preferable to give the medications twice weekly after the initial 4 to 6 weeks. During the biweekly phase, the daily dose of RIF remains the same while the INH dosage doubles to 20 to 40 mg per kilogram per dose, not to exceed 900 mg per day.

Children whose weight is more than 40 kg should receive the adult dosage regimen of 300 mg INH and 600 mg of RIF daily for the first 30 days, followed by 900 mg INH and 600 mg RIF twice weekly for the remaining 8 months. These dosages of INH and RIF should be given for the initial 2 months of a 6-month treatment regimen, with the increased dosage of INH used for the final 4 months of therapy. This combination chemotherapy can be conveniently given to children using a combination capsule containing INH, 150 mg, and RIF, 300 mg (Rifamate [Merrell Dow] or Rimatazid [Ciba]). During the twice-weekly continuation phase, two combination capsules are administered along with two 300-mg tablets of INH, making the twice-weekly doses 900 mg INH and 600 mg RIF.

Medications are preferably given early in the morning, before breakfast. Scored tablets of INH are available in 100- and 300-mg sizes. Capsules containing 100 and 300 mg of RIF are also available. For a young child who is unable to swallow tablets or capsules, tablets can be crushed or the contents removed from the RIF capsule. This small volume of medication can be mixed with a teaspoon of applesauce, jam, or soft food before it is administered. Although there have been concerns recently about the inactivation of RIF in acidic food substances such as applesauce, when these medications are added freshly each morning and not stored for prolonged periods, this regimen has been successful in our experience. The liquid preparation of INH containing 50 mg per 5 ml is available, and a similar suspension of RIF can be made by mixing 1,200 mg contained in 4 capsules of RIF in 120 ml of simple syrup. This remains stable in the refrigerator for as long as 6 weeks, but must be shaken well before each use. Capsules and tablets should always be used in preference to a liquid form of INH and RIF because of the storage difficulties.

The experience in treating tuberculous meningitis with short-course chemotherapy has been limited but successful. Meningitis is the most serious form of tuberculosis and often leaves significant residual cerebral dysfunction unless treatment is started early. If the patient has a significant loss of consciousness before therapy is initiated, no form of treatment currently available results in recovery without residua. Although INH, RIF, and PZA penetrate the cerebrospinal fluid readily and achieve concentrations well above the minimum inhibitory concentration (MIC) level for *Mycobacterium tuberculosis,* recommendation for two-drug therapy in the initial treatment of tuberculous meningitis is controversial. I would use INH, RIF, pyrazinamide, and streptomycin in the initial treatment of tuberculous meningitis in children. Because this is the most severe form of tuberculosis, with no assurance of drug susceptibility, all four drugs should be used until susceptibility studies in the patient or contacts of the patient are complete. Following the initial 4 to 6 weeks of four-drug chemotherapy, INH and RIF can be continued for the completion of the 6- to 9-month therapeutic regimen. In tuberculous meningitis, I currently recommend the total duration of 9 months of therapy because of a lack of data for the 6-month regimen.

The use of adjunctive therapy such as surgery

and corticosteroids is more commonly required in extrapulmonary tuberculosis than in pulmonary disease. Surgery may be necessary to obtain specimens for diagnosis and to treat such processes as constrictive pericarditis, spinal cord compression from miliary tuberculosis or paravertebral involvement, and abscess formation. Some experts feel that corticosteroids may be of benefit in preventing cardiac constriction from tuberculous pericarditis and in decreasing the neurologic sequelae of tuberculous meningitis. Other individuals have recommended corticosteroids for extensive pleural effusions and large obstructive lymph nodes. Although no controlled studies have proved the efficacy of corticosteroids in this regimen, I recommend corticosteroids as an adjunctive therapy in tuberculous meningitis and constrictive tuberculous pericarditis. Although uncommon in children, large obstructive lymph nodes in endobronchial tuberculosis, with significant extrinsic compression of the airway, is another disease state for which I recommend corticosteroids.

DRUG-RESISTANT ORGANISMS

A complete statement of special considerations in the treatment of tuberculosis, associated disorders, pregnancy, lactation and limitations of chemotherapy can be found in the official American Thoracic Society statement on the treatment of tuberculosis (Bass et al, 1986). Children infected with drug-resistant *Mycobacterium tuberculosis* acquire their infection from inadequately treated source cases or contacts from areas of endemic resistance. Index or source cases should be questioned thoroughly about past chemotherapy. Drug-resistant organisms are prevalent in people from Southeast Asia, the Philippines, Mexico, and other Central or South American countries. As many as 25 percent of the cultures from Asian refugees are drug resistant, and nearly half of these are resistant to several drugs. If infection with drug-resistant organisms is suspected, the best policy is to initiate treatment with four bactericidal drugs (INH, RIF, PZA, and streptomycin). Capreomycin can be used in place of streptomycin in Asian patients. After 6 to 8 weeks of daily therapy, the results of drug susceptibility testing in contacts of the patient should be available, and treatment can be continued twice weekly with two drugs to which the organism is susceptible. Older children can also be given ethambutol safely. A total of 9 months of therapy is adequate.

TREATMENT FAILURES AND RELAPSES

The most common cause of a treatment failure or suspected relapse is failure of patient compliance. Strong consideration should be given to administering therapy under direct observation in these patients. Patients who have a relapse after completing a regimen containing INH and RIF who had organisms susceptible to the drugs at the outset of treatment usually still have susceptible organisms. Thus, management of these patients generally consists of reinstitution of the INH–RIF regimen previously used. However, case contacts and isolates from contacts of the patient, as well as identification and drug susceptibility testing on the child's isolates, should be performed and the regimen modified if resistance is detected. Direct observation of therapy should be strongly considered.

ADVERSE EFFECTS OF DRUGS

Children have shown a remarkable tolerance to INH during the 30 years of its availability; the risk of INH hepatitis in patients younger than 20 years of age is currently 0 percent. A 0.3 percent incidence of INH hepatitis is currently listed for individuals between 20 and 34 years of age. Neurotoxicity may be manifest as convulsions or peripheral neuritis. Competitive inhibition of pyridoxine metabolism by INH is extremely rare in children, therefore, prophylactic use of pyridoxine is not currently recommended and rarely required. It is suggested that severely ill or malnourished children be given 25 mg of pyridoxine daily. Because of the small risk of hepatotoxicity from INH, routine liver function tests are not currently recommended. If symptoms compatible with hepatotoxicity such as malaise, anorexia, nausea, vomiting, or jaundice occur, INH therapy should be stopped and liver function studies performed. Once the patient has recovered clinically and laboratory variables are normal, INH can be slowly reintroduced to determine whether true toxicity was present. Skin rashes and gastrointestinal complaints are also managed by temporary withdrawal of INH, which often can be reintroduced. Diphenhydramine (Benadryl) can be given for skin rashes and continued throughout the reintroduction phase. Phenytoin (Dilantin) degradation can be decreased by INH, resulting in elevated blood concentrations. Dilantin concentrations in serum should be checked 2 and 6 weeks after INH has been started and the dosage decreased as necessary.

Children's tolerance of rifampin appears to be good. The experience in Arkansas has documented only 2 of 150 children with RIF toxicity. Clinical manifestations were readily detected in both cases. Rifampin uniformly causes body secretions and urine to turn bright orange, a change that is benign but occasionally frightening to children or parents. The pigment can discolor soft contact lenses. Hepatotoxicity, often associated with jaundice, has been described. Even if nausea, vomiting, or skin rash occurs, once clinical and laboratory abnormalities subside, the drug is sometimes successfully reintroduced. Drug fever during the daily phase or a flulike syndrome during the twice-weekly phase is sometimes seen. Rifampin can decrease the effectiveness of oral contraceptives and has been implicated in the interaction, with subsequent subtherapeutic drug levels of ketoconazole.

The most serious side effect of streptomycin is damage to the eighth nerve, most commonly vestibular function and less commonly the auditory branch. Nephrotoxicity, fever, and rash also occur. Capreomycin can be used in patients with organisms resistant to streptomycin because there is no cross-resistance between the two aminoglycosides. It has rarely been used in children but should be satisfactory. Side effects of the two drugs are the same. Pyrazinamide has the disadvantage of being available only in a 500-mg tablet. Hepatotoxicity occurs in 1 to 4 percent of cases, even when the drug is combined with INH and RIF. Asymptomatic hyperuricemia is common; arthralgias that occur in 1 to 7 percent of adult cases can be managed with common analgesics.

Retrobulbar neuritis is the most common and serious adverse effect of ethambutol. Symptoms include blurred vision, central scotomata, and red/green color blindness. This complication is dose-related, occurring in fewer than 1 percent of cases at a dosage of 15 mg per kilogram per day and increasing with a dosage of 25 mg per kilogram per day. Frequency of ocular effects increases in patients with renal failure, presumably because of increased serum concentrations of the drug. These renal symptoms commonly precede measurable decreases in visual acuity. Patients should be informed to report any change in vision. Generally, children who are too young for assessment of visual acuity and red/green color discrimination should be treated with ethambutol with particular caution and only after consideration of possible alternative drugs.

Obviously hepatotoxic drugs (INH, RIF, or PZA) should not be used in combination during the presence of active hepatitis. All children should be monitored clinically for adverse reactions during the period of chemotherapy. They should be instructed to look for symptoms associated with the most common adverse reactions to their medications. Patients should be seen by medical personnel at least monthly during therapy and should be specifically questioned concerning such symptoms.

MONITORING THERAPY

Although most cases of primary tuberculosis are asymptomatic, children with observed side effects should be followed closely until symptoms subside. In cases of chronic pulmonary tuberculosis of the adult type, cultures and smears for mycobacteria should be obtained every 3 weeks until three cultures are negative. Subsequently, cultures should be obtained monthly until 6 months after treatment is completed. Pulmonary infiltrates are followed with chest roentgenograms every 2 to 3 months until findings are normal. The radiographic changes of hilar adenopathy in children resolve more slowly and therefore repeat roentgenograms should be obtained no more than every 6 to 12 months. The rate of clearing of primary disease or segmental consolidation probably is not influenced by chemotherapy. Lack of a complete resolution of the chest roentgenogram is not an indication to continue chemotherapy beyond the 6- to 9-month treatment regimen.

Close supervision is necessary to monitor for drug toxicity, but also to ensure compliance with the full course of therapy. Drugs can be dispensed at weekly or monthly intervals and the patient or parent questioned about any side effects during these visits. Compliance can be evaluated by irregular clinic attendance, pill counts, and checking of the urine for the metabolite of INH and orange color of RIF.

The practicing clinician should be aware of the public health programs for tuberculosis within his or her region. All cases of tuberculosis should be reported to the appropriate public health facility, which usually provides contact investigation and bacteriologic services, and may provide medications. Public health nurses should be able to dispense drugs ordered by physicians and monitor for side effects. If direct administration of medication is necessary, it probably can be done under the supervision of the local public health facility.

PREVENTIVE TREATMENT

Children with a recently converted positive PPD reaction, normal chest roentgenograms, and normal physical examinations are considered to have tuberculous infection without disease. Patients should receive a course of INH to prevent early dissemination or subsequent development of chronic pulmonary tuberculosis. INH in a dosage of 10 to 15 mg per kilogram to a maximum of 300 mg daily for 9 months is currently recommended as preventive treatment in children. INH prophylaxis is required for children 3 years of age and younger living in a house of a smear-positive case of tuberculosis. If the child's PPD remains negative after 3 months and the index case is smear-negative on treatment, the INH can be discontinued. A newborn delivered to a mother with active pulmonary tuberculosis should also receive INH from birth until the mother is smear- and culture-negative. The infant should have a PPD skin test to determine whether he or she has become infected in utero or immediately after birth. INH can be discontinued if the parent complies with medication and is smear- and culture-negative, and the child's PPD is negative at 3 months.

I currently do not recommend the use of bacille Calmette-Guérin (BCG) vaccine within the United States because of the questionable lack of efficacy among different available lots of vaccine and the potential adverse effects of this crude preparation in children.

SUGGESTED READING

Abernathy RS, Dutt AK, Stead W, et al. Short-course chemotherapy for tuberculosis in children. Pediatrics 1983; 72:801–806.

Bass JB, Farer LS, Hopwell PC, Jacobs RF. Treatment of tuberculosis and tuberculosis infection in adults and children. Am Rev Resp Dis 1986; 134:355–363.

Jacobs RF, Abernathy RS. The treatment of tuberculosis in children. Pediatr Infect Dis 1985; 4:513–517.

TULAREMIA

RUSSELL W. STEELE, M.D.

Tularemia is a zoonotic disease that is almost always transmitted to children by infected ticks and to adults by exposure to ticks, deer flies, mites and fleas, infected animals, or ingestion of contaminated food. It has been reported throughout the United States, but the highest incidence is in the south-central region (Arkansas, Louisiana, Illinois, Tennessee, Missouri, Texas, and Virginia). Seasonal distribution in children is almost exclusively during the summer months, when environmental exposure occurs, but for adults also in the winter months, associated with rabbit and deer hunting.

Diagnosis must occasionally be made by clinical criteria alone, in highly endemic areas, because serologic confirmation cannot be achieved until the second week of illness at the earliest. Untreated, the case fatality rate is 5 to 7 percent, thereby necessitating early empiric therapy for the seriously ill patient when tularemia is part of the differential diagnosis. Clinical presentation most commonly includes fever, adenitis, and an ulcer at the site of a previous tick bite. Other manifestations are pneumonia, a typhoidal syndrome, conjunctivitis with preauricular adenitis (Parinaud's oculoglandular syndrome), and oropharyngeal infection.

The standard for diagnosis is an agglutination antibody assay that becomes positive in 98 percent of cases by 4 to 6 weeks. A titer of 1:160 or greater in serum is considered diagnostic for present or recent infection. Cultures from aspirated lymph nodes or blood may be positive; however, these organisms represent a significant laboratory hazard so should be obtained only when the appropriate personnel are forewarned that *Francisella tularensis* is a potential pathogen.

ANTIBIOTIC TREATMENT

Streptomycin remains the antibiotic of choice for all forms of tularemia, although other aminoglycosides and some third-generation cephalosporins (moxalactam, ceftazidime, ceftriaxone, and cefotaxime) demonstrate excellent in vitro activity against *F. tularensis* (Table 1). Enough clinical experience with gentamicin exists to recommend it as an acceptable alternative, but to date very few patients have been treated with the newer cephalosporins. The relapse rate in children treated with tetracycline or chloramphenicol has been high, thereby eliminating effective oral therapy. The organism is resistant to all penicillins and first- or second-generation cephalosporins (cephalothin, cefamandole, and cefoxitin). Failure of empiric therapy with these antibiotics for febrile illness often suggests the diagnosis of tularemia

A relatively short course of treatment with streptomycin, 6 days, is curative in the usual case (Table 2). Shorter duration of therapy also reduces potential ototoxicity, particularly vertigo, which commonly appears after the sixth or seventh day of therapy. Ototoxicity is cumulatively related to the total daily dosage. Twice daily dosing also allows treatment on an outpatient basis. The major shortcoming of gentamicin therapy is that dosing every 8 hours normally requires hospitalization.

For patients with impaired renal function, tetracycline, chloramphenicol, or a newer cephalosporin should be used, because neurotoxic adverse reactions

TABLE 1 MIC$_{50}$ of Antimicrobials Against *Francisella tularensis*

Antibiotic	MIC$_{50}$*
Streptomycin	2.0
Gentamicin	1.0
Tobramycin	1.0
Tetracycline	2.0
Chloramphenicol	1.0
Moxalactam	≤0.12
Ceftazidime	≤0.5
Ceftriaxone	2.0
Cefotaxime	2.0
Penicillin	>8.0
Ampicillin	>8.0

* The concentration, in micrograms per milliliter, at which 50% of the strains are inhibited.

TABLE 2 Preferred Antimicrobial Therapy for Tularemia

Streptomycin 30 mg/kg/day (maximum 2 g) div q12h (IM) for 3 days followed by 15 mg/kg/day div q12h (IM) for 3 days

or

Gentamicin 7.5 mg/kg/day (maximum 300 mg) div q8h (IV or IM) for 6 days from aminoglycosides are greatly increased in these patients. Tetracycline should be avoided in children younger than 8 years of age because this drug can cause permanent discoloration of developing teeth.

Duration of therapy must be individualized in severe cases, particularly those with pneumonia or a typhoidal presentation. The best guide for clinical decisions is the body temperature. Antimicrobial therapy should be continued until the patient has been afebrile for 5 days. This approach ensures a minimal chance of relapse while providing optimal cure rates.

SURGICAL TREATMENT

It is not necessary to drain or excise involved lymph nodes during the acute phase of illness, but in my experience about one-third of the patients who initially present with lymphadenitis progress to suppuration 1 to 3 weeks after they complete therapy. The pus is sterile at that time and should be surgically drained to avoid the scarring that may result from spontaneous rupture.

TYPHOID FEVER

FRANK E. BERKOWITZ, M.B., B.Ch., FCP (Paed) (SA)

Typhoid fever is a systemic illness caused by *Salmonella typhi* (*S. typhosa*). The following discussion also applies to an identical illness caused by *Salmonella enteritidis* serotypes paratyphi A, B, and C. Typhoid fever is a major health problem in developing countries, where proper sewage disposal and a clean water supply are lacking and hygienic standards are poor. The causative organism enters the body via the intestinal tract, penetrating the mucosa of the ileum to enter the mesenteric lymphatics and bloodstream, through which it reaches the reticuloendothelial organs. There it multiplies and reenters the circulation, at which stage clinical illness begins. The gallbladder is seeded from the blood, resulting in biliary excretion of the organism. *S. typhi* multiplies within macrophages of the reticuloendothelial system, and within the lymphoid tissue of the bowel, giving rise to many of the clinical manifestations of the disease.

The management of typhoid fever is considered under the following headings: antimicrobial therapy of the acute illness, supportive therapy, complications, carriage, nursing precautions, and prevention.

PREVENTION

Prevention of tularemia can be enhanced by limiting exposure of children to known sources of the organisms. Long-sleeved shirts, long pants, and shoes decrease the opportunity for ticks to come in contact with skin surfaces. Children who play outdoors in endemic areas should be examined frequently for embedded ticks. These may be removed with any forcepslike device, using steady traction. It is important to avoid aerosolization of potentially infected material. Older children and adults should be instructed to wear rubber gloves while cleaning wild game and to shower thoroughly after completing such activity.

Although a vaccine is available, it has not been tested for general use and has been administered only to research personnel handling the organism.

SUGGESTED READING

Baker CN, Hollis DG, Thornsberry C. Antimicrobial susceptibility testing of *Francisella tularensis* using a modified Mueller-Hinton broth. J Clin Microbiol 1985; 22:212–215.

Jacobs RF, Condrey YM, Yamauchi T. Tularemia in adults and children: a changing presentation. Pediatrics 1985; 76:818–822.

ANTIMICROBIAL THERAPY OF THE ACUTE ILLNESS

Antimicrobial therapy is the most important element of management in most cases. Adequacy of therapeutic regimens is measured by the speed of resolution of the acute febrile illness and by the rates of clinical relapse and excretion of *S. typhi* following treatment. Therapy should be continued for at least 7 days after defervescence. I prefer to continue treatment for a total of 21 days, as this appears to reduce the incidence of relapse. The results of therapeutic trials undertaken in different parts of the world are difficult to compare because different dosage regimens, routes of administration, and durations of therapy have been used. Furthermore, few studies have examined the minimal inhibitory concentrations of the causative organism to the antimicrobial agent being studied, and few have examined therapy in young children.

Typhoid fever has features of a subacute bacteremic illness, and is not usually associated with shock, unless a complication has occurred. Therefore, most patients can be given oral antimicrobial therapy from the outset. However, in patients with severe toxemia, shock, vomiting, evidence of severe enteritis, or intestinal perforation, the antimicrobial should be administered intravenously.

In typhoid fever the response to therapy is not dramatic. Fever usually subsides within 3 to 7 days after treatment is begun. In proved cases of typhoid fever, apparent failure to respond to therapy may be due to inadequate drug dosage, to a drug-resistant strain of *S. typhi,* or to another concurrent infection. The possibility of a concurrent infection is particularly important in cases of typhoid fever acquired in developing countries, where infections such as malaria and amebiasis may also have been acquired. Nosocomial infections such as phlebitis and pneumonia may also result in apparent failure to respond to therapy.

Chloramphenicol has been considered the drug of choice for many years. However, it has several disadvantages, including the precipitation of increased toxemia ("toxic crisis"), a high incidence of relapse, and the potential for causing aplastic anemia. In addition, the emergence of chloramphenicol-resistant strains of *S. typhi* has rendered this drug ineffective in some areas. Amoxicillin and trimethoprim-sulfamethoxazole are as effective as chloramphenicol in treating typhoid fever. Ampicillin has been used successfully in many cases, but is not as effective as the other drugs when given orally. Because typhoid fever occurs mainly in developing countries, where health care budgets are limited, the choice of antimicrobial agent may be determined largely by cost. Therefore, chloramphenicol and trimethoprim-sulfamethoxazole, which are cheap, may be chosen in preference to amoxicillin, which is more expensive, though safer.

Antibiotic-resistant strains of *S. typhi* have emerged in many different parts of the world. Therefore, it is important that antimicrobial susceptibility testing of clinical isolates be performed, and that resistance patterns of local strains be known.

My recommendations for the antimicrobial treatment of typhoid fever are summarized in Table 1. A range of dosages is given, based on those used in different studies. I prefer to use the larger dosage if no significant side effects occur. The studies of amoxicillin in children have used 100 mg per kilogram of body weight per day. I have used amoxicillin, my preferred drug, in a dosage of 200 mg per kilogram per day, with no undue side effects.

Of the alternative drugs that have been used, the newer cephalosporins are the most promising. These should be used when the isolate is resistant to the standard drugs, or when their use is contraindicated. Ceftriaxone, 50 to 60 mg per kilogram per day for 7 days, and cefoperazone, 100 mg per kilogram per day for 14 days, both given in two divided doses, intravenously or intramuscularly, are effective regimens.

Relapse

Relapse is characterized by recurrence of symptoms, with positive blood cultures, a few days to a few weeks after recovery from typhoid fever. A short duration of therapy predisposes to this complication. Relapse should be treated in the same way as the initial illness. However, particular attention must be given to ensuring that the causative organism is susceptible to the antimicrobial agent used, and that therapy is given at an adequate dosage for an adequate duration.

SUPPORTIVE THERAPY

Typhoid fever, being a severe systemic illness, is associated with significant catabolism, which is aggravated by a decreased food intake. Diarrhea is a common clinical feature, especially in children. It is therefore essential that adequate nutrition, fluids, and electrolytes be given. In most patients these can be provided orally. In severely dehydrated patients, fluids should be given intravenously. If it is anticipated that oral feeding will not take place within 48 hours, for example, if the patient has intestinal perforation or severe ileus, total parenteral hyperalimentation should be instituted.

Patients presenting with severe toxemia, significant mental changes, or shock, in the absence of intestinal perforation, have a high case fatality rate. The prognosis in this group is improved by the intravenous administration of dexamethasone in the dosage of 3 mg per kilogram initially, followed by 1 mg per kilogram every 6 hours for 48 hours.

TABLE 1 Recommendations for the Antimicrobial Therapy of Typhoid Fever

Route	Drug	Dosage (mg/kg/day)	Frequency	Duration (days)
Oral	Amoxicillin	100–200	q6h	14–21
Oral	TMP/SMZ*	5–10†	q12h	14–21
Oral	Chloramphenicol	50–100	q6h	14–21
Intravenous	Ampicillin (or amoxicillin)‡	200	q6h	Until oral therapy can be instituted§
Intravenous	Chloramphenicol	50–100	q6h	
Intravenous	TMP/SMZ	5–10	q12h	

* TMP/SMZ = trimethoprim-sulfamethoxazole.
† Dosage of TMP component. Dosage of up to 20 mg per kilogram per day of TMP may be used.
‡ Intravenous amoxicillin is not available in the United States.
§ TMP/SMZ should not be given intravenously for longer than 5 days.

Antipyretics such as acetominophen and salicylates should not be used, because they may result in a dramatic decrease in body temperature.

COMPLICATIONS

Typhoid fever is a multisystem disease, which can result in disturbed function of several different organ systems. The most severe complications are those affecting the intestine, namely, perforation and hemorrhage, which result from ulceration of the mucosa overlying Peyer's patches.

Intestinal Perforation

Intestinal perforation affects the distal ileum, and occasionally the proximal colon. Controversy has arisen over whether this should be treated medically or surgically. The current consensus favors surgery. Once perforation has been diagnosed, the patient should be resuscitated with fluids, electrolytes, and blood, if necessary, and submitted to surgery as soon as possible. In most cases oversewing of the perforated ulcer, and of ulcers showing signs of imminent perforation, is all that is necessary. In cases with multiple perforations, bowel diversion procedures or resection may be required. The peritoneal cavity should be generously lavaged with normal saline prior to closure. Antimicrobial therapy should be broadened to treat not only *S. typhi,* but also the normal intestinal flora such as *Escherichia coli, Bacteroides fragilis,* and streptococci. Suitable antimicrobial regimens are shown in Table 2. Cefoxitin, a cephalosporin active against bowel anaerobes, in the dosage of 100 mg per kilogram per day in four divided doses intravenously for 7 to 10 days, may be used for antimicrobial treatment of the peritonitis

TABLE 2   Antimicrobial Regimens for Treating Typhoid Fever Complicated by Intestinal Perforation*

Drug	Dosage (mg/kg/day)	Frequency	Duration (days)
Ampicillin	200	q6h IV	14–21†
+ gentamicin‡	5–7½	q8h IV or IM	7–10
+ metronidazole	50	q8h IV	7–10†
or			
Ampicillin	As above	As above	As above
+ gentamicin	As above	As above	As above
+ clindamycin	20–40	q6h IV	7–10†
or			
Chloramphenicol	50–100	q6h IV	14–21†
+ gentamicin	As above	As above	As above

* In addition to surgery (see text).

† Change to oral therapy as soon as possible. Amoxicillin should be used in preference to ampicillin once oral therapy becomes possible.

‡ In some hospitals there may be a high incidence of gentamicin resistance among enteric bacilli, so that an alternative aminoglycoside would be indicated, e.g., amikacin 15 to 20 mg per kilogram per day every 12 hours IV or IM for 7 to 10 days.

following perforation, but cannot be relied on for adequate treatment of typhoid fever.

Intestinal Hemorrhage

Intestinal hemorrhage results from erosion of blood vessels within the typhoid ulcer. It may be aggravated by a coagulopathy and thrombocytopenia. Supportive management, consisting of blood transfusion and replacement of clotting factors and platelets, is usually adequate. If bleeding is uncontrolled, surgery, consisting of undersewing of the ulcer or bowel resection, may be necessary.

Extraintestinal Complications

Encephalopathy

Many patients with typhoid fever initially have slight clouding of consciousness. Severe depression in the level of consciousness is associated with a poor prognosis. A wide range of neurologic disturbances have been described, including psychiatric, pyramidal, extrapyramidal, cerebellar, and peripheral nerve disturbances. These improve following antimicrobial therapy, but may take several weeks to do so. Convulsions, which are fairly common in young children and may be the presenting symptom, require anticonvulsant therapy.

Myocarditis

Myocarditis may manifest itself with only electrocardiographic changes, but it can result in cardiac failure, requiring inotropes, diuretics, or antiarrhythmic agents.

Anemia

Anemia may be a result of the infection itself, of intestinal bleeding, or of hemolysis in patients with glucose-6-phosphate dehydrogenase (G6PD) deficiency. In the Mediterranean variety of G6PD deficiency, hemolysis may be aggravated by chloramphenicol or TMP/SMZ treatment, so that an alternative drug should be used. If anemia is severe, a blood transfusion should be given. Iron therapy should be withheld until the patient has recovered from the infection, as it may encourage the growth of *S. typhi.*

Pneumonia

Pneumonia may be part of the primary infection, or be acquired in hospital, in which case additional antimicrobial therapy should be given.

Renal Disease

Glomerulonephritis and pyelonephritis occurring in typhoid fever do not usually require specific management. However, renal failure, which may be precipitated by shock or the hemolytic-uremic syndrome, may require specific supportive management, such as restriction of fluid, salt, and protein, or dialysis.

Hepatitis and Coagulation Abnormalities

Hepatitis and coagulation abnormalities are common, if laboratory evidence for them is sought, but they are usually subclinical.

Suppurative Complications

During the bacteremic stage of the infection, *S. typhi* may seed any organ, e.g., meninges or bone. These metastatic infections are uncommon, however, and may manifest many years after an episode of typhoid fever, or without the patient having a previous history of such an episode. They should be treated with one of the drugs used in treating typhoid fever (see Table 1), but they may also require surgical drainage.

TREATMENT OF CARRIERS

Following recovery from typhoid fever, the patient may continue to excrete *S. typhi* in the stool (or occasionally in the urine). This is usually transient, lasting for a few weeks (convalescent carriage). However, in about 3 percent of cases, mostly adults, carriage continues. Patients excreting the organism for longer than 1 year after the acute illness are termed chronic carriers. They are asymptomatic, but pose a typhoid threat to the community. Chronic fecal carriage is caused by infection of the gallbladder, which is usually chronically diseased, with excretion of organisms into the bile.

Antimicrobial therapy of chronic fecal carriers can result in elimination of carriage in up to 75 percent of cases. Regimens that have been used with some success are shown in Table 3. Because this problem is confined almost entirely to adults, pediatric dosages have not been indicated. Fecal cultures should be performed periodically for at least 1 year after treatment, to confirm that carriage has been eliminated. If medical treatment fails, and it is essential that carriage in a particular individual be eliminated, cholecystectomy should be considered. This is not without hazard, and it does not guarantee suc-

TABLE 3 Antimicrobial Regimens for Adult Chronic Fecal Carriers of *Salmonella typhi*

Drug	Dosage	Frequency	Route	Duration
Ampicillin	1 g	q6h	Oral	28 days minimum
Ampicillin	1 g	q8h	IV	14 days
Amoxicillin	2 g	q8h	Oral	28 days
TMP/SMZ*	160 mg TMP, 800 mg SMZ	q12h	Oral	3 months

* TMP/SMZ = trimethoprim-sulfamethoxazole.

cess. *Clonorchis* (*Opisthorchis*) *sinensis,* a trematode acquired in Asia, which infects the biliary tract, may predispose to chronic fecal carriage of *S. typhi*. It is diagnosed by the presence of ova in the feces, and should be treated with praziquantel, 25 mg per kilogram per dose for three doses, given in one day.

Urinary tract carriage is often associated with schistosomiasis. If ova of *Schistosoma haematobium* are present in the urine, the patient should be treated with praziquantel, 40 mg per kilogram in a single dose, or metrifonate 7.5 to 10 mg per kilogram, every other week for three doses.

A neglected area in typhoid treatment is the management of convalescent carriers. Although these patients are usually only transient carriers, they remain a threat to the community as long as they are excreting the organism. Therefore, following treatment of typhoid fever, patients should not be discharged from hospital until three fecal and urine cultures have excluded carriage. Convalescent carriers should be treated in the same manner as chronic carriers, but cholecystectomy should not be performed at this stage.

Elimination of *S. typhi* from the biliary tract requires the presence of adequate concentrations of an active antimicrobial agent in bile. Many beta-lactam agents, especially some of the newer cephalosporins, fulfill this criterion, as do trimethoprim-sulfamethoxazole and the quinolones. These should be further evaluated for their role in treating typhoid fever and typhoid carriage.

It is of the utmost importance that typhoid carriers and their family members be educated about the spread of typhoid and the importance of good personal hygiene. The family members should be considered candidates for immunization (see following).

NURSING PRECAUTIONS

Nosocomial spread of typhoid fever is rare but has been described. Enteric precautions must therefore be applied when such patients are nursed. The most important of these is vigorous handwashing following any contact with the patient or the patient's excretions. The wearing of a gown and gloves, and the use of a private room are also desirable. Because the diagnosis of typhoid fever is not usually confirmed at the time the patient is admitted to hospital, precautions against the spread of other infections presenting with fever of unknown origin should also be applied, especially if the patient has come from a tropical country.

The local health authority should be informed about any case of typhoid fever, so that the source of infection can be investigated.

PREVENTION

Prevention is primarily an engineering challenge, consisting of installation of proper sewage disposal systems and of a clean water supply. This reduces the incidence not only of typhoid, but also other enteric infections. Unfortunately, in many developing countries this is unlikely to be accomplished in the near future.

Immunization provides an alternative, though less satisfactory, solution. Two different injectable, killed whole-cell vaccines have been shown to be partially effective in preventing typhoid fever in endemic areas. The acetone-inactivated (K) vaccine is superior to the heat-inactivated phenol-preserved (L) vaccine. The former should therefore be used. It is given as two subcutaneous injections of 0.5 ml each, 1 month apart. Side effects are common, consisting mainly of local pain and fever. The paratyphoid vaccines should not be used. An oral vaccine, derived from the Ty 21a strain, an enzyme-deficient mutant, has shown promise, and an injectable vaccine derived from the capsular polysaccharide (Vi antigen) is currently being investigated.

Candidates for immunization include residents of endemic areas, travelers to such areas, household members of carriers, and laboratory workers.

SUGGESTED READING

Bitar R, Tarpley J. Intestinal perforation in typhoid fever: a historical and state-of-the-art review. Rev Infect Dis 1985; 7:257–271.

Edelman R, Levine MM. Summary of an international workshop of typhoid fever. Rev Infect Dis 1986; 8:329–349.

Hoffman SL, et al. Reduction of mortality in chloramphenicol-treated severe typhoid fever by high-dose dexamethasone. N Engl J Med 1984; 310:82–88.

Mandal BK. Typhoid and paratyphoid fever. Clin Gastroenterol 1979; 8:715–735.

Scragg J, Rubidge C, Wallace HL. Typhoid fever in African and Indian children in Durban. Arch Dis Child 1969; 44:18–28.

VARICELLA-ZOSTER VIRUS INFECTION

ANNE A. GERSHON, M.D.

Varicella-zoster virus (VZV) is the cause of two diseases, varicella and zoster. Varicella is the primary infection or first encounter with the virus, and zoster is a secondary infection, resulting from reactivation of latent VZV that developed during chickenpox. Both diseases are initially characterized by a vesicular skin eruption, which is generalized in varicella and localized and unilateral in zoster. Varicella is usually a mild, uncomplicated illness in otherwise healthy children, but it can be severe or fatal in the immunoincompetent person. Zoster most often occurs in the elderly and the immunocompromised, in whom it may also become disseminated.

TREATMENT OF VZV INFECTIONS

Most VZV infections in normal hosts require no specific therapy. The itching of varicella can be alleviated with calamine lotion or antihistamines. Aspirin should not be administered to children or adolescents with chickenpox because Reye's syndrome has been reported to follow both varicella and aspirin usage. VZV infection can be treated with calamine lotion or Burow's solution; it is characteristically mild in healthy children. Bacterial superinfections (usually caused by staphylococci or streptococci) that follow VZV infections are usually treated with an anti-staphylococcal penicillin until the offending organism is identified and antibiotic susceptibility test results are available.

In situations requiring specific antiviral therapy, acyclovir is the preferred drug for VZV infections, although it is actually licensed only for treatment of herpes simplex virus infections. Acyclovir is mainly indicated for treatment of immunocompromised patients who are at great risk to develop severe VZV infections. Until more data are available, acyclovir is best given by the intravenous route in a dosage of 500 mg per square meter per dose, three times a day (1,500 mg per square meter per day) in patients with normal renal function. The dosage of acyclovir for patients with abnormal renal function (creatinine clearance less than 50 ml per minute per 1.73 m^2) should be smaller (usually one-half to one-third) than that routinely employed, in order to prevent toxic concentrations of the drug from developing.

Varicella

Immunocompromised patients with varicella who have not been passively immunized or who have not received varicella vaccine previously (see later) should be admitted to the hospital as soon as the diagnosis of varicella is made. Children at high risk to develop severe varicella include those with an underlying malignancy (especially leukemia and lymphoma) for which they are receiving therapy, children with congenital or acquired immunodeficiency, and those receiving large dosages of steroids for any reason (1.5 mg per kilogram per day or more of prednisone or its equivalent).

Treatment with intravenous acyclovir should be started immediately, even if the patient has only a few skin lesions. Successful antiviral therapy has been associated mainly with administration of the drug within the first 3 days after onset of illness. One should not wait for a high-risk patient to develop severe disease before beginning antiviral therapy, although this means that in order to save one child many may be treated unnecessarily. It is sometimes possible, early in the course of varicella, to identify a high-risk child who will do poorly if untreated; in such cases early treatment seems to be the safest approach. Baseline chest radiographs, blood gas determinations, and serum transaminase levels should be obtained before therapy is started. Blood gases should be monitored, and mechanically assisted ventilation should be used when it is necessary. In children with an underlying malignancy, consideration should be given to temporary postponement of chemotherapy. The dosage of steroids should be decreased to physiologic levels, if possible, but stress doses may be given to severely ill children. Steroids should not be stopped abruptly.

Intravenous acyclovir therapy is usually given for 5 to 10 days, although in some instances a shorter or a longer interval may be appropriate. It is reasonable to consider discontinuing acyclovir in patients who cease developing new lesions for a period of at least 4 days, who have become afebrile, and who are clearly recovering. It is not uncommon, however, for patients in the early stages of severe varicella to appear to be stable for 1 or 2 days and then manifest new lesions, presumably secondary to another bout of viremia. Therefore, care should be taken not to stop acyclovir therapy too soon in immunocompromised patients.

Zoster

Few patients with zoster develop severe disseminated infection. Even those with disseminated zoster may have a self-limited infection. Presumably, since zoster is a secondary infection rather than a primary one, the prognosis is better for zoster in the immunocompromised than it is for varicella. Whether or not one should begin acyclovir therapy in patients with zoster can be a difficult decision because it involves hospitalization. Because acyclovir is so well tolerated, however, it seems prudent to treat most if not all zoster patients with an underlying illness causing poor immune function. The main reason for using acyclovir in such patients is to prevent dissemination (or further dissemination) of VZV. Since acyclovir is well tolerated, it should be viewed not only as a lifesaving drug but also as one that decreases morbidity. Patients with zoster who are treated heal more rapidly, experience less acute pain, and have fewer days of vesiculation than untreated patients, although postherpetic pain is not prevented. Latent infection with VZV is also not prevented or cured with any currently available antiviral drug.

The efficacy of intravenous acyclovir therapy for VZV infections is well documented. In double-blind, placebo-controlled studies of varicella in children with underlying cancer, those who received early treatment with acyclovir were less likely to develop pneumonia and more likely to survive. In comparative studies with vidarabine in similar patients there was less dissemination of virus in recipients of acyclovir. In double-blind, placebo-controlled studies of immunocompromised zoster patients, there was also less progression of disease and fewer treatment failures in those receiving acyclovir than in controls. Acyclovir has also been compared with vidarabine in immunocompromised patients with zoster; again there was less dissemination in acyclovir-treated patients, and the time for healing of zoster was shorter in patients treated with acyclovir.

VZV is not as susceptible to acyclovir in vitro, as are herpes simplex virus (HSV) I or II, and there is also considerable variability of susceptibilities of different strains of VZV to the drug. An intravenous dose of 500 mg per square meter results in blood concentrations that are significantly above levels inhibitory to VZV, but oral administration of acyclovir at the usual adult dosage for HSV (200 mg, five times a day) probably will not. Only about 20 percent of orally administered acyclovir is absorbed, and the importance of blood levels of the drug is debatable because intracellular or intravesicular levels might be of greater importance than blood levels. Since an effective dosage of *oral* acyclovir (if there is one) has not been determined for children, this strategy for treatment of potentially serious VZV in children should not be used. Patients with or at high risk for severe VZV infection should be treated with intravenous acyclovir.

Central Nervous System Infection

It is difficult to make recommendations concerning antiviral therapy for patients with central nervous system (CNS) involvement with VZV, because the underlying pathogenesis of this complication is unknown, and no controlled studies of the efficacy of antiviral therapy have been performed. Some clinicians elect to treat immunocompromised patients with VZV infections and CNS involvement but not to administer antivirals to immunologically normal patients with similar complications. This rationale is based on the likelihood that at least part of the problem in immunocompromised patients is a result of viral multiplication; this would be unlikely in immunologically normal patients. On the other hand, some physicians try a course of acyclovir in all patients with CNS complications of VZV, because the issue is controversial and the drug is unlikely to cause harm. My preference is usually to do the latter.

Adverse Effects of Drugs

Relatively common adverse effects of acyclovir include the following: phlebitis due to the high pH of the intravenous solution (in about 15 percent of patients), reversible elevation of the serum creatinine (in about 5 percent), hivelike rash (in about 5 percent), and nausea and vomiting (in about 1 percent). Elevation of serum creatinine is a result of precipitation of the drug in the renal tubules when it is administered at a high concentration. This can be prevented by allowing at least 1 hour for infusion of each dose, and providing maintenance volumes of fluids during and just preceding each infusion. Rare toxicity of acyclovir includes encephalopathic manifestations such as tremors, confusion, and agitation.

Vidarabine is now the second-line drug for treatment of VZV infections. Zoster patients treated with vidarabine fare less well than those who are given acyclovir, and vidarabine treatment is associated with a higher incidence of central nervous system toxicity. Use of vidarabine has, however, been associated with more rapid healing and lower mortality than placebo treatment, both for varicella and zoster. If for some reason acyclovir cannot be given, vidarabine should be used for high-risk patients. The dosage of vidarabine is 10 mg per kilogram per day intravenously, administered once a day over a period of 12 hours, usually for 5 days. There are no data concerning the simultaneous use of both drugs for VZV infections, and because of potential toxicity, this is not recommended.

Whether or not to administer steroids to zoster patients is a controversial issue. The aim of such treatment is to lessen the chances of developing postherpetic neuralgia without interfering with healing of vesicles. Because this complication is so rare in children, use of steroids is usually not an issue for pediatricians.

PREVENTION OF VARICELLA

Varicella-Zoster Immune Globulin (VZIG)

Zoster immune globulin (ZIG), was shown to be effective in preventing clinical varicella in healthy children exposed to a sibling with chickenpox. In studies of immunocompromised children, a larger dosage of ZIG administered within 3 days of household exposure to varicella also either modified or prevented varicella.

In the late 1970s, the efficacy of a new preparation, varicella-zoster immune globulin (VZIG), was compared with that of ZIG in a double-blind randomized fashion. VZIG was prepared not from blood of convalescent zoster patients as ZIG had been, but rather from outdated plasma that was screened for high titers of VZV antibodies. Although the titers of VZV antibody measured by various methods were somewhat lower in VZIG than they were in ZIG, both preparations were found to be equally effective in preventing severe varicella in immunocompromised children.

VZIG was licensed for use in 1981. It is produced and distributed in Massachusetts by the Massachusetts Public Health Biologic Laboratory and distributed elsewhere by the American Red Cross through local blood centers. Although VZIG is effective when administered up to 3 days after exposure, it should be given as soon as possible after the exposure. Even though optimal results cannot be expected, VZIG may also provide a benefit if given as long as 5 days after exposure; after that it should not be given. The dosage is 125 U for each 10 kg of body weight, with a maximum dosage of 625 U, intramuscularly. The cost of one vial containing 125 U of VZIG is $75. VZIG should be readministered to high-risk children who are closely reexposed to VZV 3 weeks following a first exposure for which VZIG was given.

Indications for Use of VZIG

The most important use of VZIG today is for prevention of severe varicella in children who have been closely exposed to varicella or zoster and are at high risk to develop severe or fatal varicella. This includes immunocompromised children (see earlier) and also newborn infants whose mothers have active varicella at the time of delivery. Candidates for whom VZIG is recommended by the Centers for Disease Control (CDC) in Atlanta, Georgia, are listed in Table 1.

Infants and children who are listed in the high-risk group should receive VZIG if they have had a close exposure to varicella or zoster, as indicated in Table 2. They should be considered to be susceptible to varicella if either they have no history of having had chickenpox or they are uncertain about it. It is potentially hazardous to base the decision to withhold VZIG on a positive antibody titer in an immunocompromised child who has no history of the clinical illness because of the possibility of a false-positive antibody test.

Because only about 25 percent of adults with no history of varicella are truly susceptible, and healthy

TABLE 1 Candidates for Whom VZIG is Indicated

No previous history of clinical varicella,
  and

Underlying condition:
  leukemia, lymphoma
  congenital or acquired immunodeficiency
  immunosuppressive therapy (including
    prednisone)
  newborn infant of mother with onset of varicella
    within 5 days before delivery and 2 days after
    delivery
  premature infant more than 28 weeks gestation
    whose mother has no prior history of varicella
  premature infant less than 28 weeks gestation,
    and

Significant exposure (see Table 2)

Source: Modified from MMWR 1984; 33:84–100.

TABLE 2 Indications for Use of VZIG

Continuous household contact *or*
Playmate contact, greater than 1 hour indoors *or*
Hospital contact: in same 2- or 4-bed room or
    adjacent beds in large ward; face-to-face
    contact with an infectious employee or patient
    or
Newborn contact with infected mother *and*
    within 3 days of contact (preferably given
    sooner; in some cases may give up to 5 days
    after exposure) *and*
    high risk to develop severe varicella (see Table 1)

Modified from MMWR 1984; 33:84–100.

adults are at substantially less risk to develop severe varicella than are immunocompromised children, VZIG is not indicated for adults unless they are proved to be susceptible by laboratory testing. It is therefore reasonable for adults with no past history of varicella who are likely to be closely exposed to VZV, such as medical personnel and parents of young children, to have their blood tested for VZV antibodies. Then, should a close exposure occur, VZIG could be given.

Patients with acquired immunodeficiency syndrome (AIDS) and AIDS-related complex (ARC) are another potential high-risk group for varicella. Their management should be similar to that for immunocompromised children and adults. Even those children who have been receiving intravenous globulin for treatment of AIDS should receive VZIG if there is no past history of varicella and a close exposure has occurred.

Infants whose mothers have active varicella at delivery should also receive VZIG. Specifically, infants whose mothers have the onset of chickenpox 5 days or fewer prior to delivery or within 48 hours after delivery should be passively immunized. These infants will have been infected by the transplacental route, possibly to a large inoculum of virus. This type of exposure and the immaturity of the immune system at this age probably account for the severity of varicella in these babies. Attack rates of up to 50 percent have been reported, even following administration of VZIG. Usually varicella is mild in passively immunized infants, but a minority develop severe varicella despite administration of VZIG. Passively immunized infants must therefore be watched carefully, but usually this can be done at home. Should they develop an extensive skin rash (more than 300 to 500 vesicles) or evidence of pneumonia, intravenous acyclovir should be administered.

I rarely administer VZIG to full-term infants exposed when they are more than 48 hours old. Assuming there is no shortage of VZIG for leukemic and other clearly high-risk children, VZIG could be given to infants under 1 week old if their siblings at home have active varicella and if the mother has no history of chickenpox. It might also be given to infants less than 1 week old whose mothers develop varicella. Infants whose mothers have had varicella and who are exposed to siblings or others with chickenpox are probably at little risk to develop severe varicella because they are endowed with specific maternal antibody. Similarly, infants exposed to mothers with zoster are not expected to develop severe varicella and therefore do not require prophylactic VZIG. Although the reported mortality rate from varicella in children younger than 1 year old is four times that seen in older children, both rates are exceedingly low—8 per 100,000 cases and 2 per 100,000 cases, respectively. In contrast, the mortality rate for adults and for leukemic children receiving chemotherapy is 20 to 1,000 times higher. The dose of VZIG for infants is 125 units, intramuscularly.

By 6 months of age, transplacental VZV antibody is no longer detectable in the serum of most full-term infants. Low-birth-weight infants, however, may have undetectable titers at birth. Therefore, it is recommended that newborn infants weighing less than 1,000 g or of less than 28 weeks gestation who are exposed to VZV be passively immunized, even if the mother had varicella (see Table 1). Varicella has been observed in infants with preexisting maternal transplacental antibodies when exposed to VZV. Although this antibody does not necessarily have preventive value, it can usually be expected to modify chickenpox, and this may be one reason that varicella in infants between 1 and 6 months of age is characteristically mild.

Zoster occurs despite serum antibody to VZV, and patients with zoster manifest brisk increases in VZV antibody titer. VZIG therefore should not be used either to treat or to prevent zoster, even in high-risk patients.

Varicella Vaccine

A live attenuated varicella vaccine was developed in Japan about 15 years ago. This vaccine is licensed in some European countries and in Japan, but it is not yet licensed in the United States. The vaccine is highly protective in immunocompromised children and healthy adults, and there is great interest in vaccinating healthy children on a routine basis. Not all vaccinees are completely protected, however. Some manifest a mild breakthrough illness following an exposure. However, varicella vaccine has been 100 percent effective in preventing severe varicella. It has thus far been unnecessary to use antiviral therapy in vaccinated high-risk children with a breakthrough illness. Leukemic children who are immunized have a 50 percent chance of developing a vaccine-associated rash 1 month after vaccination if they are still receiving maintenance chemotherapy; 5 percent require antiviral therapy for this rash. Vaccinees with a rash may also transmit the vaccine-type virus to about 10 percent of other varicella susceptibles with whom they have close contact. Some leukemic vaccinees also have experienced waning immunity to VZV and require booster doses of vaccine. Boosters are well tolerated.

NOSOCOMIAL VARICELLA

A combination of susceptibility testing for hospital employees, furlough of susceptible personnel during potential incubation periods, isolation of exposed susceptible children and those with active varicella, and early discharge of exposed susceptibles is usually employed. Even using this strategy, however, hospital outbreaks lasting many weeks have been reported. Routine serologic testing of all hospital staff with no prior history of varicella is strongly recommended. Because VZIG modifies rather than prevents varicella, use of VZIG in exposed hospital staff members for the purpose of controlling nosocomial varicella is not recommended. It may prolong the incubation period of varicella, and also lead to an atypical modified illness that goes undiagnosed; therefore, it may make an outbreak more difficult to control. Susceptible hospital personnel who are passively immunized should be furloughed between days 8 and 28 after an exposure; those not passively immunized may return to work after 21 days unless they develop varicella.

VARICELLA IN PREGNANCY

Varicella can be severe in pregnant women, and careful follow-up is indicated; treatment with acyclo-vir should be used in severe cases such as those complicated by pneumonia. An unusual fetal syndrome (low birth weight, skin scarring, hypoplastic limb, mental retardation) occurs in about 5 percent of infants born to women with varicella in the first or second trimester of pregnancy. Ultrasonography may be used to assess the condition of the fetus in some instances. Usually termination of pregnancy is not recommended, although each case must be individualized. As described previously, infants born to women with chickenpox at term should be passively immunized.

SUGGESTED READING

Arvin A. Oral therapy with acyclovir in infants and children. Pediatr Infect Dis 1987; 6:56–58.

Balfour H, McMonigal K, Bean B. Acyclovir therapy of varicella-zoster virus infections in immunocompromised patients. J Antimicrob Chemother 1983; 12(Suppl B):169–179.

Centers for Disease Control. Varicella-zoster immune globulin for the prevention of chickenpox. MMWR 1984; 33:84–100.

Feldman S, Robertson P, Lott L, Thornton D. Neurotoxicity due to adenine arabinoside therapy during varicella-zoster virus infections in immunocompromised children. J Infect Dis 1986; 154:889–893.

Gershon A, Steinberg S, Gelb L, et al. Live attenuated varicella vaccine: efficacy in immunocompromised children and adults. Pediatrics 1986; 78(Suppl):757–762.

Shepp DH, Dandliker PS, Meyers JD. Treatment of varicella-zoster virus infection in severely immunocompromised patients: a randomized comparison of acyclovir and vidarabine. N Engl J Med 1986; 314:208–212.

Zaia JA, Levin M, Preblud S, et al. Evaluation of varicella-zoster immune globulin: protection of immunosuppressed children after household exposure to varicella. J Infect Dis 1983; 147:737–743.

MISCELLANEOUS CONDITIONS

ACQUIRED IMMUNODEFICIENCY SYNDROME

ANTHONY B. MINNEFOR, M.D.

Infection with the retrovirus responsible for acquired immunodeficiency syndrome (AIDS) has a wide range of clinical expression—from an asymptomatic carrier state, through the AIDS-related complex (ARC), to the full-blown condition. The causative agent, designated human immunodeficiency virus (HIV), needs to be suppressed or eradicated before a "cure" can be affected. Until such time, treatment has focused on supportive therapy and management of the secondary opportunistic infections (OI) that occur. These infections are discussed in other chapters, so the emphasis in this chapter is on special aspects of such infections in AIDS patients.

GENERAL CONCEPTS

Over what is generally considered the pediatric age group, infancy through late adolescence, certain clinical features vary markedly. Opportunistic infection involving the central nervous system (CNS), for example, is rare in preschool-age children. The same is true of CNS lymphomas and Kaposi's sarcoma at any site. Conversely, invasive bacterial infections dominate and often herald the identification of HIV infection in infants. The immunologic defect is such that multiple pathogens may be present simultaneously at the same or different body sites. Similarly, histopathologic changes, e.g., granuloma formation, may not develop in response to mycobacterial infections. Comprehensive stains and cultures for the full range of potential pathogens are mandatory on all surgical specimens. Fevers may be protracted and high grade without apparent explanation, in part presumably because of reactivation of latent agents such as cytomegalovirus (CMV) and Epstein-Barr virus (EBV) or HIV itself. Dermatologic lesions occasionally reflect systemic illnesses (e.g., candidiasis, cryptococcosis) and may be atypical in appearance and/or progression (e.g., herpes simplex virus [HSV], varicella-zoster).

SUPPORTIVE CARE

The mainstays of care are nutritional support and intravenous gamma globulin (IVGG). The latter may seem paradoxical considering the striking hypergammaglobulinemia that is so characteristic in these patients. But responses to antigenic stimulation in vivo (e.g., immunization) are poor and pyogenic bacterial infections so common that immunoglobulins are obviously functionally inadequate.

Accordingly, all symptomatic cases are treated with IVGG in a dosage of 400 mg per kilogram, given every 3 to 4 weeks. The infusion is given over 3 to 4 hours by an infusion pump. This practice has been associated with an overall reduction of bacterial sepsis in this population from 45 to 1.5 percent. The IVGG has generally been very well tolerated. Type I allergic reactions can occur, and release of vasoactive enzymes may be associated with hypotension, tachycardia, flushing, nausea, vomiting, chills, and fever. Merely slowing the rate of infusion to that tolerated best by an individual patient usually suffices. Patients who fail to respond to this maneuver are premedicated with age-appropriate doses of aspirin and Benadryl the evening before and again 30 to 60 minutes before the treatment is administered. This approach, infrequently necessary, has virtually eliminated adverse reactions. One can also decrease the IVGG dosage to a more physiologic 200 mg per kilogram and administer it every 2 weeks.

The IVGG preparation I employ is Gamimune-N (5 percent solution), which is in ready-to-use liquid form. Another commonly used product is Sandoglobulin, which is lyophilized and can be made into either a 3 or 6 percent solution with reconstitution. For the purpose in question, both are equally effective and safe IVGG products. Switching randomly from one to another is inadvisable because this increases the risk of the aforementioned reactions. Conversely, one brand of IVGG may regularly cause problems in a given patient who has no difficulties with another preparation. Finally, serodiagnostic studies should be drawn before an IVGG treatment program is initiated, as the serum antibody concentrations subsequently attained render most results uninterpretable.

When standard antibiotics are thought necessary pending culture results, either cefuroxime or cefotaxime is usually given in full therapeutic dosage (150 mg per kilogram per day, given intravenously in three divided doses every 8 hours). The bacterial organisms commonly associated with invasive infections in the children (*Haemophilus influenzae, Streptococcus pneumoniae, Staphylococcus aureus,* and *Salmonella* spp.) have generally been susceptible to these drugs.

Nutritional deficiency is common and increasingly being managed by use of indwelling central lines (Broviac catheters) to administer central hyperalimentation. It is encouraging that in 22 such patients only three exit site infections have developed. Despite this acceptably low rate, common catheter-associated pathogens such as *Candida* spp. and *Staphylococcus epidermidis* must always be considered in treating catheter-dependent patients showing signs of infection.

The Centers for Disease Control (CDC) has published recommendations regarding immunization of children residing in the United States with HIV infection. Symptomatic patients should not receive any live virus or bacterial vaccine (measles-mumps-rubella [MMR] vaccine, oral poliovaccine [OPV], BCG). Inactivated poliovaccine (IPV) is advised along with diphtheria-tetanus-pertussis (DTP) vaccine and *H. influenzae* type b vaccine, in accordance with standard schedules. Children older than 6 months of age should receive annual reimmunization with inactivated influenza vaccine, and those older than 2 years of age should receive a one-time administration of pneumococcal vaccine. Following significant exposure to measles or varicella, immune serum globulin (ISG) or varicella immune globulin (VZIG), respectively, is recommended. With the exception of tuberculosis, considerable passive protection is probably provided by the regular regimen of IVGG infusions.

Asymptomatic children with HIV infection are immunized routinely, except for use of IPV, which is recommended for any child whose household members have contracted infection with HIV.

OPPORTUNISTIC INFECTIONS

Pulmonary Diseases

Lung disease, caused largely by *Pneumocystis carinii* and lymphocytic interstitial pneumonia (LIP), is by far the major cause of morbidity and mortality in pediatric cases of HIV infection. Open lung biopsy is usually the only definitive means of distinguishing between these conditions and diagnosing other less common opportunistic agents (e.g., mycobacteria, *Cryptococcus, Candida,* CMV). Certain features, however, may help guide empiric therapy. Children with *P. carinii* pneumonia (PCP) are more often febrile, with abrupt onset of severe respiratory distress associated with rales, ronchi, and wheezes. Patients with LIP have a more gradual onset, less hypoxemia and auscultatory findings, digital clubbing, generalized lymphadenopathy, and parotid enlargement. A lymphonodular infiltrate and hilar adenopathy on chest radiograph are highly predictive of LIP. If time permits, a gallium scan can be a useful adjunct in determining "hot spots" likely to yield pathogens if biopsy is contemplated.

It is prudent, however, to send sputum, tracheal, or endotracheal tube aspirates for *Pneumocystis* stains before resorting to lung biopsy or initiating empiric therapy. These specimens are positive more often than in most other compromised patients, allowing for safe, rapid diagnosis. If PCP is found or strongly suspected, trimethoprim-sulfamethoxazole (TMP/SMZ) therapy is begun (calculated as 20 mg per kilogram per day of the trimethoprim component, given intravenously in four divided doses every 6 hours), often with cefuroxime or cefotaxime when bacterial infection cannot be ruled out. If there is no response to TMP/SMZ in 72 to 96 hours, or if the condition worsens at any time, pentamidine (Pentam), 4 mg per kilogram per day given in a single daily dose intramuscularly or intravenously, is added. Both drugs are continued for a total of 14 days. Even young AIDS patients have an extraordinarily high rate of adverse reaction (rashes, fever, leukopenia, and thrombocytopenia) to TMP/SMZ.

Recurrences of PCP are so common that at the conclusion of parenteral therapy "prophylactic" treatment with oral TMP/SMZ (5 to 10 mg per kilogram of the TMP component in two divided doses) is begun in preschool patients. Treatment is maintained indefinitely or until intolerance/reactions occur. Hemograms and liver function tests should be monitored closely. Some clinicians are now using once-weekly injections of pentamidine (4 mg per kilogram). In adults the antimalarial agent Fansidar (sulfadoxine and pyrimethamine), one 500-mg tablet per week, has been used. Stevens–Johnson syndrome has occurred with this agent, and it should be discontinued if any rash or blood dyscrasias develop. In patients older than 18 years of age, dapsone (100 mg in a single dose daily) combined with trimethoprim (20 mg per kilogram per day in four divided doses), both given orally for 21 days, has been at least as effective and safe as pentamidine or TMP/SMZ for first-episode PCP. I have used dapsone, 100 mg per day, alone for secondary prophylaxis of PCP in older adolescents. Reported side effects include dose-related hemolysis, peripheral neuropathy, visual disturbances, and gastrointestinal upset. TMP/SMZ primary prophylaxis of PCP is being considered for infants who develop symptomatic HIV infection before 6 to 12 months of age. The prognosis is so poor and PCP so common in this subgroup that such an approach may be warranted.

Lung tissue of patients with LIP has revealed the genome of both EBV and HIV. The resulting diffuse lymphocytic infiltrate can cause acute and chronic pulmonary insufficiency. If patients are hypoxic with arterial oxygen tension less than 65 torr, corticosteroid therapy is begun. If the diagnosis is not based on tissue diagnosis, caution should be exercised because

CMV or other pathogens may be present. Prednisone or methylprednisolone (2 mg per kilogram per day) is given for periods of 2 to 4 weeks. Tapering of steroids may require 4 to 6 months or longer, with maintenance doses of 0.5 mg per kilogram being given over this period. Repeated courses of treatment may be necessary.

Mycobacteria are important pathogens of pulmonary and extrapulmonary disease in AIDS patients. All tissue specimens should be stained for acid-fast bacilli and cultured for mycobacteria. *Mycobacterium avium* complex is the most common mycobacterial pathogen isolated, but *M. tuberculosis* is responsible for a substantial number of cases. Since the latter organisms are far more responsive to treatment than the *M. avium* complex, standard antituberculosis drugs are given whenever mycobacteria are found in a specimen. A three-drug regimen of isoniazid (INH), 10 mg per kilogram per day (maximum 300 mg), rifampin, 10 mg per kilogram per day (maximum 600 mg), and ethambutol, 15 mg per kilogram per day is maintained for at least 12 months. In the case of *M. tuberculosis* infection, one can anticipate a response approaching that expected in non-AIDS patients.

On the other hand it is uncertain whether any intervention is effective in *M. avium* complex. For that reason, I do not initiate therapy with agents purported to be effective against this pathogen. Indeed, it is at times difficult to define precisely the clinical significance of *M. avium* complex in a given patient. When that is the case, I generally maintain the preceding regimen. Some clinicians prefer to treat with a combination of drugs they consider optimal therapy for *M. avium* complex. Generally, INH and ethambutol are combined with the investigational drug rifabutin (ansamycin, LM 427) and clofazimine. Rifabutin is distributed by the Centers for Disease Control (CDC) Drug Service (404-329-3670). The drug is provided in 150-mg capsules with a recommended once-a-day dose of 5 mg per kilogram (maximum, 300 mg). Side effects include gastrointestinal intolerance, liver function changes, leukopenia, and thrombocytopenia. Clofazimine has received approval for its leprosy indication and is now available by prescription. It is also distributed under the Orphan Drug Act by Ciba Geigy (201-277-5787). This drug is available in 50- or 100-mg capsules with a recommended once-a-day dose of 2 to 5 mg per kilogram (maximum, 200 mg). A dose-related and reversible discoloration of the skin is the most noteworthy side effect.

Gastrointestinal Diseases

Candida infection of the esophagus is the most frequent OI of the gastrointestinal (GI) tract reported to CDC in pediatric AIDS patients. Oropharyngeal and esophageal candidiasis, if inadequately controlled, exacerbates nutritional deficiency and may predispose to disseminated disease. The more severe the thrush, the greater the likelihood of esophageal involvement, although thrush may be absent. It is not usually necessary to perform esophagograms, and endoscopy is rarely done. Odynophagia is usually present, and in this setting amphotericin B treatment is empirically started. A dosage of 0.6 mg per kilogram per day is reached in several days and maintained for 1 to 2 weeks. At that point nystatin liquid, clotrimazole troches, and ketoconazole are used as detailed in the chapter on *Candidiasis*. If daily prophylaxis with one or more of these agents eventually fails, the sequence is repeated.

For children who do not respond to amphotericin B, I empirically treat for herpetic esophagitis (acyclovir, 15 to 30 mg per kilogram per day, given intravenously in three divided doses every 8 hours for 5 to 10 days).

Cryptosporidiosis is the next most common pathogen reported. This protozoan organism can be detected in stools or biopsy specimens as acid-fast–positive oocysts using a modified cold Kinyoun stain. Diarrhea can be extremely debilitating and persistent with spontaneous remissions occurring without therapy. Treatment is unsatisfactory at best. I have only used spiramycin, but other drugs have been used and are described in the chapters on parasitic diseases.

Neurologic Diseases

There is incontrovertible evidence for HIV infection of the brain. On occasion the encephalopathy is manifested by an acute meningoencephalitis picture with or without seizures. The cerebrospinal fluid examination is usually normal, but it may have slight protein elevation or pleocytosis. AIDS encephalopathy almost always occurs without concomitant opportunistic infection or malignancy. All CSF specimens should be tested for the presence of cryptococcal antigen and cultured for fungi and acid-fast bacilli (AFB) in addition to routine studies. When cryptococcal meningitis is diagnosed, intravenous amphotericin B is administered for a period of 6 weeks (0.6 mg per kilogram per day). As noted in the chapter on *Cryptococcosis,* twice-weekly doses are continued indefinitely. I do not use flucytosine in children because of the unacceptable toxicity and prefer to increase the dosage of amphotericin B. In young children, renal tubular acidosis and electrolyte imbalance are the major adverse reactions.

Even less common than cryptococcal meningitis is CNS toxoplasmosis. As described in the chapter on *Protozoan Infection,* pyrimethamine, sulfadiazine, folinic acid, and corticosteroids represent the standard regimen. The latter may be discontinued when cerebral edema resolves. The other agents need to be continued for a minimum of 6 months in most instances.

SPECIFIC PATHOGENS

The treatments of infection with HSV, VZ, and CMV are detailed elsewhere. HSV and VZ infections generally respond to the larger-dosage regimens of intravenous acyclovir given for 7 to 10 days no differently than other immunocompromised patients. It has not been necessary to institute secondary prophylaxis with oral acylovir.

At present, therapy of CMV infection is investigational. I am unaware of any formal studies in pediatric AIDS patients using DHPG (BW B759U/ganciclovir), a drug that offers promise for the therapy of serious infections.

ANTI-HIV CHEMOTHERAPY

At least two antiviral compounds directed against HIV in pediatric patients are under study. A drug with a relatively narrow therapeutic index, 3'-azido-3'deoxythymidine (AZT, Retrovir), is being used in patients with advanced disease. AZT is a competitive inhibitor of reverse transcriptase. In adults, placebo-controlled studies showed a reduction in mortality, fevers, and OI and improvement in immune responses, weight gain, and liver function tests. Side effects include a macrocytic megaloblastic anemia requiring blood transfusion, neutropenia, nausea, myalgia, headaches, and possibly neurotoxicity with seizures. AZT analogs are also being developed.

Oral ribavirin (Virazole) is being evaluated in a phase-I study of stable children with ARC. This drug can also be administered intravenously or by inhalation, it has an acceptable tolerance and safety profile even with long-term administration, and it penetrates into the CNS. The most common side effects reported are anemia and liver function changes. Preliminary data indicate that patients report decreased

TABLE 1   Considerations in the Search for Clinically Effective Anti-HIV Compounds

Oral bioavailability
Penetration of the blood–brain barrier
Acceptable toxicity with long-term use
Synergy or antagonism with combination therapy
Effects on immunologic function with or without
  immunomodulators
Equitable and expeditious distribution of drugs to
  eligible patients
Cost

night sweats, and increased appetite and activity. A general trend toward an increase in absolute number and percentage of T-helper cells has also been noted. Unresolved issues and problems to be considered in treatment of HIV infection are summarized in Table 1.

SUGGESTED READING

ACIP. Immunization of children infected with HTLV-III/LAV. MMWR 1986; 35:595–606.
CDC. Diagnosis and management of mycobacterial infection and disease in persons with human immunodeficiency virus infection. Ann Intern Med 1987; 106:254–256.
Connor EM, Minnefor AB, Oleske JM. Human immunodeficiency virus infection in infants and children. In: Jeffries et al, eds. Current topics in AIDS, Vol I. London: John Wiley & Sons, 1987; 185–209.
Rubinstein A. Pediatric AIDS. In: Lockhart JD, ed. Current problems in pediatrics, Vol XVI. Chicago: Year Book Medical Publishers, 1986; 185–209.
Rubinstein A, Morecki R, Silverman B, et al. Pulmonary disease in children with acquired immune deficiency syndrome. J Pediatr 1986; 108:498–503.

CHILDHOOD EXANTHEMS

MAXWELL STILLERMAN, M.D.

RUBELLA

Rubella is an acute mild viral infectious disease characterized by minimal or absent prodromal symptoms, a 3-day basically maculopapular rash, and lymphadenopathy, especially of the postauricular, suboccipital, and posterior cervical lymph nodes. The disease can be confused with mild measles, scarlet fever, roseola, erythema infectiosum, infectious mononucleosis (especially in patients given ampicillin), acquired toxoplasmosis, certain adenoviral and enteroviral infections, and drug eruptions. About 25 percent of the infections are subclinical. Transient joint involvement occurs occasionally in children and more frequently in adolescents. Mild thrombocytopenia is not uncommon, but hemorrhagic manifestations and encephalitis are very rare complications.

The most important consequences of rubella are intrauterine infection, especially during the first trimester of pregnancy, and its ability to produce fetal death and anomalies in the developing fetus. The most commonly described anomalies associated with congenital rubella syndrome (CRS) include growth retardation, deafness, and eye, cardiac, and central nervous system defects. Moderate and severe cases of CRS are recognizable at birth; mild cardiac involvement, partial deafness, and mental retardation may not be detected for months or years; and insulin-dependent diabetes, hypo- or hyperthyroidism, and progressive panencephalitis are late manifestations with onset occurring not until the first two decades of life or beyond.

The laboratory diagnosis of rubella, especially in the pregnant woman or in a baby in whom CRS is suspected, is most often made serologically. A fourfold rise in specific antibody titers between acute- and convalescent-phase sera or the presence of rubella-specific immunoglobulin M (IgM) antibody in a single serum specimen drawn between 1 and 2 weeks after the onset of rash or from cord blood, indicate a recent infection. Isolation of virus from nasopharyngeal and urine specimens is usually reserved for diagnosis of CRS.

Treatment

Postnatal rubella in most instances requires no treatment. No specific therapy is available. Bed rest is advisable with fever or involvement of weightbearing joints. Arthritis is usually well controlled with aspirin. For severe cases of thrombocytopenic purpura, intravenous immune globulin, corticosteroid therapy, or platelet transfusion may be indicated. A patient with rubella encephalitis should be treated the same way as a patient with measles encephalitis (see following section).

Treatment of infants born with CRS depends on which anomalies are manifest at birth and which are manifest later in life. Generally, the management of the various anomalies is the same as that used when such defects result from other diverse etiologies. Most CRS infants survive with chronic neurologic, sensory, developmental, or cardiovascular problems. Early consultation with appropriate specialists can help detect and manage these problems. Frequent periodic evaluations identify the transient, progressive, and permanent nature of recognized defects and the development of new ones. Most states and communities provide special educational and other services to help chronically handicapped children. The average lifetime expenditure associated with a CRS infant has recently been estimated to be in excess of $220,000.

Preventive Measures

Preventing intrauterine infection that may cause CRS is the goal of immunization programs (see chapter on *Immunizations*). In 1986 a record low of 500 cases of rubella and 11 cases of CRS were reported in the United States. The former represents a greater than 99 percent decline from the record number of prevaccine reported cases; the latter shows an increase of 9 CRS cases above the previous low of 2 cases annually reported for 1984 and 1985. Eight of the 11 CRS cases occurred in New York City. In spite of the low incidence of rubella, there is cause for concern for several reasons: 10 to 20 percent of post-pubertal women still lack serologic evidence of rubella immunity; only about one-tenth of all CRS cases are probably reported to the Centers for Disease Control; and thousands of the 30,000 CRS patients from the 1964 epidemic are at risk of developing late manifestations in the third decade of life.

Control Measures

All postnatal and congenital rubella cases should be promptly reported to the local health authority to permit early establishment of control measures.

Isolation

The primary aim of isolation procedures is to prevent rubella infection in susceptible women. Hospitalized patients with postnatal rubella should be managed under contact isolation precautions and placed in a private room for 7 days after onset of the rash. Contact isolation is also required for hospitalized infants suspected of having CRS. Infants with CRS should be considered contagious until they are 1 year old, unless nasopharyngeal and urine cultures after 3 months of age are negative for the virus. Isolation should be continued until the infants are ready to go home. At home, no special precautions are necessary for parents and young sibling contacts. Children with postnatal rubella should be excluded from school and day care facilities for 7 days after the rash appears.

Pregnant Contacts

When a pregnant female is exposed to rubella, especially in the first trimester, a blood specimen should be obtained immediately and tested for rubella antibody. The presence of antibody indicates that the individual is immune. Those previously determined to be immune can be reassured. If antibody is not detected, a second blood specimen should be obtained 2 weeks later. Infection can be assumed to have occurred if antibody is present in the second specimen. If the test is negative, it should be repeated 6 weeks after exposure to rubella. At that time a negative test indicates that infection has not occurred; a positive test indicates that infection did occur. To determine whether or not the index case has rubella, detection of rubella-specific serum IgM antibody indicates a recent infection. In case of natural infection early in pregnancy, abortion should be considered because of the risk of damage to the fetus.

The routine use of immunoglobulin (Ig) for postexposure rubella prophylaxis in early pregnancy is not recommended. Administration of Ig should be considered only if termination of pregnancy is not an option. Limited data indicate that Ig in a dosage of 0.55 ml per kilogram may prevent or modify infection in an exposed susceptible person, but its value has not been established. Infants with congenital rubella have been born to mothers given Ig shortly after exposure.

MEASLES

Measles is an acute highly contagious viral disease characterized by fever, conjunctivitis, coryza, cough, and a specific enanthem (Koplik spots), followed by a generalized maculopapular rash that usually appears on the fourth day of illness. It is a potentially serious disease that has not disappeared in spite of the 99 percent reduction in incidence resulting from the widespread use of measles vaccine since 1963 and the school exclusion Measles Elimination Program, which started in 1978. In 1986 measles activity was at a 6-year high, with 6,236 cases reported. The reasons for this increase are not clear, but unvaccinated preschool-age children and vaccine failure have contributed to a large number of outbreaks. Because of the low incidence of indigenous measles, serologic confirmation is important, especially in the absence of exposure to a confirmed case. The most common complications are otitis media, pneumonia, and encephalitis.

Treatment

Treatment is chiefly supportive. Bed rest is advisable during the febrile period. The diet should be liquid or soft as tolerated. When the child becomes afebrile and anorexia subsides, regular indoor activity and diet can be resumed. For patients with temperatures of 39.4°C (103°F) or greater, I prescribe small doses of acetaminophen in order not to mask the temperature, which is useful in monitoring the course of the illness. Bright lights should be avoided if photophobia is present. Coryza is unaffected by treatment and nose drops are unnecessary. The measles cough is difficult to control, and most cough medicines are not very effective.

Specific antiviral therapy is not available. Immune serum globulin (ISG) does not influence the course of the disease after symptoms appear. Prophylactic antibiotics, except in children with a history of recurrent otitis media, are of no established value and may enhance the chance of superinfection with resistant bacteria.

Complications

Optimal treatment requires an understanding and recognition of the causative agents, disease severity, host factors, and complications. Complications may result from viral replication, bacterial or viral superinfection, or both. When a bacterial complication is suspected, I select an antibiotic that is effective against the most common respiratory pathogens found in various age groups and current in the community. Group A streptococci, *Streptococcus pneumoniae, Haemophilus influenzae, Branhamella catarrhalis,* and *Staphylococcus aureus* are the bacterial pathogens found most frequently during the late winter and spring, when measles occurs. *Mycoplasma pneumoniae* in children 6 years of age and older and adenoviruses can also be secondary invaders.

For acute otitis media and/or acute purulent nasopharyngitis or sinusitis in children 6 months to 5 years of age, I prescribe amoxicillin, 40 mg per kilogram per day in three divided doses for 10 to 14 days. If no response occurs in 3 to 5 days, I reexamine the patient and culture the lesion, which may be caused by beta-lactamase–producing *H. influenzae, B. catarrhalis, S. aureus,* or in the case of otitis media, an abscess requiring drainage. If a beta-lactamase–producing microorganism is found, I change to erythromycin–sulfisoxazole (50 mg per kilogram per day of the erythromycin component in four divided doses) or amoxicillin with potassium clavulanate or cefaclor, 40 mg per kilogram per day in three divided doses.

Pulmonary complications include bronchiolitis and pneumonia. Acute viral bronchiolitis occurs mainly during the first 18 months of age and is difficult to manage (see the chapter on *Bronchiolitis and Bronchitis*). Pneumonia occurs in about 5 percent of patients, is most common and severe in children under 2 years of age, and is the leading cause of death. Secondary bacterial pneumonias are most commonly caused by *S. pneumoniae,* group A streptococcus, *S. aureus,* or *H. influenzae.* Treatment of pneumonias caused by unknown and known etiology are discussed in chapters on *Acute Pneumonia of Unknown Etiology* and *Pneumonia of Known Etiology,* respectively.

Severe croup with obstructive laryngotracheitis develops occasionally. It is an emergency that requires hospitalization and treatment by an experienced team of pediatrician, anaesthesiologist, otolaryngologist, and nurse. Constant supervision is mandatory. If restlessness, dyspnea, and tachycardia increase, intubation or tracheostomy should be performed without delay. It is hazardous to wait for extreme cyanosis and other signs of asphyxia to develop.

Symptomatic encephalitis occurs in about 0.1 percent of measles cases, usually about 4 to 6 days after the onset of the rash. Although encephalitis is a potentially crippling and fatal complication, its severity varies and the course is unpredictable. Neurologic consultation is advisable. Treatment is symptomatic. Fluid and serum electrolytes should be monitored and their disturbances corrected. Coma requires supportive medical and nursing care. The value of large doses of Ig has not been demonstrated. Evidence for the efficacy of corticosteroids is not convincing.

Modified measles following Ig administration to exposed susceptible contacts, is a mild uncomplicated illness that requires no treatment.

Atypical measles syndrome occurring in those who received the inactivated measles virus vaccine from 1963 to 1967, and are subsequently infected with wild measles virus, has no specific treatment.

Control Measures

Prompt reporting of known and suspected measles cases to the local health authority results in better outbreak control. The children should be considered contagious until 4 days after onset of the rash. In hospitals, respiratory isolation from the catarrhal stage through the fourth day of the rash is indicated. For immunocompromised patients isolation should be maintained for the duration of the illness. For household and hospital contacts the availability of Ig and live attenuated measles virus vaccine (LMVV) has obviated the need for quarantine.

Procedures for measles prevention by (1) active immunization with LMVV, (2) management of exposed susceptible contacts by passive immunization with IG followed by LMVV, and (3) management of patients for whom LMVV is contraindicated are discussed in chapters on *Immunizations* and *Infections Associated with International Travel.*

ROSEOLA

Roseola infantum is a common acute benign illness characterized by fever of several days' duration and rapid defervescence, followed by a maculopapular rash. It is most common in infants 6 to 24 months of age. Occasionally when temperatures are 40°C (104°F) or greater, convulsions may usher in the disease or a mild exudative tonsillitis may be present.

Treatment is supportive. Antimicrobial agents do not alter the course of the illness. Acetaminophen and/or phenobarbital may be given to patients with very high fever or a history of previous febrile convulsions. The management of infants whose disease is ushered in with high fever and convulsions is the same as that for any initial febrile seizure.

Isolation and control measures are not necessary.

ERYTHEMA INFECTIOSUM

Erythema infectiosum, also known as Fifth Disease, is a mild acute contagious disease occurring as epidemics among children and characterized by a typical rash that appears in three stages, usually without fever or other constitutional symptoms. The human parvovirus (HPV) B19 was implicated as the causative agent in 1983. Viremia precedes the onset of the rash. The virus has caused subclinical infections and induced aplastic crisis in patients with chronic hemolytic anemias. Maternal HPV B19 infection in pregnancy, like rubella, is one of the causes of fetal hydrops. Confirmatory diagnosis can be established by tests currently available only in research laboratories, such as serologic tests, electron microscopy, and demonstration of HPV B19 DNA by hybridization. Arthritis is an occasional and encephalitis is a rare complication in children.

Treatment is supportive.

Respiratory isolation for hospitalized patients is advised for 7 days after onset of illness.

In my opinion it is prudent to avoid contact between pregnant women and children with early erythema infectiosum. If a pregnant woman is exposed to erythema infectiosum or to a suspicious rash shown not to be caused by rubella, she should be serotested for recent infection with HPV B19. Whether the infection is confirmed or merely suspected, the fetus should be examined ultrasonically to exclude the possibility of fetal hydrops.

ENTEROVIRUS INFECTIONS

Coxsackieviruses, group A and group B, echoviruses, and enteroviruses are infectious agents commonly associated with a variety of skin manifestations, chiefly maculopapular, vesicular, or petechial. In the summer and fall they are the leading causes of exanthems, mainly in young children. The exanthems can occur alone or in combination with fever, enanthem, aseptic meningitis, respiratory, or gastrointestinal symptoms. Some virus/disease syndromes with a rash are coxsackievirus A16 and enterovirus 71 in hand-foot-and-mouth disease, echovirus type 9 in aseptic meningitis with petechiae, and echovirus type 16 in outbreaks of maculopapular rash that characterizes the Boston exanthem disease. In the differential diagnosis, bacterial and other viral diseases associated with exanthems, drug eruptions, insect bites, and miliaria should be considered. Primary diagnosis is based on virus isolation on tissue culture, suckling mice inoculation, and serologic methods.

Treatment

There is no specific therapy for enteroviral infections. Immune serum globulin may be of benefit in immunocompromised patients and has been used in severe, life-threatening neonatal infections.

Isolation of the Hospitalized Patient

Enteric precautions are indicated for 7 days after the onset of illness.

Control Measures

Particular attention should be paid to handwashing and personal hygiene.

SUGGESTED READING

American Public Health Association. Control of communicable diseases in man. 14th ed. Washington, DC: American Public Health Association, 1985.

Anand A, Gray ES, Brown T, et al. Human parvovirus infection in pregnancy and hydrops fetalis. N Engl J Med 1987; 316:183–186.

Committee on Infectious Diseases of the American Academy of Pediatrics. Report of the Committee on Infectious Diseases. 20th ed. Elk Grove Village IL: American Academy of Pediatrics, 1986.

Krugman S, Katz SL, Gershon AA, Wilfert C. Infectious diseases of children. 8th ed. St. Louis: CV Mosby, 1985.

Melnick JL. Enteroviruses: polioviruses, coxsackievirus, echoviruses and newer enteroviruses. In: Fields BN, et al. Virology. New York: Raven Press, 1985; 739–791.

NEONATAL SEPSIS

KENNETH M. BOYER, M.D.

Neonates, particularly those born prematurely, are compromised hosts. During the first months of life, they are subject to infections by a unique list of pathogens, including group B streptococci, coagulase-positive and -negative staphylococci, coliform organisms, *Listeria,* and *Candida.* Impaired localization of infections by these neonatal pathogens commonly leads to septicemia. Untreated, these infections are usually fatal. Even with current therapy, fatal outcome occurs in 20 to 30 percent of infected infants. Presenting symptoms may be vague or nonspecific, a feature that leads to "septic workups" and empiric antimicrobial therapy of the majority of infants admitted to neonatal high-risk nurseries. A discussion of therapy of "neonatal sepsis," then, must address not only the management of babies with proven bacteremic disease, but also a rational empiric approach to sick babies with a provisional or unsubstantiated diagnosis of sepsis.

The blood culture is the key microbiologic test in diagnosing neonatal sepsis. When positive for a recognized neonatal pathogen, and particularly when the culture is positive after relatively short incubation (24 hours or less) in both bottles of a set, there is little etiologic doubt. Problems arise in interpretation of "late positives" (cultures that turn positive after 48 hours), isolates of uncertain pathogenicity (e.g., alpha-streptococci or coagulase-negative staphylococci), or discordant results (only one of several culture bottles positive). Such results often imply technical errors in collection or inoculation of blood specimens, but may occasionally be the only tip to an occult infection such as an infected central venous catheter, osteomyelitis, or abscess. Thus, a broader focus than just the blood culture is generally desirable in diagnosing and managing neonatal sepsis.

I find the results of complete blood counts, particularly studies done serially, a helpful guide to the presence of bacterial infection and therapeutic response. Elevated neutrophil counts or, more impressively, an initial low count followed by a dramatic response after initiation of therapy favor bacterial etiology. An immature:total neutrophil ratio of 0.2 or more and thrombocytopenia are also helpful hematologic indicators.

Detection of group B streptococcal or *Escherichia coli* K1 polysaccharide antigens in urine by latex agglutination is a useful confirmatory adjunct to blood culture. A positive blood culture with a negative concomitant urine antigen test suggests transient bacteremia. On the other hand, positive urine antigen tests with negative blood cultures may imply occult infection (e.g., group B streptococcal osteomyelitis) or partial treatment by intrapartum therapy.

Evaluation of the baby's mother is another useful diagnostic adjunct, particularly when early-onset neonatal infection is suspected. We pediatricians need to encourage our obstetric colleagues to obtain blood cultures from febrile parturients, in addition to other cultures (e.g., urine, lochia, amniotic fluid at C-section, placental surfaces), to define maternal infections that imply intrapartum exposure of the neonate. In turn, obstetricians must communicate situations in which suspicion of intrapartum infection exists.

Most important, evaluation of the neonate for infection should include an effort to identify the extent of spread and the portal of entry. Because meningitis is a common concomitant of neonatal bacteremic infection, the lumbar puncture is a standard component of the septic workup. However, because cerebrospinal fluid (CSF) cultures are rarely positive in the absence of bacteremia, in my opinion there are a few circumstances in which a lumbar puncture can be deferred. I would defer the lumbar puncture, for example, in an intubated, asphyxiated, premature newborn whose cardiorespiratory condition is unstable or in an asymptomatic full-term baby in whom blood culture is being done solely because of maternal prolonged membrane rupture. If blood cultures are positive in such situations, subsequent reevaluation should include lumbar puncture. Even if therapy has rendered cultures negative, results of cell counts, chemistries, and antigen detection are likely to identify the baby who has meningitis. In contrast, the neonate with meningomyelocele and (shunted or unshunted) hydrocephalus may well have meningitis without a positive blood culture and warrants examination of CSF whenever infection is suspected.

The urinary tract is rarely the portal of entry for bacteremia in a neonate less than 72 hours of age. In the older baby, identification of a urinary source for gram-negative sepsis may permit early correction of a structural anomaly. Clean-catch, catheterized, or suprapubic tap urine specimens are vastly superior to bagged urine specimens for culture. In contrast to CSF specimens obtained after treatment, however, urine cultures need to be obtained before therapy to be meaningful.

Other potentially helpful bacteriologic information regarding portal of entry is often overlooked. A predominant organism in a Gram-stained gastric aspirate implies significant growth of organisms in amniotic fluid and an infectious challenge to the neonate during labor and delivery. Gram stains and cultures of tracheal aspirates obtained shortly after intubation have a high correlation with etiology in neonatal pneumonia. Intravascular catheter tips should always be cultured at the time of removal using the semiquantitative "roll-plate" technique. More than 15 colonies on the plate imply a catheter source for bacteremia. Stool cultures, if processed to identify predominant aerobic species, may be useful in guiding broad-spectrum therapy in babies with necrotizing enterocolitis. Cultures of skin lesions, including pustules, intravenous catheter exit sites, surgical wounds, or "weepy" umbilical stumps, may identify the source of bloodstream invasion or focus attention on sites that require removal of hardware, local treatment, or surgical intervention.

EMPIRIC THERAPY

Empiric therapy with combinations of antibiotics is the usual starting point in managing neonatal sepsis. As a general rule, a decision for workup is a decision for intensive parenteral treatment, despite the fact that only 5 to 10 percent of blood cultures will prove to be positive. Broad coverage of likely infecting organisms, CSF penetration, safety, and selective pressures for development of drug resistance are the key considerations in choosing regimens. Because actual dosages are tiny, drug costs are not a consideration. Factors that determine likely infecting organisms include the patient's age, birthweight, environment (home or hospital), prior courses of treatment, perinatal or nosocomial exposures to specific pathogens, the presence of hardware (e.g., catheters, drains, or endotracheal tubes), and the identification of specific sites of infection (e.g., pneumonia, meningitis, thrombophlebitis, or necrotizing enterocolitis).

Empiric therapy for early-onset sepsis (onset before age 7 days) is predicated on the origin of virtually all infecting organisms in the maternal enteric or genital flora. The usual pathogens include group B streptococci, *Escherichia coli,* enterococci, alpha-hemolytic streptococci, *Haemophilus influenzae,* and *Listeria monocytogenes.* Anaerobes are not uncommon, but positive blood cultures generally clear with or without treatment. Staphylococci, hospital "water bugs," and fungi are rare. The standard regimen for early-onset disease is ampicillin and an aminoglycoside, generally gentamicin or tobramycin. This combination not only provides broad coverage, but is synergistic against streptococci and *Listeria.* Cephalosporins, regardless of their generation, are not active against *Listeria* or enterococci and should not be used without concomitant ampicillin. Used with ampicillin, moreover, they do not offer the advantage of synergism.

Late-onset disease (onset after age 7 days) is more heterogeneous in its epidemiology and clinical presentation than early-onset, and may reflect maternal, family, community, or, most commonly, nosocomial sources for infecting organisms. Consequently, the pathogens involved cover a broad taxonomic spectrum. Bacterial infections in normal infants who have been discharged home may include late-onset group B streptococcal, *E. coli,* or listerial septicemia, local or disseminated *Staphylococcus aureus* infections, urosepsis caused by coliforms, or community-acquired *Haemophilus influenzae* type b disease. I currently recommend ampicillin and a third-generation cephalosporin (cefotaxime or ceftriaxone) for empiric therapy of occult infection in these older neonates.

The sick premature infant with a prolonged hospitalization often has had his maternally derived flora eradicated by at least one course of therapy with ampicillin and an aminoglycoside and is particularly prone to nosocomial pneumonias related to prolonged intubation, necrotizing enterocolitis when feedings are introduced, and intravenous sepsis related to central or peripheral intravascular catheters. Major pathogens include coagulase-negative and -positive staphylococci, relatively resistant coliforms including *Klebsiella* and *Enterobacter,* highly resistant opportunists such as *Pseudomonas* and *Serratia,* and *Candida.* Selection of empiric regimens for such babies is difficult, and should be individualized according to the drugs previously used to treat the infant, clinical presentation (e.g., occult infection, suspect necrotizing enterocolitis, pneumonia, or inflamed Broviac tunnel), Gram stains, surveillance cultures (e.g., throat, skin, ostomy stomas, catheter exits, or endotracheal aspirates), and annual reviews of bacterial isolates from the nursery and their sensitivities. I most frequently recommend the combinations of ampicillin, gentamicin, and clindamycin for suspected necrotizing enterocolitis, vancomycin and cefotaxime for patients with central vascular catheters or occult infection, cefotaxime and gentamicin for babies with pneumonia, and nafcillin and tobramycin for babies with skin breakdown. Empiric use of ceftazidime and amikacin is tempting, but I tend to hold these in reserve for specific bacteriologic indications or treatment failures with first-line drugs. I never treat fungal infection empirically, reserving amphotericin B and flucytosine for well-documented invasive fungal infection.

Empiric antibiotics are a therapeutic first approximation and should be stopped or modified depending on the baby's clinical course and diagnostic workup. As a general rule, empiric antibiotics should be stopped after 72 hours if cultures, clinical course, and ancillary tests do not support the diagnosis of infection. Even if blood cultures are sterile, however, treatment should be continued in focal infections and in situations in which bacterial infection continues to offer a plausible explanation for a baby's clinical status. Clinical judgment determines the fine line between the use and abuse of antibiotics in the nursery.

SPECIFIC THERAPY

Specific therapy in the septic neonate is determined by whether or not the infection can be identified as to site and the specific infecting organism(s). Therapeutic recommendations according to site are provided elsewhere in this book (e.g., chapters on *Necrotizing Enterocolitis, Suppurative Arthritis and Osteomyelitis, Bacterial Meningitis, Nosocomial Pneumonia,* and *Catheter-Associated Infections*). From the welter of currently available antibiotic alternatives, the list of drugs that can be comfortably recommended for use in the neonatal period is relatively

TABLE 1 Dosage Schedule for Antimicrobial Agents Commonly Used for Treatment of Neonatal Sepsis

| | | Dosages (mg/kg/day) and Intervals of Administration | | | |
| | | Body Weight < 2000 g | | Body Weight > 2000 g | |
Drug	Routes of Administration	Age 0–7 days	>7 days	Age 0–7 days	>7 days
Amikacin*	IV, IM	15 div q12h	22.5 div q8h	20 div q12h	30 div q8h
Amphotericin B*	IV	1 once daily†	1 once daily†	1 once daily†	1 once daily†
Ampicillin	IV, IM				
Meningitis		200 div q12h	300 div q8h	200 div q8h	300 div q6h
Other diseases		75 div q12h	100 div q8h	75 div q8h	100 div q6h
Cefotaxime	IV, IM	100 div q12h	150 div q8h	100 div q12h	150 div q8h
Ceftazidime	IV, IM	100 div q12h	150 div q8h	100 div q12h	150 div q8h
Ceftriaxone	IV, IM	50 once daily	50 once daily	50 once daily	80 once daily
Clindamycin	IV, IM	10 div q12h	15 div q8h	15 div q8h	20 div q6h
Flucytosine*	PO	100 div q6h	100 div q6h	100 div q6h	100 div q6h
Gentamicin*	IV, IM	5 div q12h	7.5 div q8h	5 div q12h	7.5 div q8h
Methicillin	IV, IM				
Meningitis		100 div q12h	150 div q8h	150 div q8h	200 div q6h
Other diseases		50 div q12h	75 div q8h	75 div q8h	100 div q6h
Metronidazole	IV	15 div q12h	15 div q12h	15 div q12h	30 div q12h
Mezlocillin	IV, IM	150 div q12h	225 div q8h	150 div q12h	225 div q8h
Oxacillin	IV, IM	50 div q12h	100 div q8h	75 div q8h	150 div q6h
Nafcillin	IV	50 div q12h	100 div q8h	50 div q8h	100 div q6h
Netilmicin*	IV, IM	5 div q12h	7.5 div q8h	5 div q12h	7.5 div q12h
Penicillin G	IV				
Meningitis		100,000 U div q12h	150,000 U div q8h	150,000 U div q8h	250,000 U div q6h
Other diseases		50,000 U div q12 h	75,000 U div q8h	50,000 U div q8h	100,000 U div q6h
Ticarcillin	IV, IM	150 div q12h	225 div q8h	225 div q8h	300 div q6h
Tobramycin*	IV, IM	4 div q12h	6 div q8h	4 div q12h	6 div q8h
Vancomycin*	IV	30 div q12h	45 div q8h	30 div q12h	45 div q8h

* Serum concentration and/or toxicity monitoring desirable.
† Gradual dosage buildup recommended. Give 0.25 mg per kilogram for 2 days, then 0.50 mg per kilogram for 2 days, then 0.75 mg per kilogram for 2 days, then 1 mg per kilogram per day maintenance. Dosage may be maintained at 0.5 to 0.75 mg per kilogram per day if flucytosine used concomitantly.

short (Table 1). A number of once-popular agents have been superseded because of limitations in spectrum, distribution, or toxicity. I would include among these carbenicillin, kanamycin, chloramphenicol, moxalactam, and virtually all first- and second-generation cephalosporins. Other recently licensed drugs have not been well studied in newborn infants and should be avoided until more information is available. Such drugs include azlocillin, piperacillin, imipenem, aztreonam, and ticarcillin-clavulanate. The third-generation cephalosporins cefotaxime, ceftriaxone, and ceftazidime, however, have been well studied in neonates and are rapidly gaining a major role in therapy. (Note that ceftazidime is the only third-generation cephalosporin with reliable activity against *P. aeruginosa.*)

Recommended drugs for babies with proven infection by the more common pathogens are summarized in Table 2. These recommendations should be considered guidelines. Because most hospital laboratories provide the clinician with susceptibility data on blood culture isolates simultaneously with (or even before) speciation, susceptibilities must be taken into account in modifying an initial empiric regimen.

A number of infecting organisms are best treated with combination therapy. Addition of gentamicin to ampicillin for treatment of listeriosis or enterococcal infection provides synergistic activity and more rapid killing of a large initial inoculum. The same synergism has been documented for group B streptococci, but I generally stop the aminoglycoside and change to "meningitic" doses of penicillin G after initial improvement. Addition of gentamicin to a semisynthetic penicillin dramatically improves bactericidal activity against "tolerant" strains of *S. aureus.* Combination therapy of infections by *Pseudomonas aeruginosa* is important, because of the emergence of resistance with single-drug treatment. The addition of flucytosine to amphotericin B for treatment of disseminated candidiasis permits smaller dosages of amphotericin (0.5 to 0.75 mg per kilogram per day) to be employed.

TABLE 2 Recommended Specific Therapy for Selected Organisms Causing Neonatal Sepsis

Organisms	Drugs of Choice	Alternatives (based on susceptibility)
Bacteroides fragilis	Clindamycin	Metronidazole; ticarcillin
Bacteroides spp	Penicillin G	Clindamycin, metronidazole
Candida albicans	Amphotericin B + flucytosine	
Citrobacter spp	Cephalosporin*	Aminoglycoside†
Enterobacter spp	Aminoglycoside	Cephalosporin; mezlocillin
Escherichia coli	Aminoglycoside	Cephalosporin; ampicillin
Haemophilus influenzae	Cephalosporin	Ampicillin
Klebsiella spp	Cephalosporin	Aminoglycoside; mezlocillin
Listeria monocytogenes	Ampicillin + gentamicin	TMP/SMZ‡
Pseudomonas aeruginosa	Ticarcillin + tobramycin	Ceftazidime; amikacin
Salmonella spp	Ampicillin	TMP/SMZ; ceftriaxone
Serratia marcescens	Aminoglycoside	Cephalosporin
Staphylococcus aureus	Semisynthetic penicillin§	Vancomycin
Staphylococcus epidermidis	Vancomycin	Semisynthetic penicillin
Streptococcus spp		
Enterococcus	Ampicillin + gentamicin	Vancomycin
Other species	Penicillin G	Ampicillin

* Cefotaxime, ceftriaxone, or ceftazidime.
† Gentamicin, tobramycin, netilmicin, or amikacin.
‡ Trimethoprim–sulfamethoxazole.
§ Nafcillin, oxacillin, or methicillin.

Duration and route of therapy are often issues, particularly in our current climate of cost-efficiency and parent–infant bonding. Isolation of a pathogen from the blood of a sick newborn mandates a minimum 10-day course of parenteral therapy, in my opinion. Longer courses of treatment are necessary for meningitis (14 to 21 days or longer, depending on organism and clinical response), osteomyelitis (4 to 6 weeks or more), and disseminated candidiasis (6 weeks, or a total dosage of 20 to 30 mg per kilogram of amphotericin B). Clinical judgment determines the duration of treatment in patients with asymptomatic bacteremia, culture-negative sepsis, antigenuria, or focal infections without bacteremia. I am always reluctant to sanction oral treatment for a newborn recovering from a serious infection because of the uncertainty of absorption of oral medication. If the infecting organism is saved in the microbiology laboratory, bactericidal activity can be monitored in blood, and the turnaround time for results is efficient, I will condone this approach in some instances. The realities of efficient laboratory testing, however, are that the laboratory must have grown the organism overnight in broth before testing, the blood sample must be obtained at the correct time interval (1 hour) after oral administration and received in the laboratory early in the morning, and the test should not overlap a weekend. Daily intramuscular ceftriaxone or home intravenous therapy with other drugs are possible alternatives to oral treatment I have used in a few cases.

SUPPORTIVE THERAPY

Major therapeutic considerations in neonatal sepsis other than antibiotics include cardiorespiratory, nutritional, and immunologic status. Blood pressure measurements are mandatory in the septic newborn. The presence of shock should prompt aggressive volume expansion with fresh frozen plasma and may require the use of pressors (see the chapter on *Septic Shock*). Disseminated intravascular coagulation is a common concomitant of septic shock and should be treated with platelet infusions in addition to fresh frozen plasma. Persistent fetal circulation, manifested by profound hypoxemia, is a common feature of early-onset group B streptococcal infection and generally requires high concentrations of inspired oxygen, mechanical ventilation, and possibly tolazoline or prostaglandins. Respiratory failure may be a consequence of the combination of birth asphyxia, neonatal pneumonia, hyaline membrane disease, and "shock lung." Babies with this combination of problems, if they survive, often become the long-term residents of neonatal nurseries with bronchopulmonary dysplasia. Aggressive early management is an important preventive measure.

Nutritional status, particularly in the infected premature infant with limited metabolic reserves, is a major consideration during a prolonged course of antimicrobial therapy. Such babies have increased nutritional demands created by thermoregulatory disturbances, cardiopulmonary stress, frequent blood drawing, and surgical procedures. Depending on the site of infection, enteral feedings are generally not introduced or are interrupted during treatment. Delays in starting parenteral nutrition and the often marginal caloric intake provided by "peripheral hyperal" generally lead to weight loss and a negative nitrogen balance at a time when reparative needs are greatest. Despite perceived infection risks, early central hyperalimentation is warranted in many of these babies.

Augmentation of the neonate's marginal supplies of white cells, antibodies, and nonspecific opsonins (e.g., complement, fibronectin) is a logical but as yet unproven adjunct to antimicrobial therapy. Fresh frozen plasma is the volume expander of choice in the nursery because of its content of IgG and IgM immunoglobulins and nonspecific opsonins. White cell transfusions, in my opinion, pose difficult logistic problems for the blood bank with only minimal benefit in terms of therapeutic outcome. The therapeutic use of intravenous gamma globulin may permit correction of deficiencies in transplacental specific immunoglobulins, enhance localization of infection, and prevent depletion of marrow neutrophil reserves. It should be recalled, however, that intravenous gamma globulin is also used to block the reticuloendothelial system in the treatment of idiopathic thrombocytopenic purpura. Therapeutic outcome may therefore strike a balance between the benefit of specific opsonins and the risk of nonspecific blockade of phagocytic capacity. Further studies are needed in this important area.

MONITORING THERAPY

Babies with clinical signs suggestive of bacterial infection deserve hospitalization in an observation unit, intensive care nursery, or pediatric ward, not in a normal nursery or at home. In addition to monitoring therapeutic response, monitoring such infants involves recognition of complications and drug toxicity.

Adequate treatment of a septic neonate generally results in a dramatic response within 24 to 48 hours, as manifested by improved activity, respiratory effort, temperature regulation, and peripheral perfusion. White blood cell counts and proportions of segmented neutrophils often rise with treatment, a short-term response that is generally a favorable sign. Babies who do not respond to treatment may have a resistant organism, an occult focus of infection, or a viral or noninfectious problem. I encourage repeating the blood culture at the first report of a positive result, to document sterilization. Measurement of serum bactericidal activity provides a more reliable indication of treatment efficacy than in vitro susceptibility tests (which are based on bacteriostatic activity). Occult bacterial infections associated with slow response or persistence of bacteremia include meningitis, osteomyelitis, abscesses (intra-abdominal, renal, brain, subperiosteal), and intravascular infections (suppurative thrombophlebitis, endocarditis). Computerized tomography, ultrasonography, and gallium scan may be helpful in identifying such problems. Disseminated neonatal herpes, in the absence of skin lesions or CNS abnormalities, can resemble bacterial sepsis. Striking elevation of serum transaminase values is a useful clue to this diagnosis. Keep in mind that the patient who does not respond to antibiotics or whose condition deteriorates during therapy may in fact have a noninfectious condition (e.g., hypoplastic left heart syndrome, pneumothorax, intraventricular hemorrhage, or intestinal obstruction).

Monitoring serum concentrations of aminoglycosides has become a standard of care in many nurseries, although the occurrence of ototoxicity and nephrotoxicity from these drugs has been difficult to study because of confounding by other conditions such as shock, asphyxia, acidosis, or hyperbilirubinemia. I recommend measurement of peak (at conclusion of intravenous infusion or 30 minutes following intramuscular injection) and trough (immediately before the next dose) concentrations in all infants with uncertain renal function or birthweights less than 1,500 g. Waiting to measure concentrations until after the third dose of drug is reasonable, in order to ensure equilibration. Target peak and trough antibiotic concentrations in serum are summarized in Table 3. Other drugs requiring measurement of serum concentrations during therapy are flucytosine and vancomycin. Vancomycin has been well studied in newborns; experience with flucytosine is anecdotal. Amphotericin B concentrations are difficult to measure and not well correlated with toxicity. Safe use of amphotericin is best monitored by serial measurements of serum potassium, urea nitrogen, creatinine, and hematologic values, and by careful documentation of urine output.

PREVENTION

The key elements in the prevention of early-onset neonatal sepsis are prevention of prematurity and obstetric management of labor and delivery. Prevention of late-onset disease can best be accomplished by giving close attention to handwashing, adhering to guidelines for isolation of communicable conditions in mothers, infants, and personnel, and minimizing antibiotic abuse (see chapter on *Nosocomial Infections in the Nursery*).

A substantial proportion of cases of early-onset group B streptococcal disease can now be anticipated and prevented by the strategy of selective intrapartum chemoprophylaxis. Administration of ampicillin during labor to mothers with prenatal group B streptococcal colonization and the obstetric risk factors of premature labor (less than 37 weeks), prolonged membrane rupture (greater than 12 hours), or intrapartum fever (greater than 37.5°C) dramatically reduced neonatal colonization and virtually eliminated

TABLE 3 Suggested Target Levels of Selected Antibiotics to Optimize Efficacy and Minimize Toxicity

Drug	Peak (µg/ml)	Trough (µg/ml)
Gentamicin	4–8	<2
Tobramycin	4–8	<2
Netilmicin	4–8	<2
Amikacin	15–25	<6
Vancomycin	15–30	?
Flucytosine	50–100	?

early-onset sepsis in a large controlled trial. The strategy involves taking cultures at prenatal visits to identify colonized mothers. The administration of prophylactic ampicillin in only a subpopulation of colonized mothers (overall, about 4 percent of parturients) exerts little selective pressure for emergence of drug resistance. I personally advocate extending this approach to the colonized mothers of infants previously infected by group B streptococci (irrespective of obstetric risk factors). I would also consider a single dose of intramuscular penicillin G at birth for normal infants born to colonized mothers without risk factors.

SUGGESTED READING

Boyer KM, Gotoff SP. Prevention of early-onset neonatal group B streptococcal disease with selective intrapartum chemoprophylaxis. N Engl J Med 1986; 314:1665–1669.

Bradley JS. Neonatal infections. Pediatr Infect Dis 1985; 4:315–320.

Hill HR. Host defenses in the neonate: prospects for enhancement. Semin Perinatol 1985; 9:2–11.

McCracken GH Jr, Nelson JD. Antimicrobial therapy for newborns. 2nd ed. New York: Grune & Stratton, 1983..

Mize CE. Starvation in the PICU. In: Levin DL, Morriss FC, Moore GC, eds. A practical guide to pediatric intensive care. 2nd ed. St Louis: CV Mosby, 1984; 382–388.

SEPTIC SHOCK

RONALD M. PERKIN, M.D.

Septic shock continues to be a major cause of death despite careful monitoring, aggressive surgery, and the use of specific antibiotic therapy. Septic shock comprises a cascade of metabolic, hemodynamic, and clinical changes resulting from invasive infection and the release of microbial toxins in the bloodstream. Historically, a distinction was made between the clinical findings and the type of invading microorganism. However, on closer analysis, it became apparent that the systemic response was independent of the type of invading organism (bacteria, virus, fungus, rickettsia); rather, it was a host-dependent response. Septic shock is a constellation of signs and symptoms that reflect multiple organ system derangements at the subcellular level. It is difficult to differentiate arbitrarily septic shock from sepsis without shock, because each appears to be a different stage in the spectrum of sepsis.

The pathogenesis of septic shock remains controversial and is probably multifactorial in origin. In addition to the organism and its toxin, a network of mediators and activators interact to produce the septic syndrome. The mediators and activators may include autonomic discharge of catecholamines; products of specific cells such as macrophages, granular leukocytes, and platelets; products of activated protein cascade systems (complement, coagulation); endogenous vasodilators and vasoconstrictors; and yet-to-be characterized myocardial and vascular depressant factors. Sepsis in a previously healthy patient should be readily correctable. However, septic shock only occasionally presents as a community-acquired disease. Rather, hospitalized patients are most at risk to develop septic shock. This population includes seriously ill surgical and medical patients who are likely to be debilitated or immunodeficient. They may have a variety of invasive devices and are often receiving antibiotic therapy.

PATHOPHYSIOLOGY AND PRESENTATION

Hemodynamic

The clinical patterns and presentations of septic shock vary considerably, depending on the dynamic interplay of the invading organism, elapsing time, and the host status. Abnormal hemodynamic responses constitute a primary hallmark of septic shock. The early stages consist of a hyperdynamic state characterized by an elevated cardiac output, a decreased systemic vascular resistance, a widened pulse pressure, an often normal systolic blood pressure, with episodic hypotension, and warm extremities on physical examination. In this stage, the syndrome can also be recognized by the presence of high fever, mental confusion, and hyperventilation, with hypocapnia and respiratory alkalosis. Although these patients are typically tachycardic and tachypneic, the vital signs and clinical examination may not reflect the severity of disease. Close neurologic examination, however, usually shows that the patients are confused or hallucinating; this is a valuable, but often neglected, clinical clue.

If sepsis is unchecked and uncorrected, steady deterioration in cardiovascular performance occurs, characterized by a decline in cardiac output, hypotension, and metabolic acidosis. It is of interest that hypotension occurs in the presence of normal or elevated cardiac output. One fundamental abnormality in patients with septic shock is an altered relationship of systemic vascular resistance and cardiac output. The patient's status deteriorates when cardiac compensation for diminishing systemic vascular resistance is lost. The progression from high to low cardiac output may happen quickly, in minutes or hours, or slowly, requiring days. The lower the cardiac output, the more likely it is that progressive lactacidemia will terminate in a fatal outcome.

Survival in septic shock has been related to the host's ability to establish and maintain a hyperdynamic cardiovascular state. In early stages, hypovolemia or myocardial dysfunction resulting from preexisting or intercurrent ventricular disease can blunt or eliminate the hyperdynamic response to sepsis. Several factors may contribute to hypovolemia, which commonly occurs in septic shock. Increased microvascular permeability, arteriolar and venular dilatation with subsequent peripheral pooling of intravascular volume, inappropriate polyuria, and poor oral intake all combine to result in a reduced effective blood volume. Fluid loss secondary to fever, diarrhea, vomiting, or sequestered third space fluid also contribute to the hypovolemia.

In some patients, without complicating preexisting heart disease, a *relative* depression in left ventricular contractility exists even in early stages. The cause of depressed contractility in septic shock is not immediately apparent. Diffuse myocardial edema, the inhibitory effects of a myocardial depressant factor, adrenergic receptor dysfunction, and impaired sarcolemmal calcium flux have all been proposed. In patients who survive, this myocardial depression is transient, lasting for 1 to 4 days, and then myocardial function returns to normal. Although right ventricular failure is uncommon in critically ill septic patients, subtle and potentially important changes in right ventricular function do occur. Impedance to right ventricular ejection may be increased as a consequence of an elevated pulmonary vascular resistance and mean pulmonary artery pressure. Humorally mediated pulmonary vasoconstriction, microembolic occlusion of the pulmonary vasculature, structural changes in pulmonary arteriolar smooth muscle with protracted lung injury, and the use of positive end-expiratory pressure all contribute to an increase in pulmonary artery pressure. Regardless of mechanism, the occurrence of pulmonary hypertension in septic patients has demonstrable effects on right ventricular performance that potentially can limit the hyperdynamic state required to ensure tissue oxygen delivery.

Metabolic

Septic shock is a syndrome characterized by abnormal use of oxygen. Although sepsis is a well-known hypermetabolic stress associated with increased oxygen consumption, deterioration of the septic process characteristically shows a fall in oxygen consumption during a period when cardiovascular function and oxygen delivery remain increased. This reduction in oxygen consumption is the result of decreased oxygen extraction and reflects a severe impairment of oxidative metabolism at a time of major metabolic and physiologic stress. The pathophysiology of inadequate oxygen consumption in septic

shock is still unclear. The most widely accepted theories to account for this oxygen debt are the redistribution of blood flow, with a consequent decrease in nutrient capillary flow, and the development of a cellular metabolic blockade at the mitochondrial level such that delivered oxygen cannot be used. More likely, a spectrum of abnormalities exists. In early stages, flow-dependent oxygen consumption is observed and a high cardiac output allows the required oxygen consumption to be maintained. As the septic shock state progresses, a failure of central venous hemoglobin desaturation occurs. The arteriovenous oxygen content then becomes inappropriately narrow for the existing level of cardiac output. This phenomenon continues, and the total body oxygen consumption falls in spite of large volumes of oxygen delivered to the periphery. Progressive deterioration in oxygen consumption and oxygen extraction portends a poor prognosis for septic shock patients.

In addition to oxygen, impaired use of other metabolic substrates has been demonstrated in septic shock. The septic event appears to hinder sequentially the utilization as energy sources of glucose, then fat, and finally protein. Late states of septic shock are characterized by abnormalities in energy availability and substrate utilization. The exact process responsible for these abnormalities is not known at this time. Metabolically, the overall picture is consistent with a progressive inhibition of substrate entry into the Krebs cycle. Multiple system organ failure is the result of this progressive peripheral energy deficit.

TREATMENT

Primary therapeutic goals for initial treatment of septic shock are rapid reversal of perfusion failure and identification and control of the infection.

The removal or control of microorganisms is the single most important principle of treatment. Antibiotic treatment is appropriate in patients with circulatory shock whenever an infectious etiology is suspected. Before broad-spectrum antibiotic therapy is initiated, blood, urine, and samples from other potentially infected sites should be sent for culture and susceptibility testing.

Improved patient survival is unlikely if the source of infection is not eradicated. Surgical drainage of closed space infections is mandatory, and a vigorous search for the infectious site is indicated in patients unresponsive to appropriate antibiotic therapy.

Cardiovascular Support

The primary goal in the initial management of septic shock is to restore hemodynamic stability. Interruption of the natural pathophysiologic progression of septic shock by controlling cardiopulmonary variables may improve the outcome. Every effort to enhance oxygen delivery to the tissues must be made.

Maximizing cardiac output and arterial oxygen content while minimizing oxygen requirements are fundamentals of management. Many studies indicate that normal ranges of cardiopulmonary variables are not necessarily optimal for children in septic shock. Establishing a hyperdynamic state, because of the high oxygen requirements and the failing oxygen extraction, may improve survival. Although maximizing cardiac output appears to be important, efforts to decrease oxygen requirements may play a role in management. The increased work of breathing commonly found in patients with shock can increase tissues oxygen consumption substantially. This problem can be overcome by using assisted ventilation and administering paralytic and/or sedative medications. Extremes in body temperature also increase oxygen requirements, therefore, efforts to maintain normothermia should be made.

Volume resuscitation is the first therapeutic measure for a decreased cardiac output. Early and effective expansion of the circulating blood volume may enhance oxygen delivery and prevent progression of the septic shock state. Central venous access should be obtained and fluid administration started. Patients with septic shock have an enormous fluid requirement caused primarily by peripheral vasodilatation and capillary leak. In some patients, blood volume restoration on the basis of central venous pressure measurements alone may be deleterious. Disparate ventricular function, abnormalities in ventricular compliance, and elevated pulmonary vascular resistance may make central venous pressure unreliable and preclude appropriate volume replacement. Placement of a thermodilution pulmonary artery catheter may be indicated in children who demonstrate a sluggish response to fluid infusion, have signs of pulmonary edema with normal central venous pressure, or show clinical or echocardiographic evidence of myocardial dysfunction. This catheter allows measurement of central venous pressure, pulmonary artery and pulmonary capillary wedge pressure, and cardiac output. It also allows calculation of oxygen consumption, oxygen delivery, systemic and pulmonary vascular resistances, and other important hemodynamic parameters. These data are invaluable in evaluating results of therapeutic interventions as well as following trends in the patient's condition.

Debate continues regarding the use of crystalloids or colloid solutions in restoring intravascular volume in the presence of septic shock. Isotonic crystalloid solution (normal saline or Ringer's lactate) may be used initially if it increases the blood volume and cardiac output; however, there is evidence that colloid solutions expand blood volume more effectively.

Although fluid administration and antimicrobial therapy remain the cornerstones of the therapeutic approach to sepsis and septic shock, patients often require therapy with inotropic agents and/or vasoactive drugs. Myocardial depression may complicate septic shock and prevent the development of optimal cardiac output, despite adequate intravascular volume. Optimal cardiac output is best judged by obtaining any or all of the following objective criteria: a state in which oxygen consumption is not flow dependent, an appropriate level of existing oxygen consumption, and absence of metabolic acidosis. In most cases, these require that cardiac output be maintained at greater than normal values.

Dopamine is frequently the initial inotropic agent of choice in septic shock because of its beta-adrenergic effects in the myocardium, its alpha-adrenergic effects in the peripheral vasculature, and its selective dopaminergic effects on renal and splanchnic vascular beds. If myocardial function is decreased and systemic vascular resistance is elevated, the combined use of dobutamine and low-dosage dopamine may be helpful. Dobutamine possesses minimal peripheral alpha-adrenergic effects, and therefore should not increase systemic vascular resistance in vasoconstricted patients.

Patients with profound hypotension and myocardial depression may not respond to large amounts of dopamine or dobutamine. In these cases, epinephrine or norepinephrine should be added. Unfortunately, use of these potent vasoconstrictors may not lead to an increase in systemic vascular resistance and arterial blood pressure. Sepsis-induced abnormalities in adrenergic receptor function, such as alpha-adrenergic receptor downregulation, and peripheral vascular adrenergic action depression may account for this poor response. New nonadrenergic inotropic agents (milrinone, amrinone) may find a place in the treatment of septic shock when severe myocardial failure is resistant to adrenergic agents. Although digoxin has been used in septic shock, it is not routinely employed because of its long half-life and narrow therapeutic-toxic range.

Electrolyte abnormalities, metabolic acidosis, hypocalcemia, hypophosphatemia, and hypoglycemia may be present in septic shock and should be treated. Correction of these biochemical aberrations helps optimize myocardial function.

Vasodilator drugs (nitroprusside, nitroglycerin, phentolamine) may be indicated in treatment if systemic vascular resistance is elevated despite inotropic and adequate volume resuscitation. Factors contributing to high systemic vascular resistance such as hypothermia, pain, and agitation should be excluded before vasodilator drugs are used.

Multiorgan Support

Shock, regardless of etiology, is a multiorgan system disease. Several complications of septic shock may arise despite antibiotic therapy and cardiovascular support. Renal failure, liver dysfunction, coagulopathy, central nervous system dysfunction, and respiratory failure have all been described and must be anticipated.

Sepsis is recognized as a leading cause of the adult respiratory distress syndrome (ARDS). The mortality of patients with septic ARDS in many reported series ranges from 80 to 90 percent. The hypoxemia seen in shock and ARDS is associated with bilateral diffuse inspiratory rales and rapidly progressive radiographic signs of interstitial and intra-alveolar infiltrates. Increased alveolar-capillary membrane permeability with exudation of protein-rich fluid into the interstitium and alveoli occurs. The initiation of diffuse lung injury has been ascribed to complement activation and leukocyte aggregation, superoxide-induced injury from release of neutrophil by-products of phagocytosis, protease release with resultant destruction of collagen, and platelet aggregation. Injury induced by prostaglandins and thromboxane also have been demonstrated. Inspired oxygen fractions more than 0.5 further contribute to lung injury and may play a role in the subsequent fibrosis that occurs in ARDS. This rapidly progressive pulmonary fibrosis is the principal impediment to late survival.

The therapy of patients with ARDS complicating shock is disappointing. However, positive end-expiratory pressure (PEEP) in conjunction with mechanical ventilation has been shown to improve respiratory function. PEEP must be carefully used so that adverse effects on cardiac output and tissue oxygen delivery do not occur. Treating hypovolemia in patients who also have ARDS is particularly difficult because the choice of fluid and the level of pulmonary capillary wedge pressure may lead to increased accumulation of extravascular lung water. Glucocorticoids, fibronectin, anticoagulants, and other experimental therapies have undergone trials in the therapy of ARDS. To date, there is no conclusive evidence of improved survival with any of these agents.

Even in the absence of ARDS, shock may be augmented by hypoventilation caused by respiratory muscle fatigue. Hyperventilation in early stages of shock, coupled with respiratory muscle ischemia from hypoperfusion, may result in profound interference with respiratory muscle function. This may result in inadequate minute ventilation, worsening of systemic acidosis, and respiratory arrest. Mechanical ventilation reverses these changes.

Nutrition

It has long been recognized that septic patients develop protein-calorie malnutrition as a principal manifestation of the mediated metabolic response. In patients who were previously malnourished or remain hypermetabolic, this rapidly developing malnutrition is believed to contribute to morbidity and mortality. However, the abnormalities in intermediary metabolism described earlier make the provision of an adequate level of metabolic support challenging. The septic process, in some unknown way, triggers a progressive sequential fuel failure. In early stages, the ability to use glucose as an energy source is limited, and fat is increasingly relied on as an energy source. In this stage, a balanced fuel mixture including relatively low quantities of glucose with at least 30 to 40 percent of the calories as lipid, and a complete amino acid profile should be used. Parenteral nutrition should be begun as soon as cardiovascular stability is achieved. In late stages of sepsis, triglyceride intolerance appears with inability to clear a standard long-chain fat load. At this point, branched-chain amino acids (BCAA) are preferentially used as a fuel source because of the abnormalities in glucose and fat utilization. As a result, the body autocannibalizes its skeletal muscle protein to obtain adequate amounts of BCAA fuel substrate. At this stage, fat administration must be adjusted on the basis of repeated assessment of fat tolerance and the use of BCAA-enriched solution may be better than a balanced amino acid solution. The mechanism for fat intolerance may be due in part to an absolute or relative carnitine deficiency. Carnitine administration in this setting may be useful.

Recent studies suggest an advantage to enteric feeding, when it is possible, because the first passage of substrate from the gut is to the liver and also involves activation of normal pancreatic hormone regulation. However, there are many instances in which sepsis occurs and effective bowel function cannot be maintained. Under these circumstances, parenteral nutrition is a necessity.

Experimental Therapies

The use of corticosteroids in the treatment of septic shock remains a controversial subject. There are many potential mechanisms for the possible beneficial actions of steroids in sepsis and shock, but most remain unproved. The most straightforward benefit of steroids would be the demonstration that sepsis and shock has produced hypoadrenalism and that replacement of adrenal corticosteroids was necessary. Although this explanation is reasonable, it does not justify the large dosages of steroids advocated in recent literature. The rationale for the use of steroids in septic shock has included the ability of these drugs to stabilize lysosomal and cell membranes, to inhibit complement-induced granulocyte and platelet aggregation, to improve myocardial performance, to modulate the release of endogenous opiates, to reverse metabolic defects involving the heart and liver, to decrease products of arachidonic acid metabolism, to prevent oxygen radical-mediated cell damage, and to decrease red blood cell oxygen affinity. Potential adverse effects include superinfection, electrolyte disturbances, hyperglycemia, gastrointestinal bleeding, psychosis, and dysrhythmias. Recent studies have not shown steroids to be efficacious in the management of septic shock. Moreover, the data suggest a larger mortality in steroid treated patients. Until further data are available to support their use, large-dosage corticosteroid therapy should probably be withheld in the septic patient.

Much interest has been generated regarding the role of naloxone in the treatment of septic shock. Naloxone is an antagonist of endogenous opiates, a group of peptides that are reported to be a pathophysiologic mediator of hypotension during sepsis. Animal studies using naloxone have shown improvement in cardiac function and reversal of hypotension. Use of naloxone in human subjects has not consistently confirmed animal studies, and serious adverse reactions have occurred. Use of naloxone in septic shock cannot be advocated at this time.

A number of pharmacologic agents and other therapies have been evaluated as adjunctive treatment in sepsis and septic shock. Such modalities of therapy include a multitude of drugs that inhibit arachidonic acid metabolism and the formation of thromboxanes, prostaglandins, and leukotrienes; exchange transfusion; white blood cell infusions; passive immunotherapy; toxic oxygen scavengers, inhibitors of myocardial depressant factor; and fibronectin administration. Although these therapies may have significant potential therapeutic usefulness, further study is required.

SUGGESTED READING

Ayres SM. New horizons conference on sepsis and septic shock. Crit Care Med 1985; 13:864–866.

Cerra FB. The systemic septic response: multiple systems organ failure. Crit Care Clinics 1985; 1:591.

Perkin RM, Lerin DL. Shock in the pediatric patient. J Pediatr 1982; 101:163, 319.

Pollack MM, Fields AI, Ruhimann UE. Sequential cardiopulmonary variables of infants and children in septic shock. Crit Care Med 1984; 12:554–559.

Zimmerman JJ, Dietrich KA. Current perspectives on septic shock. Pediatr Clin North Am 1987; 34:131–163.

FEVER AND INFECTION IN THE CHILD WITH CANCER

ARTHUR E. BROWN, M.D., F.A.C.P.

Children with cancer who are neutropenic (absolute neutrophil count less than 1,000 per cubic millimeter) and become febrile are at risk for having severe, life-threatening infection. Autopsy data from cancer centers indicate that infection is the leading cause of death among pediatric patients with leukemia. The most important factor in determining the outcome of infection in the febrile neutropenic patient with cancer is the absolute neutrophil count. Many studies have shown that the incidence of such infections is directly related to the length of time a patient is neutropenic as well as to the degree of neutropenia. Most infectious diseases and oncology experts agree that the threshold for beginning antibacterial therapy is an absolute neutrophil count of less than 1,000 per cubic milliliter. It is what happens to the absolute neutrophil count after this point that is an important prognostic factor. If the absolute neutrophil count falls quickly below 100 per cubic milliliter and remains at that nadir for more than 10 to 14 days (so-called profound and prolonged neutropenia), the risk of fatality from the infectious episode is magnified. However, if the absolute neutrophil count quickly returns to greater than 1,000 per cubic milliliter, a much more favorable outcome can be predicted.

Another important host defense that can be disrupted in the child with cancer is the integument. The skin may be broken by venipuncture, bone marrow aspirates and biopsies, lumbar punctures, and catheters inserted into the bladder and the venous and arterial tree. All such manipulations create portals of entry for resident flora that may be endogenous or newly acquired by the host in the hospital. Such newly acquired flora may well be resistant, since nosocomial bacterial organisms frequently are. Another area that often becomes disrupted is that of the mucous membranes of the gastrointestinal tract and the respiratory tree. Mucous membranes in these areas become involved in the mucositis that results from cytotoxic chemotherapy. These areas provide portals of entry, too, for bacterial and fungal organisms.

ORGANISMS CAUSING INFECTIONS

To appreciate what the therapeutic choices are for the febrile neutropenic child with neoplastic disease, one must have an understanding of the organisms most likely to cause infection in such patients. Bacterial organisms are of initial concern in the febrile neutropenic child with cancer. Although patterns of infection have been changing in the United States to an increase in gram-positive bacterial infections, including *Staphylococcus epidermidis,* the aerobic gram-negative enteric bacilli and *Pseudomonas aeruginosa* are still major pathogens against which initial empiric antibacterial therapy is directed in the febrile neutropenic patient. This need for prompt and appropriate antibacterial therapy against gram-negative rods is further reinforced when the case fatality rates in patients with septicemia caused by *E. coli, Klebsiella* species, and *Pseudomonas aeruginosa* are considered. Such high mortality rates prompt me to begin a broad-spectrum empiric regimen that covers these particular pathogens whenever there are no focal symptoms, signs, or laboratory evidence to suggest a specific microbial diagnosis, and thus a more specific therapy.

EMPIRIC ANTIMICROBIAL THERAPY

It should be stressed that the choice of empiric antimicrobial therapy is partly determined by the knowledge of the resistance patterns of the bacterial pathogens in the hospital and community in which a patient resides. Patterns of antibiotic susceptibilities may vary from hospital to hospital within a city as well as from city to city or state to state. Pediatricians must know the patterns within their community and in the hospital(s) to which they admit their patients.

I prefer a combination of an aminoglycoside and a beta-lactam antibiotic to monotherapy or to combinations of two beta-lactam agents. Currently, I use the combination of gentamicin and ticarcillin–clavulanic acid as the empiric regimen in the neutropenic febrile child with cancer. (The latter drug is not approved by the Food and Drug Administration [FDA] for children younger than 12 years of age.)

Gentamicin is given intravenously as a 2-mg-per-kilogram loading dose, followed by 5.0 to 7.5 mg per kilogram per day in divided doses every 6 to 8 hours. Adjustments in gentamicin dosing must be made for diminished renal function. Aminoglycoside serum concentrations should be monitored and adjustments made accordingly. I aim to have the trough gentamicin concentration less than 2.0 μg per milliliter and the peak concentration between 5.0 and 10.0 μg per milliliter. An alternative is tobramycin, which is given in dosages identical to those of gentamicin. Amikacin may also be considered, but the schedule is quite different because the serum half-life is longer. Amikacin may be given in a dosage of 7.5 mg per kilogram, intravenously every 8 to 12 hours. Gentamicin is the least expensive choice.

The combination of ticarcillin and clavulanic acid comes in a fixed ratio of 100 mg of the clavulanate per 3 g of the ticarcillin. Dosing is therefore calculated on the basis of the ticarcillin at 300 mg per kilogram per day, intravenously in divided doses every 4 to 6 hours. An alternative to consider is ceftazidime, administered at a dosage of 100 mg per kilogram per day, intravenously in divided doses every 8 hours.

In special circumstances, I would consider monotherapy with ceftazidime. These circumstances include the concomitant use of nephrotoxic chemotherapeutic agents such as cis-platinum. In such instances, when a child's hearing and renal function are severely impaired or even potentially impaired by using an aminoglycoside antibiotic, I use ceftazidime as a single agent. I would not do this in cases in which the child is expected to be neutropenic for an extended period of time (greater than 7 days). Also, very close supervision is required, and if the child does not appear to be responding to ceftazidime alone, an aminoglycoside is added—usually gentamicin. I do not use monotherapy for children with leukemia who are neutropenic and febrile and expected to have prolonged and profound episodes of neutropenia.

Empiric antibiotic therapy should continue until resolution of the fever and neutropenia occurs. Changes may need to be made in the original antibiotic selection based on culture and susceptibility test data that become available.

The discussion thus far has been about the starting choices of antibiotics for empiric therapy of the febrile neutropenic child with cancer. We must also consider what to do if such a patient remains febrile and still has no localizing symptoms or signs of infection that would help to make a specific microbial diagnosis. Repeated cultures are essential. In such cases usually 7 to 10 days have elapsed after antibiotics were started, and the addition of amphotericin B is now warranted because the risk of fungal superinfection is substantial. I rapidly escalate in about 24 to 36 hours from a "test" dose of 1 mg of amphotericin to the full 1 mg per kilogram per day dosage.

SPECIFIC SITES OF INFECTION

Catheter-Related Infections

The increased use of indwelling subcutaneous intravenous catheters for venous access has greatly changed many aspects of the care of the neutropenic febrile child with cancer. Gram-positive organisms such as *Staphylococcus aureus* and coagulase-negative staphylococci have become more dominant in the 1980s than previously. In our institution, very few isolates of methicillin-resistant staphylococci (MRSA) have been recovered, and I do not recommend the use of vancomycin empirically. However, I am quite aware that the situation is different elsewhere. If MRSA are a problem, one must consider adding vancomycin to the empiric regimen if a skin or soft tissue source is likely or if the child has an indwelling intravenous catheter in place.

Catheter infections are grouped into three categories: catheter-related sepsis, exit-site infection, and tunnel infection. Studies at our center indicate that removal of the catheter is not always needed to cure the child of catheter-related sepsis when there are no localizing signs. Appropriate antibiotics alone often cure catheter-related sepsis in children who do not have an exit-site infection or a tunnel infection. Removal of the catheter is generally required in patients with tunnel infections and with catheter-related sepsis that does not respond to appropriate antibiotics.

Pneumonia

Pulmonary infection is one of the most common infectious illnesses confronting the pediatrician and parents of the neutropenic febrile child with cancer. Gram-negative pneumonia in particular is among the most deadly infectious conditions. For this reason, an unexplained pulmonary infiltrate in an admission chest radiograph should be considered to be caused by gram-negative organisms and treated accordingly with a broad-spectrum combination of agents (gentamicin and either ticarcillin–clavulanic acid or ceftazidime). Continuous reassessment of the clinical situation is required, and the antimicrobial agents should be continued until the neutropenia and fever both resolve.

A new cough, fever, and pulmonary infiltrate on radiographic examination of the chest in a neutropenic patient who is already receiving broad-spectrum antibiotics suggests fungal superinfection, particularly aspergillosis. This diagnosis is best made by bronchoscopic examination with bronchial alveolar lavage and transbronchial biopsy or with an open lung biopsy. However, that is not always possible in the neutropenic patient, who usually is also thrombocytopenic. If that is the case, empiric amphotericin B therapy should be started and the dose promptly escalated to the full dose of 1 mg per kilogram per day.

Gastrointestinal Infections

Typhlitis is a syndrome seen particularly in children who have acute leukemia and are neutropenic. The presenting symptoms are those of vague abdominal pain ordinarily localizing in the right lower quadrant. Other symptoms include vomiting, diarrhea, which may be bloody, and fever. Rebound tenderness and abdominal distension are often present, but the classic peritoneal signs may be absent or blunted by steroid therapy. Conservative management with nasogastric suction, intravenous hydration, and broad-spectrum antibiotics including anaerobic coverage with either clindamycin or metronidazole should be undertaken promptly if the child is not already receiving broad-spectrum antibacterial therapy. Some advocate surgical intervention to remove the necrotic cecum and to construct a temporary ileostomy and a mucous fistula of the right transverse colon. Gastrointestinal continuity can be restored subsequently when the patient is in remission.

Diagnosis of *Clostridium difficile* toxin-related colitis is accomplished by submitting a stool specimen for toxin assay. This condition should be suspected in children receiving multiple antibiotics and/or chemotherapeutic agents. The treatment is either

oral vancomycin or metronidazole (see chapter *Antibiotic-Associated Diarrheal Syndromes*).

Perianal infections in the neutropenic patient should be treated medically with broad-spectrum intravenous antibiotics that include coverage for anaerobic bacteria (clindamycin or metronidazole) as well as local care.

Central Nervous System Infections

Meningitis is rarely a problem in neutropenic patients, but when it occurs it can be extremely difficult to treat. Meningitis caused by *Pseudomonas aeruginosa* is especially difficult, in that the patient needs an Ommaya (or similar) ventricular reservoir to achieve therapeutic levels of an aminoglycoside in ventricular fluid. Parenteral aminoglycoside therapy and an antipseudomonal penicillin should also be given.

SPECIFIC ORGANISMS CAUSING INFECTION

Fungal Infection

Fungal infections (see the chapters on specific fungal infections for detailed information) often follow a presumed or proved bacterial infection in the neutropenic febrile child with cancer. Histopathology remains the principal means of diagnosing invasive fungal infection. Amphotericin B is the treatment of choice. Invasive infections caused by *Candida* species, particularly *Candida tropicalis,* respond best to the combination of amphotericin B and flucytosine. I usually start therapy with amphotericin B and rapidly escalate to the full 1-mg-per-kilogram-per-day dosage within 24 to 36 hours and then begin oral flucytosine (100 mg per kilogram per day in divided doses every 6 hours). Children receiving flucytosine need to be monitored closely for renal dysfunction and thrombocytopenia. Serum concentrations of flucytosine should be monitored. Although no one can say exactly how long a child with invasive candidiasis, aspergillosis, or mucormycosis should be treated, they are usually treated for 6 to 8 weeks or longer.

Stomatitis caused by *Candida* is treated initially with nystatin "swish and swallow," clotrimazole troches or ketoconazole. These may be effective as long as the problem is localized. However, if the child begins to complain of retrosternal pain and difficulty swallowing, intravenous amphotericin B therapy becomes necessary to treat esophagitis.

Parasitic Infection

Pneumocystis carinii pneumonia is a preventable disease among children in the well-defined risk group of acute lymphocytic leukemia. These children should be receiving oral trimethoprim-sulfamethoxazole prophylaxis (5 mg per kilogram per day of the trimethoprim component in two divided doses for a maximum of 320 mg of trimethoprim a day). Therapy for *Pneumocystis carinii* pneumonia is with either trimethoprim-sulfamethoxazole at 20 mg per kilogram per day, given intravenously in divided doses every 8 hours or with pentamidine, 4 mg per kilogram per day as a single intravenous dose over 90 minutes. Pentamidine is painful when given intramuscularly and can cause sterile abscesses. Side effects from the intravenous administration of pentamidine include hypotension, tachycardia, and hypoglycemia and require close monitoring during the infusion (see chapter *Protozoan Infection* for details of treatment).

Viral Infections

Stomatitis and esophagitis caused by herpes simplex virus is best diagnosed by viral culture. Intravenous acyclovir (750 mg per square meter per day in divided doses every 8 hours) is recommended for neutropenic children with severe gingivostomatitis (see chapter *Herpes Simplex Virus Infection*).

PREVENTION

Scrupulous attention to proper handwashing technique by personnel and families caring for these children who are at high risk for death from infection cannot be overemphasized. Proper care of catheters by pediatricians, nurses, and parents is also essential. Continuous educational programs for children and parents are a part of our infection control program. Our neutropenic patients are on CDC-JK precautions while in the hospital. This includes an iodophor surgical soap bath daily to reduce skin colonization with *Corynebacterium* species CDC-JK.

SUGGESTED READING

Brown AE. Neutropenia, fever and infection. In: Brown AE, Armstrong D, eds. Infectious complications of neoplastic disease: controversies in management. New York: Yorke Medical Books, 1985; 19–34.
Brown AE. Management in the febrile, neutropenic patient with cancer: therapeutic considerations. J Pediatr 1985; 106:1035–1042.
Pizzo PA. Infectious complications in the child with cancer. I. Pathophysiology of the compromised host and the initial evaluation and management of the febrile cancer patient. J Pediatr 1981; 98:341–354.
Pizzo PA. Infectious complications in the child with cancer. II. Management of specific infectious organisms. J Pediatr 1981; 98:513–523.
Pizzo PA. Infectious complications in the child with cancer. III. Prevention. J Pediatr 1981; 98:524–530.
Pizzo PA. After empiric therapy: what to do until the granulocyte count comes back. Rev Infect Dis 1987; 9:214–219.

ANTIBODY DEFICIENCY STATES

RICHARD L. WASSERMAN, M.D., Ph.D.

I define an antibody deficiency state as the absence of preformed antibody specific for an infecting microorganism at the time of the infection and the inability to generate a protecting antibody in a timely fashion. The prototype antibody deficiency state is Bruton's X-linked agammaglobulinemia, a congenital immunodeficiency characterized by the complete inability to produce antibody. Other well-recognized antibody deficiencies include common variable hypogammaglobulinemia, immunoglobulin A (IgA) deficiency and combined immunodeficiencies such as severe combined immunodeficiency disease, Wiskott-Aldrich syndrome, and ataxia telangiectasia. More subtle defects of antibody production such as IgG subclass deficiency and antigen-specific unresponsiveness are now being recognized with increasing frequency. The significance of antibody deficiency in premature infants, in burn and other surgical patients, and in patients with certain malignancies remains controversial. In this chapter I discuss immunoglobulin replacement therapy and the management of infections in patients with immunoglobulin deficiency.

IMMUNOGLOBULIN REPLACEMENT

Passive immunization by the administration of gamma globulin (GG) has been available for many years. GG, prepared from pooled plasma, consists of more than 90 percent IgG, with varying amounts of IgA, IgM, and IgE depending on the method of preparation. GG therapy is useful for the replacement of IgG only. The small amounts of other immunoglobulins present in the GG preparation cannot in any way replace a deficiency in IgA or IgM. Although fresh frozen plasma does contain representative amounts of IgA and IgM, supplementation of those immunoglobulin isotypes is not recommended.

GG for intramuscular administration (IMGG) has been used for more than 30 years. Since 1982, intravenous GG (IVGG) has been available commercially in the United States. In my opinion, IVGG is now the treatment of choice for immunoglobulin replacement therapy. Although both IMGG and IVGG are prepared from the same donor pools, intramuscular administration is painful and significantly limits the total dosage that can be administered on a routine basis. The IVGG, which requires only the placement of an intravenous catheter and allows virtually unlimited dosing options, is less painful and more effective. Currently three IVGG preparations are available in the United States. At this time, no clear-cut data support the notion that one of these products is superior to the other two at the level of clinical efficacy and side effects. Therefore, I consider them to be equivalent in the treatment of humoral immunodeficiency. GG preparations available in the United States appear to be free of risk for transfusion transmitted viruses. GG is prepared from hepatitis B surface antigen (HBsAg)-negative, human immunodeficiency virus (HIV) negative donor units. In addition, the processing methods inactivate HIV. Viruses responsible for non-A, non-B (NANB) hepatitis are either inactivated during processing or neutralized by antibodies in the preparation itself, since commercial GG has not been implicated in NANB hepatitis in the United States. At this time there are no known long-term side effects of IVGG.

Dosage

I initiate GG therapy with a loading dose of 400 mg per kilogram for the first administration and 200 mg per kilogram for subsequent doses. The appropriate dosage for a given patient is that which results in a significant decrease in the frequency and severity of infection. Often patients require a maintenance dosage greater than 200 mg per kilogram. Because trough immunoglobulin concentrations in serum increase with each dose, I usually make changes at 3-month intervals. There are essentially no dosage-related side effects and, therefore, it is our routine to administer an entire vial even if that brings the dosage to above 200 mg per kilogram (e.g., a 12-kg child would require 2.4 g per dose; one brand is sold in 3.0-g vials and I would administer the entire vial).

Dosing Interval

Therapy is routinely given on an every-4-week schedule. Some patients appear to do well on an every-5-week schedule. I know of patients at other centers who receive their GG every 6 weeks. If trough serum concentrations (see following) are inadequate or the patient seems to develop problems several days or a week before the next infusion, the dosing interval can be shortened or the dose administered raised. In general, I try to avoid administering GG every 3 weeks, and I have no patients currently receiving GG more frequently than that. There are reports of patients who self-administer GG at home using a relatively small dose every week, and this could certainly be an option.

Intercurrent illness is never a reason to defer GG. I usually accelerate the schedule and give IVGG during the acute illness if a significant problem occurs more than 2 weeks after the last dose.

Serum Concentrations of Immunoglobulins

In most circumstances we follow trough serum concentrations, which we obtain on the day of administering the next dose of IVGG. The amount required for a particular patient is that which is associated with good clinical results. Most of our patients appear to do well with a trough serum concentration of IgG greater than or equal to 400 mg per deciliter. A few of our patients have had marked clinical improvement when their trough values were increased from the low 400s to greater than 500 mg per deciliter. In a patient with clearly defined humoral immunodeficiency, I would not hesitate to aim for as high a trough concentration as is needed to obtain a good clinical result. Depending on the weight of the patient, the size of the vial used, and issues relating to convenience, the dosage and interval can be adjusted to maintain whatever trough concentration one chooses.

Administration

I administer IVGG using a 23-gauge butterfly or a 22-gauge plastic catheter in those patients who are young and uncooperative. On the first administration I begin at a rate of 0.5 ml per kilogram per hour. The infusion rate is increased by 0.5 ml per kilogram per hour every 10 to 15 minutes, as long as no side effects occur. I never intentionally exceed an infusion rate of 180 ml per hour. If the first infusion takes place smoothly and without incident, I begin subsequent infusions at a faster rate.

Side Effects

Commonly reported side effects include fever, chills, myalgias, nausea and vomiting, chest "tightness," and sinus pain. These side reactions occur in approximately 3 to 5 percent of patients, and at least 90 percent of them are related to the rate of infusion. That is, if the infusion rate is slowed the side effects remit. Significant cardiovascular abnormalities such as hypertension, hypotension, or anaphylaxis occur rarely, probably with an incidence of 1:10,000 administrations or less. An anecdotal report suggests that all episodes of cardiovascular instability have occurred during the first several IVGG administrations or when more than 2 months had elapsed between infusions. I recommend that initial (see below) IVGG infusions be administered only under circumstances in which the initial management of shock is possible. Intravenous epinephrine and at least 1 liter of normal saline should be available for the emergency management of shock.

The mild side effects described here can be ameliorated or prevented by premedication with an antihistamine such as diphenhydramine and aspirin or acetaminophen. Some immunologists believe that aspirin is superior to acetaminophen in preventing these reactions. An anecdotal observation indicates that side effects are most prominent in patients who normally carry a significant antigenic burden such as patients with bronchiectasis or other chronically infected foci.

I strongly recommend that an administration log be kept for the first few doses. Carefully monitoring rate of infusion, vital signs, and side effects helps you adjust the regimen to minimize problems and still give the IVGG in a reasonable amount of time (see the Sample IVGG Administration Order Sheet in Figure 1).

Clinical Results

Appropriate GG replacement therapy should result in a significant decrease in the frequency and severity of infections among patients with humoral immunodeficiency. Usually catch-up growth and weight gain occurs in patients who have been growth retarded or underweight. It often takes several months of treatment to see a clear-cut clinical effect, and in at least one well-done study, patients did much better during the second 6 months of therapy than during the first 6 months.

Home Therapy

Home administration of IVGG is a convenient, cost-effective approach to treating patients in need of immunoglobulin replacement. Many patients or family members can be taught to start intravenous infusions and administer GG without difficulty. Since significant, life-threatening side effects seldom, if ever, occur in patients on regular maintenance therapy, home administration appears to be safe. I insist that at least six infusions be administered under direct medical supervision but that if those treatments proceed without incident, home administration is

---

DATE OF PROCEDURE: _______________________ TIME: _______________ DIAGNOSIS: _______________

WEIGHT _____________ HEIGHT _____________

BLOOD PRESSURE __________ RESP. RATE __________ TEMPERATURE __________ HEART RATE __________

1. On arrival obtain baseline height, weight, and vital signs.

2. Premedication orders:

   _____________________ PO __________ minutes prior to infusion
   _____________________ PO __________ minutes prior to infusion
   _____________________ PO __________ minutes prior to infusion

3. Start 22-gauge angiocath or 23-gauge butterfly.

4. Obtain the following lab studies: ____
   ____
   ____

5. Administer _________________________________ IVGG __________ g in __________ % solution.

   A. Begin infusion at 0.5 ml/kg/hr for the first 15 min.
   B. If no signs or symptoms of reaction increase rate to 1.0 ml/kg/hr for 15 min.
   C. If no reaction, increase rate to 2.0 ml/kg/hr for 15 min.
   D. If no reaction, increase rate to maximum of 4.0 ml/kg/hr for the duration of the infusion.

6. Monitor vital signs and physical assessment for signs of reaction every _______ minutes for the first hour, then _______.

7. If reaction occurs but there is no significant change in respiratory rate (RR < 30), heart rate (HR < 30 more than baseline) or blood pressure (BP within 10% of baseline) reduce the infusion rate to 0.5 ml/kg/hr and give:

   Diphenhydramine _______ mg _______ and acetaminophen _______ mg PO or aspirin _______ mg PO.

   If a reaction results in a significant change in vital signs:

   A. Stop infusion.
   B. Page _________________________ STAT.
   C. Start normal saline infusion at TKO rate.
   D. Draw up epinephrine (1:10,000) 0.1 ml/kg (max 0.35 ml).
   E. Draw up diphenhydramine 1.5 mg/kg (0.03 ml/kg).

Physician _________________________   Nurse _________________________

TIME	INFUSION RATE	HR	RR	BP	TEMP

Figure 1 Sample IVGG administration order sheet.

then possible. In addition to full instruction on the recognition of side effects, epinephrine and intravenous diphenhydramine must be available during the administration.

IMGG

Intramuscular GG may be used for replacement but, as noted earlier, pain and volume constraints limit its effectiveness. The routine dosage is 0.6 to 0.8 ml per kilogram every 3 weeks. I always split the dosage into at least two deep intramuscular injections, one in each upper outer quadrant of the buttocks. The addition of up to 0.05 ml of lidocaine per milliliter of IMGG to each injection will not prevent the immediate pain but may modify the discomfort at the injection site over the next few hours. Experienced recipients, especially preteenagers, often require several holders during the injections. One may elect to give weekly injections of 0.2 to 0.3 mg per kilogram. Using IMGG it is seldom possible to achieve a trough IgG concentration in serum of more than 300 mg per deciliter.

Fresh Frozen Plasma

Fresh frozen plasma (FFP) is not ideal for immunoglobulin replacement. Very large amounts of FFP are needed to achieve IgG levels comparable to those achievable using IVGG. (FFP typically contains less than 1 percent IgG; IVGG is used as a 3, 5, or 6 percent solution.) More important, the risk of transfusion-transmitted disease is equal to that of any other blood transfusion. GG, which is produced from 1,500 to 10,000 plasma donors, is likely to have a greater range of antibodies than FFP.

If FFP must be used, a panel of donors should be identified and immunized with diphtheria–tetanus toxoid, *Haemophilus influenzae* vaccine, and pneumococcal polysaccharide vaccine. Periodic plasmapheresis may be the best means of harvesting sufficient quantities of plasma from the donor group. Patients usually receive 15 to 20 ml per kilogram every 3 weeks.

IgA Deficiency

Patients with complete IgA deficiency, alone or in combination with other dysgammaglobulinemias, may develop anti-IgA antibodies when given immunoglobulin containing IgA. These anti-IgA antibodies may cause significant side effects, including potentially fatal anaphylaxis.

Although GG therapy is contraindicated in patients with selective IgA deficiency, it may be useful in patients with associated defects in IgG production. IVGG with a very small IgA concentration has been used successfully in a small number of IgA-deficient patients and would be the best means of providing immunoglobulin to these patients.

ANTIBIOTIC THERAPY IN PATIENTS WITH HUMORAL IMMUNODEFICIENCY

Patients with humoral immunodeficiency, including Bruton's agammaglobulinemia, common variable hypogammaglobulinemia, IgG subclass deficiency, and selective IgA deficiency, are subject to infections of greater frequency and severity than other children. Despite this increased incidence of infection, the location and organisms involved in such infections are not extraordinary. These patients tend to have their greatest problems with sinopulmonary infections and otitis, and the most common infecting organisms are pneumococci, streptococci, staphylococci, and *H. influenzae.*

Although these patients may demonstrate a response to antibiotics equivalent to that of a normal child, prolonged antibiotic therapy is usually required. Occasionally, larger-than-normal dosages of antibiotics are used.

Prophylaxis

I prefer to use sulfisoxazole for chronic prophylaxis in patients who require such therapy. Typically, I use 75 mg per kilogram per day in two divided doses, although a single daily dose is acceptable. I find that prophylaxis with sulfisoxazole tends not to cause fungal overgrowth, and because of its relatively narrow spectrum, there are many treatment options if a breakthrough infection occurs. An additional advantage is activity against some ampicillin-resistant *Haemophilus* and the fact that sulfa drugs penetrate well into secretions.

Acceptable alternatives to sulfisoxazole are amoxicillin, tetracycline (in older children), and trimethoprim–sulfamethoxazole. Amoxicillin and tetracycline are used in dosages of 250 or 500 mg per day, depending on the weight of the child. Trimethoprim–sulfamethoxazole is used in a dosage of 5 mg of the trimethoprim component per kilogram of body weight once daily.

Treatment

Amoxicillin, Augmentin, Ceclor, Bactrim or Septra and Pediazole are the most commonly used drugs for treatment. Routinely recommended dosages are acceptable for all of these drugs, with the exception of Ceclor, which should be administered in a dosage of 60 mg per kilogram per day.

Otitis Media

In general, otitis can be treated in the routine fashion for 10 days. The choice of antibiotics may be determined by the child's previous antibiotic exposure or myringotomy fluid culture, if appropriate. Follow-up examinations are mandatory. Recurrent otitis media is usually an indication for chronic prophylaxis (see chapter on *Otitis Media with Effusion*).

Sinusitis

Sinusitis is treated for 3 to 6 weeks. Sinusitis is usually treated with Augmentin, Ceclor, Bactrim, or Septra. Some response, as measured by a decrease in fever and a change in the character of nasal secretions, is expected within the first 4 to 7 days. Follow-up sinus roentgenograms are usually not obtained. Inadequate clinical response usually requires a change in drugs preferably to a different class of antibiotics. Significant worsening on antibiotics or failure to respond to two or more appropriate antibiotics may indicate the need for surgical intervention.

Chest Disease

The new onset of cough without any physical findings, with or without a normal chest radiograph, should be treated with amoxicillin for 5 days. Significant clinical pneumonitis with or without radiographic changes should be treated for 14 days. Focal lobar infiltrate should also be treated for a minimum of 14 days independent of a favorable clinical response. Significant clinical illness in the face of a diffuse interstitial pattern usually requires more extensive evaluation and not just oral antibiotics. Patients with chronic lung disease may require chronic prophylaxis and a more aggressive approach to antibiotic management.

Cutaneous Infections and Superficial Abscesses

Superficial infections should be drained. Adequate antistaphycoccal antibiotic coverage must always be provided. Children unable to swallow capsules should be treated with cephalexin or cefaclor. Older children may be treated with cloxacillin or dicloxacillin.

SUGGESTED READING

Buckley RH. Common variable immunodeficiency. In: Lichtenstein LM, Fauci AS, eds. Current therapy in allergy, immunology and rheumatology 1985–1986. Ontario, Canada: BC Decker, 1985; 99–102.
Morell A, Nydegger UE, eds. Clinical use of intravenous immunoglobulins. Orlando: Academic Press, 1986.

CHRONIC GRANULOMATOUS DISEASE

RICHARD L. WASSERMAN, M.D., Ph.D.

Chronic granulomatous disease (CGD) is probably the best-defined group of disorders of phagocytic cell function. The prototypic defect is an x-linked recessive deficiency of phagocyte oxidative metabolism. It is characterized by the inability of phagocytic cells to generate hydrogen peroxide and anions necessary for killing certain bacteria and fungi. Extensive biochemical and genetic heterogeneity has been described, and CGD is recognized to have many etiologies. Other portions of the host defense system and indeed most other phagocytic cell functions are normal, and the inability to eradicate the infecting microorganism results in granuloma formation—thus the name chronic granulomatous disease.

Chronic granulomatous disease should be considered in patients who have experienced recurrent infection with common, catalase-positive organisms or a single significant infection with a less common catalase-positive organism such as *Serratia marcescens* (Table 1). CGD patients are often identified following the development of a deep tissue abscess, osteomyelitis, or the finding of granulomata in lymph node biopsies performed for chronic or recurrent adenitis. The diagnosis of chronic granulomatous disease significantly alters your management approach to the acute presenting illness as well as the long-term management of your patient. In this chapter, I address chronic management, the approach to diagnosis and management of acute disease, and the management of syndromes peculiar to CGD patients.

CHRONIC CARE

The early report by Bridges et al of "a fatal granulomatous disease of childhood" describes the natu-

TABLE 1 Organisms Commonly Causing Significant Infection in CGD Patients

Bacteria	Fungi
Staphylococcus aureus	*Aspergillus* species
Salmonella species	*Candida* species
Pseudomonas cepacia	
Serratia marcescens	
Chromobacterium species	
Escherichia coli	
Klebsiella species	
Nocardia asteroides	
Mycobacterium species	
Actinomyces species	

ral history of CGD in four patients, all of whom died before reaching 6 years of age. It is clear that chronic administration of prophylactic antibiotics can modify both the frequency and the severity of infectious episodes in these patients. I have relied heavily on the use of trimethoprim–sulfamethoxazole in my patients, with good results. I recommend 10 mg of TMP per kilogram per day, in two divided doses. This regimen has been shown to be superior to use of dicloxacillin alone but not significantly different from the combination of dicloxacillin and trimethoprim in sulfa-allergic patients (Table 2). The use of both dicloxacillin and trimethoprim–sulfamethoxazole at the same time does not appear to add significantly to the efficacy of treatment. These prophylactic antibiotic regimens appear to extend the intervals between potentially life-threatening infections from about once in 12 months to about once in 40 months.

The goal of chronic therapy in CGD patients, as in other immunodeficiency patients, is normal growth and development. Therefore, I discourage parents from limiting activity and encourage full participation in sports and most outdoor activities. Because these patients are subject to infections with unusual organisms, which may pose a diagnostic and therapeutic dilemma should the child become infected, I caution against swimming in standing water such as ponds or slow moving creeks and I suggest that sneakers or other protective footwear be worn when swimming in the ocean. Breaks in the skin are cleaned in the routine fashion and then scrubbed with 3 percent hydrogen peroxide. Such wounds are left open to the air whenever possible and observed scrupulously for signs of infection. Since these patients do not have all of the normal inflammatory signs of infection, delayed wound healing is often the first clue that more aggressive intervention is necessary.

Although periodontal disease is less a problem than in certain other patients with phagocytic cell functional defects, scrupulous attention to dental hygiene is necessary. In addition to careful, daily hygiene including flossing, fluoride prophylaxis, and regular dental visits, I recommend hydrogen peroxide mouth rinse using 3 percent hydrogen peroxide mixed 1:1 with warm water, used twice a day after brushing. Intravenous antibiotic prophylaxis is necessary for all dental procedures as well as surgery (Table 3).

TABLE 2　Prophylactic Antibiotic Regimens

Drug	Daily Dosage (mg/kg)	Maximum* Dose (mg/day)
Trimethoprim–sulfamethoxazole	10 (TMP)	160
Trimethoprim plus	10	200
dicloxacillin	10	500
Trimethoprim plus	10	200
cephalexin	10	500

* Maximum dose when used for prophylaxis.

TABLE 3　Prophylactic Antibiotics for Dental and Surgical Procedures

Drug	Dosage (mg/kg)	Timing
Oxacillin*	200 IV†	30–60 min pre-, 8 hr post, 16 hr post
Plus gentamicin‡	3–5 IM or IV	30–60 min pre-, 8 hr post, 16 hr post

* Another beta-lactam antibiotic effective against *Staphylococcus aureus*, such as nafcillin or cefazolin, may be substituted. Vancomycin (10 mg per kilogram per dose) may be used in penicillin-allergic patients.
† Medications are given parenterally. If parenteral administration is not possible, then oral administration of cephalexin (25 mg per kilogram 30 to 60 minutes before the procedure is started, then 10 mg per kilogram every 6 hours for eight doses) and intramuscularly administration of gentamicin in the dosages outlined can be substitued.
‡ Amikacin or netilmicin may be substitued for gentamicin if local patterns of antibiotic susceptibility so indicate.

SUBACUTE GRANULOMATOUS INFLAMMATION

Granulomatous inflammation of both the gastrointestinal and urinary tracts has been reported in CGD patients. In general, these are not acute, life-threatening disorders, but represent a significant chronic management problem. Granulomas may form at any point along the gastrointestinal (GI) tract and, although obstruction may occur as a result of a mass effect, malabsorption syndromes, diarrhea, and abdominal pain are more common. Granulomatous urethritis and cystitis mimic urinary tract infection, but are culture-negative and not associated with pyuria. In addition to the usual symptoms of lower urinary tract infection, intense itch on urination was reported by one of my patients. Diagnostic procedures visualizing or biopsying the granulomatous lesions may be performed, but in my experience have seldom influenced the approach to therapy. Microorganisms are rarely isolated from such biopsies. I have had satisfactory results in a limited number of patients by adding antibiotics to the chronic prophylactic regimen. If there is going to be a response to a new antibiotic, one usually sees improvement within 3 or 4 days and I believe this approach is entirely arbitrary. I usually start therapy with clindamycin and then go to metronidazole or chloramphenicol. Some clinicians have used prednisone, but have reported the development of steroid dependancy with its attendant side effects, and I have not needed to use steroids.

ACUTE INFECTIONS

Discriminating simple viral infections from the early presentation of potentially serious bacterial or fungal disease may be difficult in CGD patients. Total leukocyte and differential white counts are usually less informative in CGD patients than in normal children. I have found that combining an erythrocyte sedimentation rate with a white count and differential is sometimes helpful. Therefore, I include both studies in my routine evaluation when the children are well, so that baseline values are available. Patients who develop signs of infection such as poor appetite, lassitude, malaise, and fever of more than a few days' duration, but without any focal findings are treated initially by increasing the dosage of trimethoprim–sulfa to 20 mg of TMP per kilogram per day in four divided doses. Frequently, there is improvement within 2 or 3 days, and this regimen of increased antibiotics is then continued for 2 weeks. If the presenting signs and symptoms suggest more severe illness, or if there is not a rapid resolution when the dosage of oral antibiotics is increased, I become much more aggressive in my approach to diagnosis and therapy. I do not arbitrarily change antibiotics without attempting to isolate an organism.

Patients unresponsive to an increase in trimethoprim-sulfa are admitted to the hospital and subjected to an intensive search for an etiologic organism. Antibiotic therapy is begun as soon as the initial studies are complete. I recommend ceftazidime and vancomycin as a combination that provides good coverage against catalase-positive gram-negative bacteria and staphylococci. The addition of an aminoglycoside to enhance gram-negative coverage may be considered. Imipenem is an alternative as a single drug, but it has not yet been approved for use in children younger than 12 years of age (Table 4).

SEVERE, NONFOCAL INFECTIONS

Significant infections with moderate to severe signs and symptoms, but no readily identifiable

TABLE 4   Empiric Antibiotic Therapy*

Drug	Dosage (mg/kg/day)	Interval
Recommended		
Ceftazidime plus	150	q8 h
oxacillin	200	q6 h
Vancomycin†	40	q6 h
Alternatives		
Trimethoprim-		
sulfamethoxazole	20 (TMP)	q6 h
Amikacin‡	20–30	q8 h
Imipenem§	80–100	q6 h

* Serious, life-threatening infections are more likely to be caused by gram-negative organisms. Initial empiric therapy should provide both gram-negative and staphylococcal coverage if there is no focus of infection.

† Vancomycin is recommended if methicillin-resistant *Staphylococcus aureus* is locally prevalent. Trimethoprim–sulfamethoxazole may provide some staphylococcal coverage as well as gram-negative coverage in patients who have not had recent exposure to that drug. It should not be used as a single-drug therapy unless a susceptible organism has been isolated.

‡ The addition of an aminoglycoside to enhance gram-negative coverage may be appropriate in toxic patients.

§ Imipenem may be ideal for single-drug empiric therapy because of its very broad spectrum. It is not approved for use in children younger than 12 years of age.

focus, are a common problem in these patients. Every reasonable attempt should be made to identify the site of infection and, although it is often unrewarding, a vigorous search for the infecting microorganism is always warranted.

When faced with a CGD patient who is ill and has only vague abdominal pain or no symptoms at all, the search for an infectious focus may be difficult. A chest roentgenogram and abdominal ultrasound examination are the least costly and least invasive studies and that is where I usually begin. Computerized tomography may be helpful (see following), but in the absence of any localizing signs or symptoms I have not attempted whole body scans. Although intracellular killing is defective in these patients, chemotaxis is usually intact. Therefore, gallium scans that label granulocytes that home to the infected area offer the opportunity to evaluate the whole body without the guidance of localizing clinical findings. If gallium scan is unrewarding, normal donor granulocytes obtained by leukopheresis may be radiolabeled in vitro with indium and then infused into the patient as a granulocyte transfusion. The patient is then scanned for localized radiation.

The general rule that antibiotic therapy should be withheld until a diagnosis is made and an organism identified applies to CGD patients, but must be modified in recognition of the fact that there is at best a 50 percent likelihood of obtaining a positive culture. Therefore, the severity and progression of illness must weigh heavily in the decision to initiate empiric antibiotic therapy. Obviously there can be no straightforward, simple rules or guidelines here, and the risks of delay must be balanced against the risks of empiric therapy on a case-by-case basis. Empiric therapy should provide good coverage for catalase-positive bacteria that frequently infect these patients (see Table 1). Although *Staphylococcus aureus* was the most common isolate in at least one study, gram-negative enteric rods, particularly *Salmonella*, are more frequently associated with sepsis and life-threatening infection. My first choice for treatment in the absence of an isolate would be the combination of ceftazidime and vancomycin, with added amikacin or another aminoglycoside if the patient is toxic (see Table 4).

ACUTE, LOCALIZABLE INFECTIONS

Despite the inability of CGD patients to mount a normal inflammatory response displaying the classic signs of tissue injury, there are usually some localizing clinical findings. In my experience, the most common finding is swelling, which may or may not be painful but is neither erythematous nor hot. I have seen this presentation occur primarily in the head and neck, but it may also occur in lymph nodes or in the extremities. Pulmonary infection may be manifest by cough, fever, and malaise only without auscultatory findings and with a normal plain radiograph of the chest. Intra-abdominal infections frequently result in some physical finding of a mass or organomegaly, but mild pain and tenderness may be the only clue.

When the infection is superficial and readily accessible to the surgeon or aspiration needle, the etiologic organism should be pursued with vigor. Suppurative lesions should be surgically drained, and nonsuppurative lesions should be aspirated for culture. The surgeon must be aware of the patient's defect and should plan to use more than the usual number of drains and remove them more slowly than in a normal patient.

When there are some localizing signs or symptoms, computed tomographic (CT) scan has been very helpful in precisely defining the lesion. We have identified subsegmental pneumonia in a patient with cough but no auscultatory or routine radiographic findings. In another patient, the CT scan discriminated parotitis from buccal cellulitis in a patient with bilateral, nonred, nontender cheek swelling. CT can also be helpful in identifying sinusitis in young patients. When the suspected focus of infection is axial (i.e., head and neck, chest, or abdomen), then I think CT scanning should be attempted first. Osteomyelitis should be the prime consideration for an infection in an extremity (although it may occur anywhere), and in that situation a radionuclide bone scan should be performed first.

Although the utility of a positive culture cannot be overestimated, therapy should not be delayed in a patient with systemic toxicity or involvement of crucial organs. Suppurative lesions should, of course, be aspirated or drained but, in the absence of suppuration, I usually advocate biopsy for culture. Unless there is a rapid response (within 72 hours) to empiric antibiotic therapy for pneumonia, I recommend a percutaneous needle aspiration of the affected portion of the lung. Similarly, peritoneal lavage should be performed in suspected peritonitis that does not improve rapidly. It is particularly important to continue to pursue an etiologic diagnosis after empiric therapy is initiated, unless a patient demonstrates objective evidence of improvement. Open lung biopsy is too often delayed and should be performed before the development of significant respiratory compromise.

ANTIBIOTIC THERAPY FOR SERIOUS INFECTIONS

The recognition that catalase-positive organisms pose the greatest threat to these patients is fundamental to selecting appropriate antimicrobial therapy. The susceptibility of the bacterial or fungal isolate to the specific antibiotic or antifungal being used is crucial. The fact that the granulocytes of CGD patients are capable of phagocytosis but are defective in killing means that phagocytic cells may provide a sanctuary for ingested bacteria or fungus. The antimicrobial agent must penetrate both the outer cell membrane and the lysosomal membrane of the

phagocyte to reach the target. Consequently, I choose the largest standard dosages of antibiotics and monitor serum drug concentrations when toxicity is a potential problem. Chloramphenicol penetrates membranes well, and this feature combined with a broad spectrum makes its use more attractive in these patients than in a normal host. Table 5 lists the antimicrobial agents I prefer for treatment of these patients.

The duration of antibiotic therapy is determined by the clinical response and an awareness of the sanctuary effect described previously. CGD patients always receive a more prolonged course of antibiotics than normal hosts. As a general rule, I treat serious infections with antibiotics for 1 to 3 weeks longer than I would in a normal child. If one has the luxury of having isolated the organism, and it is susceptible to oral antimicrobial therapy, then the final weeks of antibiotics may be administered orally on an outpatient basis. If one has achieved a clinical response using empiric therapy, I would continue intravenous treatment for 1 week after the granulocyte count and sedimentation rate return to normal, or for 1 week after granulocyte transfusion therapy is completed (see following).

FUNGAL INFECTIONS

Fungal infections may be difficult to identify at the initial presentation of infection. The specific immune system is normal in CGD patients. Therefore, fungal serology and delayed hypersensitivity skin testing may enable one to make a diagnosis without a

TABLE 5 Specific Antibiotic Therapy*

Drug	Dosage† (mg/kg/day)	Dosing Interval
Cephalosporins		
Ceftazidime	150	q8 h
Ceftriaxone	100	q12 h or 24 h
Penicillins		
Mezlocillin	300	q6 h
Imipenem‡	100	q6 h
Aminoglycosides		
Amikacin	30	q8 h or 12 h
Netilmicin	7.5	q8 h
Miscellaneous		
Vancomycin§	60	q6 h
Chloramphenicol	100	q6 h
Clindamycin	40	q6–8 h
Antifungals		
Amphotericin B	0.75	q24 h
Ketoconazole	10 (200 mg max.)	q24 h

* Antibiotic selection may be influenced by the site of infection. If a microorganism has been isolated, the patient should be treated with two synergistic drugs based on susceptibilities, if possible.

† Dosages indicated are meningitis-type maximum doses. Large dosages are used because of the need to deliver the drug into phagocytic lysosomes (see the text).

‡ Imipenem is an attractive choice because of its broad spectrum. It is not approved for use in children.

§ Vancomycin is recommended if methicillin-resistant *Staphylococcus aureus* is locally prevalent.

positive culture or histopathology. I do not recommend antifungal therapy in the absence of strong evidence supporting the diagnosis. Amphotericin B is the treatment of choice for most fungal infections and for all deep tissue fungal infections (see the relevant chapters).

GRANULOCYTE TRANSFUSIONS

Granulocyte transfusions may be life-saving in CGD patients with serious infections. I use granulocyte transfusion therapy unless I get a good, objective response to antibiotics within 48 to 72 hours of beginning treatment. Early initiation of granulocyte transfusions is appropriate in patients with significant systemic toxicity or involvement of the head. In the most seriously ill patients, I begin granulocyte transfusions immediately. It is certainly possible to treat adenitis, osteomyelitis, and superficial abscesses effectively without the use of granulocytes, but serious, deep tissue infections may be difficult or impossible to eradicate without the assistance of fully functional granulocytes.

The granulocytes of CGD patients will never normalize (in contrast to oncology patients on chemotherapy who experience transient neutropenia). Therefore, daily granulocyte transfusions may be needed for 3 weeks or longer. Because granulocytes must be prepared by pheresis for all but the smallest of patients, it is prudent to inform your blood bank of the possible need for granulocyte transfusions at the time of admission. Since granulocyte transfusions require a daily preparation of product, the demand for donors often exceeds the blood bank's list of volunteers. The potential need for granulocytes and the procedures involved in donation should be explained to the parents so that they can begin to recruit donors. This is particularly true for patients with less common blood types, but should be initiated for all patients because some volunteers are not suitable for donation.

Although the supporting data are scanty, I require a minimum of 1×10^9 granulocytes per kilogram or 10 ml per kilogram, whichever provides more cells, up to a full adult pheresis donor granulocyte unit (about 1 to 5×10^{10} granulocytes when donors are pretreated with steroids and hydroxyethyl starch is used during pheresis to enhance the yield). Granulocytes are administered daily and continued until at least 5 days after a satisfactory response has been achieved. My criteria for discontinuing granulocyte transfusions are normalization of the fever curve, a normal erythrocyte sedimentation rate (or at least a clear-cut trend toward normalization of at least 7 days), or objective physical findings consistent with resolution of infection.

Reactions to granulocyte transfusions are not rare. These may include chills, fever, rash, and increased discomfort at the site of infection. In the absence of side effects, the granulocyte transfusion should be administered relatively rapidly (60 minutes or less) because granulocyte function deteriorates in vitro. Untoward reactions may be minimized by slowing the infusion rate, premedicating with diphenhydramine, given intravenously (1.5 mg per kilogram), and aspirin or acetaminophen (10 mg per kilogram). Methylprednisolone (2 mg per kilogram) is used intravenously in those patients who continue to experience side effects despite adjusting the infusion rate and administering diphenhydramine and aspirin.

Granulocyte transfusions should be administered with extreme caution in patients receiving amphotericin B, especially if pulmonary infection is present or suspected. If this combination must be used, it should be carefully timed to maximize the interval between administrations, and both infusions should be given slowly.

BONE MARROW TRANSPLANTATION

Allogeneic bone marrow transplantation can effect a complete and permanent cure of the defect in chronic granulomatous disease. Several patients with CGD have been transplanted successfully, and this approach may offer normality and freedom from chronic drug administration and frequent hospitalization. As of this writing, however, allogeneic bone marrow transplantation still carries a significant risk of severe and even fatal graft versus host disease. In view of the improvement in the outcome of these patients that has been achieved through the use of prophylactic antibiotics and granulocyte transfusions, I do not recommend bone marrow transplantation in cases in which one risks trading chronic granulomatous disease for chronic graft versus host disease.

SUGGESTED READING

Bridges RA, Berendes H, Good RA. A fatal granulomatous disease of childhood. Am J Dis Child 1959; 97:387–408.

Gallin JI, Buescher ES. Disorders of phagocyte function. In: Lichtenstein LM, Fauci AS, eds. Current therapy in allergy and immunology. Toronto, Canada: BC Decker, 1983; 287–293.

Gallin JI, Buescher ES, Seligmann BE, et al. Recent advances in chronic granulomatous disease. Ann Intern Med 1983; 99:657–674.

Lazarus GM, Neu HC. Agents responsible for infection in chronic granulomatous disease of childhood. J Pediatr 1975; 86:415–417.

Leonard AS, Mulholland MW, Filipovich AH. Surgery of the immunodeficient child. Surg Clin North Am 1985; 65:1505–1525.

SURGICAL INFECTIONS

JACK H. T. CHANG, M.D.

The topic of surgical infections is too broad in scope to be covered in great detail, and specifics about management of many surgical infections can be found in other chapters of this book. This chapter addresses principles of management and provides an overview of the subject.

Three principles guide the treatment of surgical infections: (1) cultures should be obtained, if at all possible, before the initiation of antibiotic therapy; (2) abscesses require adequate drainage; (3) given time, the nth generation antibiotic will yield the nth + 1 generation organism. The procurement and the proper and timely handling of culture material are well known but poorly executed. If culture and susceptibility test results are ignored and serum antibiotic concentrations are not obtained, recurrence of infection or development of resistant organisms can result. Inflammatory infections are frequently cured by antibiotics because abundant blood supply allows antibiotic access to the inciting organisms. The presence of fluctuance indicates abscess formation. Abscesses may be contained, but they are rarely cured by antibiotic therapy alone. Drainage to an external surface with maintenance of the drainage tract until the cavity coalesceses is curative. Many abscess cavities contain septa that may compartmentalize the abscess. These walls must be mechanically ruptured to prevent recurrence. To complete drainage, most surgical procedures in children are performed with general anesthesia. Packing of the abscess cavity serves to diminish blood loss from the inflammatory surface and to maintain the drainage tract. In the absence of systemic symptoms of bacteremia and sepsis, antibiotics are unnecessary after proper abscess drainage.

Over the past decade I have used approximately ten different antibiotics (Table 1). Choice is, of course, governed by the local prevailing organisms and their individual antibiotic susceptibilities. In penicillin-sensitive patients, I substitute a cephalosporin or erythromycin.

HEAD AND NECK INFECTIONS

Furuncles and carbuncles arise from a primary folliculitis and usually contain *Staphyloccus aureus.* Simple incision and drainage with packing is performed. The packing is removed the following day and the skin kept clean and open with Q-tip applications of hydrogen peroxide twice daily, until the cavity consolidates. Antibiotic is usually not necessary.

Congenital malformations such as thyroglossal duct cyst, with connection to the foramen cecum at the base of the tongue, and second branchial cleft sinus cyst, with its opening at the base of the tonsillar pillar, are prone to infections. After the inflammation or abscess is treated with penicillin and/or by drainage, the anomaly should be surgically extirpated to prevent recurrence. Cystic hygroma infection or abscess is treated in a similar manner. The early administration of penicillin frequently aborts abscess formation. My practice is to instruct the parent to start medication as soon as inflammation is seen. Surgical removal should be tempered by the location of the hygroma and the size of the child. Overzealous surgeries have resulted in permanent neurologic damage and even limb loss.

Lymph node infections and abscesses are frequently encountered in children. While many of these infections are viral in origin, bacterial sources such as tonsillitis, pharyngitis, and dental abscesses

TABLE 1   Antibiotics Used in Surgical Patients

Antibiotic	Dosage (dose/kg/24 hr)	Organisms
Amoxicillin	40 mg q8 h	*Streptococcus,* Enterococcus group, *P. mirabilis, H. influenzae*
Ampicillin	100 mg q12 h <7 days of age 150 mg q6 h >7 days of age	*Streptococcus,* Enterococcus group
Cefazolin	100 mg q8 h	*S. aureus, Streptococcus, E. coli, P. mirabilis, Klebsiella, Enterobacter*
Cephalexin	50 mg q6 h	As cefazolin
Clindamycin	25 mg q6 h	*Bacteroides, S. aureus*
Dicloxacillin	10 mg q6 h	Penicillinase-producing *S. aureus*
Gentamicin	5 mg q12 h <7 days of age 7.5 mg q8 h >7 days of age	*Enterobacter, E. coli, K. pneumoniae, Pseudomonas*
Metronidazole	30 mg q6 h	*Bacteroides*
Nafcillin	50 mg q12 h <7 days of age 150 mg q6 h >7 days of age	Penicillinase-producing *S. aureus*
Penicillin G/V	50,000–20,000 U q6 h	*Staphylococcus, Streptococcus, P. multocida*

Note: Broad-spectrum coverage is achieved with the combination of ampicillin, gentamicin, and clindamycin.

should be sought. When the source is unknown, an antibiotic to cover *S. aureus* and group A beta-hemolytic streptococcus is used. Fluctuance dictates surgical drainage, and I do not subscribe to repeated needle aspirations. Ultrasonography has been helpful in determining the presence and location of an abscess cavity. When there is a coalescence of nodes, culture for atypical mycobacteria should be obtained. Atypical mycobacterial lymphadenopathy is treated by excision of the involved node or nodes. In the face of an abscess caused by atypical mycobacteria, I curet out all of the necrotic and involved lymph node and pack the wound open. Incomplete removal of such nodes result in prolonged drainage and recurrence.

CHEST INFECTIONS

S. aureus is the usual organism involved in infantile breast infections. Abscesses are drained through a circumareolar incision to minimize scarring and tissue damage.

Mediastinal infections are usually secondary to anastomotic leaks, endoscopic perforations, or penetrating missiles. Broad-spectrum antibiotics including anaerobic coverage is started. In the absence of pleural fluid and abscess formation, as determined by computerized tomography, and with rapid defervescence of systemic signs (fever, leukocytosis, etc.), I initially treat anastomotic leak and endoscopic perforation with antibiotics alone. Any localization of infection, progression of symptoms, or penetrating missile injuries demands drainage, usually by means of the neck or through a chest tube. This can be a highly lethal infection and the patient requires intensive observation and care.

Infected pleural effusions should be drained adequately and totally. If the infected material obtained by thoracentesis is at all thick, closed-chest tube drainage is performed using the largest tube that is comfortably accommodated by the intercostal space. The development of a trapped lung as a result of inadequate or untimely drainage denotes poor management. Although most empyemas eventually resolve, the patient usually runs weeks of fever, loses weight, and misses a good deal of school. The early and proper placement of a chest tube obviates multiple thoracenteses with their attendant risks, prevents the protracted convalescence of an empyema, and eliminates the risks of pleurectomy. Antibiotics are aimed at *Streptococcus pneumoniae, Haemophilus influenzae,* and *S. aureus* while culture results are awaited.

Lung abscesses are fortunately rare today because of prompt antibiotic therapy and are found mostly in immunosupressed patients. Indications for lobectomy include large (greater than 5 cm), thick-walled cavitary lesions unresponsive to 4 weeks of intensive antibiotic therapy, progression to empyema, or massive hemoptysis. Antibiotics are dictated by the culture results.

ABDOMINAL INFECTIONS

The two most common intra-abdominal infections encountered in the pediatric patient are necrotizing enterocolitis in the newborn and appendicitis in the child. Necrotizing enterocolitis is initially treated by a penicillin derivative and an aminoglycoside. The usual organisms involved are *Escherichia coli Klebsiella, Clostridium,* and *Streptococcus* species. Anaerobic organisms are unusual. When operative intervention is necessary, the necrotic bowel is resected and the abdominal cavity copiously irrigated. Drains are unnecessary because abscess formation is rare. Disseminated intravascular coagulopathy is best treated with a double body volume exchange transfusion.

In the patient with acute appendicitis without suspicion of perforation, I usually treat with a cephalosporin for 24 hours. Any intra-abdominal fluid found should be cultured. Suspected perforated appendicitis (high fever, marked leukocytosis, rebound tenderness, abdominal/rectal mass) is treated with a penicillin derivative, an aminoglycoside, and an antianaerobic organism drug. My choices are ampicillin, gentamicin, and clindamycin. Loculated abscesses should be drained, although some pediatric surgeons also drain free pus. Antibiotics are altered according to culture and susceptibility test results. Advancement of the drain begins on the fifth day. When the patient has been afebrile for 24 hours, intravenous antibiotics are changed to oral drugs and continued for a full 10-day course. Occasionally one encounters a patient with a successfully treated perforated appendicitis returning in a week or two with fever and the finding of a retroperitoneal phlegmon (thickening of the retroperitoneum on rectal examination) without abscess formation. Generally a full 10-day course of intravenous antibiotics is curative. Intra-abdominal abscesses usually involve *Bacteroides* species and require transvaginal, transrectal, or transabdominal drainage.

The very serious topic of necrotizing fasciitis is detailed elsewhere. Generally caused by mixed gram-positive or oral organisms above the waist and enteric organisms below the waist, this gangrenous soft tissue infection spreads along the fascial cleft between the deep and superficial fascias. With its deceptive physical findings, the patient may suffer sudden vascular collapse and death. Treatment includes broad-spectrum antibiotic coverage and wide surgical exposure and debridement of all necrotic tissue until bleeding tissue is encountered. The wound is packed open and skin grafts are used when granulating tissue develops.

PERIANAL AND PERIRECTAL INFECTIONS

Perianal and perirectal infections usually contain *S. aureus* or enteric organisms and therefore require broad-spectrum coverage. A cephalosporin is usually adequate for the cellulitis after proper drainage. Since most patients require a general anesthetic, fistulous communications to the anal crypts should be sought and if found, unroofed. Postoperative sitz bath provides both cleansing of the wound and comfort for the patient. Ischiorectal and supralevator abscesses are fortunately rare in the pediatric patient but require aggressive broad-spectrum coverage as in perforated appendicitis and drainage.

Perianal and perirectal infections are not infrequently encountered in the immunosuppressed patient. If fluctuance is not found by physical examination or by ultrasound, the infection is best treated by broad-spectrum antibiotics alone. Open wounds in such patients are extremely slow in healing and serve as a route for secondary bacterial invasion. If a perianal cellulitis is refractory to antibiotics and local care in a leukemic patient, one should perform a punch biopsy to exclude leukemic infiltration.

EXTREMITY INFECTIONS

The most common infection of the extremity is secondary to the intravenous catheter, resulting in phlebitis or thrombophlebitis. Such complications can usually be avoided by using aseptic technique, selecting the correct size catheter, and avoiding caustic solutions. Most can be treated by removing the catheter and applying local heat. Those with bacterial infection, usually *S. aureus,* require antibiotic treatment and occasionally surgical extirpation. Deep venous thrombophlebitis is discussed in another chapter.

Lymphangitis is usually secondary to a streptococcal cellulitis and presents as a red subcutaneous streak. Administration of penicillin and local heat is usually curative.

Infections of the hand should be considered serious and treated by intravenous antibiotics, heat, and elevation. This is especially true if the infection is secondary to striking an opponents teeth or from a human bite. Massive intravenous doses of penicillin are used. Drainage, if necessary, should be performed on the volar surface in flexion creases.

Paronychia and felon are usually caused by *S. aureus,* which may be penicillin resistant. I prefer to use dicloxacillin. Paronychia is drained by inserting a scalpel blade parallel to the nail in the corner of the affected side, incising the tissue laterally until the proximal corner of the nail is exposed. Packing controls the bleeding. A felon cavity can be located by transillumination of the fingertip. The incision is in the shape of a hockey stick, slightly dorsal to the lateral line (to avoid the neurovascular bundle) and parallel to the axis of the finger, extending from the lateral bony phalanx to its tip. The cavity is widely opened by a hemostat and packed. After the pack is removed, the finger is soaked twice a day and oral antibiotics are continued for 10 days.

The most dangerous infection of the hand involves the tendon sheaths. Diagnosis is made by the presence of (1) diffuse swelling of the finger, (2) volar tenderness along the course of the tendon sheath, (3) maintenance of the finger in a partial flexed position, and (4) pain in extending the affected finger. Broad-spectrum antibiotics are administered and surgical drainage is performed. Delayed or inadequate drainage results in tendon necrosis with permanent dysfunction.

Infections of the foot are frequently secondary to ingrown toenails and foreign bodies. Infected ingrown toenails can be treated with penicillin and frequent soaks. Preventing recurrence requires proper fitting shoes, avoidance of high heel shoes, daily foot care, and proper nail cutting without curving at the edges. Recurrent or refractory infections require removal of one-third of the nail with curettage of the nail bed. This is best done under general anesthesia in children. Any recurrent infections of the foot should raise the possibility of a foreign body. Multiple-angle radiographs are obtained. Unless the foreign body is very superficial, it should be approached through the dorsum or lateral surfaces, to prevent a pressure-sensitive scar. The most efficacious means of removal is under fluoroscopic control.

WOUND INFECTIONS

The guiding principles of wound care are proper debridement, copious irrigation, and the gentle approximation of tissue. Lacerations occurring within 4 to 6 hours are primarily repaired. Older injuries are closed over drains or the skin is left open to granulate. Infections of the face that drain into the cavernous sinus should be treated by intravenous penicillin. Lacerations of the mucous membranes of the mouth can usually be left alone because epithelialization occurs within 24 hours. Flaps should be loosely approximated.

Operative surgical wound infections are usually caused by *S. aureus* or streptococcus and treated by drainage and dicloxacillin or penicillin. Wound infections after intestinal surgery are usually caused by enteric organisms and as such require broad-spectrum antibiotics, including anaerobic coverage. Ampicillin, gentamicin, and clindamycin are my drugs of choice. The wounds are opened, packed, and allowed to heal by secondary intention.

Dog or cat bites should be widely debrided and copiously irrigated. Nonfacial wounds may be loosely closed over a drain. Facial wounds are closed because a postclosure infection requiring drainage will not yield a worse scar than if the wound is left open. Animal bites are treated with penicillin.

BURN INFECTIONS

Second- or third-degree burns result in a loss of integumentary integrity and the opportunity for bacterial invasion. The most common initial organism is streptococcus, and therefore penicillin is given prophylactically. Daily wound care is given with debridement of all necrotic tissue. The wound is covered by mafenide acetate cream (Sulfamylon). Skin grafting is accomplished as soon as a granulating bed is obtained. All debrided skin should be sent for culture. Clostridial and fungal infections are not uncommon after extensive burns and are responsible for burn sepsis and death (see the chapter on *Infections in Burn Patients*).

VASCULAR ACCESS LINE INFECTIONS

The use of vascular lines for nutritional support and cancer therapy, usually in the immunodepressed or immunosuppressed patient, has given rise to a 5 to 10 percent incidence of line infections. These are usually caused by *S. aureus* or *S. epidermidis*. Ideally, the line should be removed. However, I often try a course of broad-spectrum coverage including vancomycin and gentamicin and repeat a line culture at the end of 10 days. Obviously, lack of improvement, progression of symptoms, or repeatedly positive cultures mandate removal (see the chapter on *Catheter-Associated Infections*).

SUGGESTED READING

Simmons RL, Howard RJ. Surgical infectious disease. New York: Appleton Century Crofts, 1982.

FEVER WITHOUT FOCAL INFECTION IN INFANTS AND TODDLERS

EUGENE D. SHAPIRO, M.D.

The evaluation and management of febrile children is one of the most common yet one of the most difficult clinical problems that physicians who care for children face. A small proportion of young children with fever and no apparent focus of infection who do not appear to be seriously ill have occult bacteremia and, of these, some may develop focal complications such as bacterial meningitis. Controversy persists over which diagnostic tests are indicated in the evaluation of febrile children as well as whether any such children should be routinely treated with antimicrobial drugs. Because these issues are beyond the scope of this chapter, the reader is referred to other reviews for a more complete discussion.

CHILDREN FROM 4 TO 12 WEEKS OF AGE

Compared with older infants, children between 4 and 12 weeks of age are at a greater risk of serious bacterial infection, a risk that increases with higher degrees of fever and decreases with increasing age. In addition, certain bacteria that may be responsible for infections in children of this age (such as group B streptococcus and *Listeria monocytogenes*) rarely cause invasive infections in older children. Furthermore, the clinical findings commonly used to assess whether or not a child has a serious infection are less reliable in younger infants.

Infants with fever should be evaluated carefully for an identifiable focus of infection. In addition to a history and physical examination, a specimen of urine should be obtained for both urinalysis and culture because of the possibility of a urinary tract infection. Because specimens obtained by the "bag" method are easily contaminated, if either the results of the urinalysis are abnormal or antimicrobials are to be administered to the child, an uncontaminated specimen of urine should be obtained (by either suprapubic aspiration or urethral catheterization) and cultured. A culture of the blood and a complete blood cell count with differential should be obtained and, in most instances, the child should undergo a diagnostic lumbar puncture.

If the child clinically appears to be seriously ill or the results of the laboratory tests are abnormal (e.g., definite leukocytosis of more than 15,000 white blood cells per cubic millimeter), I would hospitalize the child and treat with broad-spectrum antimicrobials. I prefer ampicillin (200 mg per kilogram per day, administered intravenously in divided doses every 6 hours) and cefotaxime (150 mg per kilogram per day, administered intravenously in divided doses every 8 hours). An alternative regimen, while awaiting the results of the cultures, is ampicillin and chloramphenicol (75 mg per kilogram per day, administered intravenously in divided doses every 6 hours).

If the cultures are sterile after 48 hours of incubation and the child's condition has improved clinically, I discontinue the antimicrobials and follow the child as an outpatient. If the cultures are positive, the child should be treated based on the antimicrobial susceptibility of the bacterial pathogen and the specific type of infection.

If the child does not appear clinically to be seriously ill and the laboratory investigations are normal, I may decide to follow the child closely without administering antimicrobials. I am more likely to do this with the older infant (e.g., an 11-week-old) than with a younger one (e.g., a 5-week-old). In some instances in which close follow-up can be ensured as an outpatient, hospitalization may not be necessary. Often, however, it is necessary to hospitalize the child for close observation. If the clinical condition deteriorates or a focal infection develops, appropriate antimicrobial therapy is begun promptly.

CHILDREN FROM 12 WEEKS TO 2 YEARS OF AGE

There is even more controversy about the proper evaluation and management of the febrile child in the 12-week-to-2-year-old age group than for the younger infant. High degrees of fever are more common in children of this age than in the younger child. Most of these illnesses are caused by self-limited viral infections, but approximately 3 to 5 percent of children in this age group with a temperature greater than 39°C and no apparent focus of infection have occult bacteremia caused by *Streptococcus pneumoniae, Haemophilus influenzae* type b, or *Neisseria meningitidis* (or, occasionally, *Salmonella* species). Although most recover uneventfully, a small proportion of these children develop a serious focal complication of bacteremia such as bacterial meningitis. In children with recurrent or prolonged fever, the possibility of an infection of the urinary tract should be considered and a specimen of urine should be obtained for analysis and culture.

My approach to the child of this age with fever and no apparent focus of infection is to assess carefully the child's well-being. (McCarthy has developed clinical scales to quantify a febrile child's clinical status.) Although febrile children with an elevated white blood cell count and/or an elevated erythrocyte sedimentation rate are at an increased risk of occult bacteremia, abnormalities of these tests are not very specific because 85 percent or more of the febrile children with abnormalities of these tests do *not* have occult bacteremia. Consequently, I find that these tests are rarely clinically useful. Rather, I depend on the clinical assessment of the child to guide decisions about management.

If the child does not appear to be seriously ill (and the results of the lumbar puncture, if it is deemed to be necessary, are normal) and I can rely on good follow-up, I will manage the child with close follow-up by telephone. Although some experts recommend that young febrile children with no focus of infection and leukocytosis be routinely treated orally with antimicrobials, I believe that there is little scientifically valid evidence that such treatment prevents focal complications of bacteremia. In addition, I am concerned that antimicrobial treatment is associated with some risk of adverse side effects and makes subsequent evaluation of the patient more difficult. For example, because it is more difficult to interpret the results of analyses of the cerebrospinal fluid of children who have been taking antimicrobials, a slight pleocytosis or a bloody tap at the time of follow-up in

such children is more likely to result in hospitalization and antimicrobial therapy for possible meningitis when such action otherwise would not be necessary. Furthermore, by producing a false sense of security in the parents or the physician, it may delay follow-up evaluation of a sick child.

Although taking cultures of the blood of such children at the initial visit have become routine at some centers, it should be remembered that culture of the blood is not a therapeutic maneuver. A culture of the blood that becomes positive in 12 to 48 hours may serve as a "red flag" to ensure that appropriate follow-up is performed. However, there is no evidence that febrile children who have had their blood cultured have better outcomes, fewer subsequent outpatient visits, or fewer diagnostic tests performed subsequently.

Rarely, over an adequate period of observation the child may appear to be seriously ill, although no focus of infection can be found. In this event I hospitalize the child and treat with cefuroxime (100 mg per kilogram per day administered intravenously in divided doses every 8 hours). The combination of ampicillin and chloramphenicol is an alternative regimen. A clinical impression that the child may be septic takes precedence over other data in the decision to initiate antimicrobial therapy. Finally, if I feel uncertain about the reliability of follow-up, I may have the child remain in the office, clinic, or emergency room for several hours. This gives me the opportunity to perform serial assessments over time and thus gain a better feeling for the severity of the child's illness. On occasion, it may be necessary to hospitalize the child for observation.

One should remember that no combination of clinical assessment or laboratory tests can infallibly identify the febrile child who is at risk of a serious bacterial infection. Consequently, careful clinical follow-up is of critical importance in managing these children.

SUGGESTED READING

Dagan R, Powell KR, Hall CB, Menegus MA. Identification of infants unlikely to have serious bacterial infection although hospitalized for suspected sepsis. J Pediatr 1985; 107:855–860.

DeAngelis C, Joffe A, Wilson M, Willis E. Iatrogenic risks and financial costs of hospitalizing febrile infants. Am J Dis Child 1983; 137:1146–1149.

DeAngelis C, Joffe A, Willis E, Wilson M. Hospitalization v outpatient treatment of young, febrile infants. Am J Dis Child 1983; 137:1150–1152.

Jaffe DM, Tanz RR, Davis AT, et al. Expectant antibiotic therapy for febrile children at risk for bacteremia. N Engl J Med, in press.

Kramer MS, Mills EL, MacLellan AM, Coates PJK. Effects of obtaining a blood culture on subsequent management of young febrile children without an evident focus of infection. Can Med Assoc J 1986; 135:1125–1129.

McCarthy PL, ed. The evaluation and management of febrile children. New York: Appleton Century Crofts, 1985.

Shapiro ED. Bacteremia in the febrile child. In: Aronoff SC, ed. Advances in pediatric infectious diseases, Vol 1. Chicago: Year Book Medical Publishers, 1986; 19–35.

ANTIBIOTIC PROPHYLAXIS

JEROME O. KLEIN, M.D.

Chemoprophylaxis implies use of an antimicrobial agent in anticipation of an infectious disease. The list of uses of antimicrobial agents for prevention of infection in children continues to expand, and appropriately so. Prevention is the most efficient mode of disease management. I have identified 11 uses of chemoprophylaxis for children that are of consistent and proven value, three uses that are recommended though not yet uniformly accepted, and two uses of potential value.

Indispensable sources for new and changing recommendations about chemoprophylaxis are The Redbook (Report of the Committee on Infectious Disease of the American Academy of Pediatrics), Morbidity and Mortality Weekly Reports (prepared by the Centers for Disease Control), and The Medical Letter (published by The Medical Letter, Inc. 56 Harrison St., New Rochelle, NY 10801).

CRITERIA FOR APPROPRIATE USAGE OF CHEMOPROPHYLAXIS

- The patient is at significant risk if infection occurs.
- The organism or organisms are consistently associated with the condition to be prevented.
- The drug to be used is uniformly effective against the organism.
- Prophylactic usage of the drug is unlikely to lead to microbial resistance.
- The drug has limited side effects or toxicity.
- The drug can be administered in a convenient form and dosage for a defined period of time.

CHEMOPROPHYLAXIS OF PROVEN VALUE

For prevention of group A streptococcal infection in patients with a history of rheumatic fever the drug of choice is penicillin G; alternative: sulfonamide.

It should be recalled that sulfonamides (including trimethoprim–sulfamethoxazole) are ineffective for treatment of streptococcal pharyngitis, although they are effective for streptococcal prophylaxis. Presumably the drug prevents implantation and colonization but is unable to combat established infection.

For prevention of bacterial endocarditis in patients with congenital heart disease and in patients with rheumatic or other acquired valvular heart diseases, the specific regimens and dosage schedules are revised periodically by the American Heart Association. The most recent recommendations appear in the chapter on *Rheumatic Fever.*

For prevention of neonatal ophthalmia, the drugs of choice are 1 percent silver nitrate solution, 0.5 percent erythromycin, or 1 percent tetracycline ointments applied once to the eyes immediately after birth.

Silver nitrate solution is ineffective for prevention of ophthalmia caused by *Chlamydia trachomatis;* erythromycin and tetracycline ointments are possibly effective against *C. trachomatis* (but there are conflicting data), but efficacy for prophylaxis against the gonococcus is unproved in randomized trials. To date, however, I am unaware of reports of gonococcal ophthalmia in infants receiving erythromycin or tetracycline ointments. If gonococcal disease is more important than *Chlamydia* in your area, silver nitrate is the preferred drug. If the rate of gonococcal disease is low, erythromycin or tetracycline ointments are probably preferable.

For prevention of meningococcal disease in contacts the drugs of choice are sulfonamide for susceptible strains or rifampin for sulfonamide-resistant strains. Rifampin, 10 mg per kilogram (maximum, 600 mg), is given every 12 hours for four doses. The sulfisoxazole dosage is 500 mg daily for infants less than 1 year, 500 mg every 12 hours for children from 1 to 12 years, and 1 g every 12 hours for older children and adults. Prophylaxis is given for 48 hours.

Household, day care, and nursery contacts should receive prophylaxis. Medical personnel should receive prophylaxis only if they have had intimate exposure, such as mouth-to-mouth resuscitation, intubation, or suctioning before the patient has received antibiotic therapy. Meningococcal vaccine should also be administered because of development of late cases among contacts.

For prevention of *Haemophilus influenzae* type b disease in household and day care center contacts, with at least one contact less than 48 months of age, the drug of choice is rifampin. The dosage is 20 mg per kilogram once daily (maximum, 800 mg) for 4 days.

Most experts agree on the use of prophylaxis in the household with a child younger than 48 months of age. The incidence of invasive disease in contacts in nurseries and day care centers appears to be less than that in households, but I would provide the same degree of protection to children who are exposed in the centers. The Redbook (1986) provides alternative proposals for day care centers: begin rifampin prophylaxis when two or more cases of invasive disease have occurred among attendees within 60 days; consider usage after the first case if the day care resembles a household (children younger than 2 years of age in which contact is 25 hours per week or more).

To eliminate colonization with *Bordetella pertussis,* the drug of choice is erythromycin (40 to 50 mg per kilogram per day in divided doses every 6 hours).

Whether or not erythromycin prevents disease is uncertain, but it is of value in eradicating carriage and preventing transmission of infection.

For prevention of malaria, the drug of choice is chloroquine, and pyrimethamine–sulfadoxine for travelers to chloroquine-resistant areas if they develop a febrile illness (see the chapter on *Protozoan Infections* for dosage regimens).

The Centers for Disease Control provides the invaluable service of having experts available by telephone to discuss information related to usage of drugs for parasitic information: during business hours, you can call 404/329-3670, and 404/329-2888 on nights, weekends, and holidays.

For prevention of tuberculous infection in household members and close associates, the drug of choice is isoniazid; rifampin is recommended for isoniazid-resistant organisms (see the chapter on *Tuberculosis* for criteria for usage and regimens).

For prevention of invasive disease in patients with sickle-cell disease or asplenia, the drug of choice is penicillin V, 125 or 250 mg twice daily.

A recent study sponsored by the National Institute of Health concluded that penicillin V, given twice daily, significantly decreased the frequency of pneumococcal disease. Penicillin V is uniformly effective against *S. pneumoniae* but much less effective against *H. influenzae* type b and the meningococcus than are ampicillin or penicillin G. Patients with sickle-cell disease or asplenia are susceptible to the encapsulated bacteria that cause invasive disease: the pneumococcus, meningococcus, and *H. influenzae.* Thus, history of the use of penicillin V prophylaxis should not limit aggressive response to the febrile infant. The best results, in terms of prevention or therapy for the child with sickle-cell disease, are achieved by a liberal policy of treatment with antibiotics even for trivial infections.

For systemic infection in patients with burns, the drug of choice is penicillin G.

Invasive group A streptococcal infection may occur during the first few days after a burn occurs. Prophylactic use of penicillin G for 3 to 5 days is warranted. Topical antisepsis, including silver sulfadiazine, is of demonstrated efficacy in preventing invasive infection from the wound surface.

For prevention of surgical wound infection, controlled clinical trials have established the value of antimicrobial prophylaxis for selected procedures. Antimicrobial agents used for surgical prophylaxis should provide an adequate concentration of active drug in the tissues at the time of the procedure.

CHEMOPROPHYLAXIS TO BE CONSIDERED FOR SELECTED PATIENTS

For prevention of recurrent episodes of acute otitis media, the drugs of choice are sulfisoxazole and amoxicillin.

In 1983 Dr. Charles Bluestone and I presented a response to the problem of the child with multiple episodes of acute otitis media that I continue to favor (see Suggested Reading). We recommended consideration of chemoprophylaxis for the child who had had three documented episodes of acute otitis media in 6 months or four episodes in 12 months. Sulfisoxazole (50 mg per kilogram) or amoxicillin (20 mg per kilogram) was suggested in a once-a-day dosage schedule during the winter and spring months (when respiratory tract infections are most common) for a period of up to 6 months.

For prevention of recurrent urinary tract infections, the drugs of choice are methenamine mandelate and trimethoprim–sulfamethoxazole.

Methenamine mandelate is a suitable agent for prophylaxis because it is bactericidal in an acid medium. Trimethoprim–sulfamethoxazole (1 mg per kilogram of the trimethoprim component at bedtime) is an effective alternative for the child who has difficulty taking sufficient mandelamine to maintain an acid urine (pH 5.5 or lower).

For prevention of influenza A infection, the drug of choice is amantadine, 5 mg per kilogram per day (maximum 200 mg).

Amantadine is administered during the period of exposure and may be considered in selected children at risk if infected by influenza virus (chronic cardiac, pulmonary, metabolic, or renal disease) who have not received influenza vaccine.

CHEMOPROPHYLAXIS OF POTENTIAL VALUE

To prevent perinatal group B streptococcal infection in the neonate, investigators have proposed giving penicillin G immediately after delivery to the newborn or ampicillin to women in labor who were colonized in the genital tract. Because the highest incidence of disease and the highest mortality occur within the first 24 hours in many centers, administration of a penicillin after delivery may not be as effective as the ampicillin regimen administered during labor. Different regimens may be applicable to different settings. At present, the most important issue for pediatricians is to meet with our obstetric colleagues to define a regimen that appears most appropriate for the local hospital.

To prevent invasive disease in children with acquired immunodeficiency disease (AIDS), frequent administration of intravenous immunoglobulin and prophylactic usage of trimethoprim–sulfamethoxazole have been advocated for infants with perinatally acquired AIDS. The experience with use of either method is still too limited to be considered other than investigational (see the chapter on *Acquired Immunodeficiency Syndrome*).

SUGGESTED READING

Boyer KM, Gotoff SP. Prevention of early onset group B streptococcal disease with selected intrapartum chemoprophylaxis. N Engl J Med 1986; 314:1665–1669.
Gaston H, Verter J, Woods G, et al. Prophylaxis with oral penicillin

in children with sickle cell anemia. N Engl J Med 1986; 314:1593–1599.

Klein JO, Bluestone CD. Acute otitis media. Pediatr Infect Dis 1982; 1:66.

Shulman ST. Committee on Rheumatic Fever and Bacterial Endocarditions of the Council on Cardiovascular Diseases in the Young. Prevention of bacterial endocarditis. Pediatrics, 1985; 75:603.

Siegel JD, McCracken GH Jr, Threlkeld N, et al. Single-dose penicillin prophylaxis of neonatal group-b streptococcal disease: conclusion of a 41 month controlled trial. Lancet 1982; 1:1426–1430.

IMMUNIZATIONS

COLIN D. MARCHANT, M.D.

Immunization has had impressive effects on the health of infants and children during this century. Those who care for infants and children must be familiar with active immunization of well children and those in high-risk groups. In addition, both active and passive immunization are used in the care of those exposed to specific infectious diseases. The reader should consult the chapters on *Pertussis, Diphtheria, Influenza, Viral Hepatitis, Infection Following a Bite, Bacterial Meningitis, Childhood Exanthems, Tetanus*, and *Varicella-Zoster Virus Infection*. The recommendations that follow correspond largely to those advocated by the American Academy of Pediatrics and the Immunization Practices Advisory Committee (ACIP) of the U.S. Public Health Service. Physicians should keep abreast of changes in immunization policies that appear in the journal *Pediatrics,* and in *Morbidity and Mortality Weekly Reports*. Moreover, new vaccines such as varicella and protein-conjugated *Haemophilus influenzae* type b, are under investigation and may be released in the near future. Physicians practicing in countries other than the United States should consult policies and recommendations of appropriate advisory bodies. Clinicians are also advised to be familiar with the products they use and to read the package inserts regarding dosages and method of administration.

Of particular concern is the issue of physician liability for damages suffered from adverse effects of immunizations, specifically those attributed to pertussis vaccine. Physicians must keep the interests of children first and foremost, but must also protect themselves from liability. To reduce the likelihood of legal action, I suggest that physicians (1) obtain informed consent for all immunizations, preferably in written form, (2) maintain excellent communication with parents, (3) keep careful records of immunizations, and (4) follow guidelines outlined by regulatory bodies, such as the American Academy of Pediatrics or the ACIP.

DIPHTHERIA–TETANUS–PERTUSSIS (DTP) VACCINE

The widespread use of vaccines for prevention of diphtheria, tetanus, and pertussis has been followed by impressive reductions in the incidence of these diseases. Thus, active immunization with combined DTP vaccine is recommended for normal infants and children younger than 7 years of age (Table 1). Com-

TABLE 1 Recommended Schedules for Active Immunization

Recommended Time	Immunizations
1. Normal Infants and Children	
2 months	Diphtheria–tetanus–pertussis (DTP) and oral poliovaccine (OPV)
4 months	DTP, OPV
6 months	DTP (OPV optional)
15 months	DTP, OPV, measles–mumps–rubella (MMR)
24 months	Haemophilus b polysaccharide vaccine (HBPV)
4–6 years	DTP, OPV
14–16 years	Adult tetanus–diphtheria toxoid (Td): containing not more than 2 flocculating units of diphtheria toxoid
2. Age Less than 7 Years: Not Immunized in Early Infancy	
First visit	DTP, OPV, MMR
Interval after first visit	
1 month	HBPV (if age 24–60 months)
2 months	DTP, OPV
4 months	DTP (OPV optional)
10–16 months	DTP, OPV
Before entry into school	DTP, OPV (not necessary if DTP and OPV have already been given after age 4)
10 years after last DTP	Td
3. Age 7 Years and Older: Not Immunized in Infancy	
First visit	Td, OPV, MMR
Interval after first visit	
2 months	Td, OPV
8–14 months	Td, OPV
Age 14–16 years	Td

bined vaccine consists of diphtheria and tetanus toxoids and inactivated *Bordetella pertussis* cells as adsorbed aluminum salts. The dose is 0.5 ml, administered by intramuscular injection. In infants, the anterolateral thigh is the preferred site for administration; the deltoid is preferred in older children.

Adverse reactions to DTP vaccine are related primarily to the pertussis component (Table 2). In addition, polyneuropathy, myelopathy, and encephalopathy have occurred following administration of tetanus toxoid. Despite recent publicity of adverse reactions to pertussis vaccine, careful analysis reveals that (1) morbidity and mortality are greater from the disease in unimmunized populations than from widespread use of vaccine, (2) universal immunization has substantial cost-benefit advantage, (3) because immunization has not interrupted transmission of the organism in immunized populations, the incidence of pertussis would be expected to rise if immunization rates declined. In recent decades, falling immunization rates in both Great Britain and Japan were followed by increased mortality from pertussis. For these reasons, continued use of pertussis vaccine is in the best interests of infants and children.

Although minor reactions occur frequently they do not contraindicate further immunization with pertussis vaccine. However, infants who experience these reactions are at increased risk of similar reactions with subsequent immunization. Minor reactions can be ameliorated by the use of analgesics, such as acetaminophen during the 48 hours after inoculation. The practice of giving a reduced dosage

TABLE 2 Adverse Reactions after Administration of Pertussis Vaccine*

Reaction	Percent per Dose of Vaccine
Local reactions within 48 hours:	
Redness	7.2
Swelling	8.9
Pain	51
Systemic reactions within 48 hours:	
Fever ≥38°C (100.4°F)	47
≥40.5°C (104.9°F)	0.3
Drowsiness	32
Fretfulness	53
Vomiting	21
Anorexia	6
Persistent crying	1
High-pitched, unusual cry	0.1
Convulsions	0.06
Collapse, shocklike state	0.06
	Frequency per dose of vaccine
Encephalopathy within 7 days	1:110,000
Permanent neurologic deficit	1:310,000

* Based on data of Cody CL, Baraff LJ, Cherry JD, et al. Nature and rates of adverse reactions associated with DTP and DT immunizations in infants and children. Pediatrics 1981;68:650; and Miller DL, Ross EM, Alderslade R, et al. Pertussis immunization and serious acute neurological illness in children. Br Med J 1981;282:1595.

TABLE 3 Contraindications to Use of Pertussis Vaccine

Encephalopathy within 7 days of previous DTP immunization
Convulsion with or without fever within 3 days of DTP immunization
Persistent, unconsolable screaming or crying for 3 or more hours within 48 hours of DTP immunization
High-pitched, unusual cry within 48 hours of DTP immunization
Temperature ≥40.5°C (104.9°F) within 48 hours of DTP immunization
Allergic reaction such as anaphylaxis after DTP immunization
Evolving neurologic disorder
Recovery from culture-proved pertussis

of DTP decreases the incidence of minor adverse reactions, but it has not been established that it either reduces the rate of serious reactions or provides adequate protection against disease. This practice therefore cannot be recommended.

Serious reactions to previous DTP immunization are contraindications to administration of further doses (Table 3). Children who have had culture-proved pertussis infection need not be immunized. Children who experience either diphtheria or tetanus, however, do require subsequent immunization with diphtheria and tetanus toxoids because the natural diseases do not confer immunity. When pertussis vaccine is contraindicated, children should receive diphtheria–tetanus (DT) vaccine, containing 7 to 25 floculating units (Table 4).

In infants and children with changing neurologic signs or loss of developmental milestones, pertussis immunization should be deferred until their condition stabilizes. Children with a personal history of convulsions should not be immunized until a progressive neurologic disorder has been excluded. Those with neurologic conditions that are associated

TABLE 4 Immunization Scheduling in Special Circumstances

Pertussis Vaccine Contraindicated: Immunize with DT
  Defer DT immunization until age 1 year, since risk of these diseases is remote during the first year of life
  Give DT, followed by a second DT 2 months later, and then a third dose in 6 to 12 months
  Give a booster dose of DT before entry into school if the third dose was given before the fourth birthday
Pertussis Vaccine Deferred and then Resumed
  The number of previous doses of DTP should be determined and then additional doses given to complete the series (see Table 1)
  A fifth dose of DTP should not be given if the fourth dose was given after the fourth birthday
Populations at High Risk for Pertussis
  During epidemics or in locations with a high prevalence of disease, immunization may begin at age 2 weeks

with seizures or that may undergo neurologic deterioration should be observed to establish that their condition is stable. In these instances, pertussis immunization should be reconsidered and instituted when an evolving neurologic disorder has been excluded. The physician must also consider the risks of pertussis when considering deferrment of the immunization. If the incidence of pertussis is high, the risk of exposure is high (e.g., day care or institutional care), or the child is at increased risk for severe disease (e.g., compromised respiratory reserve), then these factors must be weighed against the risks of immunization. Static neurologic disorders, including seizure disorders, do not contraindicate immunization with pertussis vaccine. Similarly, a family history of seizure disorder or other neurologic disorder is not sufficient reason to defer pertussis immunization. Prematurity is not a contraindication to immunization, and premature infants should receive DTP at the usual postnatal ages.

POLIOVIRUS VACCINE

The incidence of poliomyelitis in developed countries has been reduced dramatically by the use of either trivalent, attenuated, oral poliovaccine (OPV) or trivalent inactivated poliovaccine (IPV) given parenterally. Both vaccines induce systemic antibody formation to poliovirus types 1, 2, and 3, whereas OPV also induces intestinal mucosal immunity. Because OPV results in the spread of live attenuated vaccine strains to nonimmunized contacts, with subsequent development of immunity, it is believed to be more effective in populations in which 100 percent immunization rates cannot be achieved. For this reason, and because OPV is simple to administer, it is the preferred vaccine for use in the United States.

Immunization with OPV normally begins at age 2 months (see Table 1), but if the risk of poliomyelitis is high, such as in an endemic area or an epidemic period, OPV can be given at the time of discharge from the newborn nursery. However, a full schedule of OPV must be given later. A minimum of 6 weeks should elapse between OPV administrations, and multiple doses are required to develop immunity to all three viral serotypes. Breastfeeding does not interfere with the development of immunity.

Rarely, OPV is associated with paralytic disease similar to that caused by wild poliovirus. The risk is estimated to be 1 per 3.2 to 8 million vaccine doses distributed. Unimmunized adult contacts and immunocompromised patients are at increased risk of paralytic disease. The risks of OPV should be explained to parents, and informed consent should be obtained.

Inactivated polio vaccine (IPV) should be given to those who refuse OPV and those with contraindications (Table 5). Pregnant females should not be immunized with either IPV or OPV unless there is a substantial risk of poliomyelitis. A primary series of

TABLE 5   Contraindications to Oral Poliovaccine

Pregnancy (theoretic risk)
Immunodeficiency diseases or
  immunosuppressive therapy
Household members with immunodeficiency
  disease, altered immune status, or
  immunosuppression
Child with a family history of
  immunodeficiency

IPV consists of three subcutaneous immunizations given at 4- to 8-week intervals followed by a fourth dose 6 to 12 months after the third dose. A booster dose should be given before entry into school and every 5 years thereafter.

Since the risk of paralytic disease is increased in unimmunized contacts of infants and children given OPV, pediatricians should consider the status of household members. Adults should be informed of the small risk of paralytic disease from administration of OPV to their infant or child. The routine schedule of OPV for the infant should not be interrupted because there is an unimmunized or partially immunized adult in the household. Partially immunized adults should receive a booster dose of IPV. Unimmunized adults should receive three doses of IPV, given at monthly intervals. This is best accomplished by giving IPV to adult household members when the infant is discharged from the hospital, followed by a second dose 1 month later and a third dose at the time of the infant's first OPV.

MEASLES–MUMPS–RUBELLA (MMR) VACCINES

Incidence of measles and mumps has declined dramatically since the introduction of universal immunization in infancy. Rubella vaccine was licensed in 1969, and since then there has been an impressive decline in the congenital rubella syndrome. All currently licensed products are live attenuated vaccines. Measles and mumps vaccines are grown in chick embryo cultures, and rubella in human diploid cells. Because effective immunity is induced with combined vaccine (MMR), there is no justification for routine childhood immunization with the individual vaccines. To ensure potency, the vaccine must be stored at 2°C or colder and protected from sunlight. A single dose of MMR, 0.5 ml given subcutaneously, is administered at 15 months of age and produces longlasting immunity. Booster doses are not required.

Fever may be observed after use of MMR. Characteristically, fever begins 6 days following immunization and lasts for several days. Transient rashes may also be observed. Measles vaccine has been associated with diffuse retinopathy. Encephalitis and encephalopathy occur following an estimated

1:1,000,000 doses of measles vaccine. Central nervous system effects are rarely observed following administration of mumps or rubella vaccine. Lymphadenopathy, neuritic symptoms, joint pain, and arthritis have been observed following use of rubella vaccine. Transient arthritis is most often observed in postpubertal females 1 to 3 weeks after immunization. Rarely, vaccine strains of rubella virus (RA27/3) have been cultured from products of conception, and congenital rubella syndrome caused by the vaccine has not been observed. Administration of mumps vaccine has been followed by unilateral nerve deafness or orchitis on very rare occasions. All of these serious reactions have been temporally associated with the use of vaccines, but a cause-effect relationship has not been proved. Furthermore, morbidity associated with the vaccine is much less than that caused by the natural disease.

Because it is possible that concurrent viral infection can interfere with the immune response, MMR should be deferred in patients who are febrile. Like other live virus vaccines, MMR and its components are contraindicated in pregnancy and in the immunocompromised host (Table 6). Unlike OPV, the attenuated viral strains of MMR are not transmitted to household contacts, and therefore pose no risk to pregnant or immunocompromised household members. Immunization should be deferred for at least 3 months in patients who have received immunosuppressive therapy. Those who have received passive immunization with immunoglobulins or transfusions should also wait 3 months before receiving MMR. Anaphylaxis to contaminants from chick embryo cultures are extremely rare. Individuals with a history of anaphylaxis from exposure to egg products should be skin tested; if the test is negative, MMR can then be given.

In epidemic situations, measles vaccine can be administered as early as 6 months of age. However, if immunization is performed before the first birthday, reimmunization at 15 months of age is indicated. Revaccination with measles vaccine should also be considered for those who have (1) received immunoglobulin with vaccine, (2) received an unknown vaccine before 1967 in the United States, (3) received inactivated measles vaccine, or (4) received inactivated measles vaccine followed within 3 months by live vaccine. Recipients of inactivated measles vac-

cine may have local reactions and fever when given measles vaccine, and in rare instances, prolonged high fever and lymphadenopathy have been observed. Because natural disease produces more serious disease than that observed in those who have received the inactivated vaccine, however, revaccination with live measles vaccine is indicated.

Since the primary purpose of rubella vaccine is to prevent the congenital rubella syndrome, it is important that efforts are made to protect women who may become pregnant. Accordingly, vaccination before puberty of girls with rubella vaccine should be actively pursued. Because the clinical diagnosis of rubella is not reliable, vaccination should not be deferred. Only those known to have received vaccine or who have documented serologic protection should not be immunized. In addition, it is advisable to immunize workers in day care centers or institutions caring for children and health care personnel, to prevent spread of the disease. Antenatal screening to determine immune status is recommended, and although the vaccine should not be given to pregnant women, postpartum immunization is advised. If Rho (D) immunoglobulin is administered postpartum, then such individuals should be retested 6 to 8 weeks later to determine if rubella vaccination has induced a serologic response. Breastfeeding is not a contraindication to rubella immunization.

HAEMOPHILUS B POLYSACCHARIDE VACCINE (HBPV)

Purified *Haemophilus influenzae* type b capsular polysaccharide vaccine is recommended for the prevention of invasive disease caused by *H. influenzae*. Efficacy is supported by a single trial in Finland, which found the vaccine to be 90 percent protective in infants 24 months of age or older. Immunogenicity of the vaccine is age related, and response is poor in early infancy. Between ages 18 and 23 months, 56 percent of infants develop anticapsular antibody. However, the efficacy of the vaccine in this age group is uncertain. Immunization with HBPV is recommended for all infants at 24 months of age, and for those up to 60 months of age if not previously immunized. Use of HBPV in infants 18 to 24 months attending day care has been recommended but is controversial. The vaccine has been criticized because its use at 24 months of age prevents only about 25 percent of invasive *H. influenzae* disease. Despite this, careful analyses have shown that this practice is cost effective. New protein conjugate vaccines that induce immunity in the first 6 months of life are under development and are expected to displace HBPV. In the meantime, active immunization with HBPV at 24 months of age is the most prudent course of action.

Local reactions are transient and rarely last 24 hours. Fever of 38.5°C or greater has been observed in fewer than 1 percent of vaccinees. Anaphylaxis is

---

TABLE 6   Contraindications to MMR

Febrile illness (defer immunization)
Pregnancy
Immunodeficiency
Immunosuppressive therapy within past 3
   months
Immunoglobulin or transfusion within past
   3 months
History of anaphylactic reaction to egg
   products or neomycin

extremely rare. Infections resulting from *H. influenzae* have been recently reported in the first few weeks after immunization. The only major contraindication is age of less than 18 months.

In addition to universal immunization at 24 months of age, those who have experienced invasive *H. influenzae* before this age should be immunized, since they may not have developed protective antibody levels because of "immunologic immaturity." Similarly, those who received HBPV at 18 to 23 months of age should be reimmunized, but no sooner than 2 months after the first HBPV. A booster response is not observed with HBPV. Those at increased risk of *H. influenzae* disease may be immunized even if older than 60 months.

IMMUNOCOMPROMISED AND IMMUNOSUPPRESSED HOSTS

The decision whether or not to immunize immunosuppressed patients must take into consideration the nature of the underlying disease and the nature and duration of immunosuppressive therapy. Some general guidelines can be followed. Immunization with live virus vaccine should not be performed until at least 3 months after immunosuppressive therapy. In some instances, a longer period is required. An exception to this general rule is the use of varicella vaccine, but this vaccine is not yet licensed in the United States. Patients receiving large dosages of steroids for more than 2 weeks should also not receive live virus vaccines. Those taking intermittent or small dosages of steroids may be immunized. As noted earlier, members of a household with immunosuppressed patients should not be given OPV, although, MMR may be given to nonimmunosuppressed household members. Inactivated vaccine should be administered to patients despite concurrent immunosuppressive therapy. An exception to this is the use of influenza vaccine during periods of lymphopenia and neutropenia (less than 1,000 cells per cubic millimeter). (See the chapter on *Influenza* for the use of influenza vaccine.)

Children with anatomic or functional asplenia, (e.g., sickle-cell disease) are at increased risk of septicemia and meningitis resulting from such organisms as *Streptococcus pneumoniae, Haemophilus influenzae* type b, and *Neisseria meningitidis.* These children should receive pneumococcal vaccine, meningococcal vacine, and HBPV at age 24 months, given at different sites. These polysaccharide vaccines are among the safest immunizing agents and produce mild local reactions and occasionally fever. Pneumococcal vaccine is composed of purified capsular polysaccharide antigens of 23 pneumococcal serotypes. These serotypes account for almost all episodes of bacteremia and meningitis in children. A single injection of 0.5 ml,

either subcutaneously or intramuscularly, is recommended. Repeat immunization may produce severe local reactions and is not recommended routinely. Quadravalent meningococcal vaccine is a purified polysaccharide vaccine containing antigens from meningococcal groups A, C, Y, and W-135. Patients with Hodgkin's disease are also at risk for bacteremia caused by *S. pneumoniae* and *H. influenzae.* They should receive pneumococcal vaccine and HBPV at age 24 months. Immunization should be performed approximately 2 weeks before chemotherapy for Hodgkin's disease, as antibody response may be suboptimal. Alternatively, patients may be immunized 3 months following chemotherapy.

With the epidemic of acquired immunodeficiency syndrome (AIDS), physicians are increasingly confronting the question of immunization practices for infants and children, either exposed to the human immunodeficiency virus or with active disease. The ACIP has recommended specific immunization policies for this group of children. Those with AIDS should not receive live virus vaccines. They should receive inactivated vaccines according to the usual schedule, including DTP, IPV, and both HBPV and pneumococcal vaccines at age 24 months. In addition, they should receive inactivated influenza vaccine after age 6 months (see the chapter on *Influenza*). Children with asymptomatic human immunodeficiency virus infection may receive MMR, as recommended for normal children. They should receive all other routine immunizations except OPV. Since OPV virus strains may cause paralytic disease in household members with AIDS, IPV should be used instead.

Children with the nephrotic syndrome should receive pneumococcal vaccine when they are 24 months of age or older. However, protection against invasive pneumococcal disease will be incomplete. Children with congenital or acquired immunodeficiency should receive inactivated vaccines, although immunologic responses may be poor. Serologic responses should be monitored in these patients to determine the optimal management of exposures at a future time.

SUGGESTED READING

Diphtheria, tetanus, and pertussis: guidelines for vaccine prophylaxis and other preventive measures. MMWR 1985; 34:405–420.

Immunization of children infected with human T-lymphotropic virus type III/lymphadenopathy associated virus. MMWR 1986; 38:595–606.

New recommended schedule for active immunization of normal infants and children. MMWR 1986; 37:577–579.

Report of the Committee on Infectious Diseases, 20th ed. Elk Grove Village, IL: American Academy of Pediatrics, 1986.

Rutledge SL, Snead OC. Neurologic complications of immunizations. J Pediatr 1986; 109:917–923.

INFECTIONS ASSOCIATED WITH INTERNATIONAL TRAVEL

PHILIP S. LARUSSA, M.D.

When a parent requests advice on precautions to be taken before traveling to another country, the physician needs to consider the following questions: What precautions are required by regulation of the countries to be visited? What additional precautions would be advisable considering the risks associated with travel to these areas? When do these precautions need to be completed in relation to the departure date? Are there any contraindications to these precautions in the individual patient?

At the initial evaluation the physician should review the child's current health problems. If ongoing care is necessary while the patient is abroad, a detailed history and management plan should be prepared for the parent to carry along. Information on referrals to physicians in the areas to be visited can be obtained from the American embassy or from a number of medical assistance programs (see the CDC publication *Health Information for International Travel:* "If medical care is needed abroad"). The next step is to review the itinerary, including all transit points and the length of stay at each location, noting whether these are rural or urban areas. It is then necessary to determine what is required by the countries to be visited. At present, the only vaccinations required for entrance into a number of countries are yellow fever and cholera vaccines. Many countries may require vaccination only if the traveler is arriving from an area where disease is currently being reported.

Check both the annual publication *Health Information for International Travel,* to determine the requirements of specific countries, and the most recent biweekly *Summary of Health Information for International Travel* (Blue Sheet) to determine where disease is currently being reported. Both of these are published by the Centers for Disease Control, Division of quarantine. Other sources of current information include the *Morbidity & Mortality Weekly Report* (section titled International Notes/Quarantine Measures), which reports changes in vaccination requirements of individual countries; the World Health Organization; the consulates of the countries to be visited; and local health departments.

A timetable should be worked out in the months before departure to allow for optimal response to vaccinations and or immune globulin. Some of the questions to be considered are how soon and for how long after immunization vaccination is considered "valid" by the countries requiring it, and whether multiple doses are necessary or whether concurrent administration of other vaccines or immune globulin will have adverse effects.

In general, multiple vaccinations, both live and inactivated, can be given simultaneously at different sites. Vaccines with similar side effects should be spaced in time, if possible. There may be an immunologic advantage to separating vaccinations with live viruses by more than one month, if they are not given simultaneously. This is also true for yellow fever and cholera vaccines.

The immune response to inactivated vaccines (bacterial and viral), toxoids, and some live virus vaccines (OPV and yellow fever) is not affected by simultaneous administration of immune globulin. Other live viral vaccines (e.g., MMR) should not be administered within 3 months of receiving immune globulin, if possible. In this situation, protection should be provided with immune globulin alone or, if the child is thought to be at high risk for serious disease, in combination with the specific vaccine. The latter approach may result in a less-than-optimal response to the vaccine. If immune globulin must be given within 14 days after administration of a live virus vaccine, the vaccination should be repeated 3 months later.

GENERAL PRECAUTIONS

Food and Drink

Food and water are the most important vectors of agents causing bacteria-, viral-, and protozoa-induced diarrhea and other illnesses that can be spread by the fecal–oral route (typhoid fever, hepatitis A and non-A, non-B, etc.). Chlorinated water does not provide protection against Giardia, ameba, and some viruses. In areas where sanitation is inadequate, it is not safe to consume beverages, including ice, made from water that has not first been boiled or to eat raw vegetables, unpeeled fruit, or undercooked seafood. Drinks made with boiled water, carbonated bottled or canned drinks, beer, and wine are usually safe to drink. Water, including water used to brush teeth, should be boiled and allowed to cool. When this is not feasible, disinfection with 2 percent tincture of iodine (5 drops per quart of clear water, let stand for 30 minutes, or 10 drops per quart of cloudy or cold water, let stand for several hours) or tetraglycine hydroperiodide tablets (following manufacturer's instructions) provides safe drinking water. Infants who are not being breast fed should be given powdered formula mixed with water that has been boiled. It would be prudent to take along a supply of oral rehydration solution packets, which can be diluted in a quart of safe water.

Flora and Fauna

If hiking or camping in rural areas is planned, it would be advisable to inquire about local hazards.

Hikers should wear clothing that covers arms and legs and high-top hiking boots to minimize the risk of contact with mosquito and tick vectors, hazardous plants, and snakes. Because animal rabies is a problem in many parts of the world, one should avoid the temptation to pet seemingly docile wild animals even at the risk of losing a coveted photographic opportunity. All animal bites should be promptly cleansed with generous amounts of soap and water. Swimming may also be risky in areas with poor sanitation or where leptospirosis or schistosomiasis is endemic.

IMMUNIZATION AND PROPHYLAXIS

Routine Immunizations

Routine immunizations should be up to date, including required boosters. The prevalence of measles, rubella, and pertussis may be higher than in the United States. In developed countries vaccination against these pathogens may not be widespread, because of either targeting of vaccines to high-risk groups or fear of vaccine complications. In developing countries, where vaccines may not be available, the prevalence of these and other preventable diseases such as poliomyelitis may be much higher than in the United States.

Diphtheria, Tetanus, and Pertussis (DTP)

Decreased protection is likely if fewer than three doses have been given. Infants and children younger than 7 years of age who remain in areas of high risk should complete the series of three DTP's at 4-week intervals. Children older than 7 years should complete the primary series or booster with Td (adult type).

Measles

Infants younger than 6 months of age are generally protected by maternally derived transplacental antibodies and need not be vaccinated earlier than the routine schedule. Infants 6 to 11 months of age should receive measles vaccine before departure and should be revaccinated with measles-mumps-rubella vaccine (MMR) at 15 months of age or, if they are still residing in a high-risk area, at 12 months of age. Infants 12 to 14 months of age can be vaccinated with MMR and need not be revaccinated.

Mumps and Rubella

Because the risk of serious disease for children is small, vaccination of those under 12 months of age is not recommended.

Polio

Children traveling to areas of high risk who have completed the primary series (three doses of oral polio vaccine [OPV] at 6- to 8-week intervals) should receive a fourth dose before departure if at least 6 weeks have passed since the primary series was completed. If the primary series has not been completed, the child should receive one dose before departure and then complete the primary series and receive the fourth dose at 4-week intervals if he or she remains in an endemic area. The World Health Organization recommends that children less than 6 weeks of age traveling to endemic areas receive a dose of vaccine before departure and proceed with the preceding schedules depending on the length of stay in the high-risk area. It is important to note that the dose given in the first 6 weeks of life does not count as part of the primary series.

Children immunized under one of these modified protocols should complete their immunizations at the standard recommended intervals once they leave the endemic area.

Requirements of Countries to Be Visited

Yellow fever and cholera are currently the only diseases for which many countries require vaccination.

Yellow fever vaccine is available only at official yellow fever vaccination centers; local state departments of health can provide their locations. Cholera vaccine can be given by any licensed physician. Documentation of vaccination is required for both yellow fever and cholera vaccinations. The appropriate information should be entered on the International Certificates of Vaccination and validated by the official vaccination center for yellow fever and for other vaccines, by any physician or city, county, or state health departments that have the "uniform stamp."

Cholera vaccine is thought to be about 50 percent effective in preventing disease for a 3- to 6-month period. It is valid for 6 months beginning 6 days after primary vaccination or on the day of revaccination if it is within 6 months of the primary immunization. Yellow fever vaccine is valid for a period of 10 years beginning 10 days after primary immunization or on the day of revaccination if it is within 10 years of the primary vaccination. The vaccine is highly effective and may afford protection for as long as 30 to 40 years.

Precautions and Exemptions

Age

Because information on safety and efficacy is lacking, children younger than 6 months of age should not receive cholera vaccine. Yellow fever vaccine associated encephalitis is most commonly linked with vaccination before the age of 4 months. For this reason, immunization of children less than 6 months of age is not recommended. Children 6 to 12 months of age should be vaccinated only if they are traveling to endemic areas.

Hypersensitivity

The growth medium used to propagate some vaccines contain components capable of provoking anaphylaxis in sensitive individuals. Persons who have a history of anaphylactoid reactions to eggs, chickens, or their feathers should not receive vaccines containing egg antigens (yellow fever, measles, mumps, or influenza vaccines) without prior skin testing and desensitization if necessary.

Other vaccines contain preservatives or antibiotics. MMR (individual or combined) contains neomycin, and OPV contains neomycin and streptomycin. Immune globulin contains trace amounts of mercury (thimerosol), which may accumulate after repeated injections.

Components of the immunizing organism may cause serious reactions. Vaccines known occasionally to provoke serious reactions include DPT, both as a combined vaccine and as individual components (the pertussis component more often than the tetanus or diphtheria component). Cholera and plague vaccines rarely provoke serious reactions. Consult the Red Book (the Report of the Committee on Infectious Diseases, American Academy of Pediatrics) for current recommendations concerning contraindications to use of pertussis vaccine.

Immunocompetence

In general, children who are immunocompromised, because of either their primary disease or its therapy, should not receive live virus vaccines.

Pregnancy

The CDC recommends that women who are likely to become pregnant during the next 3 months not be given live virus vaccines. For women traveling to high-risk areas, vaccination should be postponed until the second or third trimesters, if possible. These recommendations are based on theoretical risk, not on evidence of teratogenicity. Therefore, the physician should weigh the risk of disease against the potential risk of the vaccine. Pregnant women who are staying in areas of high endemicity for yellow fever or poliomyelitis should be vaccinated. Live virus vaccines can be safely given to children whose mothers are pregnant.

If a child is thought to be exempt from a required vaccine, either on the basis of age or medical condition, the physician should prepare a signed and dated statement on official stationery explaining the basis of the exemption.

Requirements/Country of Origin

The United States requires no vaccinations for return to the country.

Advisable Precautions

Malaria Prophylaxis

Malaria is covered in detail in another chapter, but a few guidelines are presented here to aid in advising travelers to high-risk areas. Prevention of infection involves the following precautions. Because the Anopheles mosquito feeds in evening and nighttime hours, travelers can reduce their risk, especially in rural areas where the risk of transmission is highest, by reducing outdoor excursions during these hours, wearing clothing that covers as much of the body as possible when they are outdoors, and using an effective insect repellent. The CDC recommends repellents containing N,N-diethylmetatoluamide (deet). Sleeping quarters should be screened and mosquito nets should be used to enclose the bed. The CDC recommends indoor repellents containing pyrethrum.

Deciding on the proper prophylactic regimen is predicated on the risk of malaria in a given area, the presence of chloroquine-resistant *P. falciparum* (CRPF), the length of stay, the degree of endemicity in that area, and a history of allergies to any of the medications to be used. The physician should first review the itinerary and consult *Health Information for International Travel,* to determine the overall risk and the presence of CRPF, and then choose the appropriate prophylactic course from the CDC recommended regimens and precautions outlined here:

Regimen A: Areas with little or no CRPF—chloroquine, once weekly starting 1 to 2 weeks before departure and continuing for 6 weeks after an endemic area is left.

Regimen B: Less than 3 weeks stay in areas where CRPF is endemic—in addition to chloroquine, one dose per week, a treatment dose of pyrimethamine–sulfadoxine (e.g., Fansidar) should be provided to be taken if a febrile illness develops. In this situation, it should be emphasized that chloroquine should be continued and medical care sought to evaluate the severity of infection.

Regimen C: Three weeks or longer stay in areas where CRPF is endemic—if the risk of CRPF transmission is high, the use of both chloroquine and pyrimethamine–sulfadoxine once weekly should be considered in travelers who are not allergic to sulfonamides.

Primaquine taken once daily for the last 2 weeks of the 6-week posttravel period prevents relapses due to the extraerythrocytic stages of *P. vivax* and *P. ovale.* Children at risk for glucose-6-phosphate deficiency should be tested for this deficiency before they receive primaquine. Children younger than 8 years of age should not receive tetracycline and those younger than 2 months of age should not receive sulfonamide containing compounds (e.g., Fansidar).

Hepatitis

Travelers to developing countries who venture outside the major tourist accommodations are at risk to acquire hepatitis A and non-A, non-B hepatitis through contact with contaminated water, including ice, uncooked shellfish, or fruits and vegetables that are not cooked or peeled. Avoidance of these sources is the most effective means of prevention, but this may not be feasible in rural areas over an extended period of time. In this case, prophylaxis against hepatitis A with immune globulin is recommended. For travel in a high-risk area for 3 months or less, a single injection (IM) of 0.02 ml per kilogram of body weight is sufficient. For more prolonged periods 0.06 ml per kilogram, given in divided doses of volumes appropriate to the patient's size, should be administered every 5 months. The efficacy of immune globulin in the prevention of non-A, non-B hepatitis is not known.

Traveler's Diarrhea

This is usually a self-limited disease characterized by four or five loose stools a day, lasting 3 to 4 days. It is most commonly caused by enterotoxigenic *E. coli,* but may also be caused by a variety of other bacteria, parasites, or viruses. Precautionary measures, as outlined earlier, are effective in reducing the incidence and severity of disease. Prophylactic agents including antimicrobials (TMP/SMZ, doxycycline, halogenated hydroxyquinolines), antiperistaltics (diphenoxylate, loperamide), and bismuth subsalicylate are not recommended because of associated risks, including emergence of resistant bacteria, fungal overgrowth, and allergic and toxic reactions. For treatment, see the chapter on *Traveler's Diarrhea.*

Typhoid Fever

Typhoid fever is a problem in many areas of the world where contaminated food and water cannot be avoided. Although the vaccine is not required by any country, it is 70 to 90 percent effective and is advisable for children traveling to endemic areas. The primary series consists of two doses, given 4 or more weeks apart. Boosters are required at 3-year intervals. The dosage for both the primary series and the booster is 0.25 ml for children younger than 10 years of age and 0.50 ml for those 10 years or older. Combination vaccines (TAB) offer no protection against paratyphi A and B and no advantage over typhoid vaccine for protection against *S. typhi* infection.

Postvacation Records

Because the incubation period of many diseases may be longer than the immediate posttravel period (e.g., symptoms of malaria may not appear for months afterwards), parents should be advised to include the travel itinerary in their children's medical histories.

It is not possible to discuss all the risks encountered during international travel, but it would be prudent to consult the source material listed in the Suggested Reading section or an infectious disease specialist to assess the possibility of any additional problems that may be limited to a specific or to a particular area.

SUGGESTED READING

Health Information for International Travel 1986. Atlanta, GA: U.S. Department of Health and Human Services, Public Health Service, Centers for Disease Control, Center for Prevention Services, Division of Quarantine, HHS Publication No. (CDC) 86-8280.

Morbidity & Mortality Weekly Report (MMWR). Waltham, MA: Massachusetts Medical Society.

Report of the Committee on Infectious Diseases (Red Book), 20th ed. American Academy of Pediatrics, 1986.

Summary of Health Information for International Travel (Blue Sheet). Atlanta, GA: U.S. Department of Health and Human Services, Public Health Service, Centers for Disease Control, Center for Prevention Services, Division of Quarantine, HHS Publication No. 396.

NOSOCOMIAL INFECTIONS

CATHETER-ASSOCIATED INFECTIONS

ROBERT S. BALTIMORE, M.D.

Invasion of the body with any catheter carries the risk of producing infection. The magnitude of this risk is generally related to the duration of catheterization, the type of catheter, and the care that is taken to prevent infection. Even the best care, however, will not reduce the risk of infection to zero, and it is important to recognize and treat these infections promptly to minimize infectious complications.

In this chapter the major sources of catheter-associated infections discussed are intravenous and urinary drainage catheters. Other specialized catheters, including arterial and long-term intravenous catheters, are discussed briefly. Catheters used in the central nervous system are discussed in a separate chapter in this book.

It should be kept in mind that these are almost always nosocomial infections, and principles of prevention and susceptibility are in accord with nosocomial infection epidemiology and not community acquisition. Thus, patients who require a high level of supportive care, have received broad-spectrum antibiotics, and have had major surgery are more susceptible. Pediatric patients generally have a lower incidence of nosocomial infections than adults, but the principles of care and prevention of infection are similar. Pediatric patients who require high-level intensive care have an incidence of nosocomial infections similar to that of adults.

PERIPHERAL INTRAVENOUS INFUSION CATHETERS

Peripheral intravenous infusion catheters are the major source of intravascular catheter-associated infections. It is important to recognize that these catheters can either be the cause of a localized infection, the source of a blood-borne infection, or both. Catheter complications such as extravasation and phlebitis may mimic infection but most frequently are *not* associated with infection.

Treatment of infection associated with an intravenous infusion catheter consists first of removal of the catheter and then local and systemic therapy, if needed. Immunologically normal hosts may only require removal. The chance of curing an infection without removing the device is generally not worth the risk of treatment failure and spread of the infection.

At the time that catheter-associated infection is recognized, certain attempts should be made to identify the causative organism, the point of entry into the infusion system, and the extent of the infection. The blood should be cultured with at least two separate venipunctures to minimize the chance of falsely believing a contaminant to represent a true bacteremia, and to improve the yield. The skin at the site of the cannulation should be cleaned with an antiseptic, the cannula removed, and the tip cultured, preferably by rolling it across a blood agar plate. Growth of 15 colonies or more by this method of culture strongly suggests that the catheter itself is the source of the infection. If pus can be expressed from the cannulation site, it too should be cultured and Gram stained. If there is reason to suspect the infusate as a source of infection, the infusion apparatus, the bottle or bag of infusion fluid, and the infusate should all be cultured. These cultures should be performed by hospital epidemiologists, or by specially trained clinical microbiology technicians, and not at the bedside using blood culture bottles.

Local Treatment

Appropriate local therapy depends on the findings on physical examination. If the infection appears to be only cellulitis at the site of catheter insertion, and if there are signs of phlebitis but they are mild, local therapy should consist of warm soaks and elevation of the extremity. In children, anticoagulation for phlebitis is rarely necessary. If pus can be expressed from the catheterization site, this material should be cultured and Gram stained. Simple incision and drainage should be performed if an abscess has formed. Occasionally the complication of *septic thrombophlebitis* occurs, in which the vessel is thrombosed and there is pus in the vessel. This may respond to incision and drainage of the vessel plus systemic antibiotics, but sometimes ligation and removal of the affected vessel are necessary to treat this life-threatening infection.

Systemic Treatment

Antibiotics are the main systemic treatment for intravenous catheter-associated infection. In the case of a patient who has normal immunity, has no cardiac disease or intravascular appliance, and is only moderately ill, it is appropriate to remove the catheter, treat the local inflammation, follow the patient's vital signs, and perform blood cultures serially. Systemic antibiotic treatment should be commenced if fever and other vital signs do not normalize within a few hours, if there are signs of shock or impending shock, or if the underlying clinical picture suggests that a wait of even a few hours might result in septic complications. In these cases, antibiotic treatment is begun empirically, choosing the drug(s) according to the expected species and knowledge of antibiotic susceptibilities in the particular hospital. Although organisms may enter an intravenous infusion system at any junction of the system, the entry point of the catheter through the skin is the most important and organisms responsible for infection are usually skin flora. In addition, flora from the hospital's inanimate surfaces as well as from the hands of the hospital staff may colonize this junction. In practice, *Staphylococcus aureus* and *Staphylococcus epidermidis* most commonly cause intravenous catheter infections. In addition, one may encounter streptococci (especially enterococci), coliform gram-negative rods, and non-fermenting gram-negative rods such as *Pseudomonas* and *Acinetobacter* species. Skin anaerobes such as *Propionibacterium* and fungi, especially *Candida* species, may also be involved.

Although the Gram stain of material exuded around the catheter junction may give a clue to the etiology of the infection, antibiotic treatment is usually begun empirically, before the causative organism is isolated. Choice of empiric antibiotics may vary from institution to institution, depending on endemic flora and local customs. I generally choose a combination of an antistaphylococcal penicillinase-resistant penicillin, usually oxacillin, and an aminoglycoside, generally gentamicin.

Dosages for children, maximum doses, and dose intervals are shown in Table 1. One may need to modify these recommendations if local epidemiology suggests a high frequency of an unusual organism, organisms with unusual antibiotic susceptibility, or a cluster of infections in which the suspected source is the infusion fluid. In a hospital with a substantial prevalence of methicillin-, oxacillin-, and nafcillin-resistant staphylococci, vancomycin may be chosen as the initial antistaphylococcal agent. In the treatment of serious staphylococcal infections caused by staphylococci resistant to the penicillinase-resistant penicillins, cephalosporin antibiotics may be active in vitro but have questionable efficacy. In hospitals reporting frequent isolations of gentamicin-resistant gram-negative rods, amikacin may be substituted for gentamicin. All dosages should be adjusted appropri-

TABLE 1 Parenteral Antibiotics Commonly Used for Empiric Treatment of Intravascular Catheter-Associated Infections

Antibiotic	Pediatric Patients (mg/kg)‡	Adults	Dose Interval (hours)
Oxacillin Nafcillin Methicillin	150–200	8–12 g	4–6*
Vancomycin	40	2 g	6†
Gentamicin	5–7.5	5 mg/kg	8†
Tobramycin	5–7.5	5 mg/kg	8†
Amikacin	15–30	15 mg/kg	12†
Cephalothin	100	8–12 g	4–6*
Cefotaxime	100–200	8–10 g	4–6*
Ceftazidime	100–150	3–6 g	8

The header "Daily Dosage" spans the Pediatric Patients and Adults columns.

* Frequently the shorter dose interval is used at the initiation of therapy, and then the interval is lengthened after the infection has been fully evaluated and the patient's condition has stabilized.

† Because of nephrotoxicity/ototoxicity, dosage adjustments must be made when there is renal insufficiency.

‡ These are dosages for age greater than 1 month. Dosage must be adjusted for neonates. Range is for moderate to severe infection.

ately in newborns or in patients with renal failure. Though not generally cost-effective, third-generation cephalosporins such as cefotaxime or ceftazidime may be considered as single-drug therapy for presumed intravascular catheter-associated infection. For penicillin-allergic patients, the antistaphylococcal agent of choice may be a first-generation cephalosporin such as cephalothin, or it may be vancomycin; the latter is safest in patients who have had an immediate, major reaction to a penicillin.

In the absence of an unusually high frequency of fungal intravascular catheter-associated infections, empiric antifungal agents are not recommended. If *Candida* are recovered from a culture, but the patient has improved, antifungal agents can be withheld from an immunologically normal host and cultures obtained again to see whether the *Candida* has been eliminated by normal host defenses. In a compromised host, including very-low-birth-weight infants, I generally initiate treatment with amphotericin B as soon as there has been a significant isolation of *Candida*. Continuation of therapy often depends on whether there is evidence of disseminated candidiasis. Candidal exudates in the eye grounds, cutaneous lesions, and budding yeast forms in the urine indicate disseminated infections.

If bacteria are isolated from the blood, the catheter, or the wound, empiric antibiotic therapy should be altered and one should choose the least expensive, narrowest-spectrum agent that is most effective against the isolate. In addition, the dosage of antibiotic may also need to be modified. Dosages may need to be reduced for renal failure, or increased if meningitis, an isolate with a relatively high minimum inhibitory concentration (MIC), or a low blood antibiotic concentration is present. The dosages recommended for initiation of empiric therapy are sufficiently high that they would be appropriate should further tests and observations demonstrate endocarditis to be present. Spread of infection to an endothelial focus should be a concern in any bacteremic patient, but it is more likely to occur in patients with an intravascular or cardiac appliance, a central catheter with a tip in the heart, or congenital heart disease with a high-pressure jet flow. Endocarditis as a complication of a catheter-associated infection appears to be less common in children than in adults. If the patient has prolonged fever or positive blood cultures after appropriate therapy has been instituted, in addition to considering the possibility of another infection, one must search carefully for an undrained focus of infection associated with the catheter, such as a subcutaneous abscess or septic thrombophlebitis.

The optimal duration of antibiotic treatment of intravascular catheter-associated infections has not been established. It depends on individual factors, the most important of which is an estimation of the possibility of metastatic spread of the organism because of bacteremia. If endocarditis is suspected or documented, lengthy treatment (4 to 6 weeks) is recommended. If there is an endothelial focus of infection, but it can be removed surgically, the duration of treatment may be shorter. If there has been metastatic spread of infection to a distant focus, such as osteomyelitis, meningitis, or liver abscess, treatment should be of a duration appropriate for primary infection at that focus. In the past there was so much concern about *Staphylococcus aureus* bacteremia resulting in a metastatic endothelial focus that some authorities recommended at least 1 to 2 months of antibiotic treatment. Based on reports of good outcome with short-course therapy in low-risk patients who have intravascular catheter-associated staphylococcal bacteremias, treatment for 7 to 14 days is reasonable. Low risk for complications in intravascular catheter-associated infections is generally defined by the following criteria: normal host (no valvular heart lesions, intravascular appliances, or leukopenia, and normal immune defenses), primary focus of infection easily managed, prompt response to initial therapy, causative organism susceptible to the antibiotics chosen initially, and no evidence of metastatic infectious complications during the treatment period. In addition, some experts feel that patients who do not develop staphylococcal teichoic acid antibodies are at a low risk for occult metastatic infection.

Optimal duration of treatment is even less well established for species other than staphylococci. I generally follow the same guidelines as for staphylococcal infections but use the shorter end of the range for infections caused by species that are low virulence skin flora, providing there is no evidence of a significant local or metastatic infection. This generally amounts to at least 3 to 5 days of parenteral treatment after clinical resolution of symptoms in a low-risk situation.

OTHER INTRAVASCULAR CATHETERS

The principles of treatment for peripheral intravascular catheter-associated infections are also true for treatment of infections caused by arterial catheters, pressure monitoring devices, central catheters, and umbilical artery catheters. (There are some substantial differences in the treatment of infection associated with certain long-term central catheters, which are discussed in the next section.) Complications may be more common, such as endocarditis with intracardiac infusion and monitor catheters, or they may be more difficult to diagnose, such as phlebitis of thoracic and abdominal vessels. These catheters should all be removed as a first step in treatment. Semiquantitative cultures of the catheter tips may aid in determining the etiology of the infection. Because of the difficulty in replacing central and arterial catheters, it may be reasonable on occasion to replace the whole infusion or monitoring system *except* the catheter if there is no evidence that the catheter itself, the catheter tunnel, or the vessel are infected. If symptoms quickly abate, removal of the catheter may not be necessary. If symptoms persist, or if there is sustained bacteremia, the catheter should be removed. Such an approach would be reasonable only in an otherwise normal host whose symptoms are not severe. Pressure monitor devices have been associated with a high risk of nosocomial infection; extra precautions for their use are listed in the section on Prevention of Catheter-Associated Infections.

Umbilical artery catheters have been shown to have a high rate of bacterial colonization and to be associated with infections as frequently as other catheters used in intensive care situations. Because these catheters are opened for blood gas determination as well as heparin flushes, opportunity for the introduction of microorganisms is high. Neither prophylactic antibiotics nor special care of the umbilical stump has been clearly associated with a reduction of the infection rate. The safe limit of catheter duration has never been established. In other respects the approach to infection associated with these catheters is similar to other central catheters.

INDWELLING CENTRAL CATHETERS (BROVIAC, HICKMAN, ETC.)

Management of infections associated with indwelling central catheters differs from that of other catheter-associated infections. These systems are designed to provide a physical barrier between the skin–catheter junction, where microorganisms most frequently enter the system, and the catheter tunnel. There is also a long subcutaneous tunnel between the skin end and the point of insertion into a large vessel. Most patients who have such devices are being treated for malignancies, are receiving total parenteral nutrition, or have other severe chronic diseases that make them compromised hosts. Nevertheless, as a result of treatment trials of catheter-associated bacteremia *without* removal of the catheter, it often appears to be reasonable to try to "save" the catheter by treating the patient with intravenous antibiotics delivered through the catheter.

Infection associated with this type of device can be located at the skin exit site, in the tunnel, on the catheter tip, or within the blood vessel (septic thrombophlebitis). Organisms associated with infection are similar to those that cause infection with peripheral intravascular catheters, except that *Staphylococcus epidermidis* clearly predominates, with *Staphylococcus aureus* being the next most common pathogen. In some series *Klebsiella,* enterococci, and *Candida* infections are also common. Infections with more than one species are occasionally seen. Multiple blood cultures should be performed to document whether there has been bacteremia or fungemia. In addition, we have found that simultaneously performing quantitative blood culture from blood drawn through the catheter and blood obtained through a percutaneous venipuncture at a distant site is useful in distinguishing between bacteremia originating from a vegetation on the catheter and bacteremia from another source. Colony counts many times higher from blood drawn through the catheter suggests that the catheter itself is the source.

The most important initial decision in the management of an infection associated with one of these devices is whether immediate removal of the catheter is necessary. Only limited data are available on the success rates in treating different species and different sites of infection without removal of the catheter. At this time, the following are believed to be contraindications to treatment *without* removal: frank or impending septic shock, obvious infection in the catheter tunnel, either fungal infection of the catheter itself or invasive infections around the catheter, obstruction of the catheter that does not respond to treatment with a thrombolytic agent such as urokinase, and recurrence of infection with the same strain of bacteria or fungi.

Superficial skin infection at the exit site is usually managed without removal of the catheter. If treatment without removal of the catheter is chosen, the following are indications for delayed removal of the catheter: continued fever without another source, continued signs of sepsis, continued bacteremia beyond 48 hours, purulence at the site of the catheter exit that does not respond quickly to antibiotics and local treatment, evidence of phlebitis or a vegetation that cannot be dissolved.

Generally, the choice of antibiotics follows that outlined previously for intravascular peripheral catheters with the antibiotic being delivered through the infected catheter. The predominance of *Staphylococcus epidermidis* infections and the high prevalence in many medical centers of resistance to methicillin, oxacillin, and nafcillin among this species may make vancomycin the drug of choice for empiric therapy.

One should switch to a penicillinase-resistant penicillin later if the isolate is susceptible to an antibiotic of that class, or to penicillin G if the isolate is penicillin-susceptible. Hospitals should regularly compile the susceptibility profiles of important isolates to guide practitioners in making this kind of decision. Optimal length of treatment is unknown. If the catheter is removed and there are no complications, short (i.e., 7 to 14 days) treatment is generally effective. If the catheter is not removed or if there are signs of septic emboli, septic thrombophlebitis, or concern about mural or valvular endocarditis, a longer course, of 2 to 6 weeks, should be used.

URINARY DRAINAGE CATHETER-ASSOCIATED INFECTIONS

In general, the chances that use of a urinary drainage system will result in a catheter-associated infection are related to the sterile technique used in insertion of the catheter, the quality of care in management (especially in maintaining the closure of a closed system), and the length of catheterization. Except in carefully managed, intermittent catheterization programs, infection is inevitable with catheters that remain in place for more than a few weeks. The use of prophylactic antibiotics in closed systems, administered either systemically or via the catheter, is not recommended and may result in colonization with antibiotic-resistant microorganisms.

Treatment

There are three clinical situations, each of which requires a different response: (1) the infection is diagnosed after the catheter has been removed; (2) the infection is diagnosed shortly before the expected removal of the catheter; or (3) the infection is diagnosed in a patient who is expected to require chronic catheter drainage. Whether or not the patient is symptomatic also affects treatment decisions.

1. If a patient is found to have a urinary tract infection following the removal of a catheter and is symptomatic, empiric treatment should be instituted for a hospital-acquired urinary tract infection. If only lower tract disease is suspected, but the patient is symptomatic, parenteral treatment should be begun because of the necessity of using agents that are effective against resistant hospital flora. Oral treatment may be possible later, if there is clinical response and an isolate from the urine is susceptible to an oral agent concentrated in the urine. If the Gram stain of the urine shows either gram-negative rods or no bacteria, a combination of ampicillin, 50 to 100 mg per kilogram per day in divided doses every 4 to 6 hours up to 2 to 4 g, depending on the severity of infection, plus gentamicin, 5 mg per kilogram per day in divided doses every 8 hours, is recommended. If gentamicin-resistant organisms are a concern, tobramycin,

amikacin, or a third-generation cephalosporin such as cefotaxime or ceftazidime is recommended (dosages at the lower end of the range shown in Table 1 for the treatment of intravascular catheter infections). If infection is limited to the urinary tract, dosages need only be moderate because these agents are concentrated by the kidney, except in patients with renal failure. If cultures or the Gram stain suggest *Staphylococcus,* or if the infection occurs shortly after urinary tract surgery, an appropriate antistaphylococcal penicillin or vancomycin should be added. For treatment of *Pseudomonas aeruginosa* infections, I prefer an antipseudomonal penicillin such as mezlocillin, piperacillin, or ticarcillin plus an aminoglycoside such as gentamicin. An alternative is ceftazidime, which is easier to use than aminoglycosides in patients with renal failure. If infection is uncomplicated and limited to the urinary tract, 10 days of treatment is generally sufficient. If there is significant upper tract disease, stones, obstruction, or a foreign body, surgical intervention and a longer treatment course may be necessary.

2. If asymptomatic bacteriuria is diagnosed while the catheter is still being used, removal of the catheter may be the only treatment necessary. With symptomatic infection when the catheter is expected to be removed within a few days, it is reasonable to initiate antibiotic therapy prior to its removal and to continue treatment after it is removed, according to the preceding schedule.

3. If a patient has a chronic indwelling catheter, management of infection must be individualized. It is generally not in the patient's interest to treat asymptomatic bacteriuria. The reason for this is that reinfection or recurrence is inevitable and a new infection is often caused by an organism that is less susceptible to antibiotics. Generally, treatment is reserved for symptomatic episodes and must be tailored to the antibiotic susceptibility of the patient's isolate and past responses to treatment. This is true of urethral and suprapubic catheters and of nephrosotomy drainage systems.

PREVENTION OF CATHETER-ASSOCIATED INFECTIONS

Intravascular Infusion Catheters

1. Intravenous catheters should be inserted only when clearly needed. In general, "keep open" intravenous infusions should be discouraged if they are for the convenience of the medical staff.
2. Steel needles rather than plastic catheters are generally preferred because of a lower incidence of infection.
3. Because intravenous cannulation of the lower extremities has been associated with a higher incidence of infection, this location should be avoided, if possible.

4. Cannula insertion should be performed under aseptic conditions with effective antisepsis of the skin, preferably with tincture of iodine or iodophor, ideally using sterile gloves and drapes. Cannulas inserted using less strict techniques under emergency conditions should be replaced as soon as possible after the patient is stable.
5. Cannulas should be anchored to prevent to-and-fro movement. Antibiotic ointment at the puncture site has not been proved to prevent infection, and its use is elective.
6. The infusion site should be covered with a sterile dressing and the date and time of insertion noted by writing it on the dressing.
7. Intravascular administration sets should be changed every 48 hours.
8. Peripheral intravascular cannulas should be changed every 48 to 72 hours.
9. Intravascular infusion fluid should be changed at least every 24 hours.

Arterial Pressure Monitor Catheters

1. These catheters should be calibrated and used only by specially trained staff who are aware of the risk of infection.
2. Pressure transducers should be cleaned with soap and water, rinsed, and then sterilized with ethylene oxide or glutaraldehyde between uses. Disposable chamber domes should not be reused.
3. The junctions of the system should not be opened for routine blood drawing, administration of medications, or other procedures, because each intrusion of the system increases the risk of infection.
4. Catheters and connecting equipment should be replaced frequently according to the guidelines for intravascular infusion catheters.

Urinary Catheters

1. Indwelling urinary catheters should be used only when medically indicated, and never solely for the convenience of nurses or physicians. In-and-out straight catheterization is associated with a much lower infection rate.
2. Urinary catheters should be inserted only by adequately trained individuals, preferably by a team trained for insertion and maintenance.
3. Catheters should be aseptically inserted, using sterile gloves, fenestrated drape, sponges, iodophor cleansing solution, and lubricant jelly. Catheters should be secured to prevent to-and-fro movement and urethral traction.
4. Once or twice a day, the meatal-catheter junction of catheter patients should be cleansed with an antiseptic soap, and an antimicrobial ointment may be applied.

5. A sterile closed drainage system should always be used. Any breaks in continuity of the system should be avoided. If irrigations must be performed, a triple-lumen catheter is preferred, but may not be possible in very small patients.
6. Urine for culture should be aspirated from the distal catheter using a syringe and needle after the catheter is disinfected. Other urine specimens should be obtained from the drainage bag using careful sterile technique.
7. The collecting system must be downhill, with bags always remaining below the level of the bladder.
8. Closed collecting systems should be replaced if inadvertent contamination or a break in the system occurs.
9. Routine use of antibiotic irrigation in a well-maintained *closed* system does not lower the infection rate and may predispose to more frequent infections with antibiotic-resistant microorganisms.

SUGGESTED READING

Baltimore RS. Nosocomial infections in the pediatric intensive care unit. Yale J Biol Med 1984; 57:185–197.

Iannini PB, Crossley K. Therapy of *Staphylococcus aureus* bacteremia associated with a removable focus of infection. Ann Intern Med 1976; 84:558–560.

Maki DG, Weise CE, Sarafin HW. A semiquantitative culture method for identifying intravenous-catheter-related infection. N Engl J Med 1977; 296:1305–1309.

Sheagren JN. Medical progress: *Staphylococcus aureus:* the persistent pathogen (second of two parts). N Engl J Med 1984; 310:1437–1442.

Stamm WE. Guidelines for the prevention of catheter-associated urinary tract infections. Ann Intern Med 1975; 82:386–390.

Stein JM, Pruitt BA Jr. Suppurative thrombophlebitis. A lethal iatrogenic disease. N Engl J Med 1970; 282:1452–1455.

INFECTIONS IN BURN PATIENTS

JOHN L. HUNT, M.D.
GARY F. PURDUE, M.D.

Infection is the most significant problem complicating a burn injury, accounting for 75 to 85 percent of deaths in these patients. The increased risk of infection is proportional to the extent of the burn and in part reflects a profound state of immunosuppression of both the humoral and the cell-mediated components of the immune system. The wound is an ideal site for microbial invasion and should never be considered sterile. Appropriate wound care is essential to proper patient management. This includes routine monitoring of the bacterial flora of the wound with frequent cultures, application of appropriate topical antimicrobial agent(s), expedient debridement of all necrotic tissue, and closure of the wound at the earliest possible time.

Burn depth as well as the extent of the burn, measured as a percentage of the total body surface injured, determines the severity of the injury. In spite of topical antimicrobial agents, both second- and third-degree burns can and do become infected, third-degree burns being more susceptible. The amount of necrotic tissue is obviously greater in the latter, in which case there is no possibility of spontaneous wound healing. A second-degree burn heals.

CLASSIFICATION OF BURN WOUND INFECTIONS

Colonization Only

Colonization represents a noninvasive infection. Usually only one organism predominates. The appearance of the wound is unrevealing, although slightly more exudate than normal may be evident in the dressings.

Burn Wound Invasion

The wound may exhibit a benign appearance. Quantitative biopsy and histologic examination of wound specimens are important. This is especially true for the majority of wounds infected with gram-negative organisms. The microbial invasion may be local, multifocal, or generalized.

Burn Wound Sepsis

Clinical signs and symptoms of septicemia occur in association with histologic evidence of bacteria invading viable tissue.

DETECTION AND MANAGEMENT OF WOUND INFECTION

Both qualitative and quantitative cultures are employed to monitor the bacterial flora of the wound. Cultures are taken two to three times a week or as indicated if either the gross appearance of the wound or the patient's clinical condition changes.

One culture is taken for each 15 percent total body surface burned. Qualitative cultures are used only to identify surface microbes. A RODAC plate (65 by 15 mm) is used. Growth is reported as light, less than one-fourth of the plate occupied by organisms, medium with one-fourth to one-half, and heavy with three-fourths to all of the plate occupied by organisms.

Quantitative burn wound biopsies are obtained only on third-degree burns. A 1-cm square piece of the eschar is excised down to and including underlying viable tissue. Results are reported as the number of organisms per gram of tissue. A quantitive count of 10^5 organisms per gram of tissue or greater represents a significant microbial population. The total body surface area burned must also be considered. A 70 percent burn with 10^3 organisms per gram of tissue represents just as much of a threat to developing sepsis as a 15 percent burn with 10^8 organisms. There is a delay of from 24 to 48 hours from the time of biopsy to time of reporting. During that time the log count of the wound may have doubled. The quantitative culture does not provide information as to the depth of microbial invasion. Confirmation of burn wound invasion can be determined only by histologic means.

Although the majority of organisms cause no change in the gross appearance of the eschar, there are changes in the wound that make one suspicious of wound sepsis (Table 1).

Burn wound cellulitis, which occurs with equal frequency in second- or third-degree burns, is characterized by an erysipeloid wound margin. It commonly occurs within the first week after a burn. The incidence increases in direct proportion to the size of the burn. If cellulitis is not treated, the erythema advances peripherally. The surrounding unburned skin becomes edematous and is usually only minimally tender.

Burn wound sepsis caused by *Pseudomonas aeruginosa* has a characteristic clinical appearance. The wound margins initially appear violaceous, or discrete round lesions may appear singly or in multiples anywhere—on unburned skin and healed burn. The lesions turn dark red or black, become papular, and then develop a central vesicle or bulla. Necrosis of the area occurs over 24 to 48 hours. There is rapid deterioration of the granulation tissue followed by patchy black tissue necrosis. Multiple lesions often coalesce quickly, and all lesions can be present simultaneously. This is termed ecthyma gangrenosum.

Blood cultures are of very limited value in recognizing septic complications originating in the wound. Positive cultures are often not recovered until 5 to 7 days after burn wound invasion is documented.

Generalized burn wound invasion is considered present when greater than 20 percent of the total body surface burn is infected. Septicemia is present in more than 90 percent of these patients, whereas with focal wound invasion septicemia is present in fewer than 20 percent.

Early systemic manifestations of infection are subtle at best and in the very young child are easily missed. The clinical signs of systemic sepsis include disorientation, tachycardia, hyperventilation, either hypothermia or hyperthermia, paralytic ileus, leukopenia, thrombocytopenia, and hyperglycemia. Other etiologies must be ruled out before the wound can be considered the source of the infection.

Unfortunately, a variety of factors in the burn patient can obscure these signs. Hyperthermia up to 39°C, tachycardia, and hyperventilation are a normal response in the hypermetabolic burned child. Hyperventilation can also be caused by an inhalation injury, mafenide acetate, and the pain associated with the injury. The frequent use of narcotics, and cerebral edema associated with resuscitation, affect the central nervous system. Leukocytosis may be an unreliable indicator of sepsis because there is an early postburn leukocytosis followed by leukopenia, and then a rebound leukocytosis. A leukopenia is often associated with gram-negative sepsis, but it may also be associated with the use of silver sulfadiazine burn cream.

Children commonly have a fever in the first 24 to 72 hours after the burn. A temperature of 39°C or higher may not be caused by infection. This is common with partial thickness burns—especially scald injury. If the fever continues beyond this time, is it then a preductor of infection? With children younger than 4 years, or if the burn covers more than 20 percent of the total body surface area, a temperature of greater than 39°C is not significant in identifying patients with an infection.

The type of microbes and their antibiotic susceptibilities vary from one institution to another. The early burn wound flora is usually monomicrobial with gram-positive organisms. *Staphylococcus aureus* and enterococcus predominate during the first 7 to 10 days. With the currently used topical antimicrobials, beta-hemolytic streptococci are virtually never cultured from the burn.

After the first postburn week, gram-negative pathogens begin to colonize the wound. These commonly include *Pseudomonas aeruginosa, Klebsiella,*

TABLE 1   Clinical Signs of Burn Wound Infection

Conversion of partial-thickness to full-thickness burn
Deterioration of granulation tissue
Premature separation of eschar or subeschar
　　suppuration
Focal black or brown discoloration of eschar
　　(*Pseudomonas*/fungi)
Hemorrhagic discoloration of underlying fat
　　(*Pseudomonas*/fungi)
Yellow soft eschar (*Candida*)
Vesicular lesions in both healing and healed second-
　　degree burn (virus)

TABLE 2 Common Signs and Symptoms of Burn Wound Infection

| | Type of Infecting Organism | | |
Factor	Gram-Positive	Gram-Negative	Fungal
Onset	1st week	1st week on	Late
Wound	Normal	Deterioration	Yellow, soft
Disorientation	Slight to severe	Severe	Mild
Temperature	Hyperpyrexia	Hyper/ hypothermic	Variable
WBC	Increased	Depressed	Variable
Platelets	Normal	Very depressed	Low
Ileus	Early/insidious	Severe	Mild
Hypotension	Late	Sudden/oliguria	None

Enterobacter, Proteus, Escherichia coli, Providencia, and *Acinetobacter.* Late colonizers include yeasts and fungi (Table 2).

Although invasive burn wound infection is not as common now that there are topical antibacterial agents, none sterilizes the wound. The pediatric patient with a burn of more than 30 percent is very susceptible to sepsis.

Silver sulfadiazine is the most commonly used agent of the three topical agents listed in Table 3 because of its good antimicrobial spectrum and lack of significant side effects. It is ideal for both inpatient and outpatient burns. Outpatient dressings are changed twice a day. For inpatients, an open dressing technique is used. Either no dressing is used over the cream or, in the case of very young children and infants, a single layer of gauze is used to cover the cream. For burns over 20 to 25 percent of the body, the dressing is changed three times a day.

Mafenide acetate (Sulfamylon) is very effective against *Pseudomonas.* Caution must be exercised when using it on a burn covering more than 20 percent of the body, because metabolic acidosis occurs if the compensatory hyperventilation is ineffective in countering the carbonic anhydrase inhibition caused by the drug. This is most likely to occur with a pulmonary complication (inhalation injury, bronchopneumonia, or atelectasis). It is not recommended as initial therapy on second-degree burns in children because the acid pH and high osmolarity of the drug cause intense pain.

Silver nitrate must be used with an occlusive dressing. This limits the motion of involved joints and is associated with transeschar loss of Na^+, K^+, Ca^{++}, and Cl^-. This can rapidly cause electrolyte abnormalities in very small children. The agent precipitates on the surface of the wound as silver chloride (AgCl) and therefore does not penetrate the eschar. It is a very effective agent that can be used on freshly grafted wounds.

Careful examination and culture of burn wounds are the best means of diagnosing wound infection. Unless there is a preexisting medical condition, prophylactic antibiotics, specifically penicillin, are not administered for either inpatients or outpatients.

Effective control of the microbial flora in the burn wound with topical therapy creates an eschar that is dry and hard. The color changes little after the first few days following the injury. Hemorrhage into the wound or maceration in areas of pressure (posterior portions) is commonly seen and generally does not signify infection. Eventually bacterial autolysis of the eschar occurs at the viable–nonviable interface. When this begins, the wound becomes soft and, unless timely debridement of the eschar is carried out, subeschar suppuration ensues. This commonly begins between the third and fourth week postburn. At this time wound cultures often reveal a polymicrobial bacterial flora, with one organism predominating. *Candida* species are often present. Granulation tissue now begins to appear. Although bacteria are present, healthy granulation tissue resists invasion by bacteria.

Burn wound cellulitis often has to be treated without knowledge of the organism and its antibiotic susceptibilities. Consequently, it is important to

TABLE 3 Topical Antimicrobial Agents

Agent	Chemistry	Advantages	Disadvantages
Silver sulfadiazine	1% in H_2O-miscible base	Broad-spectrum Painless Bacteriostatic	Poor penetration 10% absorbed Resistance by some *Pseudomonas* species and *Enterobacter* Early neutropenia Hypersensitivity (rare)
Mafenide	10% in H_2O miscible base	Broad-spectrum Good penetration Bacteriostatic	Painful Carbonic anhydrase inhibition Hypersensitivity (7%)
Silver nitrate	0.5% solution	Broad-spectrum Painless Bacteriostatic	No eschar penetration Electrolyte abnormalities (Na^+, K^+, Cl^-) Bulky dressing Discolors wound, environment

know the endemic microbial population of the unit and its antibiotic susceptibilities. A first-generation cephalosporin is recommended. Once the culture results are known, the drug can be changed if necessary. In the presence of a normal-appearing wound, if more than two qualitative cultures reveal moderate or heavy growth or quantitative cultures reveal more than 10^2 organisms per gram of tissue, in the absence of systemic signs of sepsis, the appropriate antibiotic is begun systemically. Because the burn wound is often colonized by more than one organism, or the endemic microbial population may have developed resistance to different antibiotics, single-agent therapy may not be adequate.

The antibiotic therapy in the burn patient is further complicated in that the half-life of aminoglycosides is decreased to 1 to 1.5 hours. This appears to be a result of both a loss of the drug through the wound and increased renal elimination concomitant with increased creatinine clearance. Peak and trough serum concentrations must be measured several times each week in these hyperdynamic, hypermetabolic patients. To minimize the renal effects, the patient's intravascular volume must be normal before and during the use of the antibiotic.

When burn wound sepsis has developed in a patient who has been treated with silver sulfadiazine, mafenide acetate is substituted. If bacteriologic data are not available, an aminoglycoside antibiotic, along with a semisynthetic penicillin, is used for gram-negative coverage and an antibiotic effective against gram-positive organisms is also added. If culture results reveal that the organism is susceptible to the semisynthetic penicillin, then subeschar clysis of that drug is begun. This technique permits delivery of a high concentration of the antibiotic into the avascular burn wound. The calculated daily dosage of the drug is diluted in 250 to 500 ml of half-normal saline. It is injected using a pediatric drip-set with a 22-gauge needle. Twenty-five milliliters is delivered into the subeschar space at 7.5-cm intervals twice a day. After 24 to 48 hours of therapy, burn wound excision, often to fascia, is performed. The wound is then covered with homograft.

The emergence of nonbacterial organisms as frequent colonizers of the burn wound is associated with the use of topical antibacterial agents. *Candida* species represent the most common of the nonbacterial colonizers, being reported in as many as 64 percent of pediatric patients. Although *Candida* usually remains confined to the wound and has a low potential for wound invasion, disseminated infection occurs in about 5 percent of patients with a mortality between 50 and 75 percent. When wound colonization is detected, a mixture is made of nystatin (30 g) in 400 g of the topical agent. If *Candida* is cultured from two organ systems, such as sputum, urine, septic vein, or blood, systemic amphotericin B therapy is begun. When the wound is the source of sepsis, burn wound excision or debridement is necessary.

Wound infections caused by broad hyphae fungi are uncommon. *Aspergillus* and *Fusarium* species tend to remain localized and are easily dealt with by local excision. The Phycomycetes invade tissue and spread rapidly along fascial planes. Vascular invasion is associated with rapid tissue necrosis. It occurs commonly in patients with uncontrolled metabolic acidosis or diabetes. Any suspicious areas of eschar (black or hemorrhagic) should be biopsied and immediate histologic examination carried out. Gross examination of the biopsy often shows fungal extension into subcutaneous tissue. Rapid culture identification of the fungi is often not possible or is unreliable. Treatment consists of excising all infected and necrotic tissue. Evidence of systemic infection or progressive and uncontrolled local disease warrants systemic administration of both amphotericin B and flucytosine. Mortality is in excess of 50 percent.

Because the burn patient has depressed cell-mediated immunity, viruses might be expected to be more than an occasional pathogen. Cutaneous clinical disease is not common, yet antibody titers to herpes viruses are elevated in up to 33 percent of pediatric patients. Most viral infections are caused by the herpes viruses, which include herpes simplex and cytomegalovirus. Unlike adults, in whom the infection is generally a reactivation of latent disease, the young pediatric patient may have a primary infection by way of blood transfusion, tissue grafting, or direct inhalation or contact exposure. The infection commonly occurs 3 to 4 weeks after the burn. The vesicles are easily ruptured and rapidly colonize with the bacterial flora on the wound, thus making early identification by microscopic examination of the scrapings or biopsy material difficult. The viral organisms commonly infect healed and healing second-degree burns. When this happens, conversion of a second-degree burn to a third-degree injury can occur in spite of topical therapy. Systemic herpes infection can involve the spleen, liver, adrenals, lung, and bone marrow.

Cutaneous lesions in the absence of systemic involvement are treated with topical acyclovir (Zovirax), a synthetic purine nucleoside analog, given every 4 hours. If there is evidence of extensive mucocutaneous lesions or extracutaneous disease, intravenous acyclovir (5 mg per kilogram every 8 hours) is necessary.

Cytomegalovirus infections are characterized by a prolonged fever, lymphocytosis without atypical lymphocytes, and rarely, anicteric hepatitis. The clinical significance, and therefore treatment, of infections with this virus remains uncertain.

OTHER SOURCES OF INFECTION

Lung

The lung is the second most common source of infection in the burned child. Pneumonias may be classified by origin of the septic insult as either airborne or hematogenous. Airborne infection (in about two-thirds of pneumonias) is characterized by nonrandom distribution, primarily in the most dependent portions of the lung, with onset usually occurring early in the hospital course. Hematogenous pneumonias arise from septic emboli from distant sources and usually have random distribution. Onset is usually later than with the airborne type.

Inhalation injury renders the patient more susceptible to pulmonary infections. Steroid treatment is not indicated for smoke inhalation in the presence of burns. This therapy has been shown to further increase the incidence of pulmonary sepsis. Although endotracheal intubation may be lifesaving, it damages the natural defenses against infection. Adequate pulmonary toilet is essential, because copious secretions and particulate matter are frequently present. Tracheostomy allows better care of the pulmonary toilet but also results in earlier bacterial colonization when performed in the immediate postburn period. Tracheostomy should be delayed until the second or third week following the burn, unless airway management problems occur earlier.

Diagnosis of pulmonary infection depends on careful evaluation of chest roentgenograms and sputum (Gram stain and culture). The infecting organisms are most often those found on the burn wound. Treatment should be based (in decreasing order of preference) on sputum cultures or, in the absence of growth, on organisms present on the wound or organisms indigenous to the ward at that time.

Cardiovascular System

Documented bacteremia can be detected in only about 50 percent of cases of clinical septicemia. Intravascular infection is minimized by recognition of the propensity of the burn patient to continue seeding the vascular system with bacteria, often from the wound itself during routine wound manipulation, debridement, and excision. All intravascular devices must be *changed every 3 days* with rotation of access sites when possible. Iatrogenic sources of infection should be evaluated continually. This includes careful examination of all catheter sites, including old percutaneous sites and cutdowns.

Right-sided bacterial endocarditis is a dreaded complication whose incidence has increased two- to threefold with more aggressive intravascular monitoring with central venous and balloon-tipped pulmonary artery catheters (Swan-Ganz). The requirement for use of these catheters and the information obtained from them must be tempered by these risks, and all catheters should be removed as soon as possible (maximum of 3 days).

Septic thrombophlebitis should be suspected when successive positive blood cultures are recovered in a patient. Specific local signs (erythema, edema, and tenderness) are absent in about 50 percent of patients, especially if the catheter site is through burn tissue. Infection may result from either percutaneous cannulation or cutdown. The most common organisms are staphylococci and those of the burn wound. Treatment is surgical opening of the suspected vein, both proximal and distal exploration, and excision of the entire segment of affected vein, proximally to the point where good back bleeding is present. However, prevention is the goal.

Central Nervous System

In contrast to the usual sources of infection in nonburned children, central nervous system infections are relatively rare, and are most frequently associated with overwhelming septicemia. Seizures are more frequently associated with electrolyte disorders than with infection. Lumbar puncture must never be performed through the burn or in proximity to it. In this case, cisternal taps are preferred. Organisms are usually the same as on the burn wound.

Genitourinary Tract

Urinary tract infections are usually the result of indwelling urinary catheters. A catheter is essential in the early postburn period and in seriously burned children. However, it should be removed as soon as the need for hourly urine output monitoring has ceased. *Candida* infections of the urinary tract in patients requiring catheterization are treated with amphotericin B bladder irrigations.

Miscellaneous Sources

All burn wounds are tetanus-prone injuries. Incomplete immunization is not protective. All unimmunized patients with major burns should receive tetanus toxoid and hyperimmune tetanus globulin (4 U per kilogram of body weight).

Otitis media is a major source of infection, with up to 8 percent of patients under 3 years developing otitis during hospitalization. Treatment is the same as in the nonburned child.

Chondritis, an infection of the cartilage of the ear, is a severe complication and one that is preventable. The ear's exposed position, poor vascularity, lack of subcutaneous tissue, and superficial location of the cartilage all contribute to the severity of the injury. Chondritis occurs in up to 25 percent of burned ears, and commonly follows superficial partial thickness burn injuries. The infection is manifested by swelling, erythema, warmth, and a gradually increasing dull pain or ache accentuated by pressure or contact on the ear. The application of mafenide acetate two to three times daily is mandatory.

Candida overgrowth of the gastrointestinal tract is a frequent accompaniment of the burn injury and its therapy. *Candida* is able to traverse the mucosa of the gut, causing candidemia. Oral and vaginal thrush is also a common complication. All children with burns over more than 10 percent of the body surface area should receive nystatin drops (400,000 U orally, twice a day) and special attention to oral hygiene.

SUGGESTED READING

Linnemann CC Jr, MacMillan BG. Viral infections in pediatric burn patients. Am J Dis Child 1981; 135:750–753.

Prasad JK, Feller I, Thomson PD. A ten-year review of *Candida* sepsis and mortality in burn patients. Surgery 1987; 101:213–216.

Pruitt BA Jr. The burn patient II. Later care and complications of thermal injury. Curr Probl Surg 1979; XVI.

Pruitt BA, DiVincenti FC, Mason AD, et al. The occurrence and significance of pneumonia and other pulmonary complications in burned patients: comparison of conventional and topical treatments. J Trauma 1970; 10:519–530.

Pruitt BA, McManus AT. Opportunistic infections in severely burned patients. Am J Med 1984; 76(3A):146–154.

Zaske DE, Sawchuk RJ, Strate RG. The necessity of increased doses of amikacin in burn patients. Surgery 1978; 84:603–608.

NOSOCOMIAL PNEUMONIA

TERRY YAMAUCHI, M.D.

A nosocomial infection is one not known to be present or incubating at the time of hospital admission. Nosocomial pneumonia in the pediatric-aged patient can be caused by a number of different microbial agents. Specific risk factors in children include respiratory therapy, surgical procedures, antibiotics, and immunocompromising conditions. Therefore, the combination of microbial etiology and specific risk factors make treatment and infection control of nosocomial pneumonia in the pediatric patient unique for the clinician.

THERAPEUTIC APPROACH

Treatment of pediatric nosocomial pneumonia is either broad spectrum or specific. Broad-spectrum antibiotic therapy is initiated for clinically suspected bacterial pneumonia when the specific etiology is unknown. To do this, it is imperative that the clinician have a good understanding of local hospital microorganisms and their antimicrobial-resistance patterns.

I prefer to initiate broad-spectrum antibiotic therapy in the pediatric nosocomial pneumonia patient. My first choice is the combination of a penicillinase-resistant penicillin, nafcillin monohydrate at 150 to 200 mg per kilogram per day, in four divided doses given intravenously or intramuscularly, plus an aminoglycoside, gentamicin sulfate at 5 to 7.5 mg per kilogram per day in three divided doses given intramuscularly or intravenously.

In hospitals with endemic methicillin-resistant *Staphylococcus aureus,* vancomycin HCl, 40 mg per kilogram per day given in four divided doses intravenously, should be substituted for nafcillin. Similarly, if your hospital has multiantibiotic-resistant microorganisms frequently associated with nosocomial infections, a third-generation cephalosporin such as cefotaxime sodium or ceftizoxime sodium, 100 to 200 mg per kilogram per day in three or four divided doses, or ceftriaxone, 100 mg per kilogram per day in two divided doses, given intravenously or intramuscularly, may be more appropriate than the aminoglycoside (Table 1). However, since *Pseudomonas aeruginosa* is a frequently encountered nosocomial pneumonia pathogen, I would continue the aminoglycoside in combination with the cephalosporin pending culture results.

Once results of cultures and susceptibility testing are available, more specific antimicrobial therapy can be undertaken.

VIRAL AGENTS

Viruses are the leading cause of nosocomial pneumonias in children. Respiratory syncytial virus (RSV), parainfluenza viruses, and the influenza viruses A and B are the major agents involved in these pneumonias.

TABLE 1 Antibiotics for Suspected Nosocomial Bacterial Pneumonia

Antibiotics	Dosage and Route
Nafcillin	150–200 mg/kg/day in four divided doses, intravenously or intramuscularly
plus	
Gentamicin	5–7.5 mg/kg/day in three divided doses, intravenously or intramuscularly
Vancomycin HCl*	40 mg/kg/day in four divided doses, intravenously
Cefotaxime†	100–200 mg/kg/day in three or four divided doses, intravenously or intramuscularly
or	
Ceftizoxime	
or	
Ceftriaxone	100 mg/kg/day in two divided doses, intravenously or intramuscularly

* May be substituted for nafcillin if methicillin-resistant *Staphylococcus aureus* are present in hospitalized patients.

† May be substituted for aminoglycoside if multiantibiotic-resistant enteric microorganisms are frequently associated with nosocomial infections in your hospital.

TABLE 2 Antiviral Agents for Suspected Nosocomial Viral Pneumonia

Antiviral Agent	Dosage and Route
Amantadine HCl	4–6 mg/kg/day in two divided doses, orally; maximum dosage in young children 150 mg/day Older children (10 yr and older), 100 mg twice a day
Ribavirin	20 mg/ml of water through a small particle aerosol generator, given 12–18 hr/day for 3 to 7 days

At present, antiviral therapy is limited to the use of amantadine for influenza A and ribavirin for RSV infection.

Amantadine hydrochloride is the antiviral agent of choice for influenza A pneumonia in infants and children. The dosage is 4 to 6 mg per kilogram per day given orally in two divided doses for 5 days. The maximum dosage in young children is 150 mg per day. Children 10 years old and over can be treated with 100 mg twice a day. Therapy is most effective with early treatment, preferably within 48 hours of onset of symptoms. I use amantadine hydrochloride even later in children with persistent respiratory difficulty during community influenza outbreaks. Although there is relatively little information regarding use of this antiviral agent in infants, a clinical trial is indicated during influenza season (Table 2).

Amantadine hydrochloride has been demonstrated to be an effective prophylactic agent for influenza A. Dosage is 4 to 6 mg per kilogram per day given orally in two divided doses. Prophylaxis must be continued for the entire duration of influenza A occurrence in the community, or if used concomitantly with immunization until natural antibody has developed, usually in 2 to 4 weeks.

Ribavirin is approved only for the treatment of RSV infections and is administered by nebulization (20 mg per milliliter of water) through a small particle aerosol generator. The drug aerosol is given for 12 to 18 hours per day for 3 to 7 days. As with amantadine, early treatment with ribavirin appears more effective than later therapy. Two precautions are necessary when using ribavirin: (1) this antiviral agent should not be administered to a patient on assisted ventilation (unless special parental consent is obtained and the respirator is closely observed for malfunction), and (2) pregnant personnel should be made aware of the teratogenic effects of ribavirin in animal models.

SUPPORTIVE CARE

Supportive care for nosocomial pneumonia centers on easing discomfort, using antipyretics, maintaining adequate oxygenation, and properly monitoring for respiratory failure and apnea.

PREVENTION

The primary means of preventing nosocomial pneumonia is to reduce acquisition of potential bacterial and viral pathogens in the upper airways, and thus reduce the possibility of aspirating these agents. Generally, handwashing, isolation procedures, prophylactic antimicrobials, and immunizations are the major mechanisms of preventing nosocomial pneumonia.

SUGGESTED READING

Hall CB. Hospital-acquired pneumonia in children: the role of respiratory viruses. Semin Resp Infect 1987; 2:48–56.
Jacobs RF. Nosocomial pneumonia. In: Donowitz LG, ed. Hospital acquired infection in the pediatric patient. Baltimore: Williams & Wilkins, in press.
Pennington JE. Hospital-acquired pneumonia. In: Wenzel RA, ed. Prevention and control of nosocomial infections. Baltimore: Williams & Wilkins, 1987; 321–334.

NOSOCOMIAL INFECTIONS IN THE NURSERY

PABLO J. SÁNCHEZ, M.D.

The incidence of nosocomial infection in the newborn nursery is approximately 1 percent, whereas in the neonatal intensive care unit (NICU), rates as high as 25 percent have been reported. When outbreaks of nosocomial disease occur in the newborn and intensive care nurseries, special control measures are usually indicated. (Dosages of antibiotics are listed in Table 1.)

STAPHYLOCOCCUS AUREUS

The prevalence of infant colonization with *Staphylococcus aureus* in the newborn nursery varies between 1.3 and 79 percent, depending on variations in nursery techniques and infection control policies. Because high colonization rates are not always associated with outbreaks of serious staphylococcal disease, routine surveillance is not indicated. Nursery epidemics are probably related to the cyclic introduction of a virulent strain, usually phage group I or II, and most recently methicillin-resistant *S. aureus*.

Presumptive evidence of an outbreak exists when two or more simultaneous cases of staphylococcal infection occur. Once an outbreak is documented, surveillance cultures should be done. The anterior

TABLE 1   Antibiotic Dosages in Newborns

| | | Dosages (mg/kg/day) and Intervals of Administration | | | |
| | | Body Weight <2,000 g | | Body Weight >2,000 g | |
Antibiotics	Routes of Administration	Age 0–7 days	>7 days	Age 0–7 days	>7 days
Acyclovir	IV				
Varicella-zoster		45 div q8h	45 div q8h	45 div q8h	45 div q8h
Amantidine*	PO				5–8 div q12h
Amikacin	IM, IV	15 div q12h	22.5 div q8h	20 div q12h	30 div q8h
Ampicillin	IV, IM				
Meningitis		100 div q12h	150 div q8h	150 div q8h	200 div q6h
Other diseases		50 div q12h	75 div q8h	75 div q8h	100 div q6h
Cefotaxime	IV, IM	100 div q12h	150 div q8h	100 div q12h	150 div q8h
Colistin sulfate	PO	15 div q8h	15 div q8h	15 div q8h	15 div q8h
Dicloxacillin	PO	25–50 div q6h	25–50 div q6h	25–50 div q6h	25–50 div q6h
Erythromycin	PO	20 div q12h	30 div q8h	20 div q12h	30–40 div q8h
Metronidazole	IV, PO	15 div q12h	15 div q12h	15 div q12h	30 div q12h
Neomycin	PO	100 div q6h	100 div q6h	100 div q6h	100 div q6h
Penicillin G, benzathine	IM	50,000 U (one dose)	50,000 U (one dose)	50,000 U (one dose)	50,000 U (one dose)
Rifampin†	PO	10 div q12h	10 div q12h	10 div q12h	10 div q12h
Trimethoprim–sulfamethoxazole‡	IV, PO		10TMP/50 SMZ div q12h		10 TMP/50 SMZ div q12h
Vancomycin	PO	10 div q6h	10 div q6h	10 div q6h	10 div q6h
Vidaribine (varicella-zoster)	IV	10 over 12h	10 over 12h	10 over 12h	10 over 12h

* One year of age or older.
† Use with caution in liver disease patients.
‡ Contraindicated in infants 2 months of age or younger, or with hyperbilirubinemia.

nares of infants and nursery personnel as well as the umbilical stump should be cultured. Antibiotic susceptibility testing and phage typing should be performed on all of the isolates. This defines the extent of colonization, as well as identifies the particular staphylococcal strain involved in the outbreak. Parents of recently discharged infants should be questioned regarding possible staphylococcal infection in their infants. This is helpful in assessing the duration and extent of the outbreak.

Colonized and infected infants should be segregated and placed in contact isolation. If it is possible, a cohort system of care should be instituted whereby infected and colonized infants are cared for by nursery personnel who have no contact with noncolonized infants. New admissions to the nursery must not be exposed to infected or colonized infants. Rooming-in with the mother may be helpful in achieving proper segregation. Nursery personnel with anterior nares colonization either should be removed from the nursery or should care only for those infants who are colonized or infected. I would treat them with bacitracin ointment or gentamicin nose drops, or, in the case of methicillin-resistant S. aureus, with trimethoprim-sulfamethoxazole and rifampin for 5 days. Individuals with staphylococcal skin lesions should not enter the nursery. Since S. aureus is most commonly transmitted from infant to infant by means of inadequately washed hands of nursery personnel, strict adherence to handwashing is the most effective means of curtailing the outbreak. Chlorhexidine-containing skin cleansers are preferable to those with iodophor because of the former's increased activity against S. aureus.

Isolation precautions should remain in effect until either all of the colonized or infected infants have been discharged to home or follow-up anterior nares and umbilical cultures are negative for the virulent strain on two separate occasions. When the outbreak involves chronically hospitalized infants, dicloxacillin can be given for 5 days in an attempt to eradicate colonization. If the S. aureus is resistant to methicillin, rifampin, and trimethoprim–sulfamethoxazole should be used (note: this treatment is not approved for use in babies less than 2 months of age). A previously colonized infant who has been discharged home and is readmitted to the hospital should be isolated until it is determined that he or she is not carrying the epidemic strain.

In a severe epidemic causing significant neonatal disease and intrafamilial spread of infection, a bacterial interference program with S. aureus 502A can be used to control colonization and disease. S. aureus 502A is administered to the anterior nares and umbilicus shortly after birth with a cotton swab moistened with broth solution containing 2 to 4 × 10^4 viable bacteria per milliliter. Its implantation prevents colonization with the virulent strain of S. aureus. Pustules and conjunctivitis have been seen in a minority of infants after implantation. Most notably, however, fatal septicemia with meningitis has been reported after insertion of an umbilical venous catheter through an umbilicus colonized with *S. aureus* 502A.

Persons involved in hospital outbreaks of staphylococcal disease should be told of the possibility of delayed disease and spread to family members. Also, since nosocomially acquired *S. aureus* infection from the nursery normally occurs at approximately 1 week of age, the physician in practice should promptly report it to the nursery of origin.

GROUP A *STREPTOCOCCUS*

Group A *Streptococcus* (GAS) can occur in epidemic form in the newborn nursery, with an approximately 2:1 colonization-to-disease ratio. The most common disease manifestation is a moist umbilicus with an unpleasant musty odor and little or no erythema of the surrounding skin. Infected circumcision site, sepsis, meningitis, primary peritonitis, and conjunctivitis have also been reported. Moreover, GAS can be transmitted to family members after discharge from the nursery.

When GAS is recovered from an infant either in the nursery or recently discharged from there, a prompt investigation is warranted. The source of the GAS can be from either the throat or skin infection of a nursery attendant or the mother's respiratory or vaginal tract. The primary site of colonization in the infant is usually the umbilicus. The probable route of transmission between infants is inadequately washed hands of nursery personnel.

All infants should have throat and umbilicus cultured for GAS. Likewise, all nursery personnel should have throat cultures performed. Nursery attendants with positive throat cultures for GAS need to be treated with an appropriate antimicrobial agent for at least 24 hours before they return to work. They should also have a repeat throat culture performed at that time to document effective therapy. Colonized infants should be segregated as a single cohort and placed in strict isolation with separate nursing care.

All colonized infants should receive an intramuscular injection of benzathine penicillin (PCN). Because the antibiotic does not penetrate well into the avascular umbilical cord, it does not completely eradicate GAS colonization. Therefore, triple dye (brilliant green, gentian violet, prolamine hemisulfate) should be applied to the umbilical cord if this was not already done at birth. A single application of triple dye to the umbilical cord is the most effective prophylactic procedure against GAS colonization; therefore, if it is not a routine procedure at the time of the outbreak, it should be instituted on all newborn admissions until the epidemic is over. Alternatively, bacitracin ointment (four times a day for 5 to 7 days) can be applied to the umbilicus. If positive colonization cultures for GAS persist, prophylactic use of PCN given intramuscularly is warranted for all new admissions.

VARICELLA

Infants in the newborn nursery and NICU can be exposed to persons with varicella, whether they be physicians, nurses, respiratory therapists, parents, siblings, or an infant with congenital varicella. In general, the rate of horizontal transmission in these circumstances is low. This is because of the passive partial immunity conferred by transplacental passage of maternal antibodies, as well as by the relatively brief exposure and lack of intimate contact that occurs in the nursery.

The potential exists for serious complications from nosocomial acquisition of varicella. Premature infants (less than 37 weeks of gestation) whose mothers lack a prior history of varicella, infants of less than 28 weeks of gestation or weighing 1,000 g or less, irrespective of maternal history for varicella, and infants with bronchopulmonary dysplasia (BPD) are all at higher risk of having a complicated course. Varicella zoster immune globulin (VZIG, 125 U intramuscularly) should be administered to these infants as soon as possible after exposure, and always within 72 hours.

Full-term newborns whose mothers have a history of chickenpox do not require VZIG because they are not at risk for serious complications. However, I would administer VZIG to a full-term infant less than 1 week of age who has a negative maternal history of varicella if there has been a significant exposure, although it is not certain that these infants are at higher risk. Alternatively, one can determine the immune status of the mother or infant, and if antibody is present, VZIG is not indicated. This should be done, however, only if results can be obtained within 72 hours of exposure.

Exposed infants should be discharged from the nursery as soon as possible, preferably before the 10th day after exposure, when they become potentially infectious. All exposed infants still in the nursery at that time need to be isolated in a separate room until 21 days after exposure if VZIG was not given, or 28 days if VZIG was administered. The incubation period in VZIG recipients may be prolonged.

New admissions to the nursery must not be in the same room as those who were exposed. This may necessitate closing the nursery to new admissions during the period of potential infectivity.

Nursery personnel with a negative history of varicella may continue to work up to 9 days after exposure, pending serologic results of immunity. If they are nonimmune, they will have to refrain from work until 21 days after exposure. Administration of VZIG to these nonimmune nursery personnel is not indicated.

If any of the high-risk infants develop varicella, I would treat them with acyclovir for 10 days. Alternatively, vidarabine could be used. The large fluid load needed with vidarabine administration makes it an impractical drug in the newborn period. (For details, see the chapter on *Varicella-Zoster Virus Infections.*)

If a second exposure occurs more than 3 weeks after administration of VZIG, another dose should be given to the high-risk infants, and isolation precautions again instituted as outlined previously.

RESPIRATORY SYNCYTIAL VIRUS

Respiratory syncytial virus (RSV) can be a significant nosocomial pathogen in the NICU, causing outbreaks of bronchiolitis and pneumonia. Nursery personnel and visitors can transmit RSV infection either directly, if they themselves are infected, or indirectly by means of their hands or contaminated fomites.

Premature infants with hyaline membrane disease or BPD are at risk of severe or fatal RSV infection. Endotracheal intubation seems to facilitate the nosocomial spread of RSV, not only by providing direct access to the lower airways, but also by disrupting the normal mucociliary flow. Infants with congenital heart disease, particularly those with cyanotic lesions or in congestive heart failure, are also at increased risk of experiencing complications. Preexisting neuromuscular disorders as well as immunodeficiency states are also associated with more severe RSV infection, resulting in increased mortality.

The index patient with RSV infection should be isolated, with careful attention given to strict handwashing, gowning, and proper disposition of secretions and contaminated equipment. Masks need to be worn only by those with upper respiratory tract infections. Gloves offer no protection because the virus can survive longer on rubber than on skin. Placing the infant in an isolette rather than in an open radiant warmer may decrease the amount of hand contact between infants.

Infants in proximity to the index patient should be carefully observed for development of RSV infection. If two or more cases occur in the same nursery, an RSV antigen detection test should be performed on nasal washings from all of the nursery patients. This procedure rapidly identifies all of the colonized and infected infants.

Infants colonized with RSV should be cohorted, with separate nursing care if possible. New admissions should be isolated from the infected and colonized infants. Nursing staff and medical personnel who have upper respiratory symptoms, if well enough to work, should be considered as infected with RSV, and be allowed to care only for already infected infants.

High-risk infants with symptomatic RSV infection should receive ribavirin in a concentration of 20 mg per milliliter of water. It is aerosolized by a generator supplied by the manufacturer and nebulized into an oxyhood, tent, mask, nasal CPAP tubing, or ventilator. It is continuously administered for 12 to 18 hours a day for 3 to 7 days, depending on clinical improvement.

Administration of ribavirin to mechanically ventilated infants can result in precipitation of the drug in the respirator tubing or at the expiratory valve, leading to inadvertently high positive end-expiratory pressures. This can be prevented by using one-way valves on the inspiratory lines, using a breathing circuit filter in the expiratory line, and continuously monitoring the infant and ventilator carefully. In rare instances, the initial administration of ribavirin is associated with a sudden and unexplained deterioration of respiratory function. If this occurs, treatment should be stopped and reinstituted with caution.

Wide variability exists in the duration of viral shedding following RSV infection in both untreated and ribavirin-treated infants. Therefore, isolation precautions should be maintained until either the infected infants have been discharged home or their nasal washings are RSV-negative.

Other respiratory viruses—namely, influenza A, echovirus II and rhinovirus—have caused nosocomial infection in nurseries. Meticulous handwashing, strict contact isolation, and cohorting are again recommended. I would treat infants 1 year of age or older who have influenza A disease with amantidine. (Note: amantadine is not approved by the Food and Drug Administration for use in newborns.) Treatment should be initiated as soon as possible after the onset of symptoms, and continued for 2 to 5 days, or until the infant is asymptomatic for 48 hours. Influenza, however, is potentially preventable. High-risk infants who remain in the nursery for a prolonged time because of BPD or congenital heart disease and who are 6 months of age or older should receive influenza vaccine. Nursery personnel, family members, and close contacts of high-risk infants should also be immunized.

RESISTANT ENTERIC GRAM-NEGATIVE BACILLI

Many outbreaks of colonization and disease caused by aminoglycoside-resistant enteric gram-negative bacilli have been reported. The mechanism of resistance is usually plasmid-mediated, with frequent use of the particular antibiotic acting as a selective pressure that encourages emergence of resistant strains.

Antibiotic susceptibility patterns of clinically important bacterial isolates should be monitored on a regular basis. If multiply resistant strains are isolated, surveillance cultures are performed. Stool and nasopharyngeal or tracheal aspirate cultures should be obtained. Infants colonized with the resistant strain must be isolated, and gown and glove precautions used. If possible, a cohort of infected and colonized infants should be established with separate nursing care. Meticulous handwashing between handling of infants is imperative. Iodophor-containing cleansers should be used because they are effective in reducing the hand-carrier rate of gram-negative organisms. Isolation precautions are continued until either the colonized infants are discharged home or two surveillance cultures taken 1 week apart show no growth of the resistant strain.

The aminoglycoside antibiotic should be changed to one to which the enteric organisms are susceptible. Doing so removes the selective pressure and allows susceptible organisms to reemerge. It is then safe to return to the original aminoglycoside regimen.

Resistance to gentamicin and kanamycin is most often seen. Amikacin is then a suitable alternative because it is a poor substrate for the bacterial enzymes responsible for the development of resistance. Substitution of the aminoglycoside with a third-generation cephalosporin—namely, cefotaxime—to control an outbreak of gentamicin-resistant *Klebsiella pneumonia* infections in an NICU resulted in the rapid emergence of *Enterobacter cloacae* resistant to cefotaxime. Since aminoglycoside resistance develops much more slowly, aminoglycosides remain, in combination with ampicillin, the preferred empiric therapy for neonatal sepsis.

DIARRHEA

Outbreaks of diarrhea in the nursery are usually caused by bacteria such as *Salmonella, Shigella, Campylobacter jejuni,* toxigenic and enteropathogenic *Escherichia coli,* or viruses such as rotavirus or coronavirus. The association of *Clostridium difficile* with neonatal enteritis remains in question, because of the high prevalence of both organism and toxin in the stools of asymptomatic infants.

When several cases of diarrhea occur in the same nursery, symptomatic infants should be placed in a single room or segregated, and cared for as a single cohort with separate nursing personnel. Asymptomatic infants exposed to those with diarrhea should also be segregated. New admissions should not be in the same room as either the infected or the exposed infants.

Strict enteric precautions should be instituted when infected and exposed infants are handled and when disposing of soiled diapers. Meticulous handwashing should be stressed, and an iodophor cleanser used. Stool cultures for bacterial pathogens should be obtained from all symptomatic infants, as well as an antigen detection test for rotavirus infection. If the facilities are available, the stool should also be examined under electron microscopy for coronavirus particles.

Any symptomatic nursery personnel should also be cultured, and, if allowed to work, they should care only for the infected infants. Epidemiologic surveillance of recently discharged infants may be helpful in defining the extent and etiology of the outbreak.

Specific therapy depends on the results of the bacterial cultures and viral studies. If *Salmonella* is isolated, the epidemic strain should be defined and antibiotic susceptibility tests performed. Stool cultures should be obtained from all exposed infants and personnel, even if asymptomatic, as well as symptomatic parents. *Salmonella* may be present in the stool before onset of diarrhea, and asymptomatic carriage may further perpetuate the outbreak. Symptomatic infants younger than 2 months of age should be treated with ampicillin, given intravenously for 5 to 7 days, if the organism is susceptible. For ampicillin-resistant strains, cefotaxime can be used. Infants older than 2 months of age require treatment only if concurrent septicemia is suspected. Nursery personnel and parents with positive stool cultures need no antimicrobial therapy, but good handwashing techniques must be reinforced.

If *Shigella* is recovered from the stool culture, I would treat with ampicillin intravenously for 5 to 7 days if the organism is susceptible, or trimethoprim–sulfamethoxazole if the infant is 2 months of age or older. If the infant is younger than 2 months of age and the organism is resistant to ampicillin, cefotaxime can be used.

Campylobacter jejuni is treated with erythromycin stearate. No specific treatment is currently available for either rotavirus or coronavirus infection. Toxigenic *C. difficile* isolated from the stool of an infant with severe bloody diarrhea and failure to gain weight may be pathogenic, and I would treat orally with either vancomycin or metronidazole for 10 days.

Enteropathogenic *E. coli* (EPEC) should be investigated as the possible cause of the outbreak if bacterial cultures and viral studies fail to implicate another pathogen. Identification of EPEC is by agglutination and immunofluorescence with type-specific sera. All infants, even if asymptomatic, should have stool specimens examined for EPEC strains. If they are found, treatment with either neomycin sulfate or colistin sulfate given orally for 5 days is indicated.

Since intermittent excretion of enteric pathogens occurs during the convalescent period, three negative stool cultures each taken 2 days apart should be obtained before enteric isolation is discontinued. An infant with rotavirus diarrhea can be taken out of isolation when stool no longer contains rotavirus antigen.

It is important to remember that if the mother has diarrhea on admission to the labor and delivery suite, enteric isolation should be extended to both the mother and infant after delivery until stool cultures are negative for enteric pathogens.

HEPATITIS A

Asymptomatic hepatitis A in infants can lead to nosocomial spread of hepatitis A virus (HAV) in the nursery. An outbreak is first suggested by the development of hepatitis A in nursery personnel. All infants, nursery personnel, and symptomatic family contacts should be screened for HAV infection. Three infant cohorts are established: (1) infected, (2) exposed, and (3) new, unexposed admissions; each has separate nursing care. Those with negative serology should receive 0.02 mg per kilogram of immunoglobulin (Ig). Enteric precautions should be initiated, and careful handwashing between infant contacts and when soiled diapers are handled is stressed.

Infected nursery personnel, even if asymptomatic, should not care for uninfected infants. Jaundiced nursery personnel should not return to work until 1 week after the onset of jaundice.

If this degree of isolation precautions is not possible, all new admissions in the 6-week period following the last identifiable case in the nursery should receive Ig prophylaxis. Enteric precautions should also be maintained for 6 weeks after the last case, or until all of the exposed and infected infants have been discharged home. Any infant transferred to another hospital before the outbreak is recognized should have serology for HAV drawn, and if it is indicative of recent infection, Ig prophylaxis and enteric precautions need to be initiated in that nursery as well. If the transferred infant is seronegative and exposure has occurred within the previous 2 weeks, Ig prophylaxis and enteric isolation are indicated only for the infant and not for the nursery.

The most effective way of preventing nursery outbreaks of nosocomial infection is by frequent and meticulous handwashing between infant contact. Once potentially infectious problems are recognized, strict adherence to infection control measures is mandatory. Table 2 lists the specific isolation precautions for diseases in the nursery.

TABLE 2　Isolation Precautions for the Newborn in the Nursery

Strict Isolation:
  Varicella in mother
Contact Isolation:
  Gonorrhea
  Herpes simplex
  Multiply-resistant bacteria (disease or colonization)
  Respiratory viruses
  Rubella
  Skin infections, funisitis, or omphalitis (staphylococcal or group A streptococcal infection)
Enteric Isolation:
  Diarrhea
  Hepatitis A in mother
  Meningitis, aseptic
  Necrotizing enterocolitis
Drainage/Secretory Isolation:
  Chlamydia
  Conjunctivitis (other than gonococcal)
  Skin infections, funisitis, or omphalitis (minor)
  Syphilis (mucosal or skin lesions)
Blood/Body Fluids Isolation:
  AIDS
  Cytomegalovirus
  Hepatitis B and non-A, non-B in mother
  Syphilis (no skin or mucosal lesions)
Routine (no isolation required):
  Candidiasis
  Meningitis, bacterial
  Sepsis
  Toxoplasmosis
  Tuberculosis
  Urinary tract infection

SUGGESTED READING

Marcy SM, Guerrant RL. Microorganisms responsible for neonatal diarrhea. In: Remington JS, Klein JO, eds. Infectious diseases of the fetus and newborn infant. Philadelphia: WB Saunders, 1983.

Nelson JD. Control of infection acquired in the nursery. In: Remington JS, Klein JO, eds. Infectious diseases of the fetus and newborn infant. Philadelphia: WB Saunders, 1983.

Siegel JD. Controlling infection in the nursery. Pediatr Infect Dis 1985; 4(S):536–541.

Young NA, Gershon AA. Chickenpox, measles and mumps. In: Remington JS, Klein JO, eds. Infectious diseases of the fetus and newborn infant. Philadelphia: WB Saunders, 1983.

DISEASES CAUSED BY PARASITES

ECTOPARASITIC INFECTIONS

DUANE L. DOWELL, M.D.

SCABIES

Scabies is a cutaneous infestation by the eight-legged mite, *Sarcoptes scabiei* var hominis. It affects people of all ages and is characterized by severe pruritus that often leads to excoriation and secondary infection or pyoderma. The diagnosis is easier in the colder months when it is not confused with insect bites. Definitive diagnosis is accomplished by demonstrating the mite or ova within a skin scraping. Application of a drop of mineral oil to a lesion and identification of a minute black dot within the lesion promote easy scraping of the stratum corneum with shavings placed on a glass slide and observed under the microscope.

Effective management involves the entire household. Explanation to the family of what the therapy will and will not do may well be more important than the treatment of the index patient. There has been concern in the literature about the potential neurologic consequences of topical therapy. This is largely a theoretical concern if appropriate instructions are understood and followed. Lindane 1 percent lotion or cream (Kwell) is the current treatment of choice, based on years of experience and ease of use.

Parents are instructed to apply the lotion to the entire body from the neck down, covering all lesions. If there are lesions on the face and eyelids, a cotton swab may be used to apply the liquid to the affected areas, taking care to avoid the eyes and mucous membranes. The solution is left on the body 8 to 12 hours or overnight and the patient is thoroughly bathed the next morning. Ginsburg and co-workers have demonstrated that peak systemic absorption occurs at approximately 6 hours and then drops rapidly. Most studies show that less than 6 hours of application results in ineffective treatment and that leaving the medication on for longer than 8 to 12 hours is neither helpful nor increases the risk of toxicity.

The medication should be applied to cool, dry skin without bathing beforehand, since systemic absorption may be enhanced in the presence of a freshly scrubbed, wet skin surface. All other close contacts should receive the same treatment because asymptomatic family members may be a source of reinfection. It is essential to inform parents of the potential for neural toxicity to emphasize the importance of a single application. At the same time, parents need to understand that persistent itching does not indicate failure of treatment. Pruritus often continues for several weeks after effective therapy. Because itching is particularly intense in scabies, it is usually helpful to prescribe an antipruritic medication. Atarax (2 mg per kilogram per day in three divided doses) or Benadryl (3 to 5 mg per kilogram per day) are effective and safe. It is prudent to limit second applications of lindane to those patients in whom the mite can be identified after therapy or those reexposed to an untreated contact.

In conjunction with the application of the scabicidal cream or lotion, all bedding and recently worn clothing should be laundered. The hot-water cycle and the use of a dryer is sufficient to kill residual organisms. Ironing or dry cleaning or storage in plastic bags for 2 weeks also eliminates viable lice. Fumigation or special treatments and sprays are not necessary and should be avoided.

LICE

Head lice infestation (pediculosis capitis) has become an increasingly widespread problem in this country over the past 10 to 15 years. School systems and day care centers must deal with the pest on a regular basis. The head louse is somewhat smaller than the body louse, which generally infests adolescents and adults in areas of concentrated body hair. The adult feeds on human blood and the mature female attaches an egg case (nit) to the hair shaft with a cementlike substance. If the diagnosis is unrecognized for a period of time, the resulting secondary excoriation and infection can be confused with seborrhea and impetigo.

A variety of effective agents are available for treatment. Kwell (1 percent lindane) shampoo has been a standby, despite some concern about its neurotoxicity. Used according to directions, it remains a safe medication. Recent studies have demonstrated superior killing power of 1 percent permethrin over 1 percent lindane. I am convinced and will henceforth recommend the pyrethrins (Nix, Rid, A-200, R&C) over lindane preparations. The pyrethrins (with the exception of Nix) share the additional advantage of being over-the-counter preparations. This makes it practical for the school nurse to identify the condition and recommend over-the-counter treatment to parents.

For the treatment of head lice, Kwell, Rid, R&C, and A-200 all are to be used as shampoos. They are applied to *dry* hair until all the hair and scalp is wet with the preparation. They should be left on for a period of 10 minutes, not more. The medication is then rinsed out with clear water. The instructions for Rid also suggest washing out with a regular shampoo. Dead lice and nits are then combed out using a special fine-toothed nit comb, usually supplied with the product. Nix is applied as a cream rinse after the hair is shampooed and rinsed. The permethrin liquid is then worked into the hair and scalp, allowed to stand for 10 minutes, and rinsed out with clear water. Body

and pubic lice can be treated in a similar manner followed by a shower or bath.

For prevention of reinfection, combs and brushes should be placed in boiling water for 10 minutes or soaked in 2 percent lysol for 1 to 2 hours. Clothing and bedding should be handled as with scabies.

SUGGESTED READING

Ginsburg CM, Lowry W. Absorption of gamma benzene hexachloride following application of Kwell shampoo. Pediatr Dermatol 1983; 1:74–76.

Lane AL. Scabies and head lice. Pediatr Ann 1987; 16:51–54.

Meinking TL, Taplin D, Kalter D, Eberle MW. Comparative efficacy of treatments for pediculosis capitus infestations. Arch Dermatol 1986; 122:267–271.

Rasmussen J. The problem of lindane. J Am Acad Dermatol 1981; 5:507–516.

ROUNDWORM INFECTIONS (NEMATODIASES)

ZBIGNIEW S. PAWLOWSKI, M.D., D.T.M.&H.

In pediatric practice the clinical importance of intestinal or tissue nematodiases is often overestimated or underestimated. An objective, individual evaluation of the clinical significance of a roundworm infection should therefore be made of each patient before his or her treatment is decided.

The nematodiases diagnosed in man may (1) be the only cause of a disease (e.g., intensive ascariasis) that requires a specific anthelmintic treatment; (2) complicate or aggravate other existing diseases (e.g., disseminated strongyloidiasis in a child with a malignant condition or under immunosuppressive therapy), requiring both treatment of the primary disease and the use of specific anthelmintics; (3) be asymptomatic and simply coexist with another disease (e.g., nonintensive trichuriasis in a child with chronic renal problems), which may not need any specific anthelmintic treatment.

It is probable, however, that the clinical significance of a particular nematode infection in a particular patient is difficult to evaluate. In such cases, which usually present vague abdominal or neurologic symptoms or some signs of skin or systemic hypersensitivity, a priori anthelmintic treatment is justified.

For practical purposes, nematode infections in humans can be categorized into three groups: (1) intestinal nematodiases, (2) tissue nematodiases, and (3) exotic and/or rare nematode infections.

Most intestinal helminthiases can be diagnosed by fecal examination; however, some infections (enterobiasis, strongyloidiasis) require the use of specific techniques (anal swabs, nematode larvae coprocultures). Tissue nematodiases, usually suspected in patients who have eosinophilia, need to be confirmed by biopsy or indirect serologic examination. Exotic infections, which occur in those who have a history of contact with endemic areas, can cause some diagnostic problems unless specialized centers are consulted.

Many nematode infections do not present a pathognomonic clinical picture, but each one has some characteristic points in its pathology and clinical symptomatology. Therefore, at least in complicated cases, a diagnosis based on the results of a laboratory examination should be considered together with all the patient's symptoms and signs; otherwise the infection itself may be successfully treated, but the patient may not improve much if he is also suffering from something else.

In multiple infections, ascariasis, if present, should be treated first with an effective broad-spectrum drug to avoid possible complications caused by the migration of *Ascaris*.

In intestinal nematodiases, the effect of treatment is usually evaluated by a microscopic examination of feces after 2 weeks; the egg production may be perturbed for about a week after unsuccessful treatment. In tissue nematodiases, it usually takes a few days before any clinical improvement can be seen.

INTESTINAL NEMATODIASES

Ascariasis

Ascariasis (large roundworm infection) requires treatment in all cases diagnosed by finding *Ascaris* eggs in the feces or when *Ascaris* worms are vomited or expelled from the anus. Even suspected cases should be treated since laboratory examination does not detect male and immature or old female worms that might migrate and/or cause complications.

Single-dose therapy with albendazole, mebendazole, levamisole, piperazine, or pyrantel given orally is effective in about 90 percent of nonintensive and uncomplicated ascariasis cases. Intensive invasions may require two courses of treatment. Pyrantel is the safest drug for ascariasis in children younger than 2 years of age. Albendazole or mebendazole is recommended in mixed *Ascaris,* hookworm, and *Trichuris* infections. In the case of intestinal obstruction caused by *Ascaris,* piperazine or pyrantel given by a nasogastric tube is preferred.

Both albendazole, 100-mg and 200-mg tablets, or a suspension containing 100 mg per 5 ml, and mebendazole, 100-mg tablets, or a suspension containing 100 mg per 5 ml are given in single doses of 200 mg, in children irrespective of age (above 2 years) between main meals. Both drugs are contraindicated in patients with blood dyscrasia, leukopenia, or severe hepatic parenchymal impairment. Adverse reactions (nausea, vomiting, abdominal pain, diarrhea) related to single-dose therapy are rare.

Levamisole, 50- and 150-mg tablets, are given orally after breakfast in a single dose of 3 to 5 mg per kilogram of body weight, 150 mg in adults. Levamisole has some immunomodulating activity and it is possible that a single anthelmintic dose can improve depressed phagocyte and T-cell functions. Prolonged treatment with large doses is under investigation in autoimmune diseases and chronic infections. A single anthelmintic dose of levamisole may cause transient nausea, abdominal pain, headache, dizziness, weakness, or skin rash, but these adverse reactions are rare.

Piperazine hexahydrate or citrate in the form of 500- and 550-mg tablets, or syrups containing 100 and 110 mg per milliliter, respectively, are given after breakfast in a single dose of 75 mg per kilogram of body weight to a maximum dose of 3.5 g. Piperazine in syrup form is preferred in ascariasis. Two days of treatment are frequently suggested, but may not be necessary. Piperazine is contraindicated in children with impaired renal or hepatic function and in neurologic conditions such as epilepsy. It is not recommended in debilitated, malnourished, or severely anemic patients. Therapeutic dosages may cause adverse reactions such as nausea, vomiting, diarrhea, abdominal pain, and headache. Transient neurotoxic reactions (vertigo, incoordination, muscular weakness, paresthesia, lethargy) are usually related to overdosage or impaired metabolism and/or elimination of piperazine in the urine. Hypersensitivity reactions to piperazine have been reported.

Pyrantel pamoate in the form of chewable tablets containing 250 mg of pyrantel base, or a suspension containing 50 mg of the base per milliliter, should be given between meals as a single dose of 10 mg of pyrantel base per kilogram of body weight. Low daily doses of 2.5 or 5 mg of pyrantel base per kilogram of body weight were successfully used for controlling ascariasis in communities. There are no contraindications to pyrantel, but caution is recommended in patients with hepatic dysfunction since transient serum glutamic-oxaloacetic transaminase (SGOT) elevations have been observed. Experience with pyrantel in children younger than 2 years of age is limited. Adverse reactions (nausea, abdominal pain, diarrhea, headache, dizziness, weakness, rash, and fever) occur occasionally and are mild and transient.

Ascariasis can also occur in several members of a family exposed to the same contaminated soil or food. *Ascaris* eggs can remain invasive for some years in soil around houses or in gardens. Indiscriminate defecation and the use of human feces as fertilizer should be strongly discouraged to prevent early reinfection. In highly endemic areas, periodic (three to four times a year) community-oriented treatment for a few years may be necessary to control ascariasis.

Treatment of intestinal obstruction, which is the most common complication in ascariasis, should be conservative. In its early stages, the obstruction is usually incomplete and often responds well to 24-hour nasogastric suction, intravenous correction of fluid and electrolyte deficits, antispasmodics, and anthelmintics. Recently, the administration of either mineral oil, 20 ml four times a day, or Gastrografin, 20 ml, has been recommended. Patients should be carefully observed, and if there is no remission within 24 to 48 hours or if signs of acute abdominal emergency or further complications occur, surgical intervention is indicated.

The simplest surgical procedure is to massage the worms from the ileum into the cecum without opening the gut. This is possible when the intestinal wall is not likely to perforate and when the bolus of worms is small and located in the terminal ileum. In cases in which the massage procedure is not possible (e.g., the intestinal wall shows visible changes, the bolus of worms is too large, or the bolus is proximally situated or difficult to unravel), resection of the obstructed segment and end-to-end anastomosis are recommended. In severely ill children, a resection with double enterostomies can be a life-saving treatment, but it may cause wound infection or disturb fluid and electrolyte balance, and require a second surgical operation after some time. Enterotomy and extraction of *Ascaris* by forceps frequently leads to wound infection, disruption of anastomosis, and peritonitis.

Treatment of biliary ascariasis should also be as conservative as possible, with antispasmodics and anthelminthics given first. Mechanical removal of *Ascaris* from the common bile duct by endoscope has been reported.

Hookworm Infection

Hookworm infections can be diagnosed easily by finding *Ancylostoma duodenale* or *Necator ameri-*

canus eggs in the feces. Species differentiation between these infections, possible only by examination of larval or adult worms, is advisable but not essential for clinical purposes.

Any case of hypochromic microcytic anemia caused by hookworm infection should be treated, as should be any case of intensive infection, which might eventually lead to anemia and hypoproteinemia. In endemic areas light infections are common and are frequently left untreated. However, the criteria for asymptomatic or symptomatic cases, and intensive or nonintensive infections, differ from one locality to another, depending on several factors, e.g., the amount of iron in the diet and the iron stores in individuals. If possible, children should be treated, especially those suffering from other diseases, to avoid any unnecessary damage to the small intestinal mucosa and the loss of iron and protein caused by hookworms.

The treatment of hookworm infections usually requires larger dosages of anthelmintics than those used for ascariasis. The cure rates after a single treatment are between 70 and 90 percent; levamisole and pyrantel are less effective against *Necator* infections.

Albendazole is given in a single dose of 400 mg for all patients over 2 years of age. Mebendazole is used in a 100-mg dose twice daily for 3 days; a single-dose treatment is less efficient. Pyrantel is given in a daily single dose of 10 mg per kilogram of body weight for 3 days. (For the contraindications and adverse reactions of these drugs, see the previous section on Ascariasis.)

Hookwork anemia can be cured temporarily with iron therapy alone; ferrous sulfate taken orally in a dosage of 1 to 3 mg per kilogram of body weight daily, before or between meals, is recommended. However, it is usual practice to give both iron and anthelmintics in hookworm anemias to remove the worms and restore the iron deficiency at the same time.

Trichuriasis

The clinical significance of *Trichuris trichiura* infections depends largely on the intensity of infection. Quantitative stool examination (e.g., by Kato-Katz thick smear technique) is useful for reaching a proper decision concerning optimal treatment. Infections with fewer than 100 *Trichuris* eggs per gram of feces are usually asymptomatic and can be left untreated; those with more than 1,000 *Trichuris* eggs per gram are frequently symptomatic and most likely to require treatment. However, it is advisable to treat any case of trichuriasis, irrespective of the intensity of infection, in a child suffering from any allergic or neurologic condition, vague abdominal problems, or anemia.

Only a few anthelmintics are effective in trichuriasis, namely, albendazole, mebendazole, and oxantel. The dosage of albendazole and mebendazole is the same as for hookworm infections. Oxantel pamoate tablets of 125 mg or suspension with 50 mg oxantel base per milliliter, are given in a single dose of 10 to 20 mg per kilogram of body weight. Oxantel may not be available in the United States. Intensive infections need treatment for 2 or 3 days. Oxantel, which is an analog of pyrantel, is free from major side effects; however, nausea, vomiting, and abdominal cramps may occur.

Intensive infections with more than 10,000 *Trichuris* eggs per gram of feces usually require two separate courses of anthelmintic therapy plus additional treatment of any concomitant infections (shigellosis, amebiasis) or deficiencies (iron, protein).

In mixed *Trichuris, Ascaris,* and hookworm infections, treatment with broad-spectrum, single-dose anthelmintics, such as albendazole, mebendazole, or oxantel–pyrantel combined, may not result in eradication of trichuriasis, but usually bring about a clinical cure by substantially reducing the intensity of the *Trichuris* infection.

Enterobiasis

Enterobiasis is the most common nematodiasis in the developed countries, but it is also a self-limiting infection that disappears within 2 months if not reintroduced. Reinfection with *Enterobius* eggs is common, however, because of autoinfection and common household transmission (e.g., infected family members, reservoir of parasite eggs in house dust).

Enterobiasis can be diagnosed in children by finding pinworms in loose stools or in the anal area or by examining anal swab specimens for *Enterobius* eggs. Treatment depends mainly on the character of the infection, which may be sporadic (worms or eggs detected occasionally), recurrent, or established (anal swabs positive almost every day). In sporadic infections, single-dose treatment is recommended; infants with sporadic enterobiasis do not require any treatment themselves, but infected family members around them do. Recurrent infections need two courses of treatment 2 to 4 weeks apart plus treatment of the infected persons in the household. Well-established infections are difficult to treat unless (1) single-dose therapy is repeated three to four times at 2- to 3-week intervals, (2) all infected family members are treated, and (3) possible sources of infection are controlled (contacts with other infected people, poor personal hygiene, dusty bedroom or kitchen). With the constant threat of reinfection (enterobiasis among teachers or in some medical staff), it is recommended that a single dose of anthelmintics be taken once every 2 or 3 months to prevent intensive enterobiasis.

Early morning showers or perianal washing, limited intake of carbohydrates, and wearing pajamas to prevent the spread of *Enterobius* eggs all reduce the risk of reinfection.

Treatment of enterobiasis is based on repeated single and small dosages of anthelmintics: 200 mg of albendazole or 100 mg of mebendazole (both irrespective of age above 2 years) and 10 mg per kilogram of body weight of pyrantel.

Currently, levamisole, piperazine, and pyrvinium are rarely used in the treatment of enterobiasis. Local treatment of skin changes around the anal area is palliative and reduces the local irritation only temporarily.

Strongyloidiasis

Strongyloidiasis is often an opportunistic infection that is clinically manifest in individuals who are immunologically deficient or debilitated because of malignant disease or immunosuppressive therapy. In many other patients, the intensity of strongyloidiasis is low although, because of constant autoinfection, *Strongyloides stercoralis* may parasitize the human host for many years. Strongyloidiasis should be excluded before immunosuppressive therapy is initiated, and immunosuppressed patients should be examined periodically for the infection. Diagnosis is based on finding *S. stercoralis* larvae in the duodenal content or feces; specific serologic tests are also useful.

Treatment for strongyloidiasis can be given either to cure intensive and/or disseminated strongyloidiasis or to prevent possible spread of infection.

Only a few anthelmintics are effective against *S. stercoralis.* Thiabendazole, 500 mg tablets, or suspension with 100 mg per milliliter, is given in a single daily dose of 25 mg per kilogram after meals for 5 days. Disseminated strongyloidiasis is treated with 25 mg per kilogram twice daily for 5 to 7 days, and a repetition of the course of treatment after at least 1 week may be necessary.

Thiabendazole has potential toxicity, the most common adverse reactions being dizziness, anorexia, nausea, vomiting, and abdominal pain. Less common are headaches, giddiness, drowsiness, and other neurologic disturbances, liver functional abnormalities, hypotensive reactions, and skin rashes. Leukopenia, crystalluria, and hematuria may occur. Some cases of erythema multiforme (Stevens–Johnson syndrome) have been associated with thiabendazole therapy in children.

Thiabendazole is not indicated for patients with renal or hepatic dysfunction; experience with thiabendazole treatment in children weighing less than 15 kg has been only limited. The therapy should be discontinued immediately in the event of any severe adverse reaction.

Albendazole had recently been found effective in strongyloidiasis in a daily dose of 400 mg for 3 days in children between 2 and 12 years of age. In the past few years, cambendazole, in a single dose of 5 mg per kilogram body weight, has been tried in the treatment of strongyloidiasis with some success. Ivermectin has been found effective in experimental strongyloidiasis in mice, but there is not enough experience with its use in humans.

Trichostrongyloidiasis

The relatively rare intestinal nematode infection of trichostrongyloidiasis can be treated successfully with pyrantel (preferably in suspension) or mebendazole, both given as single doses (see the section on Ascariasis). Treatment is repeated after a few days if necessary. Albendazole and levamisole may also be effective.

Anisakiasis

The invasion of nematode larvae of the genera *Anisakis, Contracecum, Phocanema,* and *Terranova,* penetrating the gastric or small intestine mucosa, may require surgical intervention. These larvae can also be removed from the stomach with the help of a fibrogastroscope. The anthelmintics that are effective against *Ascaris* (preferably in the form of a suspension) may be used prophylactically against anisakiasis occurring after the consumption of infected uncooked fish.

TISSUE NEMATODIASES

There are three major tissue nematodiases that are either related to atypical intestinal parasites (cutaneous larvae migrans) or have an early intestinal phase (visceral larva migrans, trichinellosis).

Cutaneous Larva Migrans Syndrome

The cutaneous larva migrans syndrome, also known as creeping eruption, is caused by the larvae of the dog and cat hookworms (*Ancylostoma braziliense* and *A. caninum*). The resulting skin changes respond well to thiabendazole, given systemically (dosage as for intensive strongyloidiasis) or topically. Individual larva migrating in the skin can be killed by freezing with an ethyl chloride spray.

Visceral Larva Migrans Syndrome

The visceral larva migrans syndrome (VLM) is caused by the larvae of the dog or cat roundworms (*Toxocara canis* or *T. cati*). The severity of the clinical picture and the possible risk of further complications caused by migrating larvae should be carefully weighed against the use of anthelmintics, which might not be safe. Much of the toxocariasis found in humans is mild and requires no specific treatment. The hepatic and pulmonary lesions respond to treatment with thiabendazole (dosage as for intensive strongyloidiasis). Both mebendazole (3 g daily for 3 weeks) and diethylcarbamazine (6 mg per kilogram of body weight daily for 3 weeks) have been used with some success.

The patient with ocular localization of *Toxocara* larvae should be referred to an ophthalmologist for specific treatment.

Trichinellosis (Trichinosis)

The treatment of trichinellosis in children depends on the intensity of infection, stage of disease, accompanying complications, and parasite strain; it may need as much as intensive care treatment initially in severe cases or as little as simple anthelmintic therapy in asymptomatic or oligosymptomatic patients. There are three types of chemotherapeutic intervention for trichinellosis in children:

1. Anthelmintic treatment against the intestinal worms in all infected cases, or even when the consumption of infected meat is suspected. Albendazole, mebendazole, and pyrantel given for 5 days in the same daily doses as for hookworm infection are usually effective.
2. Antishock, anti-inflammatory, or antiallergic treatment in the early stages of trichinellosis, depending on the severity of the case, as well as protein and electrolyte replacement therapy and treatment of pulmonary, cardiac, or brain complications in the latter stage of the disease.
3. Anthelmintic therapy (albendazole, mebendazole) against *T. spiralis* larvae in the muscle tissue is recommended only in intensive infections and those caused by the Arctic strain of the parasite.

EXOTIC NEMATODIASES

There are three large groups of exotic nematodiases: (1) those caused by *Capillaria, Angiostrongylus,* and *Gnathostoma* species, (2) filarial infections, and (3) dracunculiasis.

Capillariases, Angiostrongyliases, and Gnathostomiasis

The treatment of these infections ranges from surgical intervention, through prolonged mebendazole therapy, to nonspecific symptomatic management only. *Capillaria philippinensis* infection, which causes severe enteropathy (intestinal capillariasis) in some areas of the Philippines and Thailand, responds well to prolonged mebendazole therapy, e.g., 400 mg daily for 20 days. There is not such a good response to mebendazole in *C. hepatica* infection (hepatic capillariasis), which has a clinical picture resembling the visceral larva migrans (VLM) syndrome. The treatment for abdominal angiostrongyliasis, which occurs in Central America and has an appendicitislike symtomatology, is largely surgical.

There is no consensus on the treatment of eosinophilic meningoencephalitis caused by *Angiostrongylus cantonensis,* which is found in Hawaii, the South Pacific, and Southeast Asia. Some experts suggest 100 mg mebendazole twice daily for 5 days, but others, fearing the strong host reaction that can develop after most of the parasites are killed, suggest only symptomatic treatment while waiting for a slow natural recovery. The larvae of *Gnathostoma spinigerum,* which migrate frequently in the subcutaneous tissue or cause abdominal tumors, can be removed surgically; chemotherapy with mebendazole may be considered for pulmonary or brain localization of the parasite.

Filarial Infections

The term *filarial infections* covers lymphatic filariasis, onchocerciasis, loiasis, and some other less important or zoonotic filariases.

In children, lymphatic filariasis usually occurs in its early stages with fever, lymphadenitis, and lymphangitis. Treatment of these cases is essential to prevent later complications caused by obstruction of the lymphatic vessels.

The drug of choice remains diethylcarbamazine (DEC), 50-mg tablets or syrup with 24 mg per milliliter. The dosage of DEC differs in individual or mass treatment. For individual therapy, 2 mg per kilogram body weight are given after meals three times a day for 2 weeks. To reduce the risk of allergic reactions, gradually increasing doses is recommended: the first day, 2 mg per kilogram; the second day, 4 mg per kilogram; the third and following days, 6 mg per kilogram.

Antihistamines can also be given for the first few days. If a severe reaction occurs, the DEC doses should be reduced or stopped altogether and corticosteroid therapy started.

With DEC therapy, the microfilariae disappear quickly from the blood, but several courses of treatment may be needed to kill the adult worms. Courses of treatment (2 weeks each) can be repeated at monthly intervals and continued for a year or more if necessary.

Mass therapy with 6 mg DEC per kilogram body weight daily for 12 days or 6 mg DEC per kilogram once a year, or 50 mg weekly for 18 months has been used to reduce local *Wuchereria bancrofti* transmission, but because of commonly occurring adverse reactions the community compliance may be poor.

There are occasional adverse reactions to the DEC itself, such as headache, malaise, anorexia, and weakness. Nausea, vomiting, and drowsiness occur less frequently. Allergic reactions related to the dead parasites include fever, malaise, rash, headache, some abdominal and pulmonary symptoms, and muscle or joint pains.

Treatment of lymphatic filariasis with DEC is recommended between the exacerbations of lymphadenitis. Some caution is advised in children with renal disease or malaria.

In onchocerciasis, DEC treatment is given even more cautiously because of stronger skin and systemic allergic reactions ("Mazzotti reaction") and the risk of iridocyclitis and posterior eye segment lesions around *Onchocerca volvulus* microfilariae. Betamethasone has been recommended to ameliorate these host reactions.

The major aim of therapy should be to prevent irreversible ocular and skin lesions and to alleviate skin symptoms. Because the two drugs effective in onchocerciasis (DEC and suramin) are toxic and can precipitate severe systemic complications and permanent ocular damage, the decision regarding optimal therapy in individual cases needs careful evaluation of possible risks and benefits of therapy.

Standard treatment in children should start with a single dose of 0.5 mg per kilogram of body weight of DEC; larger doses—0.5 mg, 1 mg, and finally 2 mg per kilogram body weight, all twice daily—can be given only when adverse reactions following the first dose have subsided. It may take 7 to 14 days to reach a daily dose of 4 mg per kilogram of body weight, which should then be continued until the microfilariae disappear from the skin snips. Later, a suppressive treatment can be continued, giving a single dose of 1 to 2 mg of DEC per kilogram of body weight weekly, or radical treatment can be started with suramin, which kills the adult worms. Treatment with suramin, which is a toxic drug given intravenously, needs considerable experience and constant medical supervision. Ivermectin in a daily dosage of 50 to 100 μg per kilogram of body weight has recently been found effective. Ivermectin is not yet freely available and at present is not recommended for children younger than 5 years of age.

In onchocerciasis, surgical nodulectomy is advisable, especially when the nodules are localized on the head.

Loiasis often responds to DEC, 6 mg per kilogram of body weight daily for 7 days, repeated once a month as needed. Encephalopathy has been reported during DEC treatment.

Dracunculiasis (Dracontiasis)

Dracunculus medinensis can be removed within a few weeks by winding out every day a few centimeters of the Guinea worm situated in the subcutaneous tissue; sterile dressing and acriflavine cream are recommended to prevent bacterial infection. Quicker removal of the worm by a small surgical incision has some risk of not being complete or leading to bacterial infection. Chemotherapy with niridazole, 25 mg per kilogram of body weight daily for 10 days, or metronidazole, 25 mg per kilogram of body weight daily in three doses for 10 days, reduces the host inflammatory reaction around the worm and facilitates the mechanical removal of the parasite, but does not offer a radical cure. Dracunculiasis is an easily preventable infection because invasive larvae are transmitted by some copepods that contaminate drinking water.

LARVAL TAPEWORM INFECTIONS

JAY S. KEYSTONE, M.D., M.Sc. (CTM), F.R.C.P.(C)

ECHINOCOCCOSIS

Human hydatid disease is caused by the cystic larval stages of three species of *Echinococcus: E. granulosus* (cystic hydatid disease) of global distribution; *E. multilocularis* (alveolar hydatid disease) confined to the Northern Hemisphere; and the very rare *E. vogeli* (polycystic hydatid disease) of Central America and northern South America.

E. granulosus

Cysts are located most frequently in the liver and lungs. The slowly enlarging larval cyst is well tolerated unless it ruptures or becomes large enough to produce symptoms of a space-occupying mass. Plain roentenography readily detects lung cysts, but only calcified cysts can be demonstrated at other sites. Computerized tomography (CT) and ultrasonography are useful, not only in the detection of cysts, but also in specific diagnosis when daughter cysts are demonstrable. The sensitivity of serodiagnostic tests (IHA, IFA, ELISA) is high for liver cysts (85 percent), but low for lung cysts (50 percent). Under no circumstances should closed aspiration be attempted as a diagnostic maneuver because accidental spillage of cyst contents could cause anaphylaxis or secondary spread.

Specific Therapy

Whenever possible, surgery remains the treatment of choice. In view of the benign course of *E. granulosus* var. canadensis (seen in Canada and Arctic regions), asymptomatic individuals do not require treatment except when complications arise.

Uncomplicated cystic hydatid disease of the liver

is best managed by suction and forceps *evacuation* of cyst contents (including daughter cysts, germinal and laminated membranes) and irrigation of the cyst cavity with a scolicidal solution, followed by primary closure of the cyst, surrounding liver tissue, and abdominal cavity. Scolicidal solutions such as 5 percent cetrimide (cetyltrimethylammonium bromide) or 0.5 percent tincture of chlorehexidine gluconate (Hibitane) are left in place for 10 to 15 minutes before being removed by suction. Some surgeons have used hypertonic saline and silver nitrate (0.5 percent final concentration) for the same purpose. Formalin is no longer recommended because of the risk of shock if it diffuses out of the cyst. More difficult procedures, such as cystectomy, partial hepatectomy, and marsupialization, carry a higher risk of intra- and postoperative complications such as hemorrhage, cyst leakage, and secondary infection.

A number of different methods have been employed to minimize spillage of cyst contents and recurrence of disease during surgical manipulation of the cyst. I prefer to have a plastic sheet sewn directly to the cyst wall so that any fluid that leaks from the cyst spills onto the drape and away from the operative site.

Other authors have used a suction cone device with a cryotherm base or they pack off the area around the cyst with pads saturated in 20 percent saline. Some surgeons inject chemicals (already discussed) to inactivate protoscolices before some of the cyst fluid is extirpated. Peritoneal and pleural lavage with 0.5 percent cetrimide has been shown to be effective in diminishing the risk of dissemination following cyst rupture at surgery, although a chemical peritonitis has been reported with this procedure. If a pre- or intraoperative spill of cyst contents is suspected or documented, I recommend a 3-week course of mebendazole (Vermox), 50 mg per kilogram per day, to be taken in divided doses with food. Although this use of mebendazole is not listed in the manufacturer's official directory and has not been studied in humans, animal experiments suggest that this is a reasonable approach.

Cystic hydatid disease of the lung in many cases, can be managed by elimination of the intact cyst by the use of positive pressure ventilation to force the cyst from the surgical opening in the lung.

If the extent or location of cysts, the patient's general condition, or lack of adequate facilities make surgery impractical or impossible, mebendazole chemotherapy should be considered. In uncontrolled studies, treatment of several hundred patients with cystic hydatid disease using large dosages of mebendazole led to subjective "improvement" in 75 percent; the remainder showed evidence of disease progression or recurrence of parasite viability after treatment. Objective criteria of improvement and cure have been documented in relatively few cases.

Medical therapy of cystic hydatid disease consists of 50 to 100 mg per kilogram per day of mebendazole for a minimum of 3 months. Some authors have used as much as 200 mg per kilogram per day in an attempt to achieve peak therapeutic blood levels of mebendazole, which should reach 80 ng per milliliter (measured by radioimmunoassay or HPLC). Since absorption is enhanced when the drug is given with food (especially fatty meals), mebendazole should be given in three divided doses with meals. Repeated courses of therapy may be necessary.

Albendazole, a new benzimidazole derivative, looks more promising than mebendazole because high blood and tissue levels of the drug can be achieved. The results of preliminary studies suggest that albendazole is more effective than mebendazole in the management of cystic hydatid disease. Multiple 28-day courses of therapy separated by 14-day drug-free periods have been recommended for subjects older than 10 years of age when surgical therapy is not possible. Compassionate use of albendazole for the treatment of human hydatid disease requires approval of the Food and Drug Administration (FDA).

Monitoring Response to Therapy

Adverse reactions to mebendazole therapy generally occur within the first month and may include febrile and allergic reactions, alopecia, glomerulonephritis, and reversible leukopenia. Patients with hepatic parenchymal disease and/or biliary obstruction may achieve substantially higher blood levels of mebendazole and be at higher risk for toxicity than those with normal hepatobiliary function. Patients taking mebendazole should be monitored clinically, biochemically (liver and renal function), and hematologically (complete blood count) weekly for the first month and then every other week.

The use of mebendazole for human hydatid disease is not listed in the manufacturer's product monograph, nor has this use been approved by the FDA. Therefore, physicians must exercise their professional judgment by weighing the risks and benefits of mebendazole to determine whether or not use of the drug is appropriate in individual cases.

Follow-up

Follow-up in our unit consists of annual abdominal ultrasound examinations for at least 5 years. A chest roentgenogram and a CT scan are done at 2 or 3 years and again at 5 years to monitor for evidence of recurrence. It should be noted that a cyst cavity may remain after successful evacuation and eradication of a hepatic liver cyst. Hydatid serology may not revert to negative for several years after successful treatment.

When mebendazole has been employed, treatment is considered to have failed if there is no appreciable change in the radiologic appearance of the lesion within 9 months after the completion of therapy.

E. multilocularis

Alveolar hydatid disease differs prognostically from cystic disease since the former acts as a slow-growing, malignant, solid "parasite tumor" of liver that metastasizes to lung and brain. When the disease is present, the classic "swiss-cheese" liver calcification pattern seen on a roentgenogram of the abdomen is pathognomonic for the disease. Findings on CT scan and ultrasonography are those of an indistinct solid mass that may have a necrotic center. Hydatid serology is usually positive at high titers. Needle biopsy confirms the diagnosis. Because alveolar hydatids are essentially solid tumors, there is no risk of anaphylaxis or spillage of protoscolices.

Specific Therapy

In many cases, alveolar hydatid disease is not diagnosed until parasite invasion is well advanced and the hepatic lesion is unresectable. Complete excision offers the only hope of cure for this malignant parasitic infection. Partial resections and bilidigestive and hepatodigestive anastomoses may be carried out as palliative measures, predominantly to ensure adequate bile drainage. Alveolar hydatid disease of the lung is invariably a metastatic focus from the liver.

When the primary lesion is inoperable or metastatic spread has occurred, patients with alveolar hydatid disease require life-time mebendazole chemotherapy at 40 mg per kilogram per day in divided doses with food. Mebendazole has been shown to arrest the growth of this parasite, but apparently does not eradicate it. However, short-term therapy with albendazole was effective in killing the larval cestode in two recently published cases.

Monitoring Response to Therapy

Monitoring of adverse reactions to drug therapy should be carried out (as for cystic hydatid disease) at weekly intervals during the first month and at monthly intervals thereafter.

CYSTICERCOSIS

Cysticercosis is caused by infection with the larval form of the porcine tapeworm, *Taenia solium.* Cysticerci (larvae) can lodge anywhere in the body, but the most common areas are brain, skeletal muscle, and subcutaneous tissue.

Although the diagnosis of cerebral cysticercosis can be confirmed by brain biopsy, indirect methods are more appropriate in view of the recent availability of medical therapy. Soft tissue roentgenograms may detect 5×10-mm calcifications in muscle or subcutaneous tissue. In the CT scan, cysts appear as solid, nodular, or cystic structures of varying size, which may or may not be calcified. Serologic testing of cerebral spinal fluid and serum detects antibodies in 70 to 100 percent of cases. A definitive diagnosis can be made by biopsy of subcutaneous cysts when they are present.

Specific Therapy

Praziquantel, a new broad-spectrum antitrematode and anticestode drug, has become the treatment of choice for cysticercosis. Patients with live, viable cysts are likely to benefit from drug therapy, whereas those with old, dead, calcified cysts are not likely to improve. It is difficult to decide when and whether intervention should take place for the following reasons: (1) the natural course of the disease is variable, (2) cysts may regress spontaneously, and (3) killing of cysts may incite a detrimental inflammatory response in some patients. This final point explains why surgical therapy is the preferred treatment for ocular cysticercosis. Praziquantel is recommended only when eye surgery is not possible.

Praziquantel is administered orally (600 mg per tablet) in a dosage of 50 mg per kilogram per day in three divided doses for 14 days. Fever, headache, nausea, vomiting, meningismus, seizures, and increased intracranial pressure have been associated with therapy, most likely from a destruction of cerebral cysts and the resulting inflammatory response. Administration of corticosteroids lessens these symptoms and should be used in conjunction with praziquantel therapy in neurocysticercosis (cerebral, spinal, or ocular involvement). Prednisone, in a dosage of 2 mg per kilogram per day in divided doses to a maximum of 60 mg per day, should be started 1 or 2 days before, continued during, and for several days after treatment with praziquantel.

Metrifonate, an organophosphorous cholmesterase inhibitor, previously used to treat *Schistosomiasis hematobium,* has been shown recently to be effective in the treatment of cysticercosis. In small uncontrolled studies in Mexico, metrifonate produced subjective improvement in most patients and objective improvement in some. The drug was at least partially effective for skin, brain, and eye disease. Adverse effects were mild and transitory. Six courses of 7.5 mg per kilogram per day were given with 2-week drug-free intervals between each 5-day course. To reduce undesirable cholinergic effects, 0.5 mg of atropine was given to children before meals on treatment days. Metrifonate might be considered to be the drug of choice for cysticercus eye disease and as an alternative to praziquantel when the latter is ineffective or poorly tolerated.

Supportive therapy for neurocysticercosis has often included antiseizure medication. Steroid therapy alone has been reported to cause short-term and sometimes long-term improvement in some instances. Until the advent of praziquantel, surgical intervention was considered the only form of treatment for this disease. At present, indications for surgery might include (1) excision of surgically approachable single lesions in the parenchyma of the brain or removal of intraventricular cysts that have not responded to medical management, and (2) decompression of hydrocephalus with ventricular shunts. However, obstruction of shunts from adhesions or free-floating cysts may necessitate frequent revisions to ensure patency.

Monitoring Response to Therapy

Patients with neurocysticercosis who receive praziquantel or metrifonate therapy should be hospitalized and monitored closely for a deterioration in neurologic status.

Follow-up

Clinical and radiologic (CT scan) responses to therapy are usually apparent within 1 to 6 months after treatment. An appreciable change in serology takes place much more slowly. Annual CT scans should be carried out for several years to monitor for evidence of recurrence.

Prevention and Management of Contacts

A small proportion of patients with cysticercosis harbor the adult tapeworm (*T. solium*) when the diagnosis is made. Therefore, the patient's stools should be examined for ova, and treatment should be given when indicated. The stools of household contacts of patients infected with the adult tapeworm should also be examined.

SUGGESTED READING

Brown WJ, Voge M. Cysticercosis, a modern day plague. Pediatr Clin North Am 1985; 32(4):953–969.

Cohen Z, Stone RM, Langer B. Surgical treatment of hydatid disease of the liver. Can J Surg 1976; 19:416–420.

Langer JC, Rose DB, Keystone JS, et al. Diagnosis and management of hydatid disease of the liver. Ann Surg 1984; 199(4):412–417.

Loo L, Braude A. Cerebral cysticercosis in San Diego, a report of 23 cases and a review of the literature. Medicine 1982; 61(6):341–359.

Nash TE, Neva FA. Recent advances in the diagnosis and treatment of cerebral cysticercosis. N Engl J Med 1984; 311(23):1492–1496.

Schantz PM, Van den Bossche H, Eckert J. Chemotherapy for larval echinococcosis in animals and humans: report of a workshop. Z Parasiten 1982; 67:5–26.

Trujillo-Valdes VM, Gonzalez-Barranco D, Sandoval-Islas ME, et al. Chemotherapy of human cysticercosis using metrifonate. In: Cysticercosis: present states of knowledge and perspectives. New York: Academic Press, 1982; 219–226.

Wilson JF, Rausch RL, McMahon BJ, Schantz PM, Trujillo DE, O'Gorman MA. Albendazole therapy in alveolar hydatid disease: a report of favorable results in two patients after short-term therapy. Am J Trop Med Hyg 1987; 37(1):162–168.

ADULT TAPEWORM INFECTIONS

ANTHONY J. REID, M.D., C.C.F.P.

Adult cestode (tapeworm) infections cause few problems for their human hosts and, for the most part, are asymptomatic. Each species has a complex life cycle and is acquired in a different manner. *Hymenolepis nana* and *Taenia solium* are the only cestode infections that can be transmitted from person to person by the fecal–oral route. Hence, stool precautions should be used as a public health measure when one is treating these two infections.

Diagnosis of tapeworm infections is made by finding eggs or worm segments (proglottids) on stool examination. Since *T. saginata* and *T. solium* eggs are morphologically identical, proglottids must be used for species identification. When *Taenia* proglottids are not available for examination, it is prudent to treat the patient as though the infection were caused by *T. solium*. If eggs of *T. solium* are regurgitated or ingested, they penetrate the intestinal mucosa and develop into the larval form in tissues (cysticercosis).

To prevent this from occurring, great care must be taken in treating *T. solium* infections. A gentle purgative of magnesium sulfate or equivalent saline purge should be given 2 hours after treatment to facilitate rapid expulsion of the worm.

All tapeworms can be effectively treated with niclosamide or praziquantel. From a safety and efficacy point of view, there is little to choose between them, with two exceptions. Praziquantel is more effective against *H. nana,* and niclosamide is the preferred drug for *T. solium* infections with concomitant cysticercosis. Praziquantel has not yet been approved by the Food and Drug Administration for use against adult intestinal tapeworms. *Neither drug is recommended for children younger than 2 years of age.* Therefore, physicians must weigh the risks and benefits of the drug to determine whether use of the drug is appropriate in individual cases.

For all tapeworms except *H. nana,* the dosage of niclosamide is 1 g (single dose) for children 2 to 6 years of age and 2 g for those over 6 years. When given by weight, the dosage is 1 g (single dose) for children weighing 11 to 34 kg and 2 g for those weighing more than 34 kg. Since *H. nana* develops in the submucosa of the intestinal tract for several days, treatment with niclosamide must be prolonged. For *H. nana,* the full dosage, as stated above, is given once; then half of the dose is given daily for 5 days. Niclosamide tablets (500 mg) should be chewed or crushed and suspended in water and administered as a single dose after a light meal. Side effects such as nausea and abdominal pain are uncommon.

Praziquantel is administered orally in a single dose of 10 mg per kilogram for *Taenia saginata*, *Taenia solium*, *Diphyllobothrium pacificum*, and *Dipylidium caninum*, and 25 mg per kilogram for *Diphyllobothrium latum* and *Hymenolepis nana*. Praziquantel occasionally causes mild, transient, gastrointestinal pain and, rarely dizziness and skin rashes.

For all tapeworm infections, at least two stool samples should be examined in follow-up 1 to 2 weeks after the completion of treatment. If these stools are free of parasite ova and proglottids, patients should be reexamined 2 to 3 months later to ensure the complete eradication of these infections. The presence of eggs or proglottids on follow-up examination is an indication of drug failure, and I would re-treat with an alternative medication.

SUGGESTED READING

American Society of Hospital Pharmacists Guide. Suppl. C (Nov. 1984). Anthelminthics (section 8:08). Niclosamide (subsection 18C).

Groll E. Praziquantel for cestode infections in man. Acta Trop 1980; 37:293–296.

Warren K, Mahmoud A. Tropical and geographic medicine. Cestode infections. New York: McGraw-Hill, 1984:471.

TREMATODE INFECTIONS

EDWARD K. MARKELL, M.D., Ph.D.

The trematodes or flukes that infect humans with two exceptions (*Schistosoma mansoni* and *Fasciola hepatica*) are not indigenous to the Western Hemisphere. *Schistosoma mansoni* cannot be acquired in continental North America, although infection is transmitted in Puerto Rico and other Caribbean islands, and extensively in South America. *Fasciola,* a common parasite of sheep and cattle, is seldom found in humans. Fluke infections are seen primarily in immigrants (especially refugees from southeast Asia) and in persons who have become exposed to them during travel.

Many such infections are asymptomatic and discovered only by stool examinations performed routinely or because of symptoms from some other cause. If trematode infection is suspected, the proper type of stool examination is critical. Some laboratories do not perform stool concentrates or do not do so unless specifically requested. Stool examinations for helminth parasites cannot be considered adequate unless concentration techniques are used. To detect trematodes, the concentrate must be done by a sedimentation technique. If the alternative flotation method is used, eggs of the flukes rupture and are not recovered.

A single properly performed stool examination should be adequate for detection of liver, lung, and intestinal flukes. Several stool specimens or, for *Schistosoma haematobium,* morning urine specimens may need to be examined before eggs are detected, as they work their way intermittently through the wall of the intestine or bladder. A hatching technique can be used in which a fairly large volume of stool is diluted with water in a darkened container, and examination of a lighted area is made for the freshly hatched phototropic larvae. Hatching also occurs spontaneously if a urine specimen containing eggs of *S. haematobium* stands for several hours. Swallowed eggs of *Paragonimus* appear in the stools and they can also be found in the sputum. Schistosome eggs can be detected in samples of rectal or bladder mucosa, preferably taken from inflamed or granulomatous areas during proctoscopy or cystoscopy. The eggs are readily seen if the mucosal specimen is compressed between two slides and examined microscopically under low power. Serologic tests for schistosomiasis and paragonimiasis are available from the Parasitic Serology Division of the Centers for Disease Control (serum specimens should be sent through the State Health Department).

Praziquantel (Biltricide) has proved highly effective for the treatment of most trematode and cestode infections, with relatively few and mild side effects. It is approved by the Food and Drug Administration (FDA) only for treatment of schistosomiasis, but must be considered the drug of choice for all fluke infections except fascioliasis.

LIVER FLUKES

Clonorchis sinensis and its close relatives, *Opisthorchis viverrini* and *O. felineus,* are the most common liver flukes of humans whereas *Fasciola* is relatively uncommon in humans. However, a laboratory diagnosis of any of these parasites must be carefully assessed. Eggs of *Fasciola* found in the feces can represent a true infection, but their presence may indicate only that the patient consumed liver that was infected with these parasites. To demonstrate that an infection was spurious, additional stool specimens passed when the patient has not eaten liver for several days must be obtained. Eggs of *Fasciola hepatica* cannot be differentiated in the laboratory from those of the intestinal fluke *Fasciolopsis buski,* and if it cannot be made on the basis of travel history, such differentiation could require duodenal sampling. Eggs found in the bile indicate an infection with *Fasciola hepatica.* Eggs of *Clonorchis* and *Opisthorchis* cannot be differentiated from those of *Heterophyes* and *Metagonimus* (all four are probably reported as *Clonorchis* by the laboratory). However, the relatively innocuous intestinal flukes *Heterophyes* and *Metagonimus* are short-lived, and eggs of the *Clonorchis* type found in the stools of a patient who has been out of an endemic area for at least one year can be assumed to be those of *Clonorchis* or *Opisthorchis.* Intestinal and hepatic infection can be differentiated by examining biliary drainage obtained by duodenal intubation or by use of the duodenal string test (EnteroTest).

Praziquantel is the only effective drug for the treatment of clonorchiasis and opisthorchiasis. It is available in tablets of 600 mg, scored so that they can be broken into four segments of 150 mg each. It is taken with meals at the rate of 25 mg per kilogram of body weight, three times in a single day. The tablets should be taken with water and are bitter if retained in the mouth. Whether praziquantel is safe for children under 4 years of age has not been established, but in older children and adults the drug is well tolerated. Mild and transient side effects include (in decreasing order of frequency) malaise, headache, dizziness, abdominal discomfort, nausea, fever, and urticaria. These generally do not require treatment, although the rarely reported urticarial reactions, if accompanied by a rash, could represent hypersensitivity to the drug and contraindicate its further use. No clinically significant changes in laboratory values have been reported. Reexamination 1 year after therapy indicates some treatment failures with the single-day regimen outlined earlier. When the same dose is given for a second day, cure rates at 1 year approach 100 percent.

Early reports indicated that praziquantel was as effective against *Fasciola hepatica* as in the treatment of other trematode infections. Later studies have not borne this out, and indeed they raise the question as to whether it has any efficacy in this condition. Bithionol* is the drug of choice in fascioliasis. Dosage of Bithionol is 30 to 50 mg per kilogram of body weight on alternate days for 10 to 15 doses. The drug is administered orally after meals, and the daily dosage may be given in two or three approximately equal parts. A cure rate approaching 100 percent may be expected from this treatment.

Mild side effects are common, but seldom require interruption of therapy. Diarrhea and abdominal cramps occur frequently, but usually disappear after the first few days of therapy. Nausea and vomiting may be troublesome, but respond to symptomatic treatment and bed rest. Urticaria, skin rashes, dizziness, and headache occur in a small percentage of patients.

Emetine hydrochloride and dehydroemetine* are also effective in fascioliasis, but are considerably more toxic than Bithionol. Dehydroemetine, less toxic than emetine hydrochloride, is administered in the same manner as in amebic abscess.

LUNG FLUKES

A number of species of *Paragonimus* are found throughout the world, and several of these infect humans. A laboratory usually reports the eggs of any species of *Paragonimus* as *P. westermani;* species differentiation on the basis of eggs is difficult or impossible, as is a precise identification on geographic grounds. Treatment is the same for all species.

The preferred treatment for lung flukes is praziquantel, administered as outlined for the treatment of liver flukes, but given for 2 consecutive days. No increase in severity of the mild side effects observed with a single day's treatment should be expected with the 2-day regimen.

Good results have been obtained in Laotian refugee children with administration of the alternative drug, Bithionol, using the regimen described for treatment of fascioliasis.

BLOOD FLUKES

Praziquantel has had its most widespread use in the treatment of the schistosomiases, and only for treatment of these parasites has this drug received FDA approval. *Schistosoma mansoni* and *S. haematobium* are effectively treated with a single oral dose of 40 mg per kilogram. Cure rates range from 70 to 95 percent. Side effects of praziquantel are similar to those described in connection with its use in liver fluke infection. *Schistosoma intercalatum* is also treated with a single oral dose of 40 mg per kilogram. *Schistosoma japonicum* and *S. mekongi* infections require slightly larger dosages of 60 mg per kilogram, given as three doses of 20 mg per kilogram.

Metrifonate (Bilarcil) (not available in the United States) is effective for treatment of *S. haematobium* infections only. This agent is inexpensive compared with praziquantel and thus suitable for mass treatment programs. The drug is taken by mouth, 7.5 to 10 mg per kilogram, every other week for three doses. Metrifonate is an organophosphate, and its administration results in reversible plasma cholinesterase inhibition. Clinical tolerance to the drug is good, but nausea or vomiting, abdominal pain, headache or vertigo, and bronchospasm are oc-

---

* Obtainable in the United States only from the Parasitic Disease Drug Service, Centers for Disease Control, Atlanta, GA 30333. Telephone (404) 329-3670.

casionally reported after treatment. Cure rates are similar to those of patients treated with praziquantel.

Oxamniquine (Vansil) is an alternative agent for the treatment of *Schistosoma mansoni* infection. For infections acquired in West Africa, the Carribean, or South America, a single oral dose (best taken after the last meal of the day) of 15 mg per kilogram (20 mg per kilogram in smaller children) is usually effective; cure rates range from 80 to 90 percent. Strains of *S. mansoni* acquired in North or East Africa are less susceptible to the drug, and a similar cure rate requires dosages of 20 mg per kilogram daily for 3 days. Side effects are generally mild, and drowsiness or dizziness occurs in about 10 percent of cases; headache, fever, nausea, diarrhea, and rash occur less often. Convulsions occur rarely. A metabolite sometimes turns the urine dark, but this is of no clinical significance.

Other pharmaceutical agents besides praziquantel that are effective against *S. japonicum* and *S. mekongi* have unacceptably high toxicity or are unavailable in the United States. Niridazole (Ambilhar) is the least toxic of these alternative drugs. A dosage of 25 mg per kilogram is given orally in two divided doses daily for 7 to 10 days. Common side effects include headache, dizziness, nausea and vomiting, and abdominal cramps. Diarrhea, myalgia, arthralgia, and paresthesia are less commonly seen. Flattening or inversion of the T wave in the electrocardiogram occurs in approximately half the patients treated. A small percentage of patients have central nervous system side effects such as agitation, confusion, visual or auditory hallucinations, or localized convulsions, usually occurring between the third and fifth day of treatment. Such reactions indicate the need to interrupt therapy. A metabolite of the drug often turns the urine an orange-brown color, but this is not clinically significant.

Certain complications of schistosomal infection require other modes of therapy. The Katayama fever, seen most frequently in *S. japonicum* infections, but also occurring in the early stages of infection by the other species, is a hypersensitivity reaction to early massive infection and is marked by fever, chills, headache, abdominal pain, nausea and vomiting, diarrhea, hepatosplenomegaly, lymphadenopathy, cough, and urticaria. Mild symptoms may respond to symptomatic treatment, but corticosteroids are recommended for more severe cases. Antischistosomal treatment should be delayed until the acute symptoms subside. Spinal schistosomiasis is thought to represent localized hypersensitivity to eggs in spinal vessels and may occur early in the infection (most frequently in *S. mansoni* infection). The infection initially occurs as transverse myelitis, usually with paraplegia and loss of sphincter control. Specific antischistosomal therapy and large-dosage corticosteroid therapy must be started promptly. Laminectomy may be indicated.

After treatment, stools or urine should be rechecked periodically for 6 months to ensure that treatment has been successful.

INTESTINAL FLUKES

The intestinal trematodes include *Fasciolopsis buski* and the minute flukes *Heterophyes heterophyes* and *Metagonimus yokogawai*. Confusion associated with differentiating their eggs from those of liver flukes has already been discussed. Although a number of species of *Echinostoma* and related genera infect humans, their eggs are all similar and unlike those of nonintestinal flukes.

The preferred treatment for all these infections is praziquantel, taken by mouth with meals at the rate of 25 mg per kilogram, three times in a single day. Side effects of treatment have been listed under treatment of liver fluke infections.

An alternative drug for therapy of all the intestinal fluke infections is tetrachloroethylene. This drug is approved for human use, but is available in the United States only as a veterinary product (Nema) in capsules containing 0.2, 0.5, 1.0, 2.5, and 5 ml. The drug is contraindicated for patients with chronic gastrointestinal disorders or liver disease. Alcohol and fatty foods must be avoided for 12 hours before and 14 hours after the drug is administered. It is best to take it in the morning, withholding food but not water until 4 hours thereafter. The dosage is 0.1 to 0.12 ml per kilogram (maximum 5 ml), and it should be followed in 2 hours with a saline purge. Side effects include epigastric distress, dizziness, headache, and drowsiness. It has disulfiramlike effects if it is taken with alcohol. Hepatic necrosis has been reported rarely after its use.

Niclosamide (Niclocide), although FDA-approved for treatment of tapeworm infections only, is also effective in fasciolopsiasis. The dosage for children weighing between 11 and 34 kg is 2 tablets (1 g), for those 34 to 50 kg, 3 tablets (1.5 g), and for those over 50 kg, 4 tablets (2 g), repeated every other day for three doses. Medication should be taken after a light meal and must be thoroughly chewed and taken with water to minimize gastric irritation. For small children, the tablets are crushed to a fine powder and mixed with water. Tablets are vanilla-flavored and generally well accepted. No posttreatment purge or dietary restrictions are necessary. Side effects are mild to moderate and include nausea, vomiting, abdominal discomfort, anorexia, diarrhea, drowsiness, dizziness, and headache. These are transitory and do not require cessation of treatment. A skin rash occurs rarely.

The stool should be reexamined about a week after treatment with any of these drugs. Retreatment is seldom warranted for intestinal fluke infections (with the possible exception of fasciolopsiasis), because light infections are generally asymptomatic.

SUGGESTED READING

Davis A. Recent advances in schistosomiasis. Q J Med 1986;
58:95–110.
Harries AD, Fryatt R, Walker J, et al. Schistosomiasis in expatri-
ates returning to Britain from the tropics: a controlled study.
Lancet 1986; 1:86–88.
Johnson RJ, Jong EC, Dunning SB, et al. Paragonimiasis: diagnosis
and the use of praziquantel in treatment. Rev Infect Dis 1985;
7:200–206.
Jong EC, Wasserheit JN, Johnson RJ, et al. Praziquantel for the
treatment of Clonorchis/Opisthorchis infections: report of a
double-blind, placebo-controlled trial. J Infect Dis 1985;
152:637–640.
Knobloch J, Deldado E, Alvarez A, et al. Human fascioliasis in
Cajamarca/Peru. I. Diagnostic methods and treatment with
praziquantel. Trop Med Parasitol 1985; 36:88–90.

PROTOZOAN INFECTIONS

J. CARL CRAFT, M.D.
ANDREA J. RUFF, M.D.

MALARIA

Malaria is caused by four species of *Plasmodium: P. falciparum, P. ovale, P. vivax,* and *P. malariae.* It is endemic in tropical and subtropical areas;
however, imported cases in immigrants and travelers
are increasing in temperate areas. The infection is
transmitted from person to person by the bite of an
Anopheles mosquito or, rarely, through blood transfusion, intraveneous drug use with contaminated
needles, or transplacentally. The parasites are inoculated into the bloodstream and then travel to the liver,
where they invade the hepatocytes, initiating the exoerythrocytic phase of the disease. After variable periods of time, the organisms rupture the hepatocytes and
invade erythrocytes. The erythrocytic stage is characterized by recurrent invasion and rupture of erythrocytes, often occuring with characteristic periodicities
of 48 to 72 hours. Two species, *P. vivax* and *P. ovale,*
also have persistent organisms in the hepatocytes, which
may cause relapses if only the erythrocytic parasites
are eradicated.

All of the pathogenicity of malaria appears to be
caused by the erythrocytic organisms, and symptoms
correspond closely to the maturation and release of
the erythrocytic parasites. Symptoms of malaria typically consist of paroxysms of chills, fever, and dia-
phoresis occurring every 48 hours with *P. vivax, P.
ovale, P. vivax,* and *P. malariae* are largely susceptible to chloroquine and quinine; however, certain *P.*
odicity of the paroxysms may be absent, particularly
in children. Other signs and symptoms include myalgias, headache, nausea, vomiting, malaise, spleno-
megaly, and anemia. *P. falciparum* is capable of producing a high level of parasitemia and a much more
fulminant illness.

Patients with *P. falciparum* malaria may develop
delirium, convulsions, coma, hepatic failure, disseminated intravascular coagulation, hemoglobinuria
with renal failure, pulmonary edema, and shock.

Children between the ages of 3 months and 5 years
are particularly prone to severe *P. falciparum* infections, which impair general growth and development,
and may end fatally. The other species of malaria
typically give rise to more benign attacks, which are
usually self-limited, rarely fatal, and commonly followed by relapses. With its protean manifestations,
malaria simulates many other diseases and is often
unrecognized.

The definitive diagnosis of malaria requires the
identification of plasmodia in peripheral blood or
other tissues such as bone marrow. Morphology of
the parasites can be seen in thin blood smears, allowing for differentiation of the species. Examination of
thick smears is often necessary to detect the organisms when they are present in small numbers. Since
parasitemia may be intermittent or low, several blood
smears should be examined before the diagnosis is
excluded. Mixed infections occur in 1 to 2 percent of
cases, and the presence of one parasite does not eliminate the possibility of another species. Diagnostic
errors occur when prophylaxis with antimalarials has
altered parasite morphology or when stains other
than Giemsa are used. Serologic tests are available
through the Centers for Disease Control; however,
they cannot differentiate between current and past
infections.

Several available antimalarials effectively eradicate the different stages of plasmodia. However, in
recent years, therapy has been complicated by the
emergence of resistance to many antimalarials (Table
1). Chloroquine-resistant *P. falciparum* strains have
been encountered since 1960, and they are now
found in Southeast Asia, South America, Oceania,
the Philippines, India, and parts of Africa. Certain
strains of *P. falciparum* found in Southeast Asia are
resistant to virtually all known antimalarials. *P.
ovale, P. vivax,* and *P. malariae* are largely susceptible to chloroquine and quinine; however, certain *P.
vivax* are resistant to pyrimethamine and sulfonamides.

Chloroquine diphosphate (Aralen, Avloclor, Re-
sochin) is the drug of choice for an uncomplicated
attack of malaria caused by any plasmodia except
resistant *P. falciparum.* It works quickly against the
erythrocytic forms of plasmodia, inducing clinical
and parasitic remission within 72 hours. The pediat-

ric dosage is 10 mg base per kilogram (maximum, 600 mg base) given orally at once, followed by 5 mg base per kilogram given 6, 24, and 48 hours later. Older children and adults receive an initial dose of 600 mg base followed by 300 mg 6 hours later and 300 mg on each of the next 2 days. The drug may produce gastrointestinal discomfort, which can be minimized by taking the medication with meals. Other side effects include pruritus, skin rashes, visual blurring, scotomata, and headache. Retinopathies have been reported after prolonged use with large total doses, and in rare instances, blood dyscrasias and neurotoxicity with convulsions and psychosis have also been seen. The drug should be used with caution in patients with glucose-6-phosphate dehydrogenase deficiency. Accidental overdose of chloroquine may be fatal, and the drug should not be accessible to children. Amodiaquine (Camoquin, Flavoquine, Miaquin), a compound related to chloroquine, has also been used to treat uncomplicated acute malaria. However, because of several reports of agranulocytosis following the use of amodiaquine, we would no longer use it for the therapy of malaria.

In those areas where chloroquine-resistant *P. falciparum* is common, the treatment of choice is a combination of quinine sulfate and pyrimethamine-sulfadoxine or quinine and tetracycline. Although quinine alone can control an attack of resistant *P. falciparum,* it may fail to prevent recurrence. The addition of pyrimethamine and sulfa decreases this possibility. The dosage of quinine sulfate is 25 mg per kilogram per day (maximum, oral dose 1,950 mg per day) for 3 days. It is given orally in three divided doses, preferably with meals to lessen gastrointestinal complaints. Toxic effects of quinine include the syndrome of cinchonism with tinnitus, headache, visual disturbances, dizziness, and skin rashes. Because the drug has reportedly been associated with embryopathy and onset of premature labor, its use during pregnancy has been discouraged; however, malaria may be particularly severe during pregnancy, compromising both maternal and fetal health. For additional information regarding the use of quinine in pregnant patients with chloroquine-resistant *P. falciparum,* we suggest you contact the Centers for Disease Control (days: 404–452–4046; nights and weekends: 404–329–3644).

In addition to quinine, a single dose of pyrimethamine–sulfadoxine should be given. These drugs are available in a tablet containing 25 mg of pyrimethamine and 500 mg of sulfadoxine (Fansidar) and should be administered in the following doses: 6 to 11 months, ¼ tablet; 1 to 3 years, ½ tablet; 4 to 8 years, 1 tablet; 9 to 14 years, 2 tablets; older than 14 years, 3 tablets. Pyrimethamine is generally well tolerated; its use is occasionally associated with vomiting and with the development of blood dyscrasias and folic acid deficiency. Because experience with pyrimethamine usage in pregnancy is limited and the drug is reportedly teratogenic in some animals, its use

in pregnant women should be avoided unless absolutely necessary. Sulfonamide toxicity includes hematuria, crystalluria, and rash; persons with glucose-6-phosphate dehydrogenase deficiency may develop hemolytic anemia with the use of sulfonamides. It has generally been recommended that pyrimethamine–sulfadoxine not be used in children less than 2 months old because of their potential for developing hyperbilirubinemia.

An alternative regimen that can be used for the therapy of chloroquine-resistant *P. falciparum* infections is the combination of quinine for 3 days *plus* tetracycline, 5 mg per kilogram four times daily (maximum, 250 mg per dose) for 7 days. This combination can be used in children older than 8 years of age and is of particular value in treating infections acquired in Thailand, where *P. falciparum* is often resistant to both chloroquine and pyrimethamine-sulfadoxine. Another antimalarial, mefloquine, has been used successfully in a number of countries to treat multiply resistant *P. faciparum*. It is not currently available in this country.

Patients with severe malaria who are unable to tolerate oral medication should be treated with parenteral quinine dihydrochloride. The usual dosage is 25 mg per kilogram per day (maximum, 600 mg per dose). One-third of the dose is diluted in normal saline and given slowly over 2 to 4 hours. If there is no clinical improvement, the same dose (one-third the total daily dose) is given 8 hours later, and oral therapy is substituted as soon as possible. The daily dosage of quinine should be adjusted to one-half or one-third the usual dosage in patients with renal or hepatic failure. Intravenous quinine is associated with significant toxicity including hypotension, cardiac arrhythmias, delirium, and coma. Close monitoring of vital signs is essential during the administration of this drug. It is available from the Parasitic Diseases Division, Centers for Disease Control, Atlanta, Georgia, (days: 404–452–4046; nights and weekends: 404-329-3644). Quinidine gluconate is more widely available in many countries and has been used successfully for the therapy of severe falciparum malaria. The pediatric dosage has not been established; however, the currently recommended adult dosage is a loading dose of 10 mg per kilogram, followed by an infusion of 0.02 mg per kilogram per minute up to 72 hours. It may also have serious cardiac toxicity and should be given intravenously very slowly with ECG monitoring. Because quinidine has not been approved for the therapy of malaria in children in this country, persons desiring to use it for this purpose should contact the Centers for Disease Control for additional information (numbers as indicated). An alternative therapy used in adults is intramuscular chloroquine hydrochloride. It should be avoided in infants and children because of its greater toxicity in that age group.

In *P. ovale* and *P. vivax* malaria, additional therapy is required to eradicate the exoerythrocytic para-

TABLE 1   Treatment Regimens for Protozoan Diseases

Amebiasis (*Entamoeba histolytica*)
Asymptomatic
Drug of choice: Diloxanide furoate (CDC) 20 mg/kg/day PO div q8h × 10 days (max. 1,500 mg/day)
Alternative: Iodoquinol 30–40 mg/kg/day PO div q8h × 20 days (max. 1,950 mg/day)
  Paromomycin 30 mg/kg/day PO div q8h × 7 days (max 1,500 mg/day)
Moderate and severe colitis
Drug of choice: Metronidazole 35–50 mg/kg/day PO div q8h × 10 days (max 2,250 mg/day)
  plus
  Diloxanide furoate as above or iodoquinol as above
Extraintestinal disease
Drug of choice: Metronidazole 50 mg/kg/day PO div q8h × 10 days
  plus
  Diloxanide furoate as above or iodoquinol as above
Alternative: Dehydroemetine 1–1.5 mg/kg/day IM div q12–24h × 5 days (max. 90 mg/day) followed by
  Chloroquine 10 mg base/kg/day PO × 14–21 days (300 mg base/dose)
  plus
  Diloxanide furoate as above or iodoquinol as above

Amebic meningoencephalitis (*Naegleria, Acanthamoeba*)
Drug of choice: Amphotericin B 1 mg/kg/day IV for uncertain duration, start with test dose of 0.1 mg/kg, max. 1 mg
  plus
  Intrathecal amphotericin B 0.1–0.5 mg daily or every other day

Babesiosis (*Babesia* species)
Drug of choice: Clindamycin 20 mg/kg/day PO or IV div q6h × 7–10 days (max. 2–4 g/day)
  plus
  Quinine sulfate 25 mg/kg/day PO div q8h × 7–10 days (max. 1,950 mg/day)

Balantidiasis (*Balantidium coli*)
Drug of choice: Metronidazole 15 mg/kg/day PO div q8h × 7–10 days (max. 750 mg/day)
Alternative: Tetracycline 40 mg/kg/day PO div q6h × 10 days (max. 2 g/day)
  Iodoquinol 40 mg/kg/day PO div q8h × 20 days (max. 1,950 mg/day)

Cryptosporidiosis (*Cryptosporidium* species)
Drug of choice No proven effective therapy
Alternative: Spiramycin (FDA) 1 g/day PO div q6h (adult dose—4 g/day) for uncertain duration (may be effective)
  Furazolidone 9 mg/kg/day PO div q8h (max. 400 mg/day) for uncertain duration (may be effective)

Dientamoeba fragilis
Drug of choice:
  Children <8 y Metronidazole 15 mg/kg/day PO div q8h × 7–10 days (max. 750 mg/day)
  Children >8 y Tetracycline 40 mg/kg/day PO div q6h × 10 days (max. 2 g/day)
Alternative: Iodoquinol 40 mg/kg/day PO div q8h × 20 days (max. 1,950 mg/day)

Giardiasis (*Giardia lamblia*)
Drug of choice: Furazolidone 9 mg/kg/day PO div q8h × 10 days (max. 400 mg/day)
Alternative: Quinacrine 6 mg/kg/day PO div q8h × 10 days (max. 300 mg/day)
  Metronidazole 15 mg/kg/day PO div q8h × 10 days (max. 750 mg/day)

Leishmaniasis (*Leishmania* species)
Drug of choice: Stibogluconate sodium (CDC) 20 mg/kg/day IV, daily × 20–30 days may require 2–3 courses of therapy (max. 850 mg/day)
Alternative: Pentamidine isethionate 4 mg/kg/day IM daily × 14 days (max. 4 mg/kg/day)
  Amphotericin B 1 mg/kg/day IV for 30–60 days (max. 1 mg/kg/day)

Malaria (*Plasmodium* species)
Drug of choice:
  P. vivax, P. ovale Chloroquine 10 mg base/kg/day (max. 600 mg base/dose) PO stat, then 5 mg base/kg 6, 24, and 48 hours later (max. 300 mg base/dose), followed by primaquine 0.3 mg base/kg/day × 14 days (max. 15 mg base/day)
  P. malariae Chloroquine only as above
  P. falciparum
  Chloroquine-susceptible Chloroquine only as above
  Chloroquine-resistant Quinine 25 mg/kg/day PO div q8h × 3 days (max. 1,950 mg/day)
  plus
  Pyrimethamine–sulfadoxine (Fansidar) in a single dose: 6–11 months: ¼ tablet, 1–3 years: ½ tablet, 4–8 years: 1 tablet, 9–14 years: 2 tablets, >14 years: 3 tablets
  (Parenteral quinine is available from the CDC for IV use)
Prophylaxis
  Areas without chloroquine resistance: Chloroquine 5 mg/kg/day (max. 300 mg base/dose) PO beginning 1 week before arriving in a malarial zone and continuing for 6 weeks after last exposure
  Areas with chloroquine-resistant P. falciparum Consider use of pyrimethamine-sulfadoxine (Fansidar): 2–11 months: ⅛ tablet/week, 1–3 years: ¼ tablet/week, 4–8 years: ½ tablet/week, 9–14 years: ¾ tablet/week, >14 years: 1 tablet/week

Pneumocystis pneumonia (*Pneumocystis carinii*)
Drug of choice: Trimethoprim–sulfamethoxazole, trimethoprim 20 mg/kg/day, sulfamethoxazole 100 mg/kg/day PO div q6h × 14 days (max. 20 mg/kg TMP/100 mg/kg SMZ per day)
Alternative: Pentamidine isethionate 4 mg/kg/day IM × 14 days (max. 4 mg/kg/day)
Prophylaxis: Trimethoprim 5 mg/kg/day, sulfamethoxazole 25 mg/kg/day PO q12h until the patients immune system returns to normal

Toxoplasmosis (*Toxoplasma gondii*)
Drug of choice: Pyrimethamine 2 mg/kg/day (max. 50 mg/day) PO div q12h × 2–3 days, then 1 mg/kg/day (max. 25 mg) PO given every 1–2 days × 3 weeks (Supp. folinic acid)
  plus
  Sulfadiazine or trisulfapyrimidines 100 mg/kg/day (max. 2–6 g/day) PO div q12h × 4 weeks
  or
  Spiramycin (FDA) 100 mg/kg/day PO div q6h × 4 weeks (max. 3–4 g/day) (neonates and infants should receive the same dose divided q12h)

TABLE 1 (*continued*)

Trichomoniasis (*Trichomonas vaginalis*)	**Alternative:** Pentamidine isethionate 4 mg/kg/day IM × 10 days (max. 4 mg/kg/day)
Drug of choice: Metronidazole 15 mg/kg/day PO div q8h × 7 days (max. 750 mg/day)	
Chagas' disease (*Trypanosoma cruzi*)	Late disease with CNS involvement
Drug of choice: Nifurtimox (CDC) 5 mg/kg/day PO div q6h, increasing by 2–5 mg/kg ql–2 weeks until a maximum of 15–17 mg/kg/day is reached. Continue therapy for 3–4 months	Drug of choice: Melarsoprol (CDC), initial pediatric dose 0.36 mg/kg IV, gradually increase dosage to maximum of 3.6 mg/kg ql–5 days given over 1 month (total dose of 18–25 mg/kg in 1 month)
Sleeping sickness (*Trypanosoma gambiense, Trypananosoma rhodesiense*)	
Acute Stage	
Drug of choice: Suramin (CDC), test dose of 2 mg/kg/day, followed by 20 mg/kg/day on days 1, 3, 7, 14, and 21 (max. 1 g/dose)	

sites and prevent relapses. Primaquine phosphate given in an oral dosage of 0.3 mg base per kilogram per day for 14 days is the treatment of choice. Older children should be given 15 mg base per day for 14 days. Side effects of primaquine vary from mild gastrointestinal distress to severe hemolytic reactions in individuals with glucose-6-phosphate dehydrogenase deficiency. It may produce reversible bone marrow suppression and should not be used in patients with conditions predisposing them to granulocytopenia. Quinacrine (Atabrine) appears to potentiate the toxicity of primaquine and should not be used concurrently. Primaquine usage should also be avoided during pregnancy. *Plasmodium falciparum,* transfusion-acquired malaria, and congenital malaria do not require primaquine therapy because there are no exoerythrocytic organisms in the liver to be eradicated. Occasionally, relapses occur after appropriate chloroquine-primaquine therapy, and they should be treated with another complete course of combination therapy. Patients should have several blood smears examined for 1 month following therapy to detect recrudescence of the infection.

Supportive care is essential in the treatment of malaria to prevent many of the potentially life-threatening complications. Patients may require vigorous fluid resuscitation for shock, blood transfusions for acute severe anemia, treatment of hypoglycemia, and dialysis for renal failure. Although the use of corticosteroids had been recommended for complications such as cerebral malaria, recent evidence suggests that they might be harmful. Therefore, steroids should not be used in cerebral malaria. Whole blood exchange transfusions have been increasingly recommended for the treatment of high density parasitemia (greater than 10 to 20 percent) and/or cerebral malaria.

Prevention of malaria is possible with the regular use of chemoprophylactic agents. It is recommended that prophylaxis be started 1 week before arrival in an endemic area (so that drug toxicities can be observed before leaving the country), be taken weekly for the duration of the stay, and be continued for 6 weeks after leaving the malarious area. Because it is efficacious and relatively nontoxic, chloroquine phosphate in a dose of 5 mg base per kilogram once weekly (maximum, 300 mg base per week) is the drug of choice. Hydroxychloroquine (Plaquenil), chloroquine sulfate (Nivaquine B), and amodiaquine (Camoquin, Flavoquin, Miaquin) have all been used successfully as prophylaxis and are sometimes more readily available than chloroquine diphosphate in other countries. Because of unacceptable toxicity (occasional cases of agranulocytosis), the use of amodiaquine prophylactically is no longer indicated. Pyrimethamine (Daraprim) and chloroguanide (proguanil, Paludrine) have also been used prophylactically; however, they may be less effective than chloroquine against chloroquine-susceptible *P. falciparum.* It is generally recommended that in areas without known chloroquine resistance, these alternative agents be used only in patients who are unable to tolerate chloroquine (see Table 1).

In *P. vivax* and *P. ovale* infections, chloroquine prophylaxis may not eradicate persistent exoerythrocytic forms in the liver, leaving the patient at risk for relapse. Primaquine phosphate in a dose of 0.3 mg base per kilogram per day for 14 days prevents persistent infection. However, because the actual risk of *P. ovale* or *P. vivax* malaria in short-term travelers is low and the potential side effects from primaquine are not insignificant, routine prophylaxis of this type is no longer recommended. If travelers spend more than a few weeks in rural endemic areas with heavy mosquito exposure, prophylaxis with primaquine is warranted.

The recommended prophylaxis in areas with known chloroquine resistance is a combination of chloroquine and pyrimethamine–sulfadoxine (Fansidar, Antemal, Falcidar). Because weekly prophylaxis with Fansidar has caused severe and sometimes fatal cutaneous reactions, it is no longer recommended for all travelers to areas with chloroquine resistance. The decision to use Fansidar with chloroquine should be based on the estimated risk of acquiring a resistant *P. falciparum* infection in various geographic areas. Short-term travelers (3 weeks or less) to Africa should receive chloroquine alone as prophylaxis. They should have available pyrimethamine–sulfadoxine (25 mg pyrimethamine and 500 mg sulfadoxine) to be taken presumptively as a single dose in the event of a febrile illness in a setting where medical care is unavailable. The pediatric dose is as follows: 2 to 11 months, ¼ tablet; 1 to 3 years, ½ tablet; 4 to 8 years, 1 tablet; 9 to 14 years, 2 tablets; older than 14 years, 3 tablets—in each case the dose is given orally as a single dose. This medication is contraindicated for persons with glucose-6-phosphate dehydrogenase deficiency, infants younger than 2 months old, persons with sulfa allergies, and pregnant women.

A prolonged stay in areas with known chloroquine resistance, under conditions promoting malaria transmission, may warrant weekly use of Fansidar along with chloroquine. The prophylactic pediatric dose of Fansidar is as follows: 2 to 11 months, ⅛ tablet per week; 1 to 3 years, ¼ tablet per week; 4 to 8 years, ½ tablet per week; 9 to 14 years, ¾ tablet per week; older than 14 years, 1 tablet per week (25 mg pyrimethamine per 500 mg of sulfadoxine per tablet). Prophylaxis with Fansidar should be discontinued if any mucocutaneous signs or symptoms such as pruritus, rash, orogenital lesions, or pharyngitis develop. Alternative chemoprophylactic agents for chloroquine-resistant *P. falciparum* include proguanil and doxycycline. Proguanil is not currently available in this country; widespread resistance of *P. falciparum* to the drug may limit its usefulness in other countries. The use of daily doxycycline in a dose of 2 mg per kilogram (maximum 100 mg per day) is currently recommended for those individuals traveling to areas with chloroquine- and pyrimethamine–sulfadoxine-resistant *P. falciparum* (in particular, parts of Thailand). It has been associated with photosensitivity and should not be used in children less than 8 years old or pregnant women.

Areas where the risk of acquiring chloroquine-resistant falciparum malaria appears to be the highest include parts of Africa (particularly East Africa) and Oceania. Long-term travelers to these areas should consider use of Fansidar along with chloroquine. Travelers to China and Southeast Asia staying primarily in urban areas have little risk of acquiring malaria and do not routinely need prophylaxis. If travelers anticipate significant outdoor exposure in rural malarious areas of China and Southeast Asia, they should receive prophylaxis with chloroquine and Fansidar. Similar recommendations can be made for travelers to South America, but chloroquine prophylaxis alone is recommended for travelers to the Indian subcontinent.

As drug resistance increases, chemoprophylaxis may become less effective. Since the worldwide pattern of drug resistance to Plasmodia is constantly changing, physicians should contact the Centers for Disease Control (days: 404-452-4046; nights and weekends: 404-329-3644) for the latest recommendations regarding therapy or prophylaxis of *P. falciparum* infections. Travelers to endemic areas should always take additional measures to reduce contact with mosquitoes, decreasing the risk of malaria transmission. This includes the use of mosquito nets, insect repellent, and clothes that cover most of the body.

BABESIOSIS

Babesiosis* is a usually self-limited, malarialike disease caused in the United States by infection of human red blood cells with the protozoan parasite *Babesia microti*. Most infections are subclinical and are detected only by serologic surveys. Severe infections with fever, hemolytic anemia, hemoglobinuria, and renal failure have occurred in splenectomized adults. Symptomatic infection in the pediatric age group is rare. The diagnosis is made by examination of a Giemsa-stained thin or thick blood film for the presence of characteristic intraerythrocytic parasites and can be confirmed by hamster inoculation or by a rise in indirect immunofluorescent antibody titer.

The disease is transmitted by a bite of the small, hard-bodied tick *Ixodes dammini,* present during the summer in coastal areas and on off-shore islands of Massachusetts, Rhode Island, and New York. Other cases have followed transfusion of refrigerated or frozen-thawed blood or platelets from parasitemic but asymptomatic donors residing in endemic areas.

The illness usually resolves spontaneously and requires only symptomatic treatment. Severe infections in adults have been treated successfully by exchange transfusion. Chloroquine and other antimalarials, diminazene aceturate, and pentamidine isethionate have been administered without clear benefit. Recently, a premature infant with transfusion babesiosis was cured with clindamycin plus quinine, a combination also shown to be effective against *B. microti* infection in hamsters.

Therefore, an ill or immunocompromised patient with babesiosis should be treated with clindamycin, 20 mg per kilogram per day given orally, intravenously, or intramuscularly in four divided doses (maximum, 600 mg every 6 hours) and quinine sulfate, 25 mg per kilogram per day given orally in three divided doses (maximum, 650 mg three times a day), both for 7 to 10 days. Response to therapy can be followed by the decline in parasitemia (see Table 1).

LEISHMANIASIS

Organisms of the genus *Leishmania* are obligate intracellular parasites of two forms. The amastigote form of the protozoan is found in the mammalian host, and the flagellated promastigote is found in the insect vector (the female phlebotomine sandfly). The complex of diseases caused by protozoans in the genus *Leishmania* can be divided into three clinical types of leishmaniasis: visceral leishmaniasis (*L. don-*

---

* The author gratefully acknowledges the contribution of the section on Babesiosis by George A. Jacoby, M.D.

ovani), mucocutaneous leishmaniasis (*L. braziliensis*), and cutaneous leishmaniasis (*L. tropica* and *L. mexicana*). The manifestations of disease are determined by the parasites' invasiveness, tropism, and pathogenicity and the host immunity. The spectrum of disease can vary from a self-healing local ulcer to disseminated overwhelming disease. The sandfly vector can be found in the cracks in walls of houses and in rubbish outside the houses in endemic areas. Leishmaniasis is a zoonosis involving humans, rats, mice, gerbils, squirrels, dogs, and foxes.

Visceral Leishmaniasis (Kala-Azar)

Kala-azar is endemic in the Mediterranean basin (Spain, France, Italy, Greece, and north Africa), southern Russia, eastern India, China, east Africa (Kenya, Sudan, and Uganda), Brazil, Venezuela, and Paraguay. Outside these areas the diagnosis is frequently overlooked because of failure to consider visceral leishmaniasis in patients from endemic areas with intermittent fever, anemia, and hepatosplenomegaly. Additional confusion can be caused by the long incubation period, since clinical signs may not develop until long after the patient has left the endemic area.

The invasion of the reticuloendothelial system by the parasite accounts for the majority of symptoms. The first sign of disease is usually the appearance of a cutaneous nodule at the site of inoculation. After a 2- to 6-month incubation period, the disease starts insidiously with erratic fever, which may progress to the characteristic twice-daily elevation of temperature. Other less common symptoms include dizziness, weakness, and weight loss. Marked hepatosplenomegaly is the most characteristic physical finding. Lymphadenopathy is found in many cases, particularly in patients from Africa. As the infection becomes chronic, anemia, leukopenia with agranulocytosis, thrombocytopenia, bleeding tendencies, jaundice, hypoalbuminemia, and hyperimmunoglobulin G develop. Without treatment 75 to 90 percent of the patients die, usually from secondary infection.

Diagnosis is established by finding the parasite in tissue of the skin nodules, bone marrow, and spleen. The smears should be stained with Giemsa stain and examined for the characteristic Leishman-Donovan bodies (amastigotes) in macrophages or free organisms outside of ruptured cells. When biopsy material is negative but the diagnosis is still likely, cultures of bone marrow aspirate should be attempted using the Novy-MacNeal-Nicolle (NMN) medium. Cultures may become positive in 5 to 7 days, but must be held for 4 weeks. Serologic testing using indirect fluorescent antibody may be helpful, but cross-reactivity with other leishmania and trypanosomes can cause problems. The Montenegro skin test does not become positive until after successful treatment.

Kala-azar is treated with antimonial compounds. The pentavalent antimonials have replaced the more toxic trivalent compounds, but optimal therapy has not been developed. Sodium stibogluconate (Pentostam, Burroughs Wellcome) and meglumine antimonate (Glucantime, Rodia, Specia) have similar activity and toxicity, but differ in availability. Sodium stibogluconate is available in the United States from the Parasitic Diseases Division, Centers for Disease Control, Atlanta, Georgia (days: 404-329-3670; nights and weekends: 404-329-3644) as a 33 percent solution containing 100 mg of pentavalent antimony per milliliter. Since there is some variability in the antimonial content of the different lots of this drug, dosage is based on the antimonial content of the preparation. Sodium stibogluconate should be given in a dosage of 20 mg per kilogram per day (maximum, 850 mg of the antimonial base per day) intravenously for 20 to 30 days (for a minimum of 20 days). Intramuscular doses can be given but are not recommended because they are very painful. In patients with evidence of infection at the end of 30 days of treatment, therapy should be continued until the organism is no longer found in the bone marrow or splenic aspirations or until toxicity requires discontinuance of the drug. Relapses should be treated with a second or third 20- to 30-day course of the drug. Lack of response to three courses of drug therapy suggests resistance, and alternate chemotherapeutic agents should be tried. Patients from India and South America usually respond well to a single course; those from China and the Mediterranean areas occasionally require repeat courses; and the more resistant disease from east Africa may require as many as three courses of therapy to achieve a cure. Progress of therapy can be monitored by repeated bone marrow aspirations. In east Africa, splenic aspiration is used to follow therapy because of the higher rate of positivity (98 percent) compared with that of bone marrow (86 percent). With the coagulopathy of advanced disease, the hazards of this procedure in inexperienced hands preclude its routine use in this country.

The most common side effects of the antimonial compounds include anorexia, nausea, vomiting, malaise, myalgia, headaches, and lethargy. With larger or prolonged doses, reversible cardiac changes including ECG changes (T-wave inversions and prolonged QT interval), bradycardia, and arrhythmias can be seen. At the recommended doses more than half the patients have electrocardiographic (ECG) changes that reverse with discontinuation of the drug. More serious liver dysfunction can occur. Renal failure is not infrequent and requires discontinuation of therapy. We recommend following the patients with weekly ECGs, BUN, creatinine, SGOT, and SGPT to monitor for toxicity. Antimonial therapy should not be repeated within 2 months if any intolerance was observed with the initial course. Patients with severe cardiac, liver, or renal diseases should not be treated with antimonial compounds.

Pentamidine isethionate (Pentam, LyphoMed) can be used in patients who do not respond to, or are unable to take, antimonials. The dosage is 4 mg per kilogram per day intramuscularly for 15 days. Side effects include headache, flushing, faintness, vomiting, abdominal discomfort, hypoglycemia, and vascular collapse. (See the section on treatment of *Pneumocytosis carinii pneumonia*.)

Amphotericin B, 0.5 mg per kilogram per day or 1 mg per kilogram every other day intravenously, can be used in patients who fail to respond to other therapy. A total dosage of 15 to 20 mg per kilogram should be given. The most commonly observed adverse reactions to amphotericin include fever, nausea, vomiting, headache, myalgias, anemia, and abnormal renal function with hypokalemia and elevated serum creatinine and BUN.

Allopurinol and pyrazolopyrimidine have been shown to be effective therapy in animal models and in some anecdotal case reports. They appear to hold promise for the future, but at present should be reserved for study protocols and patients who have failed to respond to conservative therapy.

In addition to chemotherapy, supportive therapy is essential for a good response. Because many patients are malnourished, a high-caloric, high-protein diet is necessary. Patients unable to tolerate oral feedings should be given tube feedings or total parenteral nutrition until they are able to take adequate calories orally. The anemia associated with visceral leishmaniasis may require transfusions. Treatment of concurrent infections decreases the mortality significantly, as does careful evaluation for nosocomial infection. Splenectomy should be avoided except in patients with hypersplenism and/or failure of chemotherapy. Because of the possibility of relapse, patients should be followed and have repeated bone marrow aspirates for as long as 2 to 3 years after successful therapy.

Cutaneous Leishmaniasis (Old World)

Cutaneous leishmaniasis ("Oriental sore") is the disease caused by *L. tropica* and occurs throughout tropical and subtropical regions of China, India, Asia Minor, Middle East, northern Africa, and central Africa. Unlike visceral leishmaniasis and cutaneous leishmaniasis of the New World, disease caused by *L. tropica* generally is not life-threatening. The disease occurs in three different forms caused by three different subspecies. The *L. tropica major* or rural form is a zoonosis of desert rodents secondarily infecting humans entering uninhabited areas or in villages along the desert. *Leishmania tropica minor* or urban cutaneous leishmaniasis is a zoonosis involving dogs and humans in cities of the Middle East, India, and Pakistan. *L. tropica aethiopica* is a zoonosis associated with hydrax, a small African mammal, and rodents. Sporadic disease occurs in endemic areas, but occasional epidemics occur when nonimmune humans enter areas with a high prevalence of the parasite in the animal reservoir.

Clinical manifestations appear after a variable incubation period (2 weeks to 3 years). In the dry form (urban), the lesions are usually single and slowly progressing. Lesions of the moist form (rural) are generally multiple, progress rapidly, and tend to heal spontaneously after several months. The initial lesion is a small papule that increases in size. As the papule increases in size it develops a crust and then ulcerates, forming the characteristic lesion. The ulcer is shallow and circular, with raised erythematous borders and a granulating center. The granulating base of the ulcer can form a hard tumorlike growth (Montpelliere sign). Occasionally satellite lesions appear, coalescing into the original lesion. Secondary bacterial infection of these lesions is common. The ulcers heal spontaneously within several months to years, leaving flat, atrophic, depigmented scars. Diffuse cutaneous leishmaniasis starts like the other forms, but the papule does not ulcerate. Satellite lesions appear, and the organisms disseminate to distant areas of skin sites, particularly to exposed areas such as the face and extremities. These lesions progress slowly and persist for many years. Leishmaniasis recidivans is a relapsing form of cutaneous leishmaniasis found mainly in Iran. The lesions spread out with healing of the centers; in rare instances these lesions involve the mucous membranes, resulting in nasal destruction. The Montenegro skin test is negative in disseminated disease and strongly positive in leishmaniasis recidivans, suggesting immunosuppression in one and hypersensitivity to the organism in the other.

The diagnosis of cutaneous leishmaniasis is mainly based on clinical presentation. A definite diagnosis requires the finding of amastigotes in stained smears of the scrapings of ulcers or biopsies of the leading edge of the ulcer. Material from ulcers can be cultured as for *L. donovani*. Serologic responses generally are not diagnostic. The Montenegro skin test becomes positive during the course of the disease, except in diffuse cutaneous disease.

The major decision in cutaneous leishmaniasis is whether to treat or to wait for spontaneous resolution. The decision to treat is based on the location and extent of the lesion. The antimonial compounds are the main form of therapy for multiple or disseminated cutaneous leishmaniasis (Old World); however, at present there is no optimal therapeutic dosage or duration of therapy for this disease. Dosages of sodium stibogluconate ranging from 10 mg per kilogram per day to 20 mg per kilogram per day have been used for 6 to 30 days. Failures occur more frequently with the smaller-dosage and shorter-duration schedules. We recommend, in patients requiring therapy, sodium stibogluconate, 20 mg per kilogram per day (maximum dosage, 850 mg per day) given intravenously or intramuscularly for 20 to 30 days. Treatment failures should be re-treated and may require two to three courses to achieve a cure. Some physicians recommend a rest period of several weeks between courses; however, this is not based on pharmacokinetic data and it is unnecessary. In patients who have severe side effects, a rest period may be helpful to allow them to recover from the toxic effects of the drug. (See the section on kala-azar for toxicities.)

Treatment failures have been treated successfully with pentamidine and amphotericin B, using the schedules for visceral leishmaniasis. Cryotherapy and local hyperthermic therapies have been reported, but have not been subjected to well-controlled trials. Many other agents have also reportedly been successful in uncontrolled trials. These case reports are difficult to evaluate in a disease that generally resolves spontaneously.

Limited cutaneous leishmaniasis caused by *L. tropica* and *L. major* can be treated with topical therapy. Local medicinal treatments have included berberine, topical meglumine antimonate, tartar emetic, and quinacrine. These treatments appear to accelerate healing, but have not been compared with a placebo group. A recent study using 15 percent paromycin sulfate and 12 percent methylbenzethonium chloride in white soft paraffin showed marked improvement in the treated lesions over the untreated lesions on the same patient. Because of this we believe that patients with limited cutaneous leishmaniasis (Old World) can be treated with an ointment containing 15 percent paromycin sulfate and 12 percent methylbenzethonium chloride in white soft paraffin applied twice a day for 10 days.

In addition to specific therapy, local care of the wound is important. The ulcers should be kept clean and secondary bacterial infections treated promptly.

Prevention of cutaneous leishmaniasis using chemoprophylaxis is not possible because of the lack of safe, effective drugs. A form of vaccination using live cultures of *L. tropica* is practiced in the U.S.S.R., Israel, and Jordan. This method of prevention cannot be recommended at present. Control of the vector and mammalian reservoirs has been successful in limiting disease, but is not expected to eliminate the parasite or the vector.

New World Cutaneous Leishmaniasis (Mucocutaneous)

Leishmania braziliensis complex and *L. mexicana* complex are responsible for New World cutaneous leishmaniasis, which includes a spectrum of disease varying from a single cutaneous ulcer to mucocutaneous disease. These organisms produce variable syndromes through Central and South America. The disease has been reported in all countries in North and South America except for Canada, Chile, and Uruguay, but it is most prevalent in Argentina, Brazil, and Peru. The main reservoirs for this zoonosis are small forest rodents, with domestic animals providing a secondary reservoir. The vectors are both ground-dwelling and arboreal sandflies (genera *Lutzomyia* and *Psychodopygus*). These sandflies are abundant in the forest and are most likely to cause disease in humans as they invade the forest, clearing land for farms, roads, lumber, and mining.

The cutaneous manifestations of cutaneous leishmaniasis include single or multiple lesions ranging in appearance from small, dry, crusted papules to large, deep, fungating ulcers, with any combination of lesions appearing on one person. The incubation period is from 2 to 8 weeks, after which a small erythematous papule appears. This slowly evolves to become a round ulcer with raised borders, a granulating base, and an exudative center. The lesion can persist for months to years, and hypertrophic granulation tissue in these lesions can mimic neoplasms. The lesions tend to be characteristic within any given region of a country, but there is some overlap. Diffuse cutaneous lesions are rare in the New World leishmaniasis. When they do occur, they start as a small nontender papule that does not ulcerate and disseminate to other areas of the body. This anergic form of the disease is characterized by a protracted course and persistently negative skin tests.

Mucocutaneous leishmaniasis is caused by *L. braziliensis,* and the protozoa has been known to persist after the ulcer has healed. The extremely mutilating lesions of this infection usually start with involvement of the nasal mucosa. As the infection progresses, the nasal septum is destroyed, causing the nose to collapse, and perforations appear in the skin of the nose and in the soft palate. Other tissues that can be involved include the lips, tongue, buccal mucosa, pharynx, larynx, trachea, and genital mucosa. Some are involved by direct extension, but others by dissemination. Patients frequently die from either aspiration or the inability to eat.

Diagnosis is dependent on identification of the organism in tissue, culture, and hamsters. Biopsy specimens from the edge of the skin lesions should be examined using Giemsa stains. The material should also be inoculated into one of the available culture media (for *L. mexicana*) and into hamsters, since *L. braziliensis* does not grow on these media. The organism is difficult to find in the tissues of mucocutaneous infection. Because of this, a diagnosis of mucocutaneous leishmaniasis is based on the clinical presentation, a positive leishmanin test (Montenegro skin test), or the presence of antibodies to leishmania in serum. The skin test is positive in 80 to 100 percent of patients, and serology is positive in 60 to 96 percent depending on the antigen used (amastigote antigen is the best). Antibodies can be used to evaluate the success of chemotherapy, with declining titers indicating success and rising titers suggesting relapse. The decision to treat cutaneous disease is more obvious in New World leishmaniasis than in Old World leishmaniasis because of the potential of the former to develop mucocutaneous lesions. In areas where mucocutaneous disease is prevalent, all cutaneous disease should be treated. Cutaneous disease that occurs in areas outside the endemic areas for mucocutaneous disease can be observed without specific therapy unless the lesions are large or disfiguring. The drug of choice in Latin America is meglumine antimoniate (Glucantime) because it is the most widely available. There is no optimal therapeutic regimen for this disease, but meglumine antimoniate, 50 to 60 mg per kilogram per day (approximately 14 to 16.8 mg of the antimonial base) for 12 days, followed by a 15-day rest period, then a second 12-day course has been successful in uncomplicated cutaneous disease. Mucocutaneous leishmaniasis has been treated with dosages of up to 100 mg per kilogram per day (28 mg of antimonial base per kilogram per day) for 20 days. Side effects are more common with the larger doses (40 to 50 percent of the patients). Relapse rates are as high as 50 percent in some areas. Patients arriving in the United States with cutaneous leishmaniasis or mucocutaneous leishmaniasis should be treated with sodium stibogluconate, 20 mg per kilogram per day of the antimonial base (maximum, 850 mg per day) given intravenously or intramuscularly for 20 to 30 days. Repeated courses of therapy can be given immediately unless severe toxicities were present during the initial or preceding therapy. In these cases, either rest periods of 2 months or an alternative therapy may be necessary. Defining cure is difficult, but it is often helpful to follow the response with periodic serum antileishmania titers.

In patients who have relapses or who have not responded to initial therapy, amphotericin B, 0.5 to 1.0 mg per kilogram per day, given either every day or every other day, can be used. A total dosage of 15 to 20 mg per kilogram is usually effective for either cutaneous or mucocutaneous disease. Side effects include anorexia, phlebitis, fever, rashes, anemia, hypokalemia, azotemia, permanent renal impairment, cardiac arrhythmias, cardiac arrest, hypertension, hypotension, pancytopenia, peripheral neuropathy, anaphylactoid reaction, and liver failure.

At present, many new drugs are being studied, but cannot be recommended for routine therapy. Drugs that have had some success include ketaconazole, rifampin, cycloguanil pamoate, allopurinol, nifurtimox, clofazime, and benznidazole. Cryosurgery has been used for single small lesions. Hyperthermia has been used successfully for the rare disseminated cutaneous lesions.

Supportive therapy is important. Caloric intake should be maintained and, in those with severe mutilation caused by mucocutaneous disease, intravenous feedings or feeding through a nasogastric tube may be required to prevent aspiration of feedings. Plastic surgery may be necessary, but should be delayed until chances of relapse are slim, usually 1 to 2 years.

Chemoprophylaxis and vaccines are unavailable at present. Control of a zoonosis involving insect vectors and mammalian reservoirs of the forest is impossible. Ideally, humans should avoid living and working in areas near the forest edge in these endemic areas; however, the economic realities make this unlikely. Insect repellents provide limited protection for travelers to these areas, but they are unlikely to help persons remaining in these areas for prolonged periods.

AFRICAN TRYPANOSOMIASIS

African human trypanosomiasis, also known as sleeping sickness, is a disease caused by the hemoflagellate protozoa, *Trypanosoma brucei rhodesiense* and *Trypanosoma brucei gambiense.* It is restricted to parts of Africa and is transmitted by the bite of an infected tsetse fly, or, rarely, transplacentally. There are two forms of the disease, which vary somewhat in onset, severity, and duration of symptoms. The Gambian form is a chronic illness that evolves slowly over many years; the Rhodesian form is much more fulminant, often killing the patient within a few months. The first sign of infection in either form may be the development of a nodule or chancre at the site of inoculation. Several days later, fever and headache appear, followed by the development of lymphadenopathy (especially postcervical) and hepatosplenomegaly. The fever becomes intermittent, and in the Gambian form, the patient may have few additional symptoms until the parasite invades the central nervous system. At that point, individuals develop severe headaches, behavioral changes, hallucinations, tremors, and somnolence and eventually lapse into coma and die. With the Rhodesian form of the disease, cardiac involvement, weight loss, and weakness are often more pronounced, and patients die before they develop the typical neurologic symptoms of sleeping sickness.

The diagnosis is established by demonstrating the trypanosome in the blood, lymph nodes, or bone marrow. If the initial blood examination is negative, it should be repeated several times, particularly during febrile periods. Animal inoculation of the patient's blood can be helpful in cases with low parasitemia. Once the central nervous system has been invaded, the organisms can be found in the cerebrospinal fluid. Specific serologic tests are also available.

Early treatment of trypanosomiasis is essential because the prognosis is poor once central nervous system involvement develops. Without therapy, the disease is almost inevitably fatal. Before institution of therapy, a lumbar puncture should be done, and if a mononuclear pleocytosis or an elevated protein is present, the patient should be treated for central nervous system involvement. For early disease, without central nervous system invasion, suramin sodium (Bayer 205, Naphuride, Germanin, Antrypol, Naganol) is the drug of choice. Since occasional severe reactions with shock follow the injection of a full dose of this drug, a test dose of 2 mg per kilogram (100 to 200 mg for an adult) should be given first. It is given intravenously as a 10 percent solution in sterile water, and if tolerated, the patient is given 20 mg per kilogram per day (maximum, 1 g) on days 1, 3, 7, 14, and 21 for a total of five doses. Suramin is available from the Centers for Disease Control (days: 404-329-3670; nights and weekends: 404-329-3644) and it often causes mild vomiting, diarrhea, skin rashes, and paresthesias. In addition, it may cause renal damage, and a urinalysis should be checked the day after each dose. If significant albuminuria, red cells, or casts appear in the urine, treatment should be interrupted and restarted with more frequent smaller doses. Optic atrophy and blood dyscrasias have also been reported with suramin use.

If suramin is unavailable or poorly tolerated, an alternative drug used to treat the early stage of trypanosomiasis is pentamidine isethionate (Pentam, Lomidine). Like suramin, it does not cross the blood–brain barrier and is therefore of little value once central nervous system involvement has occurred. It is now available commercially as a lyophilized preparation; after reconstitution of the 300-mg vial in 3 ml of distilled water, the appropriate dosage should be withdrawn and given intramuscularly. The usual dosage is 4 mg per kilogram per day, given daily for 10 days or every other day for 20 days. Patients should be kept at rest for an hour or more after each injection because transient hypotension, vertigo, and palpitations are not uncommon. Other side effects include gastrointestinal disturbances, liver damage, delirium, and cardiotoxicity. Hypoglycemia occurs less frequently, but is an indication to discontinue the drug. Since it can also produce kidney damage, it is contraindicated in patients with underlying renal disease.

Melarsonyl (Trimelarsan, Mel W.) and Diminazene B. Vet. C. (Berenil) are other compounds that have been used with some success in the early stages of trypanosomiasis. At this time, they have not been used extensively in children and they do not appear to offer any benefit over suramin and pentamidine.

For cases with central nervous system involvement, melarsoprol (Mel B, Arsobal) appears to be the most effective drug. It is an arsenical with a narrow margin of safety when given at the required dosage. It is available from the Centers for Disease Control (days: 404-329-3670; nights and weekends: 404-329-3644) and is dispensed as a 3.6 percent solution in propylene-glycol that is unstable in contact with water and is exceedingly irritating. The initial pediatric dose is 0.36 mg per kilogram per dose given intravenously. Subsequent doses are increased gradually to the maximum of 3.6 mg per kilogram given at intervals of 1 to 5 days for a total of 9 to 10 doses. The total dosage for children is 18 to 25 mg per kilogram given over a period of 1 month. A reactive encephalopathy felt to be secondary to the release of trypanosomal antigen from dying organisms is not uncommon and is not an indication to stop the drug. Other side effects include hypertension, nausea, vomiting, diarrhea, renal damage, dermatitis, and myocardial damage.

Another agent, difluoromethylornithine (DFMO), has recently been approved for the treatment of the late stage of West African trypanosomiasis. A number of small studies done in Europe and Africa appear to indicate that it is efficacious and associated with relatively minor, reversible side effects. It is available in this country, on a compassionate basis from Merrell Dow (513-948-9111). Tryparsamide is an alternative compound used to treat late trypanosomiasis with central nervous system involvement. Like melarsoprol, it is a toxic drug, occasionally precipitating optic neuritis and atrophy. It is not currently available in the United States.

Relapses after therapy may occur, particularly following treatment with suramin if central nervous system involvement was already present. Because of this possibility, patients' cerebrospinal fluid should be reexamined 6 and 12 months after therapy. Drug resistance to multiple compounds, including suramin and pentamidine, has been reported. Overall, the prognosis is good if the disease is recognized before central nervous system involvement occurs.

Prevention of the illness requires avoidance of the insect vector through the use of insect repellents, protective clothing, and clearing of vegetation. Although chemoprophylaxis with intramuscular pentamidine or intravenous suramin has been effective, it is not generally indicated because it may suppress symptoms without eradicating the infection and may contribute to the emergence of resistant organisms.

SOUTH AMERICAN TRYPANOSOMIASIS

South American trypanosomiasis, or Chagas' disease, is caused by the protozoan hemoflagellate *Trypanosoma cruzi*. It is limited to the Western Hemisphere and is prevalent in Mexico and in Central and South America. A few autochthonous cases have been reported in the United States. The disease is primarily transmitted by reduviid bugs, although transmission transplacentally and by blood transfusion has occurred.

Although the vast majority of the individuals infected with *T. cruzi* do not develop clinically overt disease, infants and young children are more likely to be symptomatic. Acute symptoms include fever, headache, anorexia, generalized lymphadenopathy, hepatosplenomegaly, unilateral palpebral or generalized edema, and skin eruptions. Cardiac involvement with myocarditis and neurologic abnormalities with meningoencephalitis may also be present. Approximately 5 to 10 percent of the patients die with an acute attack; the remainder develop the latent form of Chagas' disease. After 10 to 40 asymptomatic years, a small percentage of those patients develop cardiomyopathy, megaesophagus, or megacolon as manifestations of chronic Chagas' disease.

Diagnosis depends on demonstration of the parasite in blood or tissue or on serologic tests. During the acute illness, trypanomastigotes can be found in the peripheral blood, whereas in the chronic stage, they are more likely to be seen in the liver, bone marrow, and spleen. Blood and other tissues can be cultured for *T. cruzi* on media such as NNN and specimens can also be inoculated into guinea pigs. During periods of low parasitemia, xenodiagnosis may be the only means by which organisms can be found. In this technique, laboratory-reared reduviid bugs are fed on the patient or his blood and several weeks later are examined for the presence of trypanosomes. Household members exposed to insect vectors should have blood cultures and serologic tests done to rule out asymptomatic infection.

Treatment of Chagas' disease is unsatisfactory. A number of compounds appear to decrease the parasitemia in acute disease, potentially decreasing the degree of dissemination. However, they do not appear to affect the ultimate course of the disease, possibly because they do not eliminate intracellular organisms. Nifurtimox (Lampit) is currently recommended for therapy of acute Chagas' disease and is available from the Centers for Disease Control (days: 404-329-3670; nights and weekends: 404-329-3644). It is given initially in a dosage of 5 mg per kilogram per day divided into four equal oral doses. Every 1 to 2 weeks the dose is increased by 2 to 5 mg per kilogram until the maximum dose is reached: 1 to 10 years old, 15 to 20 mg per kilogram per day; 11 to 16 years old, 12.5 to 15 mg per kilogram per day; older than 17 years, 8 to 10 mg per kilogram per day. It is given for a period of 3 to 4 months, and side effects include gastrointestinal distress, polyneuritis, psychosis, and hemolytic anemia in glucose-6-phosphate dehydrogenase deficient individuals. Because of side effects, many individuals are unable to complete the prolonged course of therapy with nifurtimox. Although this drug effectively decreases parasitemia in the acute illness, it does not cure the chronic disease. Benznidazole (Rochagan, Radanil) has recently been used with some success for the acute disease. The recommended dosage is 5 to 7 mg per kilogram per day, divided into two doses, given for 30 to 120 days. Side effects include nausea, peripheral neuritis, thrombocytopenia, and severe dermatitis; overall, the toxicity may be less than that produced by nifurtimox. Although benznidazole is not commercially available in this country, if nifurtimox is unavailable or not tolerated by a patient with Chagas' disease, inquiries regarding the possible use of benznidazole should be addressed to the Food and Drug Administration (FDA). Therapeutic response to these drugs should be followed by checking blood smears and cultures, documenting eradication of the organism. Serologic titers decrease with adequate therapy in the acute illness, but may remain elevated in the chronic stage. Complications such as myocarditis should be managed conservatively, and steroids should be avoided because they may lead to an intensification of the infection.

The chronic form of Chagas' disease is more difficult to treat. Although the parasites may be eradicated with nifurtimox, the organ damage is irreversible. Chronic cardiomyopathy with cardiomegaly, congestive heart failure, and arrhythmias is often refractory to supportive therapy. Diuretics may be of some use; however, inotropic agents such as digoxin are rarely effective. Megaesophagus and megacolon do not resolve with therapy and often require surgical intervention. Overall, the prognosis of symptomatic Chagas' disease is poor, and a fatal outcome is not uncommon among children with the acute disease. Given the inadequacy of current therapeutic modalities, prevention of the disease is critically important. To date, vector control and elimination of animal reservoirs have been difficult. Ultimately, prevention of human infection will probably require the development of an effective vaccine. In the meantime, particular care must be taken in endemic areas to prevent transmission by transfusion of infected blood.

TOXOPLASMOSIS

Toxoplasmosis, an infection caused by the intracellular parasite *Toxoplasma gondii,* occurs in two forms—congenital and acquired. Congenital infection is either clinically inapparent or manifested by hepatosplenomegaly, thrombocytopenia, jaundice, rash, retinochoroiditis, and neurologic abnormalities. Neurologic manifestations are being seen increasingly in patients with acquired immunodeficiency syndrome (AIDS) and most often result from the reactivation of a previously acquired infection. Acquired toxoplasmosis is usually asymptomatic or produces mild nonspecific symptoms such as fever, lymphadenopathy, and malaise. The immunocompromised host may have a more severe illness with multisystemic involvement and a fatal outcome.

The diagnosis of toxoplasmosis can be made by isolating the organism from lymph nodes, bone marrow, spleen, brain, cerebrospinal fluid, or other tissues. Specimens are inoculated into tissue culture or intraperitoneally into mice, with recovery of *Toxoplasma* organisms several weeks later. The demonstration of the tachyzoite stage of the parasite in tissues or body fluids also establishes the diagnosis. More commonly, the diagnosis is based on serologic findings. High IgM antibody titers or a rise in IgG antibody titers to a high level in any standard test establishes the diagnosis of acute infection. Elevated IgG titers persist for months to years.

Treatment of toxoplasmosis has been difficult to evaluate because of the lack of controlled trials and the variable clinical course of the disease. Currently used therapeutic agents include pyrimethamine, sulfonamides, and spiramycin. Although pyrimethamine and sulfonamides act synergistically against *T. gondii,* none of the available agents appears to eradicate the organism. It is probable that resistant tissue cyst forms persist and may initiate active infection later.

Pyrimethamine treatment is initiated with a loading dose of 2 mg per kilogram per day (maximum, 50 mg per day) given orally in two equal doses for 2 to 3 days. Maintenance therapy consists of 1 mg per kilogram per day (maximum, 25 mg per day) divided into two doses. The maintenance dose of 1 mg per kilogram can initially be given daily and then decreased to every-other-day doses for more prolonged periods of time. Since pyrimethamine is a potent folic acid antagonist, it can cause bone marrow suppression with leukopenia, anemia, and thrombocytopenia. Platelet and peripheral blood counts should be monitored twice weekly and patients should be given folinic acid in a dosage of 5 mg twice weekly for infants and 5 to 10 mg every 1 to 2 days for older children and adults to help prevent bone marrow suppression. Other less serious side effects of pyrimethamine include gastrointestinal distress, headache, and an unpleasant aftertaste. It should not be accessible to children because accidental ingestion of pyrimethamine has led to fatalities. Both folinic acid and pyrimethamine are supplied as tablets and must be pulverized and put into suspension.

Sulfadiazine or trisulfapyrimidines are given along with pyrimethamine. The usual oral dosage is 100 mg per kilogram per day (maximum, 2 to 6 g per day) divided into two doses. Adverse reactions to sulfonamides include skin rashes, hematuria, crystalluria, and, rarely, neutropenia and anemia. In individuals with glucose-6-phosphate dehydrogenase deficiency, the use of sulfonamides may produce hemolytic anemia.

Spiramycin, a macrolide antibiotic, has been used widely in other countries for the treatment of toxoplasmosis in pregnant females and infants. It is available from the Food and Drug Administration (301-443-6797 to obtain an investigator number), and the recommended pediatric dosage is 100 mg per kilogram per day, given orally in two divided doses. Older children and adults should receive 3 to 4 g per day in four divided doses. The drug is generally well tolerated, producing only occasional mild gastrointestinal discomfort, and, rarely, allergic reactions.

Therapy is not necessary for the majority of acquired *T. gondii* infections because they resolve spontaneously. Currently, treatment is recommended for patients who are likely to have significant morbidity or mortality, as in the following settings: infants with congenital clinical or subclinical infection, infants whose mothers acquired infection during pregnancy, healthy infants whose mothers have elevated antibody titers of unknown date, patients with active retinochoroiditis, infection acquired during pregnancy, infection in immunocompromised hosts, and clinically persistent or severe acquired infection.

Optimal duration of therapy has not been determined for any form of toxoplasmosis. Response to therapy is difficult to assess because the clinical course is variable and serologic markers may remain elevated for months. Infants with congenital infections should be treated with pyrimethamine, sulfon-

amide, and folinic acid for 21 days, followed by spiramycin for 4 to 6 weeks. Alternating courses of pyrimethamine–sulfa and spiramycin should be continued for a minimum of 6 months, and we generally treat for 1 year. If the congenitally infected infant has evidence of active inflammation with chorioretinitis or elevated spinal fluid protein, corticosteroids should be added to the treatment regimen. Prednisone is used in an initial dosage of 1 or 2 mg per kilogram per day in two divided doses (maximum, 75 mg per day). Once signs of inflammation have subsided, the steroids are tapered progressively to nothing. Healthy infants whose mothers acquired toxoplasmosis during pregnancy should be treated with pyrimethamine and sulfadiazine for 21 days, followed by a course of spiramycin or sulfadiazine alone. If the infant does not develop laboratory evidence of infection, no additional therapy is required. Healthy newborns delivered to mothers with elevated antibody titers and an undermined date of maternal infection should be treated with spiramycin alone until laboratory evidence for the diagnosis is definitive. If sequential antibody titers indicate a recently acquired maternal infection, infants should be treated as recommended previously.

An acquired toxoplasma infection in the immunocompetent host is treated only if there is clinically overt visceral involvement or severe or persistent symptoms. Therapy consists of pyrimethamine, sulfadiazine, and folinic acid administered for 1 to 4 months, until symptoms resolve. Ocular toxoplasmosis is treated with the same combination of drugs, usually for 1 month. Occasionally, repeated courses of therapy are required. Systemic steroids should be used if the lesions involve the macula or optic nerve head. Immunodeficient patients are at significant risk for clinically severe acute disease and relapse. They should always be treated with pyrimethamine and sulfadiazine for an acute infection, and treatment should continue for 4 to 6 weeks beyond complete resolution of all signs and symptoms. Women who acquire toxoplasmosis during pregnancy should also be treated, because there is evidence that treatment decreases the incidence of fetal infection. Two different treatment regimens have been effective, one using spiramycin alone and the other using pyrimethamine–sulfadiazine combinations after the first trimester.

Certain precautions diminish the possibility of acquiring toxoplasmosis, and they should be observed by high-risk groups such as nonimmune pregnant women and immunocompromised patients. These individuals should not eat undercooked meat, should wash their hands carefully after handling raw meat, and should avoid contact with materials that are potentially contaminated with cat feces.

PNEUMOCYSTIS CARINII PNEUMONIA

Pneumocystis carinii is an ubiquitous protozoan found in humans as well as rats, guinea pigs, mice, rabbits, dogs, foxes, goats, and sheep. The organism was first identified in undernourished infants in Europe with fatal pneumonitis. With the increased use of immunosuppressive therapy and with the AIDS epidemic, the number of cases of *P. carinii* infection has skyrocketed. Small numbers of *P. carinii* cysts are sometimes found in the lungs of patients with no clinical evidence of pneumonitis. These organisms are believed to be in a latent or inactive stage, and anything decreasing the host's immunity can activate replication of the latent organisms, causing disease. Clinically the disease is characterized by abrupt onset of fever, tachypnea, and cough, progressing to rapid intercostal retractions, nasal flaring, and ashen cyanosis. The endemic infantile form has a more insidious onset with poor feeding, diarrhea, and failure to thrive as the prominent features, followed by the gradual onset of tachypnea and cyanosis.

The diagnosis of *P. carinii* infection requires demonstration of the organism in the lung tissue of the host. Open-lung biopsy is the most reliable method of diagnosis. Transbronchial biopsy, endobronchial brush-biopsy, and transthoracic percutaneous needle aspiration of the lung parenchyma have been used, but are less dependable than open lung-biopsy. Examination of tracheal aspirates, gastric contents, sputum, and bronchopulmonary lavage are not dependable methods for diagnosis. Specimens should be stained with a cyst wall stain such as methenamine-silver nitrate method of Gomori and a trophozoite stain such as Giemsa. Serologic diagnosis has not been of value because of the high percentage of healthy individuals who have antibody titers to *P. carinii*. Detection of *P. carinii* antigen by counterimmunoelectrophoresis in the serum of infected patients has been helpful in some cases. Antigenemia has been seen in immunosuppressed patients without evidence of disease, suggesting persistence of the organism without disease.

Prophylactic treatment should be considered in any patient at risk of developing *P. carinii* pneumonia, including patients with any of the following predisposing factors: immunosuppressive drug therapy and irradiation for the management of cancer or organ transplantation, congenital immunodeficiency, malnutrition (particularly in children younger than 3 months of age), and AIDS. Trimethoprim–sulfamethoxazole (TMP/SMZ) should be given in a dosage of 5 mg of trimethoprim and 25 mg of sulfamethoxazole per kilogram per day, administered by mouth in two equal doses. The drug should be continued as long as the patient remains immunosuppressed.

Patients with clinical or biopsy-proven *P. carinii* infection should receive TMP/SMZ in a dosage of 20 mg of trimethoprim and 100 mg of sulfamethoxazole per kilogram per day, administered by mouth in four equal doses for 10 to 14 days. Intravenous TMP/SMZ is available and can be given to patients who are unable to take oral medications. TMP/SMZ has the advantages of minimal side effects, oral administration, ready availability, and low cost. The adverse effects are usually mild and include rashes, candidiasis, nausea, vomiting, and diarrhea. Less common but more serious reactions include erythema multiforme, Stevens-Johnson syndrome, toxic epidermal necrolysis, vasculitis, fever, arthralgia, hepatotoxicity, interstitial nephritis, hematuria, proteinuria, peripheral neuritis, hallucinations, and hematologic abnormalities (agranulocytosis, aplastic anemia, thrombocytopenia, leukopenia, neutropenia, hemolytic anemia, megaloblastic anemia, hypoprothrominemia, methemoglobinemia, and eosinophilia). Patients with AIDS have an increased incidence of adverse reactions to TMP/SMZ, and alternative therapy may be necessary.

Pentamidine isethionate (Pentam, LyphoMed), 4 mg per kilogram per day given intramuscularly daily for 10 to 14 days, is effective therapy for *P. carinii*. It has serious adverse effects, which include nephrotoxicity, hypoglycemia, injection-site reactions, hypotension, abnormal liver function, folic acid deficiency, hematologic abnormalities, skin rashes, and hypocalcemia. Because of these problems, pentamidine should be used only in children who are unable to tolerate TMP/SMZ or who fail to respond to TMP/SMZ therapy. Failure of therapy is usually manifested by lack of clinical improvement after 3 to 4 days of therapy or a persistently positive gallium-67 lung scan 5 to 7 days into therapy. Pentamidine is ineffective as a prophylactic drug.

Patients with AIDS may be unable to tolerate TMP/SMZ or pentamidine. Dapsone 100 mg per day and trimethoprim 20 mg per kilogram per day has been shown to be at least as effective as and better tolerated in AIDS patients than the standard therapy. Difluoromethylornithine (DFMO, eflornithine) has also been shown to be effective therapy for *P. carinii* pneumonia in AIDS patients. DFMO is not presently available, but can be obtained for compassionate use from Merrell Dow (513-948-9111) for patients who have failed to respond to or cannot tolerate other drugs. Both of these drugs should be considered as alternative therapy in children with *P. carinii* pneumonia that does not respond to TMP/SMZ or pentamidine.

In addition to antiprotozoal therapy, good supportive therapy is essential for the recovery of these patients. Care should be taken to maintain their PaO_2 at or above 70 mm Hg to prevent the severe hypoxia associated with this illness. In maintaining the PaO_2 above 70 mm Hg, it is also important to keep the inspired oxygen concentration below 50 percent to avoid oxygen toxicity whenever possible. Ventilatory support or assistance is frequently necessary.

NAEGLERIA AND ACANTHAMOEBA

Naegleria and *Acanthamoeba* (Hartmannella) are free-living amebae that cause primary amebic meningoencephalitis. *Naegleria fowleri* is more common and causes an acute fulminant disease in previously healthy children and young adults. Initial symptoms include headache, fever, rhinitis, and vomiting, progressing within a few days to confusion, stupor, nuchal rigidity, deepening coma, and death. *Acanthamoeba* organisms tend to produce a more benign, chronic form of meningoencephalitis, often in older immunocompromised patients, in whom symptoms appear over a period of months and include mental status abnormalities, seizures, focal motor deficits, and nonspecific complaints of headache, nausea, and vomiting. Although coma and death generally ensue, apparent spontaneous recovery has been reported. Keratitis and corneal ulcerations have also been caused by *Acanthamoeba,* particularly following ocular trauma.

Diagnosis is made by finding typical motile *Naegleria* organisms in cerebrospinal fluid and can be confirmed with a number of additional staining and immunologic techniques. The laboratory should be alerted of the possible diagnosis because none of the material intended for direct examination or culture should be refrigerated and, unless the amebae are specifically sought, they may be overlooked or mistaken for macrophages. *Naegleria* can also be grown on coliform-seeded agar plates. *Acanthamoeba* organisms are isolated or grown from cerebrospinal fluid less often, and diagnosis is usually made histologically by brain biopsy or at autopsy. The organisms have been cultured from corneal scrapings or biopsies. Although serologic tests are available, they are generally not helpful diagnostically. However, they may be of use in helping to differentiate the indolent form of cerebral acanthamebiasis from other chronic brain infections.

Therapy of these infections has been unsatisfactory. The drug of choice for *N. fowleri* infections is amphotericin B. It is given initially as an intravenous test dose of 0.1 mg per kilogram (maximum, 1 mg) over 3 to 4 hours. If tolerated, the dosage is increased by 0.25 mg per kilogram per day until a total daily dose of 1 mg per kilogram is reached. In life-threatening situations, the 0.25-mg-per-kilogram increments can be given successively in three or four infusions during a 12- to 24-hour period. Since *Naegleria* has persisted in the cerebrospinal fluid of patients who have received intravenous amphotericin, it is now generally recommended that they receive intrathecal therapy as well. The usual initial intrathecal dose of amphotericin B is 0.025 mg, and subsequent doses are increased until a maintenance dose of 0.1 to 0.5 mg is reached. Given the long half-life of amphotericin, the intrathecal maintenance doses can be given every other day. The most commonly observed adverse reactions to amphotericin include fever, nausea, vomiting, headache, myalgias, anemia, and abnormal renal function with hypokalemia and elevated serum creatinine and BUN. Several other drugs have been used for *Naegleria* infections without much success. One patient was successfully treated with a combination of miconazole (intrathecal and intravenous), rifampin, and amphotericin. In addition, some experimental data suggest that tetracycline potentiates the effect of amphotericin B. Although a combination of agents might prove to be more efficacious in the future, at this time, amphotericin is the drug of choice. Early diagnosis and vigorous supportive care are critical factors, but even with combination chemotherapy the prognosis is bleak. Duration of therapy has not been well established and should be based on the clinical course of the individual patient.

Acanthamoebae are susceptible to sulfonamides, clotrimazole, flucytosine, polymyxin B, and pentamidine isethionate in vitro. Clinically, most available antimicrobials have been of little use; however, one patient with chronic acanthamoebiasis appeared to respond to treatment with sulfamethazine. At this time, some physicians recommend routine use of sulfonamides along with amphotericin B for primary amebic meningoencephalitis. Most cases of *Acanthamoeba* keratitis have not responded to a variety of chemotherapeutic agents and the prognosis for saving the involved eye has been poor. Recently, several patients appear to have responded to a combination of surgical intervention and a variety of chemotherapeutic agents; current therapy includes systemic ketoconazole, topical miconazole (possibly also intravenously or subconjunctivally), and neomycin.

AMEBIASIS

Amebiasis is caused by the protozoan, *Entamoeba histolytica.* Typically, the parasite resides in the lumen of the large intestine, causing no disease; however, it is capable of invading the bowel wall and disseminating to extraintestinal sites. Although the majority of patients with amebiasis are asymptomatic, some develop mild-to-moderate symptoms with lower abdominal pain, tenesmus, and intermittent diarrhea with blood and mucus-containing feces. Amebic liver abscesses are an occasional complication in children, and symptomatology includes fever, abdominal distention, irritability, tachypnea, and hepatomegaly. Other foci are less common and include the pleura, lung, pericardium, brain, and skin.

Diagnosis of amebiasis is made by identifying the organism in the feces or in tissues obtained from lesions. Because cysts are shed intermittently in asymptomatic and mild infections, examination of multiple fecal specimens may be necessary to detect the organisms. Occasionally, inexperienced laboratory technicians misidentify white blood cells in the stool as *E. histolytica.* Serologic tests are also available; they are most likely to be positive in patients with invasive disease.

Treatment is directed toward relief of symptoms and eradication of the organisms. The choice of amebicides is based on the location and severity of the infection.

Asymptomatic intestinal infection is treated with one of the luminal amebicides that are ineffective against amebae in tissue.

Diloxanide furoate (Furamide) is our drug of choice because it is effective and the best tolerated of the luminal amebicides. The recommended dosage is 20 mg per kilogram per day (maximum, 1,500 mg per day) divided into three equal oral doses for 10 days. Flatulence is the only major side effect, with nausea, vomiting, diarrhea, and pruritus occurring less often. The drug is available for children older than 2 years of age through the Parasite Drug Service, Centers for Disease Control, Atlanta, Georgia (days: 404-329-3670; nights and weekends: 404-329-3644).

Diiodohydroxyquin or iodoquinol (Yodoxin) is also effective therapy for intestinal amebiasis and is given in a dosage of 30 to 40 mg per kilogram per day (maximum, 1,950 mg per day) divided into three equal oral doses for 20 days. Side effects include skin rash, nausea, diarrhea, cramps, and pruritus. Prolonged use of this drug has been associated with optic neuritis, optic atrophy, and peripheral neuropathy. Long-term therapy therefore, requires frequent monitoring of visual acuity. In addition, because it contains iodine it should be used with caution in patients with thyroid disease.

Paromomycin (Humatin), another agent that can be used to treat asymptomatic amebiasis, is given in a dosage of 30 mg per kilogram per day (maximum, 1,500 mg per day), divided into three equal oral doses for 7 days. Although such mild side effects as nausea, vomiting, abdominal cramps, and diarrhea occasionally occur, the major drawback of this medication is its cost.

Moderate and severe (necrotizing amebic colitis or ameboma) intestinal disease should be treated with a systemic and a luminal amebicide (generally diloxanide furoate). This combination is necessary because systemic amebicides alone may not adequately treat intestinal amebic cysts.

Metronidazole is a systemic amebicide given in a dosage of 35 to 50 mg per kilogram per day in three equally divided oral doses for 10 days. Side effects such as nausea, headache, candidal overgrowth, and a metallic aftertaste are usually mild. Less common side effects include dizziness, vertigo, ataxia, irritability, depression, paresthesias, urticaria, flushing, pruritus, dysuria, cystitis, dark urine, and reversible neutropenia. Disulfiram-like reactions can occur if alcohol is consumed within 4 days of metronidazole therapy. Although the potential carcinogenicity of metronidazole is of concern, the drug is believed to be safe when used for short courses of therapy. If oral therapy is difficult, intravenous metronidazole should be used. The dosage of metronidazole is 15 mg per kilogram, infused over an hour, followed by 7.5 mg per kilogram every 6 hours. All intravenous infusions of metronidazole should be given slowly, over 1 hour. A luminal agent such as diloxanide furoate or iodoquinol should be given along with metronidazole.

In the past, dehydroemetine in a dosage of 1.0 to 1.5 mg per kilogram per day given intramuscularly in one or two doses (maximum, 90 mg per day) or emetine in a dosage of 1 mg per kilogram per day given intramuscularly in one or two doses (maximum, 60 mg per day) were used. Both are alkaloid derivatives of ipecac and are highly effective against amebae in tissues. However, they have been associated with significant toxicity including hypotension, chest pain, cardiac arrhythmias, and dyspnea. Because of their potential toxicity, these drugs should be avoided in pediatric practice unless other amebicides have failed and the patient is unable to take oral medications or intravenous metronidazole.

Extraintestinal amebiasis generally responds well to metronidazole (50 mg per kilogram per day for 10 days) in combination with diloxanide furoate or iodoquinol. Patients usually improve symptomatically within 72 hours after the onset of therapy with metronidazole. Failure to respond and/or relapses occasionally occur and should be treated with dehydroemetine, 1.0 to 1.5 mg per kilogram per day divided into one or two equal doses intramuscularly for 5 days plus chloroquine phosphate base, 10 mg per kilogram per day for 14 to 21 days. The maximum daily dose of chloroquine base is 300 mg, and potential side effects include pruritus, vomiting, and headache. Large total dosages of chloroquine (greater than 100 g) have been associated with permanent retinal damage. A luminal amebicide should be added to this regimen.

Therapeutic aspiration of amebic liver abscesses is indicated when the lesions are large or are associated with severe localized liver tenderness or marked diaphragmatic elevation. Surgical drainage is rarely necessary, and most amebic liver abscesses heal gradually, over several months, with appropriate antiamebic therapy. Pleural involvement may require drainage through a chest tube, thoracostomy, or exploration of both thorax and abdomen.

Although amebiasis generally responds to appropriate chemotherapy, parasitologic relapses sometimes occur, and stool specimens should be checked monthly for several months after therapy. Household members should also be screened initially for possible asymptomatic infection. In highly endemic areas, asymptomatic carriers are not necessarily treated because the probability of reinfection is high. Food handlers should always be treated, and the most effective means of prevention is proper sanitation. Prophylaxis with amebicides is not recommended.

NONPATHOGENIC AMEBAE

Entamoeba coli, Entamoeba hartmanni, Entamoeba polecki, Endolimax nana, and *Iodamoeba buetschlii* are nonpathogenic amebae. Since they have not been associated with disease in humans, no treatment is necessary. They can be mistaken for *Entamoeba histolytica* by inexperienced laboratory personnel. Nonpathogenic amebae in the feces can also cause *E. histolytica* to be overlooked when both are present. In addition, because they are transmitted by feces, their presence suggests a source of fecal contamination, and a careful search for other intestinal pathogens should be conducted.

NONPATHOGENIC PROTOZOA OF THE ORAL CAVITY

Trichomonas tenax, a flagellate (rare reports of an association with lung abscesses), and *Entamoeba gingivalis,* an ameba, are oral parasites of humans. Both are related to poor oral hygiene and require no specific therapy other than an improvement in oral hygiene.

BALANTIDIASIS

Balantidium coli is the only ciliate and the largest protozoan parasitizing humans. Symptoms of infection include lower abdominal pain, nausea, vomiting, tenesmus, and cramps. Watery diarrhea occasionally becomes mucoid or bloody, lasting weeks to months. The organism is most often found in humans having a close association with pigs. Person-to-person transmission also occurs. Saline mounts of human stools may demonstrate both the trophozoites and cysts, which can be identified by their large size (sometimes with the naked eye). They can also be seen in the scrapings of ulcerations of the colonic mucosa obtained by sigmoidoscopy.

Metronidazole (Flagyl), 15 mg per kilogram per day (maximum, 750 mg per day), divided into three equal doses orally for 7 to 10 days, can be used for treatment. The advantages of metronidazole therapy include its suitability for children younger than 8 years of age, less toxicity than iodoquinol, and easy availability. Side effects in children treated for 10 days are minimal and include gastrointestinal disturbances and *Candida* overgrowth. Less common reactions include dizziness, vertigo, ataxia, irritability, depression, paresthesias, urticaria, flushing, dry mouth, pruritus, dysuria, cystitis, and dark urine. Disulfiram-like reactions can occur from alcohol consumption within 4 days of metronidazole therapy. The mutagenic and carcinogenic potential of metronidazole has never been proved in human studies.

Tetracycline, 40 mg per kilogram per day (maximum, 2 g per day), divided into four equal doses given orally for 10 days, is the preferred therapy for older children and adults. It is contraindicated in children younger than 8 years of age or in pregnant females because it stains developing tooth enamel. The advantages of tetracycline are rare toxicity, low cost, and easy availability.

Iodoquinol (Yodoxin), 40 mg per kilogram per day (maximum, 1,950 mg per day), divided into three equal doses for 20 days, is effective for treating children. Side effects include skin rash, nausea, vomiting, diarrhea, cramps, and pruritus. Prolonged use of this drug has been associated with optic neuritis and peripheral neuropathies, and requires monitoring of visual acuity. In addition, because it contains iodine, it should be used with caution in patients with thyroid disease.

Paromomycin (Humatin, Parke-Davis) has also been effective for treatment, but it is very expensive and not readily available. Prevention is by means of improved hygiene, particularly in persons who work with swine.

DIENTAMOEBA FRAGILIS

Originally classified as a nonpathogenic ameba, *Dientamoeba fragilis* has recently been reclassified as a "flagellate without flagella" because of antigenic similarities with the flagellates. The organism has only a fragile trophozoite stage and no protective cyst stage. The lack of a cyst stage in a parasite that lyses rapidly once it is passed in the feces has made the transmission of this parasite a mystery. The observation of an association of *D. fragilis* with *Enterobius vermicularis* suggested a possible means by which the trophozoites of this flagellate might survive outside the host. The transmission of *D. fragilis* in the eggs of the ubiquitous pinworm has not been proved, but is the most likely answer to the mystery.

Early investigators considered the organism nonpathogenic, but recent studies have implicated *D. fragilis* as a cause of illness. Children are more frequently symptomatic than adults. They have nonspecific gastrointestinal symptoms including diarrhea, abdominal distention, nausea, vomiting, and weight loss. The diagnosis is often difficult because of the fragility of the parasite, and it is made only if very fresh or preserved fecal specimens are examined. This may account for the low prevalence of this parasite in many surveys. In patients with more chronic gastrointestinal symptoms, a careful search of fresh or preserved specimens for the trophozoites of *D. fragilis* can be rewarding.

Metronidazole (Flagyl) is our drug of choice for the treatment of *D. fragilis* infections. It comes in 250-mg tablets, which have a mildly unpleasant aftertaste when crushed into a suspension for small children. The advantages of metronidazole are a short treatment course and ready availability. Side effects in children are minimal and include gastrointestinal disturbances and *Candida* overgrowth. Less common reactions include moderate depression of white blood cell counts, dizziness, vertigo, ataxia, irritability, depression, paresthesias, urticaria, flushing, dry mouth, pruritus, dysuria, cystitis, and dark urine. Disulfiram-like reactions can occur from alcohol consumption within 4 days of metronidazole therapy. The mutagenic and carcinogenic potential of this drug is probably overstated and only mildly worrisome in patients given a short course of therapy. The dosage is 15 mg per kilogram per day (maximum, 750 mg per day), divided into three equal doses given orally for 10 days.

Iodoquinol (Yodoxin), formerly diidohydroxyquin, is available in 210-mg and 650-mg tablets and is frequently listed as the drug of choice for the treatment of *D. fragilis* infections. The drawbacks of this drug are its lack of availability in local pharmacies and its required 20-day course of therapy. Adverse reactions are not uncommon and include rashes, urticaria, pruritus, nausea, vomiting, abdominal cramps, diarrhea, and pruritus ani. Less frequent reactions include fever, chills, headache, vertigo, and enlargement of the thyroid. Optic neuritis, optic atropy, and peripheral neuropathy have been associated with prolonged courses of this drug. For treatment failures with metronidazole or intolerance to other drugs, we give iodoquinol, 40 mg per kilogram per day, divided into three equal doses given orally for 20 days (maximum, 1,950 mg per kilogram per day).

Tetracyclines are contraindicated in children younger than 8 years of age and in pregnant females (because of the permanent discoloration of the developing teeth), but in older children and adults they are an inexpensive alternative to metronidazole. Tetracycline hydrochloride, 40 mg per kilogram per day, divided into three equal doses given orally for 10 days (maximum, 2 g per day), can be used in children older than 8 years of age and in nonpregnant adults. It is preferable to iodoquinol and less expensive than metronidazole for the treatment of older children and adults.

GIARDIASIS

Giardia lamblia is the most common intestinal parasite in the world. It is found more frequently in children than in adults. *G. lamblia* is easily spread from person to person, but it can also cause epidemics through water-borne outbreaks.

The clinical spectrum of giardiasis ranges from asymptomatic infestation to severe failure to thrive and malabsorption. Adults and older children often have no symptoms or very mild symptoms. Young children often have diarrhea, but abdominal distention and bloating are the most common complaints. The diagnosis of giardiasis depends on demonstrating the parasite in feces, duodenal fluid, or mucosal biopsy of duodenum. Microscopic examination of feces is the least sensitive of these methods and there is marked variability among laboratories. Because of the potential trauma and discomfort associated with duodenal aspiration or biopsy, these methods should be reserved for patients with persistent symptoms and negative examinations of multiple stools. Recently, counterimmunoelectrophoresis and ELISA testing for *G. lamblia* fecal antigen have been shown to be as sensitive as duodenal aspiration in making the diagnosis, but these tests are not generally available.

Although treatment of *G. lamblia* infections results in prompt improvement of acute symptoms in most patients, some symptoms may persist for 1 to 2 weeks despite appropriate therapy. At present, there is no ideal therapy for all children with this organism. Because of this, it is important to understand the currently effective agents so that one can choose the most appropriate therapy for any given situation.

Furazolidone (Furoxone) is the drug of choice for treating small children, because it is the best tolerated in children under 5 years of age. It is available in 100-mg tablets and as an oral suspension of 50 mg per 15 ml. The taste is acceptable to most children, and the cure rates are from 80 to 100 percent. Because the concentration is expressed as 50 mg per 15 ml instead of the customary 5 ml, a common error is to prescribe one-third the needed dose; this probably accounts for many supposed therapeutic failures. Side effects are minimal in children and include mild gastrointestinal disturbances, reversible hypersensitivity reactions, occasional hemolysis in patients with glucose-6-phosphate dehydrogenase deficiency, rashes, and brown discoloration of the urine. Disulfiram-like reactions can result from alcohol consumption within 4 days of furazolidone treatment. (It should be remembered that elixirs contain alcohol.) Adults receiving monoamine oxidase inhibitors in addition to furazolidone can experience hypertensive crises and flushing reactions with severe headaches. In addition, tyramine-containing foods (broad beans, yeast extract, strong unpasteurized cheese, beer, wine, pickled herring, and chicken livers), indirect-acting sympathomimetic amines (phenylephrine and ephedrine), and amphetamines can precipitate similar reactions. An increased incidence of mammary tumors has been observed in rats given massive doses of furazolidone for prolonged periods.

Because it is available as an acceptable oral suspension and because of the demonstrated efficacy observed in children younger than 5 years of age, we recommend furazolidone as the drug of choice for young children. The dosage of furazolidone is 9 mg per kilogram per day (maximum, 400 mg per day), divided into three equal doses given orally for 10 days.

Quinacrine hydrochloride (Atabrine) is available only as 100-mg tablets. The taste is horrid, particularly when it is dissolved in a suspension, and it cannot be masked by flavorings. Efficacy in adults and older children able to take tablets is 90 to 100 percent. Approximately 30 percent of children younger than 5 years of age taking quinacrine have nausea and vomiting, and many refuse to take the drug. The frequency of side effects reduces the efficacy to 60 percent in children younger than 5 years. In addition, 78 percent of the children developed yellow discoloration of their skin during therapy. Psychosis associated with quinacrine is rarely recognized in children, but it is not uncommon in adults. They must be warned of this side effect and instructed to stop therapy if they or their family and friends note changes in their mental well-being. Quinacrine can also cause a mild disulfiram-like reaction. No mutagenic or carcinogenic effects have been demonstrated with quinacrine and related compounds. Because of the difficulties in treating young children, we do not recommend quinacrine for them unless the cost is important. Quinacrine hydrochloride, 6 mg per kilogram per day (maximum dose, 300 mg per day), divided into three equal doses given orally for 10 days is less expensive than furazolidone therapy.

Metronidazole (Flagyl) is available only as 250-mg tablets. When it is made into a suspension the taste is unpleasant because of the metallic aftertaste. Efficacy of metronidazole in giardiasis varies from 50 percent for some single-dose regimens to 97 percent for a 7- to 10-day course of therapy. Side effects in children after 10 days of therapy are minimal and include gastrointestinal disturbances and *Candida* overgrowth. Less common reactions include dizziness, vertigo, ataxia, irritability, depression, paresthesias, urticaria, flushing, dry mouth, pruritus, dysuria, cystitis, and dark urine. Disulfiram-like reactions can occur from alcohol consumption within 4 days of metronidazole therapy. Metronidazole is rapidly absorbed from the gastrointestinal tract, concentrates in gonadal tissue, and crosses the placenta. Mutagenic studies in bacteria show definite potential for mutation at low doses. In animals, normal therapeutic concentrations of metronidazole given over a prolonged period increased the incidence of mammary tumors. In humans, no evidence for cancer associated with metronidazole therapy has been uncovered. Because of the carcinogenic potential, the lack of FDA approval for treatment of giardiasis in children, and the relatively bad taste, we do not routinely use metronidazole in children. For treatment failures or when there is intolerance to other medications, we prescribe metronidazole in a dosage of 15 mg per kilogram per day (maximum dose, 750 mg per day), divided into three equal doses orally for 10 days.

Tinidazole, ornidazole, and nitrimidazine are new anti-*Giardia* medications, but none is currently available in the United States. They are similar in efficacy and side effects to the chemically related drug, metronidazole. Therapeutic regimens of 1 to 3 days are effective in adults at a cost of increased side effects. Since side effects are even more common in children, the benefits probably do not outweigh the potential problems except in special situations involving compliance.

Appropriate treatment of symptomatic patients with giardiasis is clearly advantageous. Treatment of the asymptomatic person infected with *G. lamblia* is not as clear. Indications for treatment are the potential for malabsorption and growth retardation in the growing child and the high rate of spread among diapered infants and toddlers. Because of these concerns,

young children should be treated regardless of symptoms. Asymptomatic older children and adults do not require therapy unless the threat of transmission is high, as with food handlers, large families, and homosexuals.

Dealing with giardiasis in the day care center is particularly difficult. Ideally, all children in a day care setting should be treated when a symptomatic index case of *G. lamblia* infection is found. In practice, this is almost impossible to accomplish because of the cost and difficulty in ensuring that all children are treated and that they all start and complete the medication at the same time. Treating only those found to be infected after surveying all the children's feces for cyst excretion has been recommended. This is difficult because of the expense, the delay between obtaining the stool samples, test results, and starting medication, and the inability of most laboratories to make the diagnosis in all infected patients. The incidence of *G. lamblia* infection in most day care centers is 10 to 30 percent in the absence of symptomatic cases. With our present understanding of the epidemiology, eliminating this parasite from all day care centers in the United States would require an enormous expenditure of time and money. The prudent approach for the present appears to be to treat only symptomatic cases and to ignore the asymptomatic.

Symptomatic giardiasis in the pregnant female is a complex situation. The teratogenic effects of anti-*Giardia* medications in humans are unknown. Because of the potential harm to the fetus, therapy with metronidazole, furazolidone, and quinacrine is contraindicated. Paromomycin (Humatin, Parke-Davis), a nonabsorbable aminoglycoside, is recommended for treatment of severe symptomatic giardiasis in the pregnant female. Symptomatic improvement can be expected in 80 to 90 percent of pregnant patients treated with an oral dose of 250 mg given three times a day for 1 week. In more than 50 percent of cases, *G. lamblia* is not eliminated from the feces, but the majority remain asymptomatic despite continued parasitosis. At present there are no controlled studies to substantiate this recommendation. We have used paromomycin is several pregnant females with severe symptoms secondary to giardiasis and have seen clinical improvements.

Prevention of *G. lamblia* infection is difficult because of the sturdiness of cysts. The primary method of transmission is person-to-person and this can be prevented by maintaining good hygiene. In day care centers, good handwashing habits, care in the disposal of waste, and adequate bathroom facilities usually prevent spread of infection. Prevention of water-borne outbreaks depends on maintaining quality water purification facilities and sewage disposal facilities. Campers and backpackers are at risk of developing giardiasis if they drink from streams and lakes. Purification of small quantities of water by means of iodination tablets, 3- to 5-μm filtration devices, and 10 minutes of boiling are reliable methods for obtaining safe drinking water while camping. Travelers are also a risk while visiting countries where water quality is less well maintained by the local governments. By drinking only boiled water, bottled carbonated drinks, or alcoholic beverages and eating adequately cooked food, most travelers can be protected.

TRICHOMONIASIS

Trichomonas vaginalis is frequently found in the urogenital systems of adult males and females, but it is uncommon in prepubertal children with the exception of newborn females. The trophozoites of *T. vaginalis* prefer the conditions present in the estrogenic vagina, but can be found in prepubertal children. Males are frequently asymptomatic, but can have dysuria associated with this organism. In the female, symptoms are common and include dysuria, vaginal itching and burning, and a foamy yellowish green discharge with a foul odor. Younger children and infants may have only a profuse watery discharge. The diagnosis is generally made by finding the motile organisms in wet mounts of vaginal fluid, prostatic fluid, or sedimented freshly passed urine. Stained smears of vaginal fluid and scrapings are unreliable because of the distortion of the trophozoites. Cultures for *T. vaginalis* is the most sensitive method of detection, but generally is not available in most laboratories. The diagnosis of *Trichomonas* infections in children other than infants and sexually active teenagers should make the physician consider sexual abuse.

No therapy is necessary for the newborn who acquires *T. vaginalis* from the maternal birth canal. The infection is self-limited and resolves as the maternal estrogen effect decreases. Older children and adolescents should be treated with metronidazole (Flagyl); 15 mg per kilogram per day (maximum, 750 mg per day), divided into three equal doses given orally for 10 days. Vaginal suppositories can be used in addition to oral therapy, but do not meet with good patient compliance. Side effects in children after 10 days of therapy are minimal and include gastrointestinal disturbances and *Candida* overgrowth. Less common reactions include dizziness, vertigo, ataxia, irritability, depression, paresthesias, urticaria, flushing, dry mouth, pruritus, dysuria, cystitis, and dark urine. Disulfiram-like reactions can occur from alcohol consumption within 4 days of metronidazole therapy. The mutagenic and carcinogenic potential of metrondiazole has never been proved in human studies.

NONPATHOGENIC INTESTINAL FLAGELLATES

Trichomonas hominis, Chilomastix mesnili, Enteromonas hominis, and *Retortamonas intestinalis* are nonpathogenic flagellates found in the feces of humans. They have not been proved to cause disease in humans and do not require therapy. They can be confused with pathogenic flagellates of the intestinal and urogenital tracts. The presence of these nonpathogenic flagellates in the feces does indicate poor hygiene, and when they are found in symptomatic patients, a careful search for other pathogens is warranted.

ISOSPORA BELLI AND ISOSPORA HOMINIS

Isospora species are parasites of the small intestine of humans. They are most frequently found in the feces of persons from tropical areas, but have been reported in temperate climates. They often cause symptoms including anorexia, nausea, abdominal pain, and diarrhea lasting for 1 to 2 months. The illness is generally self-limited, but in immunocompromised hosts it can become chronic. Finding the oocysts of *I. belli* or *I. hominis* in the feces confirms the diagnosis, but the oocysts and sporocysts are transparent and can be easily overlooked. The oocysts have also been mistaken for *Giardia lamblia* by inexperienced laboratory technicians. Pyrimethamine, sulfadiazine, trimethoprim-sulfamethoxazole, and furazolidone have been reported to be effective therapy, but all lack supportive data from clinical trials. Symptomatic improvement can occur with bismuth subsalicylate (Pepto-Bismol). The toxicities are similar to that of aspirin, and inadvertent toxic concentrations can be given when aspirin and Pepto-Bismol are given together. Preventive measures consist of improved hygiene as recommended for giardiasis.

SARCOCYSTIS

Sarcocystis species is a parasite found in the intestines of carnivorous animals and encysted in the muscles of sheep, cattle, horses, and swine. Humans can be the definitive or intermediate host. *Sarcocystis* can be found in striated and cardiac muscle at autopsy or biopsy, but is not felt to be associated with illness. The intestinal infection in humans may be associated with diarrhea and abdominal pain. In the rare patient with persistent symptoms, trimethoprim-sulfamethoxazole, pyrimethamine, and sulfadiazine may be effective therapy. Because infection results from eating uncooked meat or excreta from infected animals, it can be prevented by using care in cleaning and preparing meat and eating only well-cooked foods.

CRYPTOSPORIDIOSIS

Cryptosporidium is an intestinal protozoa, recognized in recent years as a significant cause of diarrhea in humans. Initially it was believed to be a cause of disease in animal handlers and immunosuppressed patients, but cryptosporidiosis is now being recognized with increasing frequency in normal hosts. Numerous reports have implicated *Cryptosporidium* as a cause of diarrhea among children attending day care centers. The infection appears to be transmitted by fecal–oral spread, and symptoms consist of profuse watery diarrhea, occasionally associated with abdominal cramps, nausea, vomiting, and low-grade fever. In persons with normal immune function, the diarrhea is self-limited, generally lasting 1 to 2 weeks. Immunodeficient patients may have more severe diarrhea with enormous fluid losses, and the symptoms often become chronic, lasting months to years.

For many years diagnosis required examination of intestinal biopsies; however, it is now known that oocysts are shed in the feces and can be detected with a variety of stains, including iodine, fluorescent auramine-rodamine, and modified Kinyoun acid-fast stains. Serologic diagnosis using indirect immunofluorescence is also available; however, its sensitivity and specificity remain to be defined.

Patients with cryptosporidiosis and normal immune function improve without specific therapy and require only supportive treatment. Immunocompromised patients often develop more protracted symptoms, which do not respond well to most forms of therapy. A variety of chemotherapeutic agents have been used, including clindamycin, quinine, pentamidine, trimethoprim–sulfamethoxazole, metronidazole, pyrimethamine–sulfa, furazolidone, and spiramycin. Furazolidone, 9 mg per kilogram per day in three divided oral doses (maximum, 400 mg per day), has been reported to suppress symptoms in two patients without eradicating the organism. Spiramycin, available from the Food and Drug Administration (301-443-4310 to obtain an investigator number), given in a dosage of 1 g per day (in two to four divided doses) in children and 3 to 4 g per day in adults, has produced clinical improvement, both with and without eradication of the parasite. Both drugs are relatively nontoxic in children, producing mild gastrointestinal disturbances and, occasionally, allergic reactions. In rare cases, furazolidone also produces hemolytic anemia in neonates and individuals with glucose-6-phosphate dehydrogenase deficiency and has a disulfuram-like reaction with alcohol.

During the past few years a number of additional chemotherapeutic agents such as DFMO, bovine transfer factor, trimetrexate, recombinant interleukin-2, and amprolium have been used to treat cryptosporidiosis in immunocompromised hosts. Some have produced unacceptable toxicity and none is currently recommended as standard therapy for cryptosporidiosis. To date, no antibiotic has consistently suppressed symptoms or eradicated *Cryptosporidium* in immunocompromised patients. The most effective therapy for cryptosporidiosis in these patients has been reversal of the immune deficiency (i.e., stopping immunosuppressive therapy when possible). At present, a trial of spiramycin or furazolidone is probably indicated for patients who are likely to remain immunosuppressed. For those immunosuppressed patients who continue to be symptomatic despite therapy, a trial of DFMO, available on a compassionate basis from Merrill Dow (513-948-9111), might be considered.

BLASTOCYSTIS HOMINIS

Once considered to be a yeast, *Blastocystis hominis,* more recently has been classified as a protozoan in the subphylum Sporozoa. It is found in the stools of as many as 25 percent of patients, but is only rarely the cause of symptoms. When symptoms can be attributed to *B. hominis,* they consist of persistent mild diarrhea. The diagnosis is made by finding the organism in feces by routine methods. Some care should be taken in diluting the sample with water since the organism may lyse. There is no specific therapy and the illness is generally mild and self-limited. Prevention is dependent on maintaining good hygiene.

---

* The authors gratefully acknowledge the contribution of the section on Babesiosis by George A. Jacoby, M.D.

SUGGESTED READING

Anabwani GM, Dimiti G, Ngira JA, et al. Comparison of two dosage schedules of sodium stibogluconate in the treatment of visceral leishmaniasis in Kenya. Lancet 1983; 1:210–212.

Apted FIC. Present status of chemotherapy and chemoprophylaxis of human trypanosomiasis in the Eastern Hemisphere. Pharmacol Ther 1980; 11:391–413.

Bruce-Chwatt LJ, ed. Chemotherapy of malaria. Geneva: World Health Organization Monograph Series, No 27, 1986.

Bryceson ADM. Diffuse cutaneous leishmaniasis in Ethiopia: II. Treatment. Trans R Soc Trop Med Hyg 1970; 64:369–379.

Campbell WC, Rew RS, eds. Chemotherapy of parasitic diseases. New York: Plenum Press, 1986.

Centers for Disease Control. Update: treatment of cryptosporidiosis in patients with acquired immunodeficiency syndrome (AIDS). MMWR 1984; 33(9):117–119.

Craft JC. Giardiasis in children. In: McCracken GH, Nelson JD, eds. Clinical reviews in pediatric infectious diseases. Toronto, Canada: BC Decker 1985; 129–142.

Craft JC, Murphy TV, Nelson JD. Furazolidone and quinacrine: comparative study of therapy of giardiasis in children. Am J Dis Child 1980; 135:164–166.

Crofts MAJ. Use of amphotericin B in mucocutaneous leishmaniasis. J Trop Med Hyg 1976;79:111.

Culbertson CG. Amebic meningoencephalitis. Antiobiot Chemother 1981; 30:28–53.

DeHovitz JA, Pape JW, Boncy M, Johnson WD Jr. Clinical manifestations and therapy of Isospora belli infection in patients with the acquired immunodeficiency syndrome. N Engl J Med 1986; 315:87–90.

Drugs for parasitic infections. Med Lett Drugs Ther 1986; 28(706):9–18.

Dupont HL, Sullivan PS. Giardiasis: the clinical spectrum, diagnosis and therapy. Pediatr Infect Dis 1986; 5:S131–138.

Evans DA. African trypanosomiasis. Antibiot Chemother 1981; 30:272–287.

Gombert ME, Goldstein EJ, Benach JL, et al. Human babesiosis. JAMA 1982; 248:3005.

Gutteridge WE. Existing chemotherapy and its limitations. Br Med J 1985; 41(2):162–168.

Haffar A, Boland FJ, Edwards MS. Amebic liver abscesses in children. Pediatr Infect Dis 1982; 1(5):322–327.

Hart A, Baxby D. Management of cryptosporidiosis. J Antimicrob Chemother 1985; 15(1):3–4.

Health information for international travel, 1985. Atlanta, U.S. Department of Health and Human Services, Public Health Service. Centers for Disease Control. HHS Publication No (CDC) 85-8280, 1985.

Hirst LW, Green WR, Merz W, et al. Management of *Acanthamoeba kerititis;* a case report and review of the literature. Ophthalmology 1985; 91:1105–1111.

Hughes WT. Current concepts: *Pneumocystis carinii* pneumonia. N Engl J Med 1977; 297:1381–1383.

Hughes WT, Feldman S, Chaudharg SC, et al. Comparison of pentamidine isethionate and trimethoprim-sulfamethoxazole in the treatment of *Pneumocystis carinii* pneumonia. J Pediatr 1978; 92:285–291.

Hughes WT, McNabb PL, Makres TD, Feldman S. Efficacy of trimethoprim and sulfamethoxazole in the prevention and treatment of *Pneumocystis carinii* pneumonitis. Antimicrob Agents Chemother 1974; 5:289–293.

Jacoby GA, Hunt JV, Kosinski KS, et al. Treatment of transfusion-transmitted babesiosis by exchange transfusion. N Engl J Med 1981; 303:1098–1100.

Katz M. Treatment of protozoan infections: malaria. Pediatr Infect Dis 1983; 2(6):475–480.

Knight R. The chemotherapy of amoebiasis. J Antimicrob Chemother 1980; 6:577–593.

Leoung GS, Mills J, Hopewell PC, et al. Dapsone-trimethoprim for *Pneumocystic carinii* pneumonia in the acquired immunodeficiency syndrome. Ann Intern Med 1986; 105:45–48.

Lossick JG. Treatment of *Trichomonas vaginalis* infection. Rev Infect Dis 1982; 4(Suppl):S801–818.

Luft BJ, Remington JS. Toxoplasmosis of the central nervous system. In: Remington JS. Swartz MN, eds. Current clinical topics in infectious diseases, Vol 6. New York: McGraw-Hill, 1985.

Maisonneuve H, Faber C, Piens MA, et al. Congenital toxoplasmosis. Tolerance to the pyrimethamine-sulfadoxine combination. 24 cases. Presse Med 1984; 13(14):859–862.

Markell EK, Udkow MP. Blastocystis hominis: pathogen or fellow traveler? Am J Trop Med Hyg 1986; 35:1023–1026.

Marsden PD. Current concepts in parasitology: leishmaniasis. N Engl J Med 1979; 300:350–352.

Rein MF. Current therapy of vulvovaginitis. Sex Transm Dis 1981; 8:316–321.

Remington JS, Desmonts G. Toxoplasmosis. In: Remington JS, Klein JO, eds. Infectious diseases of the fetus and newborn infant. Philadelphia: WB Saunders, 1983.

Report of the informal meeting on the chemotherapy of visceral leishmaniasis UNDP/World Bank/WHO Special Programme for Research and Training in Tropical Diseases. Brasilia, July 1979.

Report of the informal meeting on the chemotherapy of visceral leishmaniasis UNDP/World Bank/WHO Special Programme for Research and Training in Tropical Diseases. Nairobi, Kenya, June 1982.

Revised recommendations for preventing malaria in travelers to areas with chloroquine resistant *Plasmodium falciparum.* MMWR 1985; 34:185–190, 195c.

Ribeiro-dos-Santos R, Rassi A, Koberle F. Chagas' disease. Antibiot Chemother 1980; 30:115–134.

Sands M, Kron MA, Brown RB. Pentamidine: a review. Rev Infect Dis 1985; 7:625–634.

Simon MW, Wilson HD. The amebic meningoencephalitides. Pediatr Infect Dis 1986; 5:562–569.

Soave R, Armstrong D. Cryptosporidium and cryptosporidiosis. Rev Infect Dis 1986; 8(6):1012–1023.

Spencer MJ, Garcia LS, Chapin MR. Dientamoeba fragilis: an intestinal pathogen in children? Am J Dis Child 1979; 133:390–393.

Thompson Jr JE, Forlenza S, Verma R. Amebic liver abscess: a therapeutic approach. Rev Infect Dis 1985; 7(2):171–179.

Taelman H, Schechter PJ, Marcelis L, et al. Difluoromethylornithine, an effective new treatment of Gambian trypanosomiasis. Am J Med 1987; 82:607–614.

WHO. The African Trypanosomiases. Technical Report Series 635, Geneva: World Health Organization, 1979; 1–96.

Wittner M, Rowin KS, Tanowitz HB, et al. Successful chemotherapy of transfusion babesiosis. Ann Intern Med 1982; 96:601–604.

APPENDIX
CDC GUIDELINES FOR INFECTION CONTROL IN HOSPITAL PERSONNEL

DISEASE	PRIVATE ROOM?	MASKS?	GOWNS?	GLOVES?	INFECTIVE MATERIAL	APPLY PRECAUTIONS HOW LONG?	COMMENTS
Abscess, etiology unknown							
Draining, major	Yes	No	Yes if soiling is likely	Yes for touching infective material	Pus	Duration of illness	Major = no dressing or dressing does not adequately contain the pus.
Draining, minor or limited	No	No	Yes if soiling is likely	Yes for touching infective material	Pus	Duration of illness	Minor or limited = dressing covers and adequately contains the pus, or infected area is small, such as a stitch abscess.
Not draining	No	No	No	No			
Acquired immunodeficiency syndrome (AIDS)	Yes if patient hygiene is poor	No	Yes if soiling is likely	Yes for touching infective material	Blood and body fluids	Duration of illness	Use caution when handling blood and blood-soiled articles. Take special care to avoid needlestick injuries. If gastrointestinal bleeding is likely, wear gloves if touching feces. (Acquired immune deficiency syndrome [AIDS]: precautions for clinical and laboratory staffs. MMWR 1982; 31:577–580.)
Actinomycosis, all lesions	No	No	No	No			
Adenovirus infection, respiratory in infants and young children	Yes	No	Yes if soiling is likely	No	Respiratory secretions and feces	Duration of hospitalization	During epidemics patients believed to have adenovirus infection may be placed in the same room (cohorting).
Amebiasis							
Dysentery	Yes if patient hygiene is poor	No	Yes if soiling is likely	Yes for touching infective material	Feces	Duration of illness	
Liver abscess	No	No	No	No			
Anthrax							
Cutaneous	No	No	No	Yes for touching infective material	Pus	Duration of illness	
Inhalation	No	No	Yes if soiling is likely	Yes for touching infective material	Respiratory secretions may be	Duration of illness	

DISEASE	PRECAUTIONS INDICATED				INFECTIVE MATERIAL	APPLY PRE-CAUTIONS HOW LONG?	COMMENTS
	PRIVATE ROOM?	MASKS?	GOWNS?	GLOVES?			
Arthropodborne viral encephalitides (eastern equine, western equine, and Venezuelan equine encephalomyelitis, St. Louis and California encephalitis.)	No	No	No	No			
Arthropodborne viral fevers (dengue, yellow fever, and Colorado tick fever)	No	No	No	Yes for touching infective material	Blood	Duration of hospitalization	
Ascariasis	No	No	No	No			
Aspergillosis	No	No	No	No			
Babesiosis	No	No	No	Yes for touching infective material	Blood	Duration of illness	
Blastomycosis, North American, cutaneous or pulmonary	No	No	No	No			
Botulism							
Infant	No	No	No	No			
Other	No	No	No	No			
Bronchiolitis, etiology unknown in infants and young children	Yes	No	Yes if soiling is likely	No	Respiratory secretions	Duration of illness	Various etiologic agents, such as respiratory syncytial virus, parainfluenza viruses, adenoviruses, and influenza viruses, have been associated with this syndrome (Committee on Infectious Diseases, American Academy of Pediatrics. 1982 Red Book); therefore, precautions to prevent their spread are generally indicated.
Bronchitis, infective etiology unknown							
Adults	No	No	No	No	Respiratory secretions may be		
Infants and young children	Yes	No	Yes if soiling is likely	No	Respiratory secretions	Duration of illness	
Brucellosis (undulant fever, Malta fever, Mediterranean fever)							
Draining lesions, limited or minor	No	No	Yes if soiling is likely	Yes for touching infective material	Pus	Duration of illness	Limited or minor = dressing covers and adequately contains the pus, or infected area is very small.
Other	No	No	No	No			

DISEASE	PRECAUTIONS INDICATED				INFECTIVE MATERIAL	APPLY PRECAUTIONS HOW LONG?	COMMENTS
	PRIVATE ROOM?	MASKS?	GOWNS?	GLOVES?			
Burn wound (see separate section on Care of Patients with Burns)							
Campylobacter gastroenteritis	Yes if patient hygiene is poor	No	Yes if soiling is likely	Yes for touching infective material	Feces	Duration of illness	
Candidiasis, all forms, including mucocutaneous (moniliasis, thrush)	No	No	No	No			
Cat-scratch fever (benign inoculation lymphoreticulosis)	No	No	No	No			
Cellulitis,							
Draining, limited or minor	No	No	Yes if soiling is likely	Yes for touching infective material	Pus	Duration of illness	Limited or minor = dressing covers and adequately contains the pus, or infected area is very small.
Intact skin	No	No	No	No			
Chancroid (soft chancre)	No	No	No	No			
Chickenpox (varicella)	Yes	Yes	Yes	Yes	Respiratory secretions and lesion secretions	Until all lesions are crusted	Persons who are not susceptible do not need to wear a mask. Susceptible persons should, if possible, stay out of room. Special ventilation for the room, if available, may be advantageous, especially for outbreak control. Neonates born to mothers with active varicella should be placed on isolation precautions at birth. Exposed susceptible patients should be placed on isolation precautions beginning 10 days after exposure and continuing until 21 days after last exposure. See CDC Guideline for Infection Control in Hospital Personnel for recommendations for exposed susceptible personnel.
Chlamydia trachomatis infection							
Conjunctivitis	No	No	No	Yes for touching infective material	Purulent exudate	Duration of illness	
Genital	No	No	No	Yes for touching infective material	Genital discharge	Duration of illness	

DISEASE	PRECAUTIONS INDICATED				INFECTIVE MATERIAL	APPLY PRE-CAUTIONS HOW LONG?	COMMENTS
	PRIVATE ROOM?	MASKS?	GOWNS?	GLOVES?			
Respiratory	No	No	No	Yes for touching infective material	Respiratory secretions	Duration of illness	
Cholera	Yes if patient hygiene is poor	No	Yes if soiling is likely	Yes for touching infective material	Feces	Duration of illness	
Closed-cavity infection							
Draining, limited or minor	No	No	Yes if soiling is likely	Yes for touching infective material	Pus	Duration of illness	Limited or minor = dressing covers and adequately contains the pus, or infected area is very small.
Not draining	No	No	No	No			
Clostridium perfringens							
Food poisoning	No	No	No	No			
Gas gangrene	No	No	Yes if soiling is likely	Yes for touching infective material	Pus	Duration of illness	
Other	No	No	Yes if soiling is likely	Yes for touching infective material	Pus	Duration	
Coccidioidomycosis (valley fever)							
Draining lesions	No	No	No	No	Draining may be if spores form		
Pneumonia	No	No	No	No			
Colorado tick fever	No	No	No	Yes for touching infective material	Blood	Duration of hospitalization	
Common cold							
Adults	No	No	No	No	Respiratory secretions may be		
Infants and young children	Yes	No	Yes if soiling is likely	No	Respiratory secretions	Duration of illness	Although rhinoviruses are most frequently associated with the common cold and are mild in adults, severe infections may occur in infants and young children. Other etiologic agents, such as respiratory syncytial virus and parainfluenza viruses, may also cause this syndrome (Committee on Infectious Diseases, American Academy of Pediatrics. 1982 Red Book); therefore, precautions to prevent their spread are generally indicated.

| DISEASE | PRIVATE ROOM? | PRECAUTIONS INDICATED | | | INFECTIVE MATERIAL | APPLY PRECAUTIONS HOW LONG? | COMMENTS |
		MASKS?	GOWNS?	GLOVES?			
Congenital rubella	Yes	No	Yes if soiling is likely	Yes for touching infective material	Urine and respiratory secretions	During any admission for the 1st year after birth unless nasopharyngeal and urine cultures after 3 months of age are negative for rubella virus.	Susceptible persons should, if possible, stay out of room. Pregnant personnel may need special counseling (see CDC Guideline for Infection Control in Hospital Personnel).
Conjunctivitis, acute bacterial (sore eye, pink eye)	No	No	No	Yes for touching infective material	Purulent exudate	Duration of illness	
Conjunctivitis, *Chlamydia*	No	No	No	Yes for touching infective material	Purulent exudate	Duration of illness	
Conjunctivitis, gonococcal							
Adults	No	No	No	Yes for touching infective material	Purulent exudate	For 24 hours after start of effective therapy	
Newborns	Yes	No	No	Yes for touching infective material	Purulent exudate	For 24 hours after start of effective therapy	
Conjunctivitis, viral and etiology unknown (acute hemorrhagic and swimming pool conjunctivitis)	Yes if patient hygiene is poor	No	No	Yes for touching infective material	Purulent exudate	Duration of illness	
Coronavirus infection, respiratory							
Adults	No	No	No	No	Respiratory secretions may be		
Infants and young children	Yes	No	Yes if soiling is likely	No	Respiratory secretions	Duration of illness	
Coxsackievirus disease	Yes if patient hygiene is poor	No	Yes if soiling is likely	Yes for touching infective material	Feces and respiratory secretions	For 7 days after onset	
Creutzfeldt-Jakob disease	No	No	No	Yes for touching infective material	Blood, brain tissue, and spinal fluid	Duration of hospitalization	Use caution when handling blood, brain tissue, or spinal fluid. (Jarvis WR. Precautions for Creutzfeldt-Jakob disease. Infect Control 1982; 3:238–239.)

DISEASE	PRECAUTIONS INDICATED				INFECTIVE MATERIAL	APPLY PRE-CAUTIONS HOW LONG?	COMMENTS
	PRIVATE ROOM?	MASKS?	GOWNS?	GLOVES?			
Croup	Yes	No	Yes if soiling is likely	No	Respiratory secretions	Duration of illness	Because viral agents, such as parainfluenza viruses and influenza A virus, have been associated with this syndrome (Committee on Infectious Diseases, American Academy of Pediatrics. 1982 Red Book), precautions to prevent their spread are generally indicated.
Cryptococcosis	No	No	No	No			
Cysticercosis	No	No	No	No			
Cytomegalovirus infection, neonatal or immunosuppressed	No	No	No	No	Urine and respiratory secretions may be		Pregnant personnel may need special counseling (see CDC Guideline for Infection Control in Hospital Personnel).
Decubitus ulcer, infected							
Draining, major	Yes	No	Yes if soiling is likely	Yes for touching infective mterial	Pus	Duration of illness	Major = draining and not covered by dressing or dressing does not adequately contain the pus.
Draining, minor	No	No	Yes if soiling is likely	Yes for touching infective material	Pus	Duration of illness	Minor or limited = dressing covers and adequately contains the pus, or infected area is very small.
Dengue	No	No	No	Yes for touching infective material	Blood	Duration of hospitalization	
Diarrhea, acute—infective etiology suspected (see gastroenteritis)	Yes if patient hygiene is poor	No	Yes if soiling is likely	Yes for touching infective material	Feces	Duration of illness	
Diphtheria							
Cutaneous	Yes	No	Yes if soiling is likely	Yes for touching infective material	Lesion secretions	Until 2 cultures from skin lesions, taken at least 24 hours apart after cessation of antimicrobial therapy, are negative for *Corynebacterium diphtheriae*	
Pharyngeal	Yes	Yes	Yes if soiling is likely	Yes for touching infective material	Respiratory secretions	Until 2 cultures from both nose and throat taken at least 24 hours apart after cessation of antimicrobial therapy	

DISEASE	PRIVATE ROOM?	MASKS?	GOWNS?	GLOVES?	INFECTIVE MATERIAL	APPLY PRE-CAUTIONS HOW LONG?	COMMENTS
Diphtheria Pharyngeal (cont.)						are negative for *Corynebacterium diphtheriae*	
Echinococcosis (hydatidosis)	No	No	No	No			
Echovirus disease	Yes if patient hygiene is poor	No	Yes if soiling is likely	Yes for touching infective material	Feces and respiratory secretions	For 7 days after onset	
Eczema vaccination (vaccinia)	Yes	No	Yes if soiling is likely	Yes for touching infective material	Lesion secretions	Duration of illness	
Encephalitis or encephalomyelitis, etiology unknown, but infection suspected (see also specific etiologic agents; likely causes include enterovirus and arthropodborne virus infections)	Yes if patient hygiene is poor	No	Yes if soiling is likely	Yes for touching infective material	Feces	Duration of illness or 7 days after onset, whichever is less	Although specific etiologic agents can include enteroviruses, arthropod-borne viruses, and herpes simplex, precautions for enteroviruses are generally indicated until a definitive diagnosis can be made.
Endometritis							
Group A *Streptococcus*	Yes if patient hygiene is poor	No	Yes if soiling is likely	Yes for touching infective material	Vaginal discharge	For 24 hours after start of effective therapy	
Other	No	No	Yes if soiling is likely	Yes for touching infective material	Vaginal discharge	Duration of illness	
Enterobiasis (pinworm disease, oxyuriasis)	No	No	No	No			
Enterocolitis (see also necrotizing enterocolitis)							
Clostridium difficile	Yes if patient hygiene is poor	No	Yes if soiling is likely	Yes for touching infective material	Feces	Duration of illness	
Staphylococcus	Yes if patient hygiene is poor	No	Yes if soiling is likely	Yes for touching infective material	Feces	Duration of illness	
Enteroviral infection	Yes if patient hygiene is poor	No	Yes if soiling is likely	Yes for touching infective material	Feces	For 7 days after onset	
Epiglottitis, due to *Haemophilus influenzae*	Yes	Yes for those close to patient	No	No	Respiratory secretions	For 24 hours after start of effective therapy	

| DISEASE | PRECAUTIONS INDICATED | | | | INFECTIVE MATERIAL | APPLY PRECAUTIONS HOW LONG? | COMMENTS |
	PRIVATE ROOM?	MASKS?	GOWNS?	GLOVES?			
Epstein-Barr virus infection, any, including infectious mononucleosis	No	No	No	No	Respiratory secretions may be		
Erysipeloid	No	No	No	No			
Erythema infectiosum	Yes	Yes for those close to patient	No	No	Respiratory secretions	For 7 days after onset	
Escherichia coli gastroenteritis (enteropathogenic, enterotoxic, or enteroinvasive)	Yes if patient hygiene is poor	No	Yes if soiling is likely	Yes for touching infective material	Feces	Duration of hospitalization	
Fever of unknown origin (FUO)							Patients with FUO usually do not need isolation precautions; however, if a patient has signs and symptoms compatible with (and is likely to have) a disease that requires isolation precautions, use those isolation precautions for that patient.
Food poisoning							
Botulism	No	No	No	No			
Clostridium perfringens or *welchii* food poisoning)	No	No	No	No			
Salmonellosis	Yes if patient hygiene is poor	No	Yes if soiling is likely	Yes for touching infective material	Feces	Duration of illness	
Staphylococcal food poisoning	No	No	No	No			
Furunculosis— staphylococcal							
Newborns	Yes	No	Yes if soiling is likely	Yes for touching infective material	Pus	Duration of illness	During a nursery outbreak, cohorting of ill and colonized infants and use of gowns and gloves are recommended.
Others	No	No	Yes if soiling is likely	Yes for touching infective material	Pus	Duration of illness	
Gangrene							
Gas gangrene (due to any bacteria)	No	No	Yes if soiling is likely	Yes for touching infective material	Pus	Duration of illness	
Gastroenteritis							
Campylobacter species	Yes if patient hygiene is poor	No	Yes if soiling is likely	Yes for touching infective material	Feces	Duration of illness	

| DISEASE | PRECAUTIONS INDICATED | | | | INFECTIVE MATERIAL | APPLY PRE-CAUTIONS HOW LONG? | COMMENTS |
	PRIVATE ROOM?	MASKS?	GOWNS?	GLOVES?			
Clostridium difficile	Yes if patient hygiene is poor	No	Yes if soiling is likely	Yes for touching infective material	Feces	Duration of illness	
Cryptosporidium species	Yes if patient hygiene is poor	No	Yes if soiling is likely	Yes for touching infective material	Feces	Duration of illness	
Dientamoeba fragilis	Yes if patient hygiene is poor	No	Yes if soiling is likely	Yes for touching infective material	Feces	Duration of illness	
Escherichia coli (entero-pathogenic, enterotoxic, or enteroinvasive)	Yes if patient hygiene is poor	No	Yes if soiling is likely	Yes for touching infective material	Feces	Duration of illness	
Giardia lamblia	Yes if patient hygiene is poor	No	Yes if soiling is likely	Yes for touching infective material	Feces	Duration of illness	
Rotavirus	Yes if patient hygiene is poor	No	Yes if soiling is likely	Yes for touching infective material	Feces	Duration of illness or 7 days after onset, whichever is less	
Salmonella species	Yes if patient hygiene is poor	No	Yes if soiling is likely	Yes for touching infective material	Feces	Duration of illness	
Shigella species	Yes if patient hygiene is poor	No	Yes if soiling is likely	Yes for touching infective material	Feces	Until 3 consecutive cultures of feces taken after ending antimicrobial therapy are negative for infecting strain	
Unknown etiology	Yes if patient hygiene is poor	No	Yes if soiling is likely	Yes for touching infective material	Feces	Duration of illness	
Vibrio parahaemolyticus	Yes if patient hygiene is poor	No	Yes if soiling is likely	Yes for touching infective material	Feces	Duration of illness	
Viral	Yes if patient hygiene is poor	No	Yes if soiling is likely	Yes for touching infective material	Feces	Duration of illness	
Yersinia enterocolitica	Yes if patient hygiene is poor	No	Yes if soiling is likely	Yes for touching infective material	Feces	Duration of illness	

| | | PRECAUTIONS INDICATED | | | | APPLY PRE- | |
DISEASE	PRIVATE ROOM?	·MASKS?	GOWNS?	GLOVES?	INFECTIVE MATERIAL	CAUTIONS HOW LONG?	COMMENTS
German measles (rubella) (see also congential rubella)	Yes	Yes for those close to patient	No	No	Respiratory secretions	For 7 days after onset of rash	Persons who are not susceptible do not need to wear a mask. Susceptible persons should, if possible, stay out of room. Pregnant personnel may need special counseling (see CDC Guideline for Infection Control in Hospital Personnel).
Giardiasis	Yes if patient hygiene is poor	No	Yes if soiling is likely	Yes for touching infective material	Feces	Duration of illness	
Gonococcal ophthalmia neonatorum (gonorrheal ophthalmia, acute conjunctivitis of the newborn)	Yes	No	No	Yes for touching infective material	Purulent exudate	For 24 hours after start of effective therapy	
Gonorrhea	No	No	No	No	Discharge may be		
Granulocytopenia	No	No	No	No			Wash hands well *before* taking care of patient (see separate section on Care of Severely Compromised Patients).
Granuloma inguinale (donovaniasis, granuloma venereum)	No	No	No	No	Drainage may be		
Guillain-Barré syndrome	No	No	No	No			
Hand, foot, and mouth disease	Yes if patient hygiene is poor	No	Yes if soiling is likely	Yes for touching infective material	Feces	For 7 days after onset	
Hemorrhagic fevers (for example, Lassa fever)	Yes with special ventilation	Yes	Yes	Yes	Blood, body fluids, and respiratory secretions	Duration of illness	Call the State Health Department and Centers for Disease Control for advice about management of a suspected case.
Hepatitis, viral							
Type A (infectious)	Yes if patient hygiene is poor	No	Yes if soiling is likely	Yes for touching infective material	Feces may be	For 7 days after onset of jaundice	Hepatitis A is most contagious before symptoms and jaundice appear; once these appear, small, inapparent amounts of feces, which may contaminate the hands of personnel during patient care, do not appear to be infective. Thus, gowns and gloves are most useful when gross soiling with feces is anticipated or possible.

| DISEASE | PRIVATE ROOM? | PRECAUTIONS INDICATED | | | INFECTIVE MATERIAL | APPLY PRE-CAUTIONS HOW LONG? | COMMENTS |
		MASKS?	GOWNS?	GLOVES?			
Type B ("serum hepatitis"), including hepatitis B antigen (HBsAg) carrier	No	No	Yes if soiling is likely	Yes for touching infective material	Blood and body fluids	Until patient is HBsAg-negative	Use caution when handling blood and blood-soiled articles. Take special care to avoid needle-stick injuries. Pregnant personnel may need special counseling (see CDC Guideline for Infection Control in Hospital Personnel). Gowns are indicated when clothing may become contaminated with body fluids or blood (for example, when blood splattering is anticipated). If gastrointestinal bleeding is likely, wear gloves if touching feces. A private room may be indicated if profuse bleeding is likely to cause environmental contamination.
Non-A, Non-B	No	No	Yes if soiling is likely	Yes for touching infective material	Blood and body fluids	Duration of illness	Currently, the period of infectivity cannot be determined.
Unspecified type, consistent with viral etiology							Maintain precautions indicated for the infections that are most likely.
Herpangina	Yes if patient hygiene is poor	No	Yes if soiling is likely	Yes for touching infective material	Feces	For 7 days after onset	
Herpes simplex (*Herpesvirus hominis*)							
Encephalitis	No	No	No	No			
Mucocutaneous, disseminated or primary, severe (skin, oral, and genital)	Yes	No	Yes if soiling is likely	Yes for touching infective material	Lesion secretions from infected site	Duration of illness	
Mucocutaneous, recurrent (skin, oral, and genital)	No	No	No	Yes for touching infective material	Lesion secretions from infected site	Until all lesions are crusted	
Neonatal (see comments for newborn with perinatal exposure)	Yes	No	Yes if soiling is likely	Yes for touching infective material	Lesion secretions	Duration of illness	The same isolation precautions are indicated for infants delivered (either vaginally or by cesarean section if membranes have been ruptured for more than 4–6 hours) to women with active genital herpes simplex infections. Infants delivered by cesarean section to women with active genital herpes simplex infections before and probably within 4–6 hours after membrane rupture are at minimal risk of develop-

DISEASE	PRIVATE ROOM?	PRECAUTIONS INDICATED			INFECTIVE MATERIAL	APPLY PRE-CAUTIONS HOW LONG?	COMMENTS
		MASKS?	GOWNS?	GLOVES?			
Herpes simplex Neonatal (cont.)							ing herpes simplex infection; the same isolation precautions may still be indicated, however. (American Academy of Pediatrics Committee on Fetus and Newborn. Perinatal herpes simplex virus infections. Pediatrics 1980; 66:147–149. Also: Kibrick S, Herpes simplex infection at term. JAMA 1980;243:157–160.)
Herpes zoster (varicella-zoster),							
Localized in immunocompromised patient, or disseminated	Yes	Yes	Yes	Yes for touching infective material	Lesion secretions and possibly respiratory secretions	Duration of illness	Localized lesions in immunocompromised patients frequently become disseminated. Because such dissemination is unpredictable, use the same isolation precautions as for disseminated disease. Persons who are not susceptible do not need to wear a mask. Persons susceptible to varicella-zoster (chickenpox) should, if possible, stay out of room. Special ventilation for the room, if available, may be advantageous, especially for outbreak control. Exposed susceptible patients should be placed on isolation precautions beginning at 10 days after exposure and continuing until 21 days after last exposure. See CDC Guideline for Infection Control in Hospital Personnel for recommendations for exposed susceptible personnel.
Localized in normal patient	Yes if patient hygiene is poor	No	No	Yes for touching infective material	Lesion secretions	Until all lesions are crusted	Persons susceptible to varicella-zoster (chickenpox) should, if possible, stay out of room. Roommates should not be susceptible to chickenpox.
Histoplasmosis at any site	No	No	No	No			
Hookworm disease (ancylostomiasis, uncinariasis)	No	No	No	No			
Immunocompromised status	No	No	No	No			Wash hands well *before* taking care of patients (see separate section on Care of Severely Compromised Patients).

DISEASE	PRIVATE ROOM?	PRECAUTIONS INDICATED MASKS?	GOWNS?	GLOVES?	INFECTIVE MATERIAL	APPLY PRE-CAUTIONS HOW LONG?	COMMENTS
Impetigo	Yes if patient hygiene is poor	No	Yes if soiling is likely	Yes for touching infective material	Lesions	For 24 hours after start of effective therapy	
Infectious mononucleosis	No	No	No	No	Respiratory secretions may be		
Influenza							
Adults	No	No	No	No	Respiratory secretions may be		In the absence of an epidemic, influenza may be difficult to diagnose on clinical grounds. Most patients will have fully recovered by the time laboratory diagnosis is established; therefore, placing patients with suspect influenza on isolation precautions, although theoretically desirable, is simply not practical in most hospitals. During epidemics, the accuracy of clinical diagnosis increases, and patients believed to have influenza may be place in the same room (cohorting). Amantadine prophylaxis may be useful to prevent symptomatic influenza A infections in high-risk patients during epidemics.
Infants and young children	Yes	No	Yes if soiling is likely	No	Respiratory secretions	Duration of illness	In the absence of an epidemic, influenza may be difficult to diagnose. During epidemics, patients believed to have influenza may be placed in the same room (cohorting).
Jakob-Creutzfeldt disease	No	No	No	Yes for touching infective material	Blood, brain tissue, and spinal fluid	Duration of hospitalization	Use caution when handling blood, brain tissue, or spinal fluid. (Jarvis WR, Precautions for Creutzfeldt-Jakob disease. Infect Control 1982; 3:238–239.)
Kawasaki syndrome	No	No	No	No			
Keratoconjunctivitis, infective	Yes if patient hygiene is poor	No	No	Yes for touching infective material	Purulent exudate	Duration of illness	
Lassa fever	Yes with special ventilation	Yes	Yes	Yes	Blood, body fluids, and respiratory secretions	Duration of illness	Call the State Health Department and Centers for Disease Control for advice about management of a suspected case.
Legionnaires' disease	No	No	No	No	Respiratory secretions may be		
Leprosy	No	No	No	No			

DISEASE	PRECAUTIONS INDICATED				INFECTIVE MATERIAL	APPLY PRE-CAUTIONS HOW LONG?	COMMENTS
	PRIVATE ROOM?	MASKS?	GOWNS?	GLOVES?			
Leptospirosis	No	No	No	Yes for touching infective material	Blood and urine	Duration of hospitalization	
Listeriosis	No	No	No	No			
Lyme disease	No	No	No	No			
Lymphocytic choriomengitis	No	No	No	No			
Lymphogranuloma venereum	No	No	No	No	Drainage may be		
Malaria	No	No	No	Yes for touching infective material	Blood	Duration of illness	
Marburg virus disease	Yes with special ventilation	Yes	Yes	Yes	Blood, body fluids, and respiratory secretions	Duration of illness	Call the State Health Department and Centers for Disease Control for advice about management of a suspected case.
Measles (rubeola) all presentations	Yes	Yes for those close to patient	No	No	Respiratory secretions	For 4 days after start of rash, except in immuno-compromised patients with whom precautions should be maintained for duration of illness	Persons who are not susceptible do not need to wear mask. Susceptible persons should, if possible, stay out of room.
Melioidosis, all forms	No	No	No	No	Respiratory secretions may be, and, if a sinus is draining, drainage may be		
Meningitis							
Aseptic (nonbacterial or viral meningitis) (also see specific etiologies)	Yes if patient hygiene is poor	No	Yes if soiling is likely	Yes for touching infective material	Feces	For 7 days after onset	Enteroviruses are the most common cause of aseptic meningitis.
Bacterial, gram-negative enteric, in neonates	No	No	No	No	Feces may be		During a nursery outbreak, cohort ill and colonized infants, and use gowns if soiling is likely and gloves if touching feces.
Fungal	No	No	No	No			
Haemophilus influenzae, known or suspected	Yes	Yes for those close to patient	No	No	Respiratory secretions	For 24 hours after start of effective therapy	
Listeria monocytogenes	No	No	No	No			
Neisseria meningitidis (meningococcal), known or suspected	Yes	Yes for those close to patient	No	No	Respiratory secretions	For 24 hours after start of effective therapy	See CDC Guideline for Infection Control in Hospital Personnel for recommendations for prophylaxis after exposure.

DISEASE	PRECAUTIONS INDICATED				INFECTIVE MATERIAL	APPLY PRE-CAUTIONS HOW LONG?	COMMENTS
	PRIVATE ROOM?	MASKS?	GOWNS?	GLOVES?			
Pneumococcal	No	No	No	No			
Tuberculous	No	No	No	No			Patient should be examined for evidence of current (active) pulmonary tuberculosis. If present, precautions are necessary (see tuberculosis).
Other diagnosed bacterial	No	No	No	No			
Meningococcal pneumonia	Yes	Yes for those close to patient	No	No	Respiratory secretions	For 24 hours after start of effective therapy	See CDC Guideline for Infection Control in Hospital Personnel for recommendations for prophylaxis after exposure.
Meningococcemia (meningococcal sepsis)	Yes	Yes for those close to patient	No	No	Respiratory secretions	For 24 hours after start of effective therapy	See CDC Guideline for Infection Control in Hospital Personnel for recommendations for prophylaxis after exposure.
Molluscum contagiosum	No	No	No	No			
Mucormycosis	No	No	No	No			
Multiply-resistant organisms,* infection or colonization.†							
Gastrointestinal	Yes	No	Yes if soiling is likely	Yes for touching infective material	Feces	Until off antimicrobials and culture-negative	In outbreaks, cohorting of infected and colonized patients may be indicated if private rooms are not available.
Respiratory	Yes	Yes for those close to patient	Yes if soiling is likely	Yes for touching infective material	Respiratory secretions and possibly feces	Until off antimicrobials and culture-negative	In outbreaks, cohorting of infected and colonized patients may be indicated if private rooms are not available.
Skin, Wound, or Burn	Yes	No	Yes if soiling is likely	Yes for touching infective material	Pus and possibly feces	Until off antimicrobials and culture-negative	In outbreaks, cohorting of infected and colonized patients may be indicated if private rooms are not available
Urinary	Yes	No	No	Yes for touching infective material	Urine and possibly feces	Until off antimicrobials and culture-negative	Urine and urine-measuring devices are sources of infection, especially if the patient (or any nearby patients) has indwelling urinary catheter. In outbreaks, cohorting of infected and colonized patients may be indicated if private rooms are not available.

*The following multiply-resistant organisms are included:
1) Gram-negative bacilli resistant to all aminoglycosides that are tested. (In general, such organisms should be resistant to gentamicin, tobramycin, and amikacin for these special precautions to be indicated.)
2) *Staphylococcus aureus* resistant to methicillin (or nafcillin or oxacillin if they are used instead of methicillin for testing).
3) *Pneumococcus* resistant to penicillin.
4) *Haemophilus influenzae* resistant to ampicillin (beta-lactamase positive) and chloramphenicol.
5) Other resistant bacteria may be included if they are judged by the infection control team to be of special clinical and epidemiologic significance.

†Colonization may involve more than 1 site.

DISEASE	PRECAUTIONS INDICATED				INFECTIVE MATERIAL	APPLY PRE-CAUTIONS HOW LONG?	COMMENTS
	PRIVATE ROOM?	MASKS?	GOWNS?	GLOVES?			
Mumps (infectious parotitis)	Yes	Yes for those close to patient	No	No	Respiratory secretions	For 9 days after onset of swelling	Persons who are not susceptible do not need to wear mask.
Mycobacteria, nontuberculous (atypical)							
Pulmonary	No	No	No	No			
Wound	No	No	Yes if soiling is likely	Yes for touching infective material	Drainage may be	Duration of drainage	
Mycoplasma pneumonia	No	No	No	No	Respiratory secretions may be		A private room may be indicated for children.
Necrotizing enterocolitis	No	No	Yes if soiling is likely	Yes for touching infective material	Feces may be	Duration of illness	In nurseries, cohorting of ill infants is recommended. It is not known whether or how this disease is transmitted; nevertheless, gowns are recommended if soiling is likely, and gloves are recommended for touching feces.
Neutropenia	No	No	No	No			Wash hands well *before* taking care of patient (see separate section on Care of Severely Compromised Patients).
Nocardiosis							
Draining lesions	No	No	No	No	Drainage may be		
Other	No	No	No	No			
Norwalk agent gastroenteritis	Yes if patient hygiene is poor	No	Yes if soiling is likely	Yes for touching infective material	Feces	Duration of illness	
Orf	No	No	No	No	Drainage may be		
Parainfluenza virus infection, respiratory in infants and young children	Yes	No	Yes if soiling is likely	No	Respiratory secretions	Duration of illness	During epidemics, patients believed to have parainfluenza virus infection may be placed in the same room (cohorting).
Pediculosis	Yes if patient hygiene is poor	No	Yes for close contact	Yes for close contact	Infested area	For 24 hours after start of effective therapy	
Pertussis ("whooping cough")	Yes	Yes for those close to patient	No	No	Respiratory secretions	For 7 days after start of effective therapy	See CDC Guideline for Infection Control in Hospital Personnel for recommendations for prophylaxis after exposure.

DISEASE	PRECAUTIONS INDICATED				INFECTIVE MATERIAL	APPLY PRE-CAUTIONS HOW LONG?	COMMENTS
	PRIVATE ROOM?	MASKS?	GOWNS?	GLOVES?			
Pharyngitis, infective, etiology unknown							
Adults	No	No	No	No	Respiratory secretions may be		
Infants and young children	Yes if patient hygiene is poor	No	Yes if soiling is likely	No	Respiratory secretions	Duration of illness	Because adenoviruses, influenza viruses, and parainfluenza viruses have been associated with this syndrome (Committee on Infectious Diseases, American Academy of Pediatrics. 1982 Red Book), precautions to prevent their spread are generally indicated.
Pinworm infection	No	No	No	No			
Plague							
Bubonic	No	No	Yes if soiling is likely	Yes for touching infective material	Pus	For 3 days after start of effective therapy	
Pneumonic	Yes	Yes	Yes if soiling is likely	Yes for touching infective material	Respiratory secretions	For 3 days after start of effective therapy	
Pleurodynia	Yes if patient hygiene is poor	No	Yes if soiling is likely	Yes for touching infective material	Feces	For 7 days after onset	Enteroviruses frequently cause infection.
Pneumonia							
Bacterial not listed elsewhere (including gram-negative bacterial)	No	No	No	No	Respiratory secretions may be		
Chlamydia	No	No	No	Yes for touching infective material	Respiratory secretions	Duration of illness	
Etiology unknown							Maintain precautions indicated for the etiology that is most likely.
Fungal	No	No	No	No			
Haemophilus influenzae							
Adults	No	No	No	No	Respiratory secretions may be		
Infants and children (any age)	Yes	Yes for those close to patient	No	No	Respiratory secretions	For 24 hours after start of effective therapy	
Legionella	No	No	No	No	Respiratory secretions may be		

DISEASE	PRIVATE ROOM?	PRECAUTIONS INDICATED			INFECTIVE MATERIAL	APPLY PRE-CAUTIONS HOW LONG?	COMMENTS
		MASKS?	GOWNS?	GLOVES?			
Meningococcal	Yes	Yes for those close to patient	No	No	Respiratory secretions	For 24 hours after start of effective therapy	See CDC Guideline for Infection Control in Hospital Personnel for recommendations for prophylaxis after exposure.
Multiply-resistant bacterial	Yes	Yes for those close to patient	Yes if soiling is likely	Yes for touching infective material	Respiratory secretions and possibly feces	Until off antimicrobials and culture-negative	In outbreaks, cohorting of infected and colonized patients may be necessary if private rooms are not available.
Mycoplasma (primary atypical pneumonia, Eaton agent pneumonia)	No	No	No	No	Respiratory secretions may be		A private room may be useful for children
Pneumococcal	No	No	No	No	Respiratory secretions may be for 24 hours after start of effective therapy		
Pneumocystis carinii	No	No	No	No			
Staphylococcus aureus	Yes	Yes for those close to patient	Yes if soiling is likely	Yes for touching infective material	Respiratory secretions	For 48 hours after start of effective therapy	
Streptococcus, group A	Yes	Yes for those close to patient	Yes if soiling is likely	Yes for touching infective material	Respiratory secretions	For 24 hours after start of effective therapy	
Viral (see also specific etiologic agents)							
Adults	No	No	No	No	Respiratory secretions may be		
Viral Infants and young children	Yes	No	Yes if soiling is likely	No	Respiratory secretions	Duration of illness	Viral pneumonia may be caused by various etiologic agents, such as parainfluenza viruses, influenza viruses, and, particularly, respiratory syncytial virus, in children less than 5 years old (Committee on Infectious Diseases, American Academy of Pediatrics. 1982 Red Book); therefore, precautions to prevent their spread are generally indicated.
Poliomyelitis	Yes if patient hygiene is poor	No	Yes if soiling is likely	Yes for touching infective material	Feces	For 7 days after onset	
Psittacosis (ornithosis)	No	No	No	No	Respiratory secretions may be		

DISEASE	PRIVATE ROOM?	PRECAUTIONS INDICATED			INFECTIVE MATERIAL	APPLY PRE-CAUTIONS HOW LONG?	COMMENTS
		MASKS?	GOWNS?	GLOVES?			
Q fever	No	No	No	No	Respiratory secretions may be		
Rabies	Yes	Yes for those close to patient	Yes if soiling is likely	Yes for touching infective material	Respiratory secretions	Duration of illness	See CDC Guideline for Infection Control in Hospital Personnel for recommendations for prophylaxis after exposure.
Rat-bite fever (*Streptobacillus moniliformis* disease, *Spirillum minus* disease)	No	No	No	Yes for touching infective material	Blood	For 24 hours after start of effective therapy	
Relapsing fever	No	No	No	Yes for touching infective material	Blood	Duration of illness	
Resistant bacterial (see multiply-resistant bacteria)							
Respiratory infectious disease, acute (if not covered elsewhere)							
Adults	No	No	No	No	Respiratory secretions may be		
Infants and young children							Maintain precautions indicated for the bacterial or viral infections that are most likely.
Respiratory syncytial virus (RSV) infection, in infants and young children	Yes	No	Yes if soiling is likely	No	Respiratory secretions	Duration of illness	During epidemics, patients believed to have RSV infection may be placed in the same room (cohorting). The use of masks has not been recommended since they have proven ineffective in controlled studies.
Reye syndrome	No	No	No	No			
Rheumatic fever	No	No	No	No			
Rhinovirus infection, respiratory							
Adults	No	No	No	No	Respiratory secretions may be		
Infants and young children	Yes	No	Yes if soiling is likely	No	Respiratory secretions	Duration of illness	
Rickettsial fevers, tickborne (Rocky Mountain spotted fever, tickborne typhus fever)	No	No	No	No	Blood may be		
Rickettsialpox (vesicular rickettsiosis)	No	No	No	No			

DISEASE	PRIVATE ROOM?	PRECAUTIONS INDICATED MASKS?	GOWNS?	GLOVES?	INFECTIVE MATERIAL	APPLY PRE-CAUTIONS HOW LONG?	COMMENTS
Ringworm (dermatophytosis, dermatomycosis, tinea)	No	No	No	No			
Ritter's disease (staphylococcal scalded skin syndrome)	Yes	No	Yes if soiling is likely	Yes for touching infective material	Lesion drainage	Duration of illness	
Rocky Mountain spotted fever	No	No	No	No	Blood may be		
Roseola infantum (exanthem subitum)	No	No	No	No			
Rotavirus infection (viral gastroenteritis)	Yes if patient hygiene is poor	No	Yes if soiling is likely	Yes for touching infective material	Feces	Duration of illness or 7 days after onset, whichever is less	
Rubella ("German measles") (see also congenital rubella)	Yes	Yes for those close to patient	No	No	Respiratory secretions	For 7 days after onset of rash	Persons who are not susceptible do not need to wear a mask. Susceptible persons should, if possible, stay out of room. Pregnant personnel may need special counseling (see CDC Guideline for Infection Control in Hospital Personnel).
Salmonellosis	Yes if patient hygiene is poor	No	Yes if soiling is likely	Yes for touching infective material	Feces	Duration of illness	
Scabies	Yes if patient hygiene is poor	No	Yes for close contact	Yes for close contact	Infested area	For 24 hours after start of effective therapy	
Scalded skin syndrome, staphylococcal (Ritter's disease)	Yes	No	Yes if soiling is likely	Yes for touching infective material	Lesion drainage	Duration of illness	
Schistosomiasis (bilharziasis)	No	No	No	No			
Shigellosis (including bacillary dysentery)	Yes if patient hygiene is poor	No	Yes if soiling is likely	Yes for touching infective material	Feces	Until 3 consecutive cultures of feces, taken after ending antimicrobial therapy, are negative for infecting strain	
Smallpox (variola)	Yes with special ventilation	Yes	Yes	Yes	Respiratory secretions and lesion secretions	Duration of illness	As long as smallpox virus is kept stocked in laboratories, the potential exists for cases to occur. Call the State Health Department and Centers for Disease Control for advice about management of a suspected case.

| DISEASE | PRIVATE ROOM? | PRECAUTIONS INDICATED | | | INFECTIVE MATERIAL | APPLY PRE-CAUTIONS HOW LONG? | COMMENTS |
		MASKS?	GOWNS?	GLOVES?			
Sporotrichosis	No	No	No	No			
Spirillium minus disease (rat-bite fever)	No	No	No	Yes for touching infective material	Blood	For 24 hours after start of effective therapy	
Staphylococcal disease (*S. aureus*)							
Skin, wound, or burn infection							
Major	Yes	No	Yes if soiling is likely	Yes for touching infective material	Pus	Duration of illness	Major = draining and not covered by dressing or dressing does not adequately contain the pus.
Minor or limited	No	No	Yes if soiling is likely	Yes for touching infective material	Pus	Duration of illness	Minor or limited = dressing covers and adequately contains the pus, or infected area is very small.
Enterocolitis	Yes if patient hygiene is poor	No	Yes if soiling is likely	Yes for touching infective material	Feces	Duration of illness	
Pneumonia or draining lung abscess	Yes	Yes for those close to patient	Yes if soiling is likely	Yes for touching infective material	Respiratory secretions	For 48 hours after start of effective therapy	
Scalded skin syndrome	Yes	No	Yes if soiling is likely	Yes for touching infective material	Lesion drainage	Duration of illness	
Toxic shock syndrome	No	No	Yes if soiling is likely	Yes for touching infective material	Vaginal discharge or pus	Duration of illness	
Streptobacillus moniliformis disease (rat-bite fever)	No	No	No	Yes for touching infective material	Blood	For 24 hours after start of effective therapy	
Streptococcal disease (group A *Streptococcus*)							
Skin, wound, or burn infection							
Major	Yes	No	Yes if soiling is likely	Yes for touching infective material	Pus	For 24 hours after start of effective therapy	Major = draining and not covered by dressing or dressing does not adequately contain the pus.
Minor or limited	No	No	Yes if soiling is likely	Yes for touching infective material	Pus	For 24 hours after start of effective therapy	Minor or limited = dressing covers and adequately contains the pus, or infected area is very small.
Endometritis (puerperal sepsis)	Yes if patient hygiene is poor	No	Yes if soiling is likely	Yes for touching infective material	Vaginal discharge	For 24 hours after start of effective therapy	

| DISEASE | PRIVATE ROOM? | PRECAUTIONS INDICATED | | | INFECTIVE MATERIAL | APPLY PRECAUTIONS HOW LONG? | COMMENTS |
		MASKS?	GOWNS?	GLOVES?			
Pharyngitis	Yes if patient hygiene is poor	No	No	No	Respiratory secretions	For 24 hours after start of effective therapy	
Pneumonia	Yes	Yes for those close to patient	Yes if soiling is likely	Yes for touching infective material	Respiratory secretions	For 24 hours after start of effective therapy	
Scarlet fever	Yes if patient hygiene is poor	No	No	No	Respiratory secretions	For 24 hours after start of effective therapy	
Streptococcal disease (group B *Streptococcus*), neonatal	No	No	No	No	Feces may be		During a nursery outbreak, cohorting of ill and colonized infants and use of gowns and gloves is recommended.
Streptococcal disease (not group A or B) unless covered elsewhere	No	No	No	No			
Strongyloidiasis	No	No	No	No	Feces may be		If the patient is immunocompromised and has pneumonia or has disseminated disease, respiratory secretions may be infective.
Syphilis							
Skin and mucous membrane, including congenital, primary, and secondary	No	No	No	Yes for touching infective material	Lesion secretions and blood	For 24 hours after start of effective therapy	Skin lesions of primary and secondary syphilis may be highly infective.
Latent (tertiary) and seropositivity without lesions	No	No	No	No			
Tapeworm disease							
Hymenolepis nana	No	No	No	No	Feces may be		
Taenia solium (pork)	No	No	No	No	Feces may be		
Other	No	No	No	No			
Tetanus	No	No	No	No			
Tinea (fungus infection dermatophytosis, dermatomycosis, ringworm)	No	No	No	No			
"TORCH" syndrome (If congenital forms of the following diseases are seriously being considered, see separate listing for these diseases: toxoplasmosis, rubella, cytomegalovirus, herpes, and syphilis.)							

DISEASE	PRIVATE ROOM?	PRECAUTIONS INDICATED			INFECTIVE MATERIAL	APPLY PRE-CAUTIONS HOW LONG?	COMMENTS
		MASKS?	GOWNS?	GLOVES?			
Toxoplasmosis	No	No	No	No			
Toxic shock syndrome (staphylococcal disease)	No	No	Yes if soiling is likely	Yes for touching infective material	Vaginal discharge and pus	Duration of illness	
Trachoma, acute	No	No	No	Yes for touching infective material	Purulent exudate	Duration of illness	
Trench mouth (Vincent's angina)	No	No	No	No			
Trichinosis	No	No	No	No			
Trichomoniasis	No	No	No	No			
Trichuriasis (whipworm disease)	No	No	No	No			
Tuberculosis							
Extrapulmonary, draining lesion (including scrofula)	No	No	Yes if soiling is likely	Yes for touching infective material	Pus	Duration of drainage	A private room is especially important for children.
Extrapulmonary, meningitis	No	No	No	No			
Pulmonary, confirmed or suspected (sputum smear is positive or chest X-ray appearance strongly suggests current [active] TB, for example, a cavitary lesion is found), or laryngeal disease.	Yes with special ventilation	Yes if patient is coughing and does not reliably cover mouth	Yes if gross contamination of clothing is likely	No	Airborne droplet nuclei	In most instances the duration of isolation precautions can be guided by clinical response and a reduction in numbers of TB organisms on sputum smear. Usually this occurs within 2–3 weeks after chemotherapy is begun. When the patient is likely to be infected with isoniazid-resistant organisms, **Apply** precautions until patient is improving and sputum smear is negative for TB organisms.	Prompt use of effective antituberculous drugs is the most effective means of limiting transmission. Gowns are not important because TB is rarely spread by fomites, although gowns are indicated to prevent gross contamination of clothing. For more detailed guidelines refer to "Guidelines for Prevention of TB Transmission in Hospitals" (1982), Tuberculosis Control Division, Center for Prevention Services, Centers for Disease Control, Atlanta, GA, (HHS Publication No. [CDC] 82-8371) and CDC Guideline for Infection Control in Hospital Personnel. In general, infants and young children do not require isolation precautions because they rarely cough and their bronchial secretions contain few TB organisms compared to adults with pulmonary TB.

DISEASE	PRIVATE ROOM?	PRECAUTIONS INDICATED			INFECTIVE MATERIAL	APPLY PRE-CAUTIONS HOW LONG?	COMMENTS
		MASKS?	GOWNS?	GLOVES?			
Skin-test positive with no evidence of current pulmonary disease (sputum smear is negative, X-ray not suggestive of current [active] disease)	No	No	No	No			
Tularemia							
Draining lesion	No	No	Yes if soiling is likely	Yes for touching infective material	Pus may be	Duration of illness	
Pulmonary	No	No	No	No	Respiratory secretions may be		
Typhoid fever	Yes if patient hygiene is poor	No	Yes if soiling is likely	Yes for touching infective material	Feces	Duration of illness	
Typhus, endemic and epidemic	No	No	No	No	Blood may be		
Urinary tract infection (including pyelonephritis), with or without urinary catheter	No	No	No	No			See multiply-resistant bacteria if infection is with these bacteria. Spatially separate infected and uninfected patients who have indwelling catheters (see CDC Guideline for Prevention of Catheter-associated Urinary Tract Infection).
Vaccinia							
At vaccination site	No	No	Yes if soiling is likely	Yes for touching infective material	Lesion secretions	Duration of illness	
Generalized and progressive, eczema vaccinatum	Yes	No	Yes if soiling is likely	Yes for touching infective material	Lesion secretions	Duration of illness	

DISEASE	PRECAUTIONS INDICATED				INFECTIVE MATERIAL	APPLY PRE-CAUTIONS HOW LONG?	COMMENTS
	PRIVATE ROOM?	**MASKS?**	**GOWNS?**	**GLOVES?**			
Varicella (chickenpox)	Yes	Yes	Yes	Yes	Respiratory secretions and lesion secretions	Until all lesions are crusted	Persons who are not susceptible do not need to wear a mask. Susceptible persons should, if possible, stay out of the room. Special ventilation for the room, if available, may be advantageous, especially for outbreak control. Neonates born to mothers with active varicella should be placed on isolation precautions at birth. Exposed susceptible patients should be placed on isolation precautions beginning 10 days after exposure and continuing until 21 days after last exposure. See CDC Guideline for Infection Control in Hospital Personnel for recommendations for exposed susceptible personnel.
Variola (smallpox)	Yes with special ventilation	Yes	Yes	Yes	Respiratory secretions and lesion secretions	Duration of illness	Call the State Health Department and Centers for Disease Control for advice about management of a suspected case.
Vibrio parahaemolyticus gastroenteritis	Yes if patient hygiene is poor	No	Yes if soiling is likely	Yes for touching infective material	Feces	Duration of illness	
Vincent's angina (trench mouth)	No	No	No	No			
Viral diseases							
Pericarditis, myocarditis, or meningitis	Yes if patient hygiene is poor	No	Yes if soiling is likely	Yes for touching infective material	Feces and possibly respiratory secretions	For 7 days after onset	Enteroviruses frequently cause these infections.
Respiratory (if not covered elsewhere)							
Adults	No	No	No	No	Respiratory secretions may be		
Infants and young children	Yes	No	Yes if soiling is likely	No	Respiratory secretions	Duration of illness	Various etiologic agents, such as respiratory syncytial virus, parainfluenza viruses, adenoviruses, and, influenza viruses, can cause viral respiratory infections (Committee on Infectious Diseases, American Academy of Pediatrics. 1982 Red Book); therefore, precautions to prevent their spread are generally indicated.

DISEASE	PRIVATE ROOM?	PRECAUTIONS INDICATED MASKS?	GOWNS?	GLOVES?	INFECTIVE MATERIAL	APPLY PRE-CAUTIONS HOW LONG?	COMMENTS
Whooping cough (pertussis)	Yes	Yes for those close to patient	No	No	Respiratory secretions	For 7 days after start of effective therapy	See CDC Guideline for Infection Control in Hospital Personnel for recommendations for prophylaxis after exposure.
Wound infections							
Major	Yes	No	Yes if soiling is likely	Yes for touching infective material	Pus	Duration of illness	Major = draining and not covered by dressing or dressing does not adequately contain the pus.
Minor or limited	No	No	Yes if soiling is likely	Yes for touching infective material	Pus	Duration of illness	Minor or limited = dressing covers and adequately contains the pus, or infected area is very small, such as a stitch abscess.
Yersinia enterocolitica gastroenteritis	Yes if patient hygiene is poor	No	Yes if soiling is likely	Yes for touching infective material	Feces	Duration of illness	
Zoster (varicella-zoster),							
Localized in immunocompromised patient or disseminated	Yes	Yes	Yes	Yes for touching infective material	Lesion secretions	Duration of illness	Localized lesions in immunocompromised patients frequently become disseminated. Because such dissemination is unpredictable, use the same isolation precautions as with disseminated disease. Persons who are not susceptible do not need to wear a mask. Persons susceptible to varicella-zoster (chickenpox) should, if possible, stay out of the room. Special ventilation for room, if available, may be advantageous, especially for outbreak control. Exposed susceptible patients should be placed on isolation precautions beginning 10 days after exposure and continuing until 21 days after last exposure. See CDC Guideline for Infection Control in Hospital Personnel for recommendations for exposed susceptible personnel.
Localized in normal patient	Yes if patient hygiene is poor	No	No	Yes for touching infective material	Lesion secretions	Until all lesions are crusted	Persons susceptible to varicella-zoster (chickenpox) should, if possible, stay out of room. Roommates should not be susceptible to chickenpox.
Zygomycosis (phycomycosis, mucormycosis)	No	No	No	No			

A

Abdominal sepsis, 71–73
Abscess
  Bezold, 9
  of brain, 138–141
  of breast, neonatal, 108–109
  epidural
    cranial, 141
    spinal, 142
  infection control in, 347
  intra-abdominal, 71–73
  of liver, 70–71
    amebic, 340
  of lung, 51–52, 281
  prostatic, 154–155
  renal and perirenal, 153–154
  in retropharyngeal space infection, 35
  subgaleal, 141
Absidia, in zygomycosis, 177
Acanthamoeba, 328, 338–339
Accutane. *See* Isotretinoin
N-Acetylcysteine, in cystic fibrosis, 54
Acid applications, in warts, 116
Acinetobacter
  in bite wound infections, 110
  in burn wound infections, 303
  in catheter-associated infections, 297
  in pneumonia, 63
Acne, 102–105
Actinobacillus actinomycetemcomitans, in
  endocarditis, 126
Actinomyces, 183
  in sialadenitis, suppurative, 30
Actinomycosis, 183–185
  infection control in, 347
Acyclovir
  adverse effects of, 248–249
  in burn wound infections, 304
  in cytomegalovirus infection, 191
  dosage in newborns, 308
  in herpes simplex infection, 149, 195,
    198–199
  in mononucleosis, 183
  in varicella-zoster infections, 247
Adenitis
  cervical, 22
  mycobacterial, 217
Adenovirus
  enteric, in diarrhea, 84
  and infection control, 347
  in keratitis, 15
  in pneumonia, 56, 65–66
Aeromonas, in diarrhea, 79
AIDS, 252–255
  cryptococcosis in, 173
  cytomegalovirus infection in, 191–192
  immunization policies in, 291
  infection control in, 347
  opportunistic infections in, 253–254
  periodontal disease in, 23
  Pneumocystis carinii pneumonia in,
    337–338
  prevention of infections in, 286
  sialadenitis in, 29

toxoplasmosis in, 336
Albendazole
  in ascariasis, 315
  in enterobiasis, 317
  in hookworm infection, 316
  in hydatid disease, 320
  in strongyloidiasis, 317
  in trichinellosis, 318
  in trichuriasis, 316
Albuterol, in pertussis, 46
Allopurinol, in kala-azar, 332
Aluminum chloride, in erythrasma, 117
Amantadine
  dosage in newborns, 308
  in influenza, 49–50
  in influenza prevention, 286
  in laryngotracheitis, 39
  in nosocomial pneumonia, 307
  in viral CNS infections, 145
Amebiasis, 328, 339–340
  diarrhea in, 82–83
  infection control in, 347
Amebic meningoencephalitis, 328,
  338–339
Amikacin
  in cerebrospinal fluid shunt infection,
    147
  dosage in newborns, 308
  in fever and neutropenia with cancer,
    269
  in infections with chronic granulomatous
    disease, 277, 278
  in intra-abdominal sepsis, 72, 73
  in intravascular catheter-associated
    infections, 297
  in keratitis, 16
  in mediastinits, 67
  in meningitis, 135
  in mycobacterial infections,
    nontuberculous, 218
  in necrotizing enterocolitis, 86
  in neonatal sepsis, 261, 263
  in nocardiosis, 216
  in pneumonia, 59, 60
  in streptococcal endocarditis, 124
Amodiaquine, in malaria prophylaxis, 329
Amoxicillin
  clavulanic acid with. *See* Augmentin
  in cystitis, 163
  diarrhea from, 88
  in endocarditis prevention, 127
  in epididymitis, 157
  in epiglottitis, 43
  in gonorrhea, 158, 159
  in otitis media, 5
  in pneumonia, 60
  in pyelonephritis, 162
  in sinusitis, 11
  in surgical patients, 280
  in typhoid carriers, 246
  in typhoid fever, 244
Amphotericin B
  in amebic meningoencephalitis, 328, 339
  in aspergillosis, 164–165

in blastomycosis, 167
in candidiasis, 169
chloramphenicol and sulfadiazine with.
    See "Gold dust" powder
in coccidioidomycosis, 172
in cryptococcosis, 173
diarrhea from, 88
in endocarditis, 126
in endophthalmitis, 20
in fever and neutropenia with cancer,
    270
in histoplasmosis, 176–177
in infections with chronic granulomatous
    disease, 278
in kala-azar, 328, 332
in keratitis, 16
in leishmaniasis, 333, 334
liposomal, 165, 177
in liver abscess, 71
in neonatal sepsis, 261
in phaeohyphomycosis, 178
in sporotrichosis, 178
in suppurative arthritis, 94
in zygomycosis, 177
Ampicillin
  in bite wound infections, 110
  in brain abscess, 140
  in cystitis, 163
  in diarrhea, 80
  diarrhea from, 88
  dosage in newborns, 308
  in endocarditis prevention, 127
  in epiglottitis, 42
  in gonorrhea, 158
  in intra-abdominal sepsis, 72, 73
  intrapartum use of, 263–264, 286
  in listeriosis, 210–211
  in meningitis, 135
  in necrotizing enterocolitis, 86
  in neonatal sepsis, 261
  in osteomyelitis, 96
  in pneumonia, 59, 60
  in prostatitis, 154
  in pyelonephritis, 162
  in streptococcal endocarditis, 124
  in suppurative arthritis, 94
  in surgical patients, 280
  in syphilis, 230
  in tularemia, 242
  in typhoid carriers, 246
  in typhoid fever, 244
  in umbilical sepsis, 107
Amrinone, in myocarditis, 129
Ancylostomiasis, 315, 317
  infection control in, 358
Anemia, in typhoid fever, 245
Aneurysm, coronary artery, in Kawasaki
  syndrome, 203
Angina
  Ludwig, 28
  Vincent, infection control in, 369, 371
Angiostrongyliasis, 318
Animal bites, infections from, 109, 282
Anisakiasis, 317